Compendium of
MCQs in UROLOGY
Maximum MCQs

(Master Key for Aspiring Urologists)

Fifth Edition

Dr Parag Gupta
MBBS, MS
MCh (Urology), SGPGIMS, LKO

PEEPEE PUBLISHERS AND DISTRIBUTORS (P) LTD.®

Compendium of MCQs in Urology
Maximum MCQs

Published by
Pawaninder P. Vij and Anupam Vij

Peepee Publishers and Distributors (P) Ltd.
Head Office: 160, Shakti Vihar, Pitam Pura, Delhi-110 034 (India)

Correspondence Address:
7/31, First Floor, Ansari Road, Daryaganj
New Delhi-110 002 (India)
Ph: 41512412, 23246245, 9811156083
e-mail: peepee160@yahoo.co.in
e-mail: peepee160@gmail.com
www.peepeepub.com
join us on f facebook.com/pp.publishers

First Edition: 2012
Fifth Edition : 2021

ISBN: 978-81-8445-284-6

To
My parents in recognition of their
inspiring guidance!
My wife, Dr Pratibha, who cooperated with me,
first during my MCh preparation
and then for preparing this book!
My son Prakhar and daughter Pushti
for their unconditional support!

The woods are lovely, dark and deep,
    But I have promises to keep,
And miles to go before I sleep,
    And miles to go before I sleep.

—Robert Frost

PREFACE TO THE FIFTH EDITION

As a general resident, I became dismayed by the bulk of material that the general surgeon was expected to know. There is need of a book which can guide through examination. Theoretical content is adequately covered by abundant excellent textbooks but there exist need for an MCQ book.

Trainees fail to clear exam in spite of excellent practical skills due to lack of MCQ book. Leading textbook Campbell Urology is in four large volumes. Through this book I have highlighted the important points and made MCQs from book. MCQs are followed by explanation.

I have also compiled examination papers of previous years and added around 1500 questions in this new edition, so that examinee know what is expected from them. Answers are also provided in this edition. My sincere thanks to the readers, who pointed out the mistakes and we tried to correct all of them. Every effort is made not to make mistake but human beings make mistakes. If reader find any mistakes they can mail me at *drparaggupta1@yahoo.co.in.*

With this book I have also introduced Urology Essentials for quick revision of urology text.

Happy reading and good luck to all.

Dr Parag Gupta, MCh

PREFACE TO THE FIRST EDITION

During my preparation for the urology entrance examination, I felt the need of a book which can guide me through my preparation. Theoretical content is adequately covered by an abundance of excellent textbooks but there is an existing lacuna in MCQ books. Through this book I have made an effort to fill the void in MCQ format. Each stem of the MCQ is a question in itself. Reader should know each of the choice individually. Each MCQ is followed by an explanation so as to provide the reader with an idea of important topics.

I have compiled examination question papers of previous years so that the reader can know what to expect. I have tried to avoid repetition but still some questions are bound to crop up again and again. They are only meant to reinforce the point. In this edition I was not able to provide answers to examination questions but hope will be able to provide in next edition. I have provided the question bank which is a gold mine for students and the search for answers will develop a further interest in subject.

With this book I am also introducing little The Golden Book of Urology for quick revision of Urology.

I have made all possible attempts to keep the mistakes to minimum but if you find any mistakes or need any clarification you can mail me at drparaggupta1@yahoo.co.in. Any contribution in the form of questions would be duly acknowledged.

Happy reading and good luck to you all!!

Dr Parag Gupta

ACKNOWLEDGEMENTS

It would not have been possible for me to bring out this edition without the help of:

Dr. Sanjay Surekha who gave me all the questions and whose patient yet persistent urgings made me bring out this book.

My heartfelt thanks to Dr Jeetendra Rathore, specialist and senior residents Dr Gyvi and Dr Nikunj of Department of Urology, St Stephens Hospital for their indispensable help and support.

And…Most of all, my publisher and my friend, **Mr. Pawaninder P Vij,** Director Peepee Publishers and Distributors (P) Ltd., for making this book a reality.

Last but not the least **to all my teachers** of school (Hansraj Model School), MBBS (Stanley Medical College), MS (University College of Medical Sciences) and MCh (Sanjay Gandhi Institute of Medical Sciences) who made me a successful doctor.

Dr Parag Gupta

CONTENTS

IMPORTANT MCQs

CHAPTER

1

Clinical Decision Making

1. **The number of per high-power microscopic field which corresponds to colony count of 10^5/ml should be:**
   (a) 3 (b) 5
   (c) 10 (d) 20
2. **The specificity of dipstick nitrite testing for bacteriuria is:**
   (a) 40% (b) 60%
   (c) 80% (d) 90%
3. **Urine osmolality usually varies between:**
   (a) 10 and 200 mOsm/l
   (b) 50 and 500 mOsm/l
   (c) 50 and 1200 mOsm/l
   (d) 100 and 1000 mOsm/l
4. **The most common cause of cloudy urine is:**
   (a) Bacterial cystitis
   (b) Urine overgrowth with yeast
   (c) Phosphaturia
   (d) Significant proteinuria
5. **Bacteriuria without pyuria suggests:**
   (a) Infection (b) Colonization
   (c) Tuberculosis (d) Contamination
6. **All of the following may lead to a granular contracted kidney *except:***
   (a) Benign nephrosclerosis
   (b) Chronic pyelonephritis
   (c) Chronic glomerulonephritis
   (d) Diabetes mellitus
7. **RBC cast in the microscopic examination of the urine indicates:**
   (a) Acute pyelonephritis
   (b) Acute glomerulonephritis
   (c) Chronic glomerulonephritis
   (d) Nephrotic syndrome
8. **The most sterile method for urine collection is:**
   (a) Sample taken via per urethral catheter
   (b) Clean take from the urine bag
   (c) Midstream clean catch urine
   (d) Suprapubic aspiration
9. **All of the following increase specific gravity of urine *except:***
   (a) Diabetes insipidus
   (b) Inappropriate secretion of ADH
   (c) Diabetes mellitus
   (d) Decreased fluid intake
10. **Osmolality of Iohexol radio contrast media is:**
    (a) 640 (b) 320
    (c) 1530 (d) 290
11. **What percentage of rise in serum creatinine above baseline is defined as contrast induced nephropathy?**
    (a) 10% (b) 5%
    (c) 25% (d) 40%
12. **Telescopes with..... degree lens are utilized for inspection of bladder neck.**
    (a) 0 degree (b) 30 degree
    (c) 70 degree (d) 120 degree

13. In dysuric patients, an appropriate threshold value for defining significant bacteriuria is ..... of a known pathogen.

(a) 10^2 (b) 10^3

(c) 10^4 (d) 10^5

14. The diagnosis of retrograde ejaculation is confirmed by identification of:

(a) 15-20 sperm/HPF in a centrifuged specimen of post ejaculation urine

(b) 20-25 sperm/HPF in a centrifuged specimen of post ejaculation urine

(c) 5-10 sperm/HPF in a centrifuged specimen of post ejaculation urine

(d) 10-15 sperm/HPF in a centrifuged specimen of post ejaculation urine

15. The term superscan used for:

(a) Bone scan showing extensive metastasis in carcinoma prostate

(b) X-ray pelvis showing extensive metastasis in carcinoma prostate

(c) MRI pelvis showing extensive metastasis in carcinoma prostate

(d) PET scan showing lung metastasis in carcinoma prostate

16. Upper urinary tract imaging is recommended in evaluation of men with LUTS in all *except:*

(a) Hematuria

(b) History of urolithiasis

(c) History of urinary tract surgery

(d) Enlarged prostate

17. Water in T1W MRI is:

(a) Dark (b) Bright

(c) Hypointense (d) None of the above

18. Which statement regarding MRI is correct?

(a) Water appears dark in T1W and bright in T2W

(b) Fat appears dark in T1W and bright in T2W

(c) Fat appears dark in T1W and dark in T2W

(d) Water appears bright in T1W and bright in T2W

19. Contrast used in USG:

(a) Omnipaque (b) Sonovue

(c) Pnuevue (d) Hypaque

20. Current editor in chief of Gold Journal is:

(a) W Partin (b) Usterling

(c) Klein (d) Javier C

21. Best position to visualize ureter in IVU:

(a) Supine (b) Prone

(c) Upright (d) Oblique

22. Frequency of USG probe decreases when:

(a) Depth of penetration decreases

(b) Depth of penetration increases

(c) Image become more hypoechoic

(d) Image become less hypoechoic

23. Favourable urinary indices are all *except*:

(a) Osmolarity <210

(b) Na>100

(c) Cl<110

(d) α microglobulin < 10

24. True about inulin:

(a) Difficult to administer and measure

(b) Cheap

(c) Not ideal for GFR measurement

(d) Is a glucose polysaccharide

25. Cornbach's coefficient is 90%:

(a) Higher interconsistency reliability

(b) Higher accuracy

(c) Higher precision

(d) Lower reliability

Mention True and False respective to each statement. (Q. No. 26 to 62)

26. Normal urine analysis includes:

(a) Osmolality 50-300 moles

(b) pH 4.5-8
(c) Sp Gravity 1.001-1.020
(d) Phosphaturia most common cause of cloudy urine
(e) Microscopic hematuria is >3RBC/HPF

27. Hematuria:
(a) Initial hematuria due to urethral cause
(b) Initial hematuria most common cause from prostatic urethra
(c) Terminal hematuria is from bladder neck
(d) Total hematuria from bladder
(e) Terminal hematuria from upper tract

28. Hematuria with proven low grade non-muscle invasion carcinoma of bladder:
(a) Urgent cystoscopy is indicated
(b) IVP before cystoscopy
(c) USG is useful
(d) Cystoscopy should be delayed till urine cytology reports
(e) CT is more useful than USG

29. Hounsfield unit in CT:
(a) Stone:- 0 to + 100
(b) Fat:-50
(c) Air:-1000
(d) Water:- +500
(e) Typical CTKUB exposes 10 mSv

30. Regarding TRUS:
(a) Probe frequency is 7 MHz
(b) Fifty percent non-palpable, < 1 cm tumor cannot be detected by TRUS
(c) Most of hypoechoeic lesion on TRUS is carcinoma
(d) TRUS can detect microscopic extracapsular extension
(e) TRUS can be used for the planning of brachytherapy

31. Foley's catheter:
(a) It is self-retaining catheter
(b) Three-way may have better drainage than two-way of same size
(c) Orifice at the tip of catheter
(d) Three-way better for traction
(e) Three-way catheter bulb capacity is 30-50 ml

32. SPSS:
(a) Statistical package for scientific soft care
(b) Initial release in 1968
(c) Latest SPSS–21 version (August 2012)
(d) It has 2D table structures, where rows represent cases and the columns represent measurements
(e) Developer is IBM corporation

33. Regarding hematuria:
(a) Normal is ≤ 3RBC/HPF
(b) Morphological features can determine the site of origin
(c) Microscopic examination of centrifuged sample can differentiate between hematuria, hemoglobinuria and myoglobinuria
(d) Healthy, adult excretes upto 150 mg of protein in urine daily
(e) Hematuria of nephrologic origin is frequently associated with casts in the urine and almost always associated with significant proteinuria

34. Contrast media:
(a) LOCM eliminate carboxyl group but add hydrophilic hydroxyl groups at the organic side chain positions
(b) Contrast media reactions may be dose dependent or idiosyncratic
(c) LOCM made to increase excretion
(d) 5–7 times osmolarity in HOCM as compared to LOCM
(e) LOCM do not ionise in the solution

35. IVP:

(a) There is clear advantage in visualization of the urinary tract with bowel preparation

(b) Dehydration may improve imaging quality

(c) Fifty to 100 ml of contrast medium is given through an 18- or 19-gauge needle

(d) Nephrogram phase appears in 5 to 7 minutes

(e) Compression device may be attached, which distends the collecting system and allows better visualization of the pelvis and ureters

36. Hematospermia:

(a) Usually resolve spontaneously

(b) TRUS can find significant pathology

(c) Can occur after a prolonged period of sexual abstinence

(d) Caused by nonspecific seminal vesiculitis

(e) Severe HTN can cause hematospermia

37. Hematuria:

(a) Initial hematuria–urethra

(b) Painless hematuria–bladder malignancy

(c) Terminal hematuria–bladder neck

(d) Total hematuria–bladder pathology

(e) Vermiform clots–upper tract

38. Catheter:

(a) 1 French $\rightarrow$ 0.33 mm

(b) Catheter sizes refer to the inner circumference of the catheter

(c) For a given outer circumference, two-way catheters have a larger luminal size for urinary drainage than three-way catheters

(d) Foley catheter is straight tip

(e) Coude catheter is curved tip

39. About contrast:

(a) All iodinated contrast are HOCM

(b) Conventional contrast media are HOCM

(c) LOCM were made to increase excretion

(d) 5 to 7 times the osmolarity in HOCM as compared to LOCM

(e) LOCM do not ionise in the solution

40. IVP:

(a) Contract dose – 5-10 ml/kg

(b) Nephrogram – 1-2 minutes

(c) Pelvicalyceal phase – 5 min

(d) Single shot IVP – 5 min

(e) IVP – Investigation of choice in trauma

41. Regarding urinary analysis:

(a) Urine pH–(4.5– 8)

(b) Urine S.G–(1.001–1.020)

(c) Glitter's cell–Erythrocytes

(d) Microscopic hematuria–more than 3 RBC

(e) Tamm-Horsfall mucoprotein is always present in urine

42. Regarding urinary analysis:

(a) Hyaline cast may not be pathological

(b) Tubular cast always significant

(c) Most common yeast is candida albicans

(d) Most common cause of cloudy urine – phosphaturia

(e) WBC casts can be present in ATN

43. Thirty years old patient with extreme flank pain:

(a) Renal colic is a common cause

(b) Obstruction without fever immediate drainage required

(c) NCCT is investigation of choice

(d) IVU should be preferred at the time of pain

(e) Acute appendicitis can be one of the differential diagnosis

44. Thirty years old male with hematuria and bilateral flank mass with hypertension:

(a) Smoking is the most common history

(b) Bladder tumor with bilateral ureteric orifice obstruction is the most likely cause

(c) USG is the first investigation
(d) If bilateral renal cyst present then captopril renography is to be done
(e) Common anomalies associated with disease is berry aneurysms, colonic diverticulas and MVP

45. Regarding CT scan:
(a) Fat is typically of 50 HU
(b) CT KUB has exposure of 10 MSV
(c) HU for water is zero
(d) HU for air is 0 to -100
(e) HU for stone is 0 to 100

46. Regarding urine analysis:
(a) Urine for AFB–morning fresh sample needed
(b) Even in patients with high-grade tumors, however, urinary cytology may be falsely negative in 20%
(c) False-positive cytology may occur in 1% to 12% of patients
(d) To evaluate for a possible infection in a female, a catheterized urine sample should always be obtained
(e) All urine samples should be examined within 1 hour of collection

47. Twenty years boy fall from height, blood at meatus:
(a) RGU to be done immediately
(b) Gentle attempt of Foley's catheterization
(c) SPC is best
(d) After hemodynamic stability, endoscopic alignment
(e) Perineal urethroplasty will be mostly required

48. Hematuria:
(a) > 3 RBC/HPF – Microscopic hematuria
(b) Glitter cell is RBC
(c) RBC casts are from glomerular bleeding
(d) Renal tubular epithelial cells are normal finding
(e) Hyaline cast is not always pathological

49. Urine:
(a) Cloudy urine is most commonly due to phosphaturia
(b) pH (5.5 – 6.5)
(c) If not possible to examine the urine promptly, it should be refrigerated at 5°C
(d) Urine pH has no relation to serum pH
(e) In metabolic alkalosis urine is alkaline

50. Urine:
(a) Sp. gravity (1.010 – 1.030)
(b) Can be stored at 5°C for 24 hours before examination
(c) Normal osmolarity (50 – 1200 mosm/l)
(d) Osmolarity reflects renal concentrating ability
(e) Fix specific gravity of 1.035 indicates renal disease

51. Proteinuria:
(a) Normal protein excretion is 60–150 mg/dl
(b) Most common protein is albumin
(c) Overflow proteinuria occurs in the absence of any underlying renal disease
(d) Not dependent on hydration status
(e) Transient proteinuria mostly resolves spontaneously

52. IVU:
(a) Diuretic IVU is as sensitive as diuretic renogram
(b) In large parenchymal mass IVU is as sensitive as CT scan
(c) In systemic hypertension persistent nephrogram occurs
(d) Diuretic renogram (DTPA) is done for renal scarring
(e) Delayed nephrogram is seen in ureteric obstruction

53. TRUS:
(a) Probe of 7 MHz
(b) Most hypoechoic lesion are carcinoma

(c) Precisely evaluate microscopic extracapsular extension
(d) Clinically impalpable > 1 cm hypoechoic lesion are not detected in 50% of cases
(e) Used for planning of brachytherapy

54. Chronic hypercalcemia seen in:
(a) Multiple myeloma
(b) Immobilization
(c) Sarcoidosis
(d) Hypoalbuminemia
(e) Alcoholism

55. Regarding sutures:
(a) Vicryl half life–7-12 days
(b) PDS–Monofilament
(c) Prolene–Monofilament and ever lasting
(d) PDS–Half life 28 days
(e) Catgut is preserved in alcohol

56. Regarding drains:
(a) Sump drain used for draining peritonitis
(b) Suction drain used for abscess and debris
(c) Drain guarantees against collection
(d) Sump drain used for deep peritoneal abscess
(e) Suction drain is preferred in retroperitoneum

57. Regarding IV fluids:
(a) 0.9% saline→ Na^+=154 Cl^- =154
(b) 0.9% saline→ Na^+=154 Cl^- =85
(c) RL→ Na^+=130 Cl^- =109
(d) RL→ Na^+=154 Cl^- =154
(e) 3% saline→ Na^+=513 meq/l

58. Radionuclide scan:
(a) Increase risk of cancer in later life
(b) Emits gamma rays
(c) Emits α rays
(d) Emits β rays
(e) Emits $\alpha + \beta$ rays

59. Regarding strontium:
(a) Decays to sellinum 92
(b) When taken up by metastatic cells immediately metabolized
(c) Main toxicity hematologic
(d) Dose dependent platelet reduction
(e) Detoxify in liver

60. Catheter:
(a) IF=0.66 mm
(b) IF=0.33 mm
(c) IF=0.36 mm
(d) Coude catheters are specifically designed to help bypass areas of the male urethra that are difficult to negotiate with a straight catheter
(e) Self-retaining catheters are–Pezzer and Malecott catheters

61. Regarding preoperative risk in non-cardiac patient:
(a) Maximum risk with history of MI in first 3 months
(b) Perioperative arrhythmia is uncommon in normal patient
(c) Recent history of CHF increases chances of perioperative pulmonary edema
(d) In aortic, peripheral vascular surgery and abdominal surgery the risk is same
(e) Recent episode of MI increases the cardiac risk

62. Antibiotic prophylaxis:
(a) Best when given within 2 hours after surgery
(b) Prophylaxis given upto 48 hours
(c) Cephalosporin is drug of choice in procedures
(d) Vancomycin is best drug for gram +ve bacteria
(e) Operation significantly causes immunosuppression

Which of the following statement is correct?

63. Contrast associated with renal dysfunction:

(a) All are derived from a 2,4,6 tri-iodinated benzene ring
(b) HOCM is more associated
(c) LOCM is more associated
(d) HOCM have an osmolality that is five times greater than physiologic osmolality of body cells
(e) LOCM have an osmolality that is same or slightly higher than physiologic osmolality

64. Urinary cast:

(a) Hyaline cast–may not have pathological significance
(b) RBC cast is diagnostic of glomerulonephritis
(c) WBC is seen in acute pyelonephritis
(d) Fatty cast is seen in nephrotic syndrome
(e) Tamm-Horsfall mucoprotein–basic matrix of all renal casts

65. Which of the following is false?

(a) Chest X-ray–0.2 mSv
(b) Pelvic radiographs–2 mSv
(c) Bone scan–5 mSv
(d) MRI–10 mSv
(e) CT–20 mSv

66. WBC cast seen in:

(a) Lipiduria
(b) Hypothyroidism
(c) Acute interstitial nephritis
(d) Acute GN
(e) Acute pyelonephritis

67. Red urine caused by all *except*:

(a) Phenothiazine (b) Phenytoin
(c) Rifampicin (d) Phenolphthalein
(e) Triamterine

68. Causes of brown urine:

(a) Riboflavin (b) Porphyria
(c) Metronidazole (d) Rifampicin
(e) Indicanuria

69. Agent causing green-blue urine:

(a) Indigo carmine
(b) Biliverdin
(c) Amitriptyline
(d) Urobilinogen
(e) Pyridium

70. Which of the following is contraindicated for iodinized contrast?

(a) Age >65 years
(b) NIDDM
(c) Creatinine >2 mg/dl
(d) Hypertension
(e) Hyperuricosuria

71. Contrast associated renal damage – associated with:

(a) NIDDM
(b) Dehydration
(c) Sensitivity to iodinated contrast
(d) Hypertension
(e) Hyperuricemia

72. Self retaining catheter:

(a) Pezzer (b) Malecot
(c) Nelaton (d) Brasher
(e) Foley's

73. For long-term catheterization best material:

(a) Silicon (b) Latex
(c) PVC (d) Teflon
(e) Polyurethane

74. Safe in 1st trimester of pregnancy:

(a) USG (b) MR urography
(c) IVP (d) CT urography
(e) Radionuclide scan

75. 'HASTE' term used in:

(a) MR urography (b) CT urography
(c) IVP (d) Bone scan
(e) X-Ray KUB

76. Urologist awarded noble prize:

(a) Huggins (b) F. Marshall
(c) Huge H. Young (d) W. Forssmann
(e) Joseph Murray

77. Contrast study should be done with caution in:

(a) >65 years age
(b) Pulmonary hypertension
(c) IDDM
(d) Hyperthyroidism
(e) Patient on metformin

78. Indication of retrograde pyelogram:

(a) Radiolucent calculus
(b) Ureteric stricture
(c) Abnormal anatomy of ureterovaginal fistula
(d) Mapping before endoscopic procedure
(e) Evaluation of hematuria, in lieu of IVU

79. Self retaining catheter:

(a) Malecot (b) Pezzer
(c) Foley's (d) Robinson
(e) Coude

80. Ionic LOCM is:

(a) Iopamidol (b) Iohexol
(c) Ioversol (d) Ioxaglate

81. Regarding nephrogenic systemic fibrosis, not true is:

(a) Common at GFR >30
(b) Due to gadolinium contrast
(c) Presentation from 2 days - 3 months
(d) Pruritus and skin thickening

82. Chemical shift associated with:

(a) NMR spectroscopy
(b) CT scan
(c) PET
(d) DTPA

83. UPOINT classification includes all *except*:

(a) Urinary (b) Prostate
(c) Neurologic (d) Infection

84. Karnofsky scale:

(a) Divided into 5% categories
(b) 70% – normal activity with some difficulty
(c) Can be used for children
(d) Primary purpose of its development was to allow physicians to evaluate a patient's ability to survive chemotherapy for cancer

85. Twelve years old presented with reddish urine. Mother brings him to the OPD. No RBC in urine .... sample is obtained and centrifuged. Supernatant was pink.

(a) Serum to r/o hemoglobinuria
(b) Serum to r/o myoglobinuria
(c) Urine to r/o myoglobinuria
(d) Essential hematuria

86. Bacteriophage are:

(a) Eukaryocytes
(b) Megakaryocytes
(c) NK cells killing bacteria
(d) Virus

87. Bold and diffusion weighted are associated with:

(a) MRI (b) CT
(c) USG (d) PET

88. MRI spectrography in Carcinoma prostate:

(a) Citrate (b) Choline
(c) FDG (d) Gadolinium

89. Non ionic contrast:

(a) Barium sulphate (b) Iohexol
(c) Na Diatrizoate (d) Ioxaglate

90. Renal scanning for scarring due to reflux:

(a) DMSA (b) DTPA
(c) CLEC (d) MAG3

91. CECT scan for carcinoma colon, develops pain in bilateral flank with extravasation of contrast. Diagnosis and management:

(a) Bilateral fornix rupture and conservative management
(b) Bilateral contrast nephropathy and N-acetyl cysteine
(c) Bilateral renal rupture and exploration
(d) Bilateral PUJ avulsion

92. Ascorbic acid cause false positive test for:

(a) Glucose (b) RBC
(c) Proteins (d) Vitamin D

93. Neurogenic systemic fibrosis is caused by:

(a) Gadolinum (b) Diatrizoate
(c) Iohexol (d) Ioversol

94. Glitter cells in urine are:

(a) Spermatozoa
(b) Candida albicans
(c) Fresh leucocytes
(d) Transitional cells

95. Highest incidence for contrast reaction is seen in patients with:

(a) History of allergic reaction
(b) Skin sensitivity just before IV contrast
(c) Azotemia
(d) Renal failure due to DM

96. Normal urine pH:

(a) 6.5 – 7.5 (b) 5.5 – 6.5
(c) 6.5 – 7.0 (d) 4.5 – 5.5

97. Catheter used for complete RGP:

(a) Olive tip (b) Bulb tip
(c) Round tip (d) Spiral lip

98. Brodney clamp is used in:

(a) RGU (b) MCU
(c) RGP (d) Nephrostogram

99. F-15 scan is:

(a) Duplex real time doppler
(b) CT
(c) Fat adjusted MRI
(d) Dynamic renal radionuclide scan

100. Best to measure renal plasma flow:

(a) DTPA (b) DMSA
(c) MAG3 (d) Ga scan

101. Which one is not cleared by glomerular filtration?

(a) DTPA
(b) DMSA
(c) MAG3
(d) DTPA and DMSA

102. 1 mm is:

(a) 3F (b) 2F
(c) 1F (d) 0.3F

103. Isosthenuria is:

(a) Fixed specific gravity of urine
(b) Fixed osmolality of urine
(c) Osmolarity of urine same as that of serum
(d) Continuously variable osmolarity

104. Hounsfield value of water is:

(a) –10 (b) 10
(c) 0 (d) 100

105. Post-obstruction, recovery of renal function is assessed by:

(a) DMSA (b) DTPA
(c) MAG3 (d) USG

106. Dose of IVP:

(a) 1 unit/kg (b) 4 unit/kg
(c) 2 unit/kg (d) 3 unit/kg

107. False statement:

(a) No need of FNAC before radical nephrectomy
(b) If CT value <-20 HU indicates oncocytoma
(c) If there is 15 HU enhancement on CT, then RCC to be ruled out
(d) In 14% of AMLs, fat cannot be identified with CT

108. Which of the following is useful for renal scars?

(a) DMSA (b) MAG3
(c) DTPA (d) MDP

109. Photoactive porphyrins emit which color fluorescence?

(a) Blue (b) Green
(c) Red (d) White

110. Microscopic urine examinations cannot detect:

(a) Protein (b) Cells
(c) Crystals (d) Casts

111. The following isotopes and indications for use are correct *except*:

(a) Tc99m DTPA–Function and drainage of kidney
(b) Tc99m DMSA–Renal parenchymal imaging
(c) Tc99m pertechnetate–Seminoma with metastases
(d) I^{131} MIBG–Neuroblastoma

112. Normal levels of daily protein excretion in adults:

(a) 50-80 mg (b) 80-150 mg
(c) 100-200 mg (d) <50 mg

113. Following reagent is used for the detection of protein on urinary dipstick test:

(a) Peroxidise
(b) Red azo dye
(c) Indoxyl
(d) Tetrabromophenol blue

114. Leucocyte esterase test depends on:

(a) Double oxidative reaction
(b) Oxidation of diazonium salt by indoxyl
(c) Diazotisation to form red azo dye
(d) Calorimetric reaction with sodium nitroprusside

115. SI unit of absorbed dose of radiation:

(a) Gray (b) Roentgen
(c) Sieverts (d) Rads

116. Most commonly transducer used in TRUS:

(a) 2 MHz (b) 3 MHz
(c) 5 MHz (d) 7 MHz

117. Adult effective dose of radiation who are exposed to CT KUB without and with contrast is:

(a) < 0.1 mSv (b) 0.1 to 1 mSv
(c) 1 to 10 mSv (d) 10 to 30 mSv

118. Following is not a mechanism of action of idiosyncratic anaphylactoid reactions due to intravascular iodinated contrast media:

(a) Release of vasoactive substances including histamine
(b) Activation of physiologic cascades including complement, kinin, coagulation and fibrinolytic systems
(c) Activation of cholinesterase
(d) Patient's anxiety

119. When compared to silicon, catheters made up of latex are:

(a) Less cost
(b) Less tissue reactivity
(c) Less bacterial adherence
(d) Less incidence of UTI

120. **Following catheter is used during difficult catheterisation in males:**

(a) Robinson (b) Council
(c) Coude (d) Whistle tip

121. **One French (1F) equals to:**

(a) 0.33 mm in circumference
(b) 3.3 mm in circumference
(c) 0.33 mm in diameter
(d) 3.3 mm in diameter

122. **MRI scan should be avoided in which of the following situations?**

(a) In diabetic and hypertensive aged adults
(b) In pregnancy
(c) In claustrophobic patients
(d) In patients with a known history of allergic diathesis

123. **The most common cause of glomerular hematuria is:**

(a) IgA nephropathy
(b) Mesangioproliferative glomerulonephritis
(c) Membranous glomerulonephritis
(d) Focal segmental proliferative glomerulonephritis

124. **The following conditions causes cloudy urine *except*:**

(a) Phosphaturia
(b) Chyluria
(c) Pyuria
(d) Ingestion of sulfasalazine

125. **Dysmorphic erythrocytes urinary sediment indicate:**

(a) Glomerular tubular disease
(b) Proximal tubular disease
(c) Distal tubular disease
(d) Collecting duct disease

126. **Urinary crystals precipitated in acidic urine include the following *except*:**

(a) Calcium oxalate
(b) Uric acid
(c) Cystine
(d) Calcium phosphate

127. **Posterior urethra is better visualized by:**

(a) Ascending urethrogram
(b) Micturating cystourethrogram
(c) Cystography
(d) CT cystogram

128. **99mTc DMSA scan is used to:**

(a) Assess GFR
(b) Identify renal scar
(c) Detect malignancy
(d) Delineate obstruction

129. **Causes of sterile pyuria include all *except*:**

(a) Cancer (b) TB
(c) Stone (d) E. coli infection

130. **99mTc - MDP may be used for:**

(a) Diuresis renography
(b) Bone scanning
(c) Detection of renal scarring
(d) Detection of VU reflux

131. **The most common cause of glomerular hematuria is:**

(a) Nephrotic syndrome
(b) Acute glomerulonephritis
(c) IgA nephropathy
(d) Systemic lupus erythematosus

132. **Hematospermia commonly results from:**

(a) Genitourinary tuberculosis
(b) Carcinoma prostate
(c) Acute bacterial prostatitis

(d) Non-specific inflammation of prostate and seminal vesicle

133. Cloudy urine is most common in:
(a) Phosphaturia
(b) Alkaline urine
(c) Chyluria
(d) Acidic urine

134. Glitter cells are:
(a) Fresh leukocyte
(b) Old leukocyte
(c) Fresh RBC
(d) Old RBC

135. Acidic urine commonly associated with all *except*:
(a) Ca PO_4
(b) Calcium oxalate monohydrate
(c) Uric acid
(d) Calcium oxalate dihydrate

136. All of the following radiopharmaceutical is excreted by glomerular filtration *except*:
(a) DTPA (b) MAG-3
(c) DMSA (d) Na iothalamate

137. Water—HU in non-contrast CT:
(a) +10 (b) -10
(c) 0 (d) +40

138. Pyuria in females is defined as:
(a) > 5 WBC/HPF (b) > 1 WBC/HPF
(c) > 10 WBC/HPF (d) > 15 WBC/HPF

139. Contrast medium for MRI:
(a) Gadolinium (b) Iothalamate
(c) Urograffin (d) Saline

140. Investigations safe in pregnancy:
(a) USG, MRI and MAG3 Urography
(b) USG, CT, IVU
(c) USG, IVU, MRI
(d) CT, MRI, USG

141. Renogram done for:
(a) Visualization of kidney not seen in IVP
(b) Individual function of the kidney
(c) Definitive investigation for RVH
(d) To evaluate etiology of CRF

142. Radiotherapy effect in utero is classified as:
(a) Teratogenic and mutagenic
(b) Stochastic and no-stochastic
(c) Growth retardation
(d) Small for age

143. Tracer used to measure GFR in patients with renal dysfunction is:
(a) DTPA (b) DMSA
(c) MAG-3 (d) IVP

144. Dose of contrast used in IVP:
(a) 1 U/Kg (b) 2 U/Kg
(c) 4 U/Kg (d) < 1 U/Kg

145. 'Glitter cells' are:
(a) Old leucocytes
(b) Oval fat macrophages
(c) Deformed RBC's
(d) Fresh leucocytes

146. Best investigation for visualisation of renal cortical scar:
(a) Tc 99 DMSA (b) Tc 99 DTPA
(c) IVP (d) USG

147. 5 bacteria/HPF equals to:
(a) 100/ml (b) 1000/ml
(c) 10000/ml (d) 100000/ml

148. Bulbo cavernous reflex can be elicited by all *except:*
(a) Finger in the rectum
(b) Squeezing of glans
(c) Squeezing of clitoris
(d) Squeezing of scrotum

149. How is leukocyte esterase detected by dipstick urinalysis?

(a) Peroxidase

(b) Red azo dye

(c) The production of indoxyl and oxidation of a diazonium salt

(d) Tetrabromophenol blue dye

150. Dysmorphic red blood cells in the urine is seen in:

(a) Transitional cell carcinoma of the bladder

(b) IgA nephropathy

(c) Transitional cell tumor of renal pelvis

(d) Collecting duct carcinoma

151. Not used in Renal scan:

(a) DMSA (b) DTPA

(c) MAG-3 (d) MOP

(e) EC

152. Not a principle of ALARA:

(a) Distance

(b) Time

(c) Surgeon protection

(d) Temperature

153. In the evaluation of hematuria:

(a) The chances of significant pathology increases with the degree of hematuria

(b) Initial hematuria is usually secondary to upper tract malignancy

(c) Cut off for significant hematuria is greater than ten red blood cells per HPF

(d) Most common cause of older men with gross hematuria is BPH

154. Identify the correct statement regarding LUTS:

(a) Postvoid dribbling is effectively managed by shaking the penis at the end of micturition

(b) BPH causes more of obstructive symptoms and prostate cancer causes more of storage symptoms

(c) Nocturia may be due to congestive heart failure

(d) IPSS questionnaire differentiates BPH from other causes of urinary symptoms

155. Regarding urinalysis:

(a) Leukocyt esterase is produced by lymphocytes

(b) Gram negative bacteria convert nitrites to nitrates

(c) Most common cause of false positive leukocyte esterase test is contamination

(d) Specificity of nitrite dipstick for bacteriuria is more than 90%

156. Lowest osmolality is seen in which of the radio contrast medium?

(a) Iodixanol

(b) Iopamidol

(c) Ioversol

(d) Meglumine diatriazoate

157. The following regarding retrograde pyelography is correct:

(a) If the entire ureter is not seen on a static view, it is abnormal

(b) Contrast should not be diluted for RGP

(c) Open ended catheters are not used for retrograde pyelography

(d) Albarran deflector is useful in difficult orifices

158. Acoustic enhancement in renal cyst is suggestive of:

(a) Hypervascularity

(b) Infection

(c) Clear fluid

(d) Malignancy

159. For imaging solid renal lesions using MRI, which of the following statements is correct?

(a) At least 30% increased signal intensity is required to classify as malignant

(b) MRI differentiates oncocytoma from renal cell carcinoma

(c) CT is superior to MRI to evaluate calcified complex cysts

(d) Angiomylipomas enhance with gadolinium

160. Which characteristic describes how sensitive the changes over time are detected, while evaluating health related quality of life (HRQOL)?

(a) Responsiveness

(b) Content validity

(c) Construct validity

(d) Reliability

161. Highest risk from radiation exposure for a fetus is:

(a) Preimplantation to 15 weeks gestation

(b) 7 weeks – 14 weeks organogenesis

(c) 14 weeks – 20 weeks of growth

(d) 32 weeks – 40 weeks of maturation

162. Crystalluria is not seen with:

(a) Acyclovir

(b) Tenofovir

(c) Triamterene

(d) Uric acid nephropathy

(e) Ethylene glycol poisoning

163. In formula for calculation of serum osmolality the sum of following osmotically active agents is taken:

(a) Albumin

(b) Creatinine

(c) Sodium

(d) Urea

(e) Glucose

164. MRI true is:

(a) T1 fat bright, water dark

(b) T1 fat dark, water bright

(c) T2 fat bright, water dark

(d) T2 fat dark, water bright

(e) T2 fat and water bright

165. Chemotherapeutic agents which are nephrotoxic:

(a) Cyclophosphamide

(b) Dorzolamide

(c) Doxorubicine

(d) Mitomycin C

(e) Methotrexate

166. Which are not manure to improve urine cast identification?

(a) Discard first morning sample and use second sample

(b) Examine in bright light

(c) Centrifuge at low speed

(d) Urinary alkalinization

(e) Examine at edge of cover slip

167. About glomerular hematuria false are:

(a) Biopsy is not helpful

(b) It can present with hematuria without proteinuria and RBC cast

(c) MPGN does not cause glomerular hematuria

(d) IgA nephropathy is not a cause of glomerular hematuria

(e) Identification by dismorphic RBC, RBC cast and proteinuria

ANSWERS

1.	B	35.	FTTFT	69.	ABC	103.	A	137.	C
2.	D	36.	TFTTF	70.	ABCDE	104.	C	138.	A
3.	C	37.	TTTTT	71.	ABCDE	105.	B	139.	A
4.	C	38.	TFTTT	72.	ABE	106.	C	140.	A
5.	B	39.	FTFFT	73.	A	107.	B	141.	B
6.	D	40.	TTTFF	74.	AB	108.	A	142.	A
7.	B	41.	TTFTT	75.	A	109.	C	143.	C
8.	D	42.	TTTTT	76.	ADE	110.	A	144.	B
9.	A	43.	TFTFF	77.	ABDE	111.	C	145.	D
10.	A	44.	FFTFT	78.	ABCDE	112.	B	146.	A
11.	C	45.	FTTTF	79.	ABC	113.	D	147.	D
12.	D	46.	TTTTT	80.	D	114.	B	148.	D
13.	A	47.	TTTTF	81.	A	115.	B	149.	C
14.	D	48.	TFTFT	82.	A	116.	D	150.	B
15.	A	49.	TTTFT	83.	B	117.	D	151.	D
16.	D	50.	TTTFF	84.	D	118.	C	152.	D
17.	A	51.	TTFFT	85.	A	119.	A	153.	A
18.	A	52.	FFTFT	86.	D	120.	C	154.	C
19.	B	53.	TTFTF	87.	A	121.	C	155.	D
20.	C	54.	TTTTT	88.	B	122.	C	156.	C
21.	B	55.	FTTTT	89.	B	123.	A	157.	D
22.	B	56.	TFFTT	90.	A	124.	D	158.	A
23.	B	57.	TFTFT	91.	A	125.	A	159.	C
24.	A	58.	TTFFF	92.	A	126.	D	160.	D
25.	A	59.	TFTTF	93.	A	127.	B	161.	A
26.	TTTTT	60.	FTFTT	94.	C	128.	B	162.	B
27.	TFTTF	61.	TTFTT	95.	C	129.	D	163.	CDE
28.	TFTFT	62.	FFTFT	96.	B	130.	B	164.	A
29.	TTTFT	63.	ABDE	97.	B	131.	C	165.	ADE
30.	TTFFT	64.	ABCDE	98.	A	132.	D	166.	ABCD
31.	TFFTT	65.	ABD	99.	D	133.	A	167.	ACD
32.	TTTTT	66.	CDE	100.	C	134.	A		
33.	TTTTT	67.	BD	101.	C	135.	A		
34.	TTFFT	68.	BC	102.	A	136.	B		

CHAPTER

2

Basics of Urologic Surgery

1. **Which of the following is an absorbable suture?**
   (a) Silk (b) Polyester
   (c) Polypropylene (d) Polyglycolic acid

2. **Da Vinci robotic system degree of freedom:**
   (a) 5 (b) 6
   (c) 7 (d) 8

3. **Which is first generation hand assisted device?**
   (a) SILS (b) Omniport
   (c) Handport (d) Gelport

4. **Instrument used in LESS:**
   (a) Triport (b) Intromit
   (c) Omniport (d) Pneumo sleeve

5. **While creating pneumoperitoneum by Veress needle, sudden bradycardia of 20 bpm, next step should be:**
   (a) Withdraw the needle as needle is in the bowel and desufflate
   (b) Due to peritoneal stretch, desufflate
   (c) Due to decreased venous return, will become normal after a while, continue with the procedure
   (d) Due to vascular injury, call for assistance and repair

6. **In retroperitoneoscopy laparoscopic surgery space is developed in:**
   (a) Posterior pararenal space
   (b) Anterior pararenal space
   (c) Lateral
   (d) Median

Mention True and False respective to each statement (Q. No. 7 to 21)

7. **Regarding TPN:**
   (a) Measure source of energy fat
   (b) 1 gm nitrogen -6.25 protein
   (c) Gram +ve cocci is cause of catheter induced infection
   (d) Air embolism is potentially fatal
   (e) Hyperglycemia in euglycemic patients suggest sepsis

8. **Laser in urology:**
   (a) CO_2 wavelength–6000 nm
   (b) Nd:YAG (8 – 10) mm depth penetration
   (c) Argon can be used by fibres in cystoscopy
   (d) Nd:YAG vaporization is more than that of holmium
   (e) T_1 renal pelvic TCC–CO_2 laser can be used

9. **Lymphocele:**
   (a) Within 7 days of surgery
   (b) 33-50% after pelvic LND
   (c) CT can differentiate between urine and lymphocele
   (d) Active intervention is required in most of cases
   (e) If intervention is required percutaneous aspiration alone is not sufficient

10. **TPN:**
    (a) 1 gm N_2-6.25 gm protein
    (b) In central venous catheter, sepsis is most commonly due to gram -ve organism
    (c) Air embolism–fatal complication

(d) Energy source is mainly lipid
(e) Sepsis is suggested when normoglycemic shows glucose intolerance

11. Pneumo Retroperitoneoscopy:
(a) Initial port incision is at the tip and 2 inches below 12th rib
(b) Generally three ports are placed in a line, hence an "I" configuration
(c) Posterior port is placed at the junction of the lateral border of the paraspinal muscles and the 12th rib
(d) Inadvertent peritoneotomy during retroperitoneoscopy interfere with steps of the procedure, and conversion to a transperitoneal laparoscopic approach is considered
(e) Anterior port is placed at the anterior axillary line, subcostally

12. Trendelenberg position:
(a) Head down 15 - 30°
(b) Leg down 30 - 45°
(c) Can cause respiratory compromise
(d) To assist in the filling and distension of the upper central veins when placing a central line
(e) Used for hypovolemic shock

13. Regarding laser:
(a) CO_2 wavelength–10,600 nm
(b) CO_2 laser can be used for superficial T1 renal pelvic lesion
(c) Nd:YAG cause more vaporization than Hol:YAG
(d) Argon laser can be delivered through fiberoptic flexible scope
(e) Nd:YAG-penetration 8–10 mm

14. Retroperitoneoscopy:
(a) Occurrence of an inadvertent peritoneotomy during retroperitoneoscopy does not usually interfere with the subsequent steps of the procedure
(b) First port placed 2 inches below 12th rib
(c) Genitofemoral nerve is most important landmark for ureter identification
(d) Balloon dilation in the posterior pararenal space facilitates the creation of a working space for retroperitoneal
(e) Patient is placed in the true, 90 degree lateral decubitus position with the body at a right angle to the table

15. Lymphocele:
(a) Within 3 days of surgery
(b) 33-50% after pelvic LND
(c) CT can differentiate between urine and lymphocele
(d) No active intervention is required in most of cases
(e) If intervention is required percutaneous aspiration alone is not sufficient

16. Respiratory acidosis:
(a) Clinical effects of elevated pCO_2, which are separate from acidosis per se, include elevated intracranial pressure, tachycardia, central depression
(b) Failure of ventilation decreases pH
(c) Receptors for CO_2 is in hypothalamus
(d) Main stimulus is decrease PO_2 for respiration
(e) pH and pCO_2 is low

17. Pneumoperitoneum:
(a) More than 15 mm of Hg oligouria is common
(b) To begin, insufflator pressure is set at 15 mm Hg with a rate of gas flow of 1 L/min
(c) The 14-gauge Veress needle cannot deliver flow rates greater than 2 L/min
(d) Most commonly, CO_2 is used as the insufflant because
(e) Capnography measures end tidal CO_2

18. Regarding lasers:
(a) T_1 renal pelvic TCC–CO_2 laser can be used
(b) CO_2 laser wavelength–10,600
(c) Nd:YAG more vaporization than holmium
(d) Argon laser can be delivered by fiberoptics cystoscope
(e) CO_2 laser–Penetration upto 10 mm

19. Regarding lymphocele:
(a) CT scan can differentiate between lymphoma and urinoma
(b) Occurs in 50% cases of pelvic lymphadenopathy
(c) Resolve by conservative management
(d) Most of them are asymptomatic
(e) If infected open drainage is often necessary

20. CT scan:
(a) Conventional measures volume
(b) Helical measures tissue
(c) Helical gives 3-D image
(d) In conventional resolution and picture quality better
(e) Best modality for detection of RCC and renal trauma

21. Regarding lymphocele:
(a) CT scan can differentiate between lymphocele and urinoma
(b) Occurs in 50% of cases with pelvic lymphadenopathy
(c) Resolves by conservative management
(d) Most of them are asymptomatic
(e) Mostly present within 3 days

Which of the Following Statement is Correct ?

22. With increasing pneumoperitoneum pressure parameter which increases is:
(a) Mean arterial pressure
(b) End tidal CO_2
(c) PCO_2
(d) GFR
(e) Heart rate

23. Contraindication for laparoscopic kidney procedure:
(a) Coagulopathy
(b) Abdominal wall infection
(c) >7 cm tumor
(d) Cardiorespiratory disease
(e) Extensive abdominal surgery

24. Absolute contraindication for laparoscopic surgery:
(a) Severe cardiopulmonary disease
(b) Hypovolemic shock
(c) Previous abdominal surgery
(d) Obesity – weight > 85 kg
(e) Uncorrected coagulopathy

25. Which one is 2nd generation?
(a) Omniport (b) Handport
(c) Intromit (d) Pneumo sleeve

26. Maximum fibrinogen content:
(a) Tisseel (b) Coseal
(c) Floseal (d) Bioglue

27. Retroperitoneoscopy space made at:
(a) Posterior pararenal space
(b) Anterior pararenal space
(c) Lateral pararenal space
(d) Medial pararenal space

28. Most common reason for conversion from laparoscopic to open is:
(a) Bleeding
(b) Adhesions
(c) Anomalous artery
(d) Not able to progress

29. During pneumoperitoneum which statement is not true?
(a) Max flow through Veress–2 1/min

(b) O_2 can cause explosion
(c) Most common gas used as insufflant – NO
(d) Most commonly selected pressure for performing laparoscopy is 15 mm Hg

30. Surgeon performing laparoscopic surgery for benign lesion of kidney with no consent for open conversion. Aortic injury during trocar placement:
(a) Has to repair aorta without taking consent
(b) Surgery in first place was not justified
(c) Inform next to kin, take consent for repair of aorta and then repair
(d) Inform next to kin and go ahead with repair

31. During laparoscopic access, which is not true?
(a) Beginning-pressure set at 15 mm Hg with rate of gas flow of 1 liter/min
(b) Once safe entry achieved flow rate by Veress needle can be increased to maximum of 5 liter/min
(c) Overall, the most commonly selected pressure for performing laparoscopy is 15 mm Hg
(d) Most common gas used as insufflant–CO_2

32. All included in SIRS *except*:
(a) Temperature > 38°C
(b) Temperature < 36°C
(c) TLC> 4000 and < 12000
(d) Pulse rate > 90

33. Size of standard resectoscope:
(a) 18 Fr (b) 22 Fr
(c) 26 Fr (d) 32 Fr

34. Nd: YAG laser is:
(a) Solid (b) Liquid
(c) Gas (d) Semisolid

35. Robotic surgery maximally used for:
(a) Radical prostatectomy
(b) Pyeloplasty
(c) Nephrectomy
(d) Cystectomy

36. Electrosurgical bowel injury not a risk when:
(a) Direct activation
(b) Coupling to another instrument
(c) Capacitive coupling
(d) During pneumoperitonium

37. Graveyard of urologist:
(a) Retroperitoneal fossa
(b) Retropubic fossa
(c) Intraperitoneal space
(d) Supradiaphragmatic space

38. The only organ in the abdomen to have paradoxical increase in perfusion during pneumoperitoneum:
(a) Adrenals (b) Liver
(c) Pancreas (d) Kidneys

39. Advantages of rigid endoscopes are all *except:*
(a) Larger working channel
(b) Larger lumen allows for improved irrigant flow
(c) Improved image quality due to presence of rod lens system
(d) Ability to deflect the endoscope tip

40. Urethral catheter specially designed to help bypass the areas of male urethra that are difficult to negotiate:
(a) Robinson's catheter
(b) Council catheter
(c) Coude catheter
(d) Malecot's catheter

41. Advantage of rigid endoscopes are the following *except*:
(a) Larger working channel
(b) Larger lumen for water flow
(c) Better visualization due to fiberoptic system
(d) Easier to manipulate

42. In 18 Fr catheter, outer diameter is:
(a) 2mm (b) 4mm
(c) 6mm (d) 8mm

43. Long-term catheterization most compatible material:

(a) Latex (b) Silicone
(c) Polyurethane (d) Rubber

44. Inappropriate strategy to reduce surgical stress response:

(a) Epidural analgesia
(b) Complete bed rest
(c) Minimal invasive surgery
(d) Minimal preoperative starvation

45. All *except* one is the component of Ebb response:

(a) Insulin (b) Catecholamine
(c) Cortisol (d) Aldosterone

46. "Urologist's graveyard" is:

(a) Retroperitoneal space
(b) Retropubic space
(c) Supraduodenal fossa
(d) Pyriform fossa

47. 1F (French) equals to:

(a) 0.33 mm in circumference
(b) 3.3 mm in circumference
(c) 0.33 mm in diameter
(d) 3.3 mm in diameter

48. Best position for per rectal examination of prostate:

(a) Supine (b) Prone
(c) Left lateral (d) Knee chest

49. What frequency of transducer is used during transrectal ultrasound?

(a) 3.5 MHz (b) 4.5 MHz
(c) 5.5 MHz (d) 7.5 MHz

50. Which is not a handport?

(a) Extriport (b) Gelport
(c) Omniport (d) Lap disc

51. Common injured vessel in endourologic procedures:

(a) Anterior segmental artery
(b) Posterior segmental artery
(c) Medial segmental artery
(d) Lateral segmental artery

52. Stain for eosinophilia:

(a) Giemsa (b) AFB
(c) H and E (d) Malachite

53. Highest level of evidence is available favouring which of the following, to be done before urological procedures?

(a) Antibiotic prophylaxis for open nephrectomy
(b) Bowel preparation for radical cystectomy
(c) Antithrombotic therapy in those with coronary stents
(d) Skin preparation before urethral instrumentation

54. For laparoscopic pneumoperitoneum, when is helium preferred?

(a) Parkinson's disease
(b) Chronic respiratory disease
(c) Thalassemia
(d) Polycythemia vera

55. Questionnaired used to measure sexual functioning in women is:

(a) ICS questionnaire
(b) FSFI questionnaire
(c) ADAM questionnaire
(d) Mebust questionnaire

56. Color code of 16 Fr Foley's catheter:

(a) Magenta (b) Orange
(c) Yellow (d) Green
(e) Red

ANSWERS

1.	D	13.	TFFTF	25.	A	37.	B	49.	D
2.	C	14.	TTFTT	26.	A	38.	A	50.	A
3.	C	15.	FFTTF	27.	A	39.	D	51.	B
4.	A	16.	TTTFF	28.	A	40.	C	52.	C
5.	B	17.	TTTTT	29.	C	41.	D	53.	B
6.	A	18.	FTFTF	30.	B	42.	C	54.	B
7.	FTFTT	19.	FFTFT	31.	B	43.	B	55.	B
8.	FFTFF	20.	FFTFT	32.	C	44.	C	56.	B
9.	FFTFF	21.	FFTTF	33.	C	45.	D		
10.	TTTFT	22.	ABC	34.	A	46.	B		
11.	TTTFT	23.	AB	35.	A	47.	C		
12.	TFTTF	24.	E	36.	D	48.	D		

CHAPTER 3

Infection and Inflammation

1. **Acute pyelonephritis is the most likely diagnosis in a patient with:**
   (a) Bacteriuria and pyuria
   (b) Focal scar in renal cortex
   (c) Chills, fever and flank pain
   (d) Fever, chills and dysuria

2. **Most recurrent urinary tract infections in females are:**
   (a) Complicated
   (b) Reinfection
   (c) Due to bacterial resistance
   (d) Due to hereditary susceptible factors

3. **Phase variation of bacterial pili:**
   (a) Occurs only in vitro
   (b) Affects bacterial virulence
   (c) Refers to change in pili length
   (d) Is characteristic of pyelonephritis E. coli

4. **The long-term effect of recurrent urinary tract infections is:**
   (a) Minimal (b) Renal scarring
   (c) Hypertension (d) V-U reflux

5. **The anti-proliferative factor (APF) is produced in:**
   (a) Bladder urothelial cells
   (b) Glomeruli
   (c) Transitional urothelial cells in upper tract
   (d) Mast cells

6. **The nidus for Michaelis-Gutmann body is:**
   (a) Renal papillae
   (b) Bacterial fragments
   (c) Calcium crystals
   (d) Macrophages

7. **Majority of patients with chronic pyelonephritis will present with:**
   (a) No symptoms
   (b) Flank pain
   (c) Recurrent febrile illness
   (d) Hypertension

8. **Which of the following fruit juices helps in preventing U.T.I.?**
   (a) Grape (b) Raspberry
   (c) Cranberry (d) Orange

9. **Which of the following is an ideal drug for empirical treatment of uncomplicated UTIs?**
   (a) Aminoglycosides (b) Fluoroquinolones
   (c) Cephalosporins (d) Nitrofurantoin

10. **Which of the following is a source of bacterial persistence?**
    (a) Sexual activity
    (b) Fecal colonization
    (c) Struvite calculus
    (d) Increased post void residue

11. **Renal thyroidization is seen in:**
    (a) Chronic pyelonephritis
    (b) Acute pyelonephritis
    (c) Emphysema
    (d) Xanthogranulomatous pyelonephritis

12. **Michaelis-Gutmann bodies are pathognomonic of:**
    (a) Malacoplakia
    (b) Xanthogranulomatous pyelonephritis
    (c) Chronic pyelonephritis
    (d) Acute pyelonephritis

13. The mortality rate of Fournier gangrene approximately:
(a) 50% (b) 80%
(c) 5% (d) 20%

14. Drug causing epididymitis:
(a) Ampicillin (b) Metrogyl
(c) Amiodarone (d) Phenytoin

15. Interstitial cystitis most commonly associated with:
(a) Irritable bowel syndrome
(b) Allergies
(c) Fibromyalgia
(d) Depression

16. All are true about chancroid *except:*
(a) It affects men three times more often than women
(b) Painful, non-indurated ulcer
(c) Inguinal adenopathy, that is typically bilateral
(d) Incubation period ranges from 1 to 21 days

17. In HIV acute infection, HIV RNA can be detected from day:
(a) 12 (b) 26
(c) 5 (d) 29

18. The most common intrascrotal pathology in AIDS is:
(a) Epididymitis (b) Orchitis
(c) Testicular atrophy (d) Testicular abscess

19. Granulomatous changes of the epididymis have been associated with:
(a) Tuberculosis (b) BCG treatment
(c) Sarcoidosis (d) All of the above

20. In CT evaluation of a possible renal abscess:
(a) Cortical attenuation is diagnostic
(b) Striations are characteristic
(c) Delayed renal views 2-3 hours later may be needed
(d) All of the above

21. Most common organism for community acquired UTI:
(a) E coli (b) Pseudomonas
(c) Proteus (d) Staphylococcus

22. Which one of the following is most common cause of painless recurrent hematuria in a 60 years old male in India?
(a) Genitourinary tuberculosis
(b) BPH
(c) Bladder malignancy
(d) BPH with bladder stone

23. True about emphysematous pyelonephritis is:
(a) Can be treated by drainage and antibiotic
(b) Type II gas extending in parenchyma
(c) Klebsiella most common organism
(d) Mortality low in most of the cases

24. Renal thyroidization:
(a) CPN (b) APN
(c) XGPN (d) Renal abscess

Mention True and False respective to each statement (Q. No. 25 to 66)

25. Risk factor for bacteriuria and renal damage in children:
(a) Race and ethnicity (b) Gender
(c) Genetics (d) Scarring
(e) Age of child

26. Pyelonephritis:
(a) Proteus is enterobacteriaceae
(b) Hematogenous is most common
(c) Reflux is essential
(d) In emphysematous pyelonephritis E coli is the most common organism
(e) In xanthogranulomatous pyelonephritis proteus is the most common organism

27. Regarding GUTB:
(a) PUJ most common site in ureter
(b) Ureteric infection by hematogenous spread
(c) Testicular infection by epididymis
(d) Epididymitis usually persists as slowly enlarging mass
(e) Penile tuberculosis never occurs

28. GUTB:
(a) Dose of isoniazid is to be decreased if creatinine > 2
(b) Fresh early morning urine sample should be cultured
(c) M. tuberculosis–doubling time of 15 to 20 hours
(d) If AFB (–)ve that rule out GUTB
(e) Ureteric stricture of 2 cm with kidney function < 10% best is end to end anastomosis

29. UTI:
(a) Pyuria defines as > 5 RBC/HPF
(b) E.coli is most common organism in acute pyelonephritis
(c) IVU is investigation of choice in emphysematous pyelonephritis
(d) Routine microscopy positive for pus cell is gold standard for diagnosis of UTI
(e) Asymptomatic bacteriuria in elderly requires no antibiotic treatment

30. Fournier's gangrene:
(a) Fusobacterium may be associated
(b) Paraphimosis may be risk further
(c) Secondary hypercalcemia may be associated
(d) Testis is usually involved
(e) Mortality <5%

31. Regarding UTI:
(a) More common in post menopausal women
(b) TMP-SMZ abolishes gut and vaginal anaerobic flora
(c) Nitrofurantoin does not alter the bowel flora
(d) Acute pulmonary reaction is not uncommon with NFT
(e) Intermittent self medication by females in recurrent UTI is not useful

32. Regarding xanthogranulomatous pyelonephritis:
(a) Proteus is the most common organism involved
(b) Frozen section cannot make diagnosis
(c) Diagnosis is usually made postoperative
(d) Associated with nephrolithiasis, infection and obstruction
(e) Involves perinephric fat and adjacent tissues

33. Genitourinary TB:
(a) Most common age group is in childhood
(b) Microscopic hematuria is present in 50% of patients
(c) Early morning urine sample for AFB is good
(d) Surgery can be done after 12 weeks of treatment
(e) Most common site of stricture is UVJ

34. GUTB:
(a) INH, R, Z, S are bacteriostatic
(b) Dose modification is required with rifampicin in renal failure
(c) Globus minor is the most commonly involved
(d) Rarely occurs below the age of 5 years
(e) Nephrectomy is indicated for extensive disease involving the whole kidney, together with hypertension and UPJ obstruction

35. Emphysematous pyelonephritis:
(a) Most common gas produced is methane
(b) Air fluid level indicates poor prognosis
(c) Grade IV is bilateral emphysematous PN
(d) Grade I is emphysematous pyelitis only
(e) Presence of streaky or mottled gas has a mortality of 50-60%

36. Genital ulcers:
(a) LGV is diagnosed from ulcer by identifying Chlamydia trachomatis
(b) Vaginal discharge in candidiasis is thick and curdy
(c) Herpes is diagnosed from vesicles on an erythematous base that doesn't follow a neural distribution
(d) Vaginal epithelium is resistant to infection with N. gonorrhoeae but cervix is not
(e) Strawberry vulva is seen with toxoplasmosis

37. Acute pyelonephritis:
(a) Triad–flank pain, pyrexia, vomiting
(b) Staph. saprophyticus causes UTI in 10% of young females
(c) Patients who relapse after initial 14-day course of therapy usually are cured by 6 weeks of antibiotics
(d) Asymptomatic E. coli cultures from urinary diversion should be treated with antibiotics for 14 days
(e) CT scan is used to evaluate patients who do not respond after 24 hours of therapy

38. Genitourinary TB:
(a) Involves in early childhood
(b) Radiological findings forms minor criteria
(c) Microscopic hematuria is present in > 80%
(d) AFB is easily detected in early morning sample
(e) Kidney is usually the primary organ infected in urinary disease

39. Emphysematous pyelonephritis:
(a) Air fluid level is good prognostic factor
(b) Methane is most significant gas
(c) Thrombocytosis is poor prognostic factor
(d) Grade I only pyelitis
(e) Grade IV is bilateral

40. UTI:
(a) Fecal reservoir may cause ascending infection through urethra
(b) Pyelonephritis commonly hematogenous in origin
(c) For pyelonephritis, VUR is mandatory
(d) S. saprophyticus is present in young sexually active girl in more than >50%
(e) Proteus belongs to enterobacteriaceae family

41. Inflammatory myofibroblastic tumor (IMT):
(a) Also known as inflammatory pseudotumor
(b) Essential criterion are spindle myoepithelial cell proliferation and lymphocytic infiltrate
(c) Anaplastic lymphoma kinase (ALK) is a good marker for IMT
(d) Biopsy is the gold standard for diagnosis
(e) Radiation is the treatment of choice

42. Funguria in children:
(a) Candida is most common
(b) Usually stone associated
(c) Change of catheter will not help
(d) Parenteral nutrition leads to funguria
(e) Asymptomatic funguria do not require treatment

43. Treatment of asymptomatic bacteriuria is required in:
(a) Pregnancy
(b) Premenopausal non-pregnant
(c) Spinal cord injured patient
(d) Indwelling catheter
(e) Urological intervention

44. Regarding UTI:
(a) For uncomplicated lower UTI–3-4 days antibiotic is appropriate
(b) In young sexually active female–staph saprophyticus is causative organism in 10%
(c) Orthotopic neobladder–asymptomatic bacteriuria–14 days antibiotic is given
(d) Self started therapy–fluoroquinolones is ideal
(e) In female, a catheterized urine sample should be obtained to evaluate infection

45. Regarding treatment of UTI:
(a) Penicillin can be given at any trimester of pregnancy
(b) Fluoroquinolones can be given at any trimester of pregnancy
(c) Nitrofurantoin is rapidly excreted in urine
(d) TMP-SMX has been the most widely used antimicrobial agent for treatment of acute UTI
(e) Antimicrobial resistance is influenced by duration and amount of antimicrobial agent used

46. Acute pyelonephritis characterized by:
(a) Triad of flank pain, pyuria and decreased renal function
(b) Phase variation is important in virulence
(c) 'O' serotype most important bacterial virulence factor
(d) Flank pain is diagnostic
(e) It may have no morphological/functional components

47. Regarding GUTB:
(a) Urine fresh sample required
(b) For urine AFB preferably 3 samples are examined
(c) Absence of AFB in urine rules out GUTB
(d) INH should not be given in patient with serum creatinine > 2.0 mg/ml
(e) 2 cm ureteric stricture with 10% ipsilateral renal function, ureteroureterostomy should be done

48. Malakoplakia:
(a) Usually present in early twenties
(b) Usually present with bladder irritability and hematuria
(c) Biopsy is diagnostic
(d) Lesion is characterized by large histiocytes
(e) Michaelis-Gutmann bodies may be absent in early malacoplakia and are not necessary for the diagnosis

49. Pregnancy and UTI:
(a) Kidney ↑ by 1 cm in size
(b) Asymptomatic bacteriuria should be treated
(c) GFR ↑ by 10%
(d) RBF increases by 10% transiently
(e) Investigate if serum creatinine > 0.8 mg %

50. Pregnancy and UTI:
(a) Hydronephrosis due to progesterone
(b) Penicillin and cephalosporine is drug of choice
(c) TMP-SMX is indicated in 1st and 3rd trimester
(d) NFT contraindicated throughout pregnancy
(e) Pyelonephritis develops in 1-4% of all pregnant women

51. Regarding Fournier's gangrene:
(a) Mortality 20%
(b) Advanced cases present with testicular necrosis
(c) Plain film of the abdomen may be helpful in identifying air
(d) Anaerobic and aerobic synergy occurs
(e) Hypocalcemia is due to chelation of Ca^{+2}

52. Regarding UTI:
(a) Gallium most sensitive to diagnose acute pyelonephritis
(b) Fluoroquinolones ideal agent in uncomplicated cystitis
(c) In female and uncomplicated cystitis– Antibiotics should be given for 10 days
(d) Upper tract imaging usually not done in recurrent cystitis
(e) USG is the best modality for pyonephrosis

53. Screening of asymptomatic bacteria:
(a) Done in elderly and children
(b) Mandatory in pregnancy
(c) Mandatory in all patients with catheter
(d) Mandatory in all patients with CIC
(e) Mandatory in all patients undergoing TURP

54. Xanthogranulomatous pyelonephritis:
(a) Stone is uncommon
(b) More common in female
(c) Focal is more common than generalised
(d) E. coli and proteus is more common
(e) Usually bilateral

55. Bacteriuria depends upon:
(a) Age (b) Sex
(c) DM (d) Significant VUR
(e) Genitourinary tract abnormality

56. Asymptomatic bacteriuria:
(a) In pregnancy should be treated
(b) Spinal trauma patient should be treated
(c) Catheterized patient should be treated
(d) Young premenopausal and non-pregnant female should be treated
(e) In elderly should be treated

57. Regarding chyluria:
(a) Present in 20% patients of filariasis
(b) Serum lipid decreases
(c) 5% silver nitrate used as sclerosant
(d) IVP diagnostic
(e) Human is the only host for filariasis

58. Schistosomiasis:
(a) Schistosoma hematobium is one of the three species causing schistosomiasis in human
(b) Rare in human
(c) Urinary examination is not helpful
(d) Most morbidity caused by acute disease
(e) Resides in retrovesical venous plexus

59. Regarding septic shock:
(a) IL6 released by PMN and phagocytes
(b) TNF released by PMN and phagocytes
(c) Inulin like growth factor released by PMN and phagocytes
(d) TNF is regarded as a central mediator of pathophysiologic changes associated with sepsis
(e) The prime initiator of gram-negative bacterial septic shock is endotoxin, an LPS component of the bacterial outer membrane

60. In pregnant female:
(a) Asymptomatic bacteriuria should be treated
(b) Increase risk of UTI → prophylaxis throughout pregnancy
(c) Trimethoprim is contraindicated in 1st trimester
(d) Nitrofurantoin contraindicated throughout pregnancy
(e) Penicillin and cephalosporin are drug of choice

61. Renal abscess:
(a) In pre antibiotic era – Most common etiology was staphylococcus
(b) Now-a-days retrograde spread is most common
(c) Anerobic infections does not cause renal abscess
(d) The number of echoes depends on the amount of cellular debris within the abscess
(e) Actinomyces and candida infection is seen in immunocompromised

62. Prostatodynia:
(a) Caused by reflux of urine in prostate
(b) Alpha-blocker is most effective treatment
(c) A bacterial prostatitis
(d) It is categorized as 3B
(e) White blood cells (and/or bacteria) in expressed prostatic secretions, post-prostatic massage urine sediment (VB3), semen, or histologic specimens of prostate gland

63. Regarding UTI:
(a) Asymptomatic bacteriuria infected with age in men and women is a linear trend
(b) Prolonged antibiotic prophylaxis in recurrent UTI decreases incidence
(c) Fik-mediated binding to the bladder epithelium is the initial step in the intricate cascade of events leading to UTIs
(d) Mannose sensitive pili pyelonephritogenic
(e) Increased adherence of pathogenic bacteria to vaginal epithelial cells as the first demonstrable biologic difference that could be shown in women susceptible to UTI

64. Emphysematous pyelonephritis:
(a) Only adult cases reported till date
(b) Extension of severe pyelonephritis

(c) Proteus is most common organism
(d) IVU has got no role
(e) Classical triad is fever, vomiting and flank pain

65. Regarding emphysematous pyelonephritis:
(a) Occurs only in adult
(b) Klebsiella most common
(c) No use of IVP
(d) Extension of severe pyelonephritis
(e) Mortality is near 40%

66. Regarding renal infection:
(a) Staph aureus spreads by hematogenous route
(b) For ascending infection lymphatics plays predominant role
(c) Reflux is necessary for recurrent pyelonephritis
(d) Most UTI are due to fecal microbes
(e) CT scan is sensitive for focal subacute nephritis

Which of the following statement is correct?

67. Commonly used drug for prophylaxis of UTI in renal transplant patient is:
(a) Nitrofurantoin
(b) Ciprofloxacin
(c) Trimethoprim + sulfamethoxazole
(d) Amoxicillin + clavulinic acid

68. Cranberry juice–not a mechanism of action:
(a) Acidify urine
(b) Secrete IgA
(c) IL-6
(d) Bacterial adherence
(e) Inhibit hemagglutination of E. coli

69. Fever with chills, flank pain accompanied with bacteriuria and pyuria. True is:
(a) Start broad spectrum antibiotic
(b) Pigtail drainage has good prognosis
(c) Urgent management if possible
(d) Order NCCT immediately
(e) Suspect EPN

70. True about UTI:
(a) Bacterial persistence is due to infection by same organism
(b) Antibiotic prophylaxis decreases risk of recurrence
(c) 50% of female will have UTI in the lifetime
(d) Probability increases with repeated number of UTI
(e) Anaerobic facultative organism from bowel is most common cause

71. GUTB:
(a) Bladder is primary site
(b) Most common by lymphatic route
(c) Prostate and penile urethra most common site
(d) Testis is always affected by direct spread from epididymis
(e) UV junction is the most common site in ureter

72. UTI in pregnancy–safe antibiotic:
(a) Ampicillin
(b) Cotrimoxazole
(c) Cephalosporin
(d) Ciprofloxacin
(e) Tobramycin

73. Which antibiotic does not have anti-pseudomonas activity?
(a) Colistin
(b) Imipenem
(c) Amoxclav
(d) Ceftazidime
(e) Cefoperazone-sulbactum

74. Chronic bacterial prostatitis:
(a) Antimicrobial treatment mainstay
(b) Doxycycline/macrolide is first line treatment
(c) Fluoroquinolones is second line treatment
(d) Prostatic massage improves results
(e) α-blocker is adjuvant treatment

75. Treatment options for acute prostatitis:
(a) Antibiotics
(b) Analgesics
(c) Sitz bath
(d) Urethral catheterisation
(e) Prostatic massage

76. Not a part of DOTS in TB:
(a) INH (b) Rifampicin
(c) Ethambutol (d) Streptomycin
(e) Thiacetazone

77. Gonococcal urethritis not useful in diagnosis:
(a) Urethral itching
(b) Purulent urethral discharge with blood
(c) Frequency and urgency
(d) Dysuria
(e) Fever with chills

78. Antimicrobial not effective against pseudomonas:
(a) Norflox (b) Ciplox
(c) Clotrimoxazole (d) Nitrofurantoin
(e) Piperacillin

79. Malacoplakia false is:
(a) MG body pathognomonic
(b) Abnormal macrophage function against bacterial infection
(c) Only involve kidney
(d) Malacoplakia of renal parenchyma leads to renal vein thrombosis
(e) Malacoplakia means hard plaque

80. Bacteriuria true:
(a) Asymptomatic bacteria in pregnancy – no treatment
(b) Chronic catheterization–long-term prophylaxis is required
(c) Elderly men and women – bacteriuria very common
(d) Inevitable in chronic catheterization
(e) Spinal cord injury patients–long-term catheterization leads to bacteriuria

81. Interstitial cystitis – false is:
(a) Premalignant
(b) Associated with inflammatory bowel disease
(c) HPE to rule out other diseases
(d) Glomerulation or hydrodistention is diagnostic
(e) NMP-22 for follow-up

82. Painful genital ulcer seen in:
(a) Herpes (b) Chancroid
(c) Syphilis (d) LGV
(e) Gonorrhea

83. Urine abnormality present in glomerulonephritis are:
(a) Proteinuria
(b) Casts
(c) Pedal edema
(d) Microscopic hematuria
(e) Dysmorphic RBC

84. Uneventful postoperative day 4 with Candida albicans 10^4 CFU in urine–what all is done?
(a) Remove indwelling catheter
(b) IV amphotericin and fluconazole
(c) Discontinue broad spectrum antibiotics
(d) Improve nutritional status
(e) Only observation

85. Which of the following is contraindicated in pregnancy?
(a) INH (b) Streptomycin
(c) Rifampicin (d) Pyrazinamide
(e) Ethambutol

86. Interstitial cystitis symptoms–all *except*:
(a) Nocturia (b) Frequency
(c) Urgency (d) Hematuria
(e) Suprapubic pain

87. UTI prophylaxis in female done with:
(a) Nitrofurantoin (b) Norflox
(c) Trimethoprim (d) Ampicillin
(e) Amoxycillin

88. ATT acting intracellularly:
(a) INH (b) Rifampicin
(c) Ethambutol (d) Pyrazinamide
(e) Streptomycin

89. Vasal calcification seen in:
(a) Syphilis
(b) TB

(c) Schistosomiasis
(d) Hyperparathyroidism
(e) Sarcoidosis

90. Fungal bezoar caused by:
(a) Candida albicans (b) T. glabarata
(c) Zygomycosis (d) Aspergillosis
(e) Coccidiodomycosis

91. ATT – contraindicated in pregnancy:
(a) INH (b) Rifampicin
(c) Streptomycin (d) Ethambutol
(e) Pyrazinamide

92. Post unilateral nephrectomy, asymptomatic patient with urine C/S positive for candida – treatment:
(a) Stop broad spectrum antibiotics
(b) Removal of catheter
(c) IV amphotericin B
(d) Systemic fluconazole
(e) Intravesical amphotericin B

93. Antibiotic dose modification not require in renal failure:
(a) Cloxacillin (b) Gentamicin
(c) Cephalexin (d) Ampicillin
(e) Aztreonam

94. Prophylactic antimicrobial agents are:
(a) Nitrofurantoin (b) Norflox
(c) Ampicillin (d) Septran
(e) Cefazolin

95. Regarding emphysematous pyelonephritis which is not correct?
(a) N2 production
(b) More in diabetics
(c) Most common organism – E. coli
(d) All cases in adults
(e) Female > male

96. Bladder biopsy in genitourinary TB is done in all *except*:
(a) Bilateral HDUN
(b) Renal damage in IVP
(c) Obstruction at lower end of ureter with tubercular ulcer in bladder
(d) Suspicious of malignancy
(e) All cases of sterile pyuria

97. In acute epididymitis most common etiology in sexually active male is:
(a) E. coli
(b) C. trachomatis and N. gonorrhoeae
(c) H influenzatis
(d) Streptococcus

98. Abnormality in prostatitis:
(a) Lymphocytic infiltration in acini
(b) Lymphocytic infiltration in stroma
(c) Neutrophilic infiltration in acini
(d) Neutrophilic infiltration in stroma

99. Phase variation what is true?
(a) Reversible
(b) Only in vivo
(c) Specific for pyelonephric E. coli
(d) Change in length

100. Urinary candidiasis:
(a) Most catheterized patients with persistent candiduria are asymptomatic
(b) Blood cultures are helpful and yield positive results in 90% of cases of disseminated infection
(c) A potassium hydroxide smear is useful for direct demonstration of fungal cells
(d) Fluconazole is considered a first-line agent in non-neutropenic patients with candidemia

101. HIV all are true *except*:
(a) ELISA > 99% sensitivity
(b) ELISA > 98% positive predictive value
(c) Western blot highly specific
(d) In all STD, HIV should be done

102. Treatment of prostatitis are all *except*:
(a) NSAIDS, should improve the inflam-

matory parameters within the prostate and possibly result in a reduction of symptoms

(b) In absence of anatomic deformity and abscess, 2-4 weeks treatment given

(c) 2nd and 3rd gen cephalosporins are 1st line of treatment

(d) α-adrenergic blockade may diminish intraprostatic ductal reflux

103. Forty four years old has a testicular pain with recent onset. On examination testicular swelling was present and cord was tender:

(a) Torsion - antibiotics

(b) Epididymo-orchitis - antibiotics

(c) Epididymo-orchitis - surgery

(d) Torsion - surgery

104. Sixty years old patient had dysuria, fever with chills and back pain. On examination tender prostate next action:

(a) Antibiotics

(b) TRUS guided prostate biopsy

(c) PSA test immediately

(d) Admit for TURP

105. Time interval between 1st episode of UTI and recurrent UTI:

(a) > 1 week

(b) 2 weeks to 15 weeks

(c) < 2 weeks > 15 weeks

(d) < 1 week

106. Nitrofurantoin not active against:

(a) Enterococcus (b) Staph aureus

(c) E coli (d) Proteus

107. Most common cause of glomerular hematuria:

(a) IgA nephropathy

(b) SLE

(c) MSGN

(d) Membranous GN

108. Parasite which most commonly causes lymphatic filariasis:

(a) Wucheria bancrofti (b) Brugia malai

(c) Loa loa (d) Brugia timori

109. ATT which acts through DNA dependent RNA polymerase:

(a) Rifampicin (b) Isoniazid

(c) Pyrizinamide (d) Ethambutol

110. Regarding ethambutol true is:

(a) Optic neuritis is most serious symptom

(b) Reversible

(c) Occurs within few days

(d) Dose dependent

111. 68 years male present with fever 1 week with WBC > 18000, acinetobacter +ve > 10^5 colony, CT-upper pole ill-defined mass. USG shows internal echos with ring sign. Diagnosis is:

(a) Renal abscess

(b) Pyelonephritis

(c) RCC

(d) Infected HDN

112. First site to be involved in genitourinary TB:

(a) Renal parenchyma (b) Upper ureter

(c) Lower ureter (d) Bladder

113. Drug of choice for interstitial cystitis:

(a) DMSO

(b) Pentosan polysulfate

(c) Heparin

(d) Amitryptiline

114. Indications for nephrectomy in TB:

(a) Extensive diseases of kidney

(b) Non-functioning kidney with calcification

(c) Non-functioning kidney with HTN

(d) Non-functioning kidney with RCC

115. LGV-incubation period is:

(a) 0–3 days (b) 3–30 days

(c) 2 weeks (d) 9–90 days

116. Incidence of bacteriuria in elderly:
(a) 20% in men and 10% in women
(b) 20% in women and 10% in men
(c) 20% each in men and women
(d) 10% each in men and women

117. Most common bacteria for XGPN:
(a) E coli (b) Proteus
(c) Klebsiella (d) Pseudomonas

118. DOC for NGU:
(a) Erythromycin (b) Ofloxacin
(c) Azithromycin (d) Ceftriaxone

119. Most common site of stricture in GUTB:
(a) PUJ
(b) VUJ
(c) 5 cm above VUJ
(d) 5 cm below PUJ

120. Young women sexually active, 10% of UTI is caused by:
(a) Staph. saprophyticus
(b) Staph. epidermidis
(c) Pneumococcus
(d) Staph. fecalis

121. Asymptomatic bacteriuria treated with:
(a) Young women
(b) Children
(c) Older females
(d) Pregnant females

122. Reservoir of cryptococcus after HIV treatment in meningitis:
(a) Prostate (b) Renal
(c) Bladder (d) Testis

123. Regarding Kaposi sarcoma false is:
(a) In the patient with AIDS, the underlying immune deficiency predisposes the host to Kaposi's sarcoma by a factor of 7
(b) Tumor of the reticuloendothelial system
(c) Human herpesvirus 8
(d) Treatment is directed toward palliation

124. Single episode of candiduria, the major associated illnesses is with:
(a) DM
(b) Hypothyroidism
(c) Malignancy
(d) Collagen vascular disease

125. Optic neuritis found with:
(a) Ethambutol (b) INH
(c) Rifampicin (d) Pyrazinamide

126. INH hepatotoxicity:
(a) Resolves with discontinuation
(b) B_{12} is treatment
(c) Seen in 5-10% of patients
(d) Occurs in a week of starting therapy

127. Best radiological investigation of GUTB:
(a) CT (b) IVP
(c) MRI (d) USG

128. True about interstitial cystitis all *except*:
(a) Epithelial permeability is defective
(b) Mast cell inflammation may be involved
(c) Neurogenic inflammation is one cause
(d) Heparin (GAG) covers the bladder surface

129. Golf hole ureter:
(a) Schistosomiasis
(b) High grade VUR
(c) Tuberculosis
(d) All of the above

130. UTI most common in males than females, true is:
(a) <1 year of age (b) >1 year of age
(c) <50 years of age (d) >50 years of age

131. Which of the following is not true of perinephric or renal abscess?
(a) CT is not diagnostic
(b) Carbuncle is a collection of purulent material confined to the renal parenchyma

(c) Common in diabetic and VUR
(d) Pyuria and bacteriuria may not be evident

132. Urea splitting bacteria most commonly is:
(a) Proteus (b) Klebsiella
(c) E. coli (d) Pseudomonas

133. Rare site for tuberculosis is:
(a) Kidney (b) Bladder
(c) Prostate (d) Ureter

134. Drug that can be used in pregnancy:
(a) Ceftriaxone (b) Ofloxacin
(c) Ciprofloxacin (d) Doxycycline

135. In uncomplicated gonococcal urethritis not used is:
(a) Ceftriaxone (b) Ofloxacin
(c) Doxycycline (d) Ciprofloxacin

136. Causative organism of LGV:
(a) C. granulomatosis (b) H. ducreyi
(c) C. trachomatis (d) T. pallidum

137. Cystometry findings in interstitial cystitis are:
(a) Normal capacity
(b) Normal compliance
(c) Low compliance
(d) Detrusor instability

138. Renal papillary necrosis is seen in all *except*:
(a) Analgesic nephropathy
(b) Diabetic GN
(c) Pyelonephritis
(d) Glomerulonephritis

139. Gonococcal urethritis incubation period is:
(a) 0–3 days (b) 3–10 days
(c) 2 weeks (d) 9–90 days

140. The most common organism causing endocarditits after urologic procedure is:
(a) E coli (b) Pseudomonas
(c) Enterococcus (d) Candida

141. Which of the non-lymphatic microfilaria causes hanging groin?
(a) Loa loa
(b) Onchocerca volvulus
(c) Dacrofilaria
(d) Mansonella

142. The following lesions and causative organisms are correct *except*:
(a) Chancre – Treponema pallidum
(b) Chancroid – Hemophilus ducreyi
(c) Granuloma inguinale–Chlamydia trachomatis
(d) Condyloma acuminata–Human papilloma virus

143. Name an ATT that has to be avoided in an HIV patient due to drug interaction with antiviral therapy:
(a) INH (b) Rifampicin
(c) Pyrazinamide (d) Ethambutol

144. Which of the following is false about bladder pain syndrome (BPS) or interstitial cystitis?
(a) Female to male ratio 5:1
(b) Fluctuating course of disease without long term sequel
(c) No effect on pregnancy outcome
(d) Hunner's ulcer seen more commonly in males

145. Anti proliferative factor (APF) is a marker of:
(a) Acute prostatitis
(b) Neurogenic bladder
(c) Interstitial cystitis
(d) Bladder cancer

146. Following drugs are contraindicated during pregnancy *except*:
(a) Fluoroquinolones
(b) Cefaclor
(c) Chloramphenicol
(d) Tetracyclines

147. A man who is evaluated for sexually transmitted disease (STD) is unlikely to have chlamydia infection if exposure to sexual partner is more than:

(a) 15 days (b) 30 days
(c) 45 days (d) 60 days

148. Reiter's syndrome includes all *except:*

(a) Prostatitis (b) Urethritis
(c) Conjunctivitis (d) Arthritis

149. Treatment regimen for uncomplicated cystitis in asymptomatic adult women:

(a) 3 days (b) 5 days
(c) 7 days (d) 10 days

150. Michaelis-Gutmann bodies found in:

(a) Xanthogranulomatous pyelonephritis
(b) Chlamydia infection
(c) Interstitial cystitis
(d) Renal malakoplakia

151. Which of the following drugs is the best prophylactic agent for prevention of implantation of spilled protoscolices for hydatid disease?

(a) Metronidazole (b) Mebendazole
(c) Praziquantel (d) Flubendazole

152. Which of the following condition is not a component of Reiter's disease?

(a) Urethritis (b) Uveitis
(c) Arthritis (d) Cholangitis

153. In which of the following group of patients is screening for asymptomatic bacteriuria recommended?

(a) Diabetic women
(b) Patients with spinal cord injury
(c) Patients with indwelling urethral catheters
(d) Prior to urologic interventions

154. Which of the following organism is most commonly associated with infection stones?

(a) Proteus (b) Klebsiella
(c) Pseudomonas (d) Staphylococcus

155. Preferred regimen for uncomplicated cystitis in women is:

(a) Single-dose therapy
(b) 3-day therapy
(c) 7-day therapy
(d) 10-day therapy

156. Classic triad of clinical presentation of emphysematous pyelonephritis consists of the following *except*:

(a) Fever (b) Vomiting
(c) Flank pain (d) Pneumaturia

157. Moderate benefit in chronic pelvic pain syndrome is associated with:

(a) Alpha adrenergic blockers
(b) Anti-microbial agents
(c) Anti-inflammatory agents
(d) Phytotherapies

158. ATT which acts through DNA dependent RNA polymerase:

(a) Rifampicin (b) Ethambutol
(c) Pyrizinamide (d) Cycloserine

159. Classical triad of emphysematous pyelonephritis is:

(a) Fever, vomiting and flank pain
(b) Fever, vomiting and dysuria
(c) Pain, vomiting and hematuria
(d) Pain, fever and hematuria

160. Most common early reliable clinical indication of septicemia:

(a) Fever
(b) Hyperventilation
(c) Shock
(d) Chills

161. 85% community acquired UTI and 50% hospital acquired UTI caused by:
(a) Proteus (b) E. coli
(c) Staphylococcus (d) Klebsiella

162. Prostate develops from:
(a) UGS
(b) Mesonephric duct
(c) Mullerian duct
(d) Ureteric bud

163. Thyroidization of kidney seen in:
(a) Amyloidosis of kidney
(b) Chronic pyelonephritis
(c) Acute pyelonephritis
(d) Acute glomerulonephritis

164. Unusual cause of UTI:
(a) Salmonella
(b) Staph epididymis
(c) Streptococci
(d) Klebsiella

165. Most common cause of chyluria in our country:
(a) Filariasis
(b) Tuberculosis
(c) Retroperitoneal fibrosis
(d) Pelvic radiation

166. M. tuberculosis, with a doubling time of:
(a) 15-20 seconds (b) 15-20 minutes
(c) 15-20 hours (d) 15-20 days

167. Most common site of gonococcal urethral stricture:
(a) Membranous (b) Prostatic
(c) Bulbar (d) Penoscrotal

168. Which of the following is transmitted by water?
(a) Hepatitis A (b) Hepatitis B
(c) Hepatitis C (d) HIV

169. Highest risk of HIV infection:
(a) Splash of blood on face
(b) Intravenous drug abuse
(c) Needle injury while suturing on non-dominant arm
(d) Diathermy burn

170. Which of the following is reliable clinical sign for diagnosis of acute pyelonephritis?
(a) Tenderness (b) Pyuria
(c) Frequency (d) Hypertension

171. Periurethral abscess can extend upto:
(a) Chin
(b) Clavicle
(c) Inguinal region
(d) Umbilicus

172. Hunner's ulcer is characteristically seen in:
(a) Interstitial cystitis
(b) Emphysematous pyelonephritis
(c) Xanthogranulomatous pyelonephritis
(d) Malakoplakia

173. Best investigation for emphysematous pyelonephritis is:
(a) CT (b) X-ray KUB
(c) USG (d) MRI

174. Tuberculosis most commonly involves which part of epididymis?
(a) Head
(b) Globus minor
(c) Globus major
(d) All parts are affected equally

175. Calcification of vas and seminal vesicles occur in all *except:*
(a) DM
(b) Tuberculosis
(c) Hyperparathyroidism
(d) Chronic inflammatory processes

176. Drug safe in pregnancy:
(a) Cephalosporin
(b) Fluoroquinolones
(c) Chloramphenicol
(d) Nitrofurantoin

177. Basal calcification is seen with all *except:*
(a) Aging (b) DM
(c) Tuberculosis (d) Leprosy

178. Most common organism for UTI is:
(a) Gram positive cocci
(b) Gram negative cocci
(c) Gram negative bacilli
(d) Anaerobes

179. "Gold-hole" ureter is seen in:
(a) Rhabdomyosarcoma of the bladder
(b) Urethral duplication
(c) VUR
(d) Exstrophy bladder

180. Age when urinary infection is more in male than in female:
(a) Less than 1 year
(b) More than 50 years
(c) <1 year and > 50 years
(d) More than 60 years

181. True about the etiology of interstitial cystitis are all *except:*
(a) Mast cell release
(b) Neuropathic
(c) Defect in epithelial lining of bladder surface glycosaminoglycans
(d) Heparin (GAG) is found on the bladder surface normally

182. Most common cause of epididymo-orchitis is E. coli in all subgroups, *except:*
(a) Pediatrics
(b) Sexually active <35 years
(c) Elderly
(d) Homosexual men
(e) Men performing anal intercourse

183. DM with gas in parenchyma, most unlikely pathogen:
(a) Staph. viridans
(b) Klebsiella
(c) E. coli
(d) Candida albicans
(e) Clostridium

184. Best investigation for emphysematous pyelonephritis is:
(a) CT (b) X-ray KUB
(c) USG (d) MRI
(e) Needle aspiration

185. At what age men will have more UTI than girls?
(a) <1 year (b) <2 years
(c) After 15 years (d) After 50 years

186. In dysuric females significant bacteriuria is defined as when colony count is more than:
(a) 100/ml (b) 1000/ml
(c) 10000/ml (d) 100000/ml

187. False regarding emphysematous pyelonephritis:
(a) Caused by clostridium welchii
(b) Not seen in type 1 diabetics
(c) H_2, CO_2 gases are formed
(d) Obstruction is present in 25% of cases

188. Following is not a factor in the etiology of XGP:
(a) Nephrolithiasis
(b) Obstruction
(c) Infection
(d) Immunodeficiency

189. False about TB epididymitis:
(a) Usually acquired through spread from vas deferens
(b) Presents with acute scrotum
(c) Diagnosis is by culture of sinus discharge
(d) Not a primary site of genitourinary tract TB

190. Chronic pyelonephritis is best diagnosed by:
(a) USG (b) IVP
(c) CT scan abdomen (d) Tc99 DMSA

191. Enterobacteriaceae are:
(a) Aerobic gram +ve
(b) Aerobic gram -ve
(c) Anaerobic gram +ve
(d) Anaerobic gram -ve

192. Which of the following type of adhesion molecules is associated with pyelonephritis in the general population?
(a) Type 1 mannose sensitive pili
(b) Direct adhesion
(c) Type S pili
(d) Type 1 mannose resistant pili

193. Xanthogranulomatous pyelonephritis is associated with all of the following *except:*
(a) Intraparenchymal gas formation
(b) Renal calculi
(c) Chronic urinary tract infection
(d) Involved kidney is non-functional

194. The cell most likely to play central role in the pathogenesis of interstitial cystitis is:
(a) Granulocyte (b) Lymphocyte
(c) Mast cell (d) Eosinophil

195. The gas seen in emphysematous pyelonephritis is:
(a) Nitric oxide
(b) Carbon dioxide
(c) Nitrogen
(d) Free oxygen radicals

196. Which one of the following statements is not correct?
(a) All pregnant women should be screened for bacteriuria
(b) Asymptomatic bacteriuria in pregnancy does not require treatment
(c) Bacteriuria may predispose to pyelonephritis during pregnancy
(d) Pyelonephritis occurs in 20-40% of pregnant women with bacteriuria

197. Not pathological in pregnancy:
(a) Lower l/3rd ureter dilatation
(b) Dilation of left pelvicalyceal system
(c) Increase in size of kidney
(d) Difference in size 1.7 times
(e) Increase urinary frequency

198. Treatment regimen for uncomplicated cystitis in asymptomatic adult women:
(a) 3 dahys (b) 5 days
(c) 7 days (d) 10 days
(e) 14 days

199. Long-term prophylaxis in UTI includes all *except*:
(a) Trimethoprim
(b) Sulfamethoxazole
(c) Cotrimoxazole
(d) Cefuroxime
(e) Nitrofurantoin

200. Colistin is used in all *except*:
(a) Klebsiella
(b) Pseudomonas
(c) Acinetobacter
(d) Metallo beta-lactamase
(e) Proteus

201. Glomerular hematuria is suggested by:
(a) WBC cast
(b) Dysmorphic RBC
(c) HTN
(d) Worm thread like clots
(e) Fever with hematuria

202. The development of bacteriuria:
(a) 1% per day of catheterization
(b) 2% per day of catheterization
(c) 5% per day of catheterization
(d) 10% per day of catheterization

203. Poor prognostic factor in fetal urine is all *except:*
(a) Osmolarity >200
(b) Chloride < 90

(c) Beta 2 microglobulin >4 mg/l
(d) Sodium > 100

204. Alkaline urine in UTI suggests infection due to:
(a) Escherichia coli
(b) Enterococcus
(c) Beta-hemolytic streptococcus
(d) Proteus vulgaris

205. Regarding urinary tract infections:
(a) Most common mode of pyelonephritis is hematogenous spread
(b) E. coli is the most common cause of hospital acquired UTI
(c) Type 1 pili are immunogenic, thus promoting bacterial clearance
(d) Type 1 pili are expressed only on pathogenic E. coli

206. Antimicrobial prophylaxis is mandatory in which one of the following procedures?
(a) Catheter removal
(b) Diagnostic cystoscopy
(c) Urodynamics
(d) TRUS guided prostate biopsy

207. Which of the following is correct regarding the use of nitrofurantoin in the treatment of urinary tract infections?
(a) Nitrofurantoin is ideal choice for outpatient treatment of pyelonephritis
(b) Nitrofurantoin causes minimal alteration of bowel flora
(c) Highest risk of adverse pulmonary reactions with nitrofurantoin is in children
(d) Nitrofurantoin has the lowest GI adverse effects of all chemoprophylaxis

208. UPOINT clinical classification system is used in the management of:
(a) Chronic pelvic pain syndrome
(b) Dyspareunia
(c) Stress urinary incontinence
(d) Recurrent urolithiasis

209. Which of the following is correct regarding interstitial cystitis?
(a) Men are more commonly affected than women
(b) Affected men are often young
(c) Women with IC have higher incidence of adverse pregnancy outcome
(d) IC is not premalignant

210. Non-tender groin lymphadenopathy is encountered in:
(a) Primary syphilis
(b) Genital herpes
(c) Chancroid
(d) Lymphogranuloma

211. In Reiter's syndrome:
(a) There is strong association with HLA A3
(b) The lesions are distinctly different from psoriasis
(c) The lesions are often preceded by an episode of urethritis or GI infection
(d) Topical steroids can be used

212. Which one of the following is true in the diagnosis of urinary tuberculosis?
(a) Quantiferon gold test is diagnostic of urinary tuberculosis
(b) Genexpert detects resistance to isoniazid
(c) Cystoscopic biopsy is always indicated in confirming the diagnosis
(d) Nucleic acid amplification tests have high sensitivity as well as specificity

213. Which one is not associated with increased mortality in Fournier Gangrene?
(a) Infection originated from periurethral region
(b) Infection originated from colorectal region
(c) Diabetes
(d) Alcoholism
(e) Involvement of deep tissue with shock

214. All are causes of periurethral abscess:
(a) Bladder stones

(b) Gonorrhea
(c) Prostatic stents
(d) Per urethral catheterization
(e) Urethral stricture

215. XGPN all are true *except*:
(a) Extrarenal extension rare
(b) Small kidney
(c) Stone present in >75%
(d) Chronic infection
(e) Nonfunctioning or poorly functioning kidney

216. Antipseudomonal are all *except*:
(a) Amoxy + clav
(b) Cefoperazone + salbactum
(c) Colistin
(d) Cefiazidime
(e) Imipenam

217. Which of the following are not risk factor for acute prostatic abscess?
(a) Long-term periurethral catheter
(b) Diabetes mellitus
(c) Post-transplant status with immuno-suppression
(d) TRUS biopsy
(e) BPH

218. Treatment of acute prostatitis:
(a) Sitz bath
(b) Per urethral Foley's catheter
(c) Antibiotics
(d) Anti-inflammatory
(e) Prostatic massage

219. EPN common organism:
(a) Pseudomonas (b) Candida
(c) E. coli (d) C. jejuni
(e) Clostridium

220. Causes of genital ulcer:
(a) Chancroids (b) Genital herpes
(c) Secondary syphilis (d) Tertiary syphilis
(e) LGV

221. UTI in adult female, false are:
(a) 10% have at least 1 episode per year
(b) Peak incidence is 25-30 years age group
(c) Genetic predisposition is noted
(d) 75-90% occurs in sexually active females
(e) 60% have recurrent UTI

222. Asymptomatic bacteriuria in pregnant women should be treated. What is the reason?
(a) Causes neonatal sepsis
(b) Causes postpartum sepsis and renal failure
(c) Progresses to acute pyelonephritis more frequently
(d) Causes abortion or still birth

223. Which blood group phenotype in women is associated with recurrent UTI?
(a) ABO-group (b) p-group
(c) Le(a-b-) (d) Le(a-b+)

224. Plasmid mediated bacterial resistance has not been reported in one of the drugs given below:
(a) Sulfonamides (b) Nitrofurantoin
(c) Fluoroquinolones (d) Tetracycline

225. Which is the bad prognostic indicator of emphysematous pyelonephritis on CT scan?
(a) Presence of fluid levels
(b) Presence of streaky or mottled gas
(c) Presence perirenal fluid
(d) Presence of gas in the collecting system

226. A 25 years old women in her 3rd trimester of pregnancy found to have asymptomatic bacteriuria, what is the drug of choice to treat?
(a) Nitrofurantoin (b) Sulfisoxazole
(c) Erythromycin (d) Cephalosporins

227. Which is the anti-tuberculus drug that do not act on intracellular bacteria?
(a) INH (b) Rifampicin
(c) Pyrazinamide (d) Ethambutol

ANSWERS

1. C	26. TFFTT	51. TFTTT	76. E	101. B
2. B	27. FFTTF	52. FTFFT	77. CE	102. C
3. B	28. FTTFF	53. FTFFT	78. CD	103. B
4. A	29. TTFFT	54. FTFTF	79. CE	104. A
5. A	30. TTTFF	55. TTTTT	80. CDE	105. B
6. B	31. TFTTF	56. TFFFF	81. ADE	106. D
7. A	32. TTTTT	57. TTTTT	82. AB	107. A
8. C	33. FTFTT	58. TTFFT	83. ABDE	108. A
9. B	34. FTTTT	59. TTTTT	84. ACD	109. A
10. C	35. FTTTT	60. FFTFT	85. ABC	110. C
11. A	36. TTTTF	61. TTFTT	86. D	111. A
12. A	37. FTFFF	62. TTTTT	87. ABC	112. A
13. D	38. FTFFT	63. TFTFT	88. ABD	113. A
14. C	39. FFFTT	64. TTFTT	89. BCD	114. B
15. B	40. TFFFT	65. TFTTT	90. AD	115. B
16. C	41. TTTTF	66. TFFTT	91. ABD	116. B
17. A	42. TFFTT	67. C	92. AB	117. B
18. C	43. TFFFT	68. ABC	93. AE	118. C
19. D	44. TFFTT	69. ACE	94. ABCDE	119. B
20. C	45. TFTTT	70. AD	95. A	120. A
21. A	46. FTFFT	71. DE	96. ABE	121. D
22. C	47. TFFFF	72. AC	97. B	122. A
23. A	48. FTTTT	73. C	98. B	123. A
24. A	49. TTFFT	74. ADE	99. A	124. A
25. FTTTT	50. TTFFT	75. ABCD	100. B	125. A

126. A	148. A	170. A	192. D	214. BDE
127. A	149. A	171. B	193. A	215. AB
128. D	150. D	172. A	194. C	216. A
129. D	151. C	173. A	195. B	217. E
130. A	152. D	174. B	196. B	218. ACD
131. A	153. D	175. C	197. C	219. C
132. A	154. A	176. A	198. A	220. ABE
133. C	155. B	177. D	199. B	221. DE
134. A	156. D	178. B	200. E	222. C
135. C	157. A	179. C	201. B	223. D
136. C	158. A	180. A	202. D	224. C
137. B	159. A	181. D	203. B	225. B
138. D	160. B	182. B	204. D	226. A
139. B	161. B	183. C	205. C	227. B
140. C	162. A	184. A	206. D	
141. B	163. B	185. A	207. B	
142. C	164. A	186. A	208. A	
143. B	165. A	187. A	209. D	
144. D	166. C	188. D	210. D	
145. C	167. C	189. A	211. C	
146. B	168. A	190. B	212. B	
147. D	169. B	191. D	213. D	

CHAPTER 4

Molecular and Cellular Biology

1. Which of the following is true about polymorphisms? They:

(a) Are sporadic mutations

(b) Usually have functional significance

(c) Can alter gene expression

(d) Rarely occur in normal population

2. Pro-apoptotic BCL-2 family members function by:

(a) Digesting the mitochondria

(b) Increasing the mitochondrial membrane permeability

(c) Directly activating executioner caspase

(d) Increasing nuclear membrane permeability

3. Which of the following mediates the TP53-induced apoptosis?

(a) CD 95 receptor

(b) APAF-l/caspase-9

(c) BCL-2

(d) TP_{21}^{CIP}

4. The regulatory proteins at the G_2M check-point primarily respond to:

(a) Hypoxia

(b) Nutrient poor environment

(c) DNA damage

(d) Cytokines

5. Pan T cell marker:

(a) CD 1 (b) CD 2

(c) CD 3 (d) CD 4

6. Immunosuppressant IL is:

(a) 1 (b) 6

(c) 10 (d) 16

7. A patient has recurrent hematuria, underwent Turp earlier. USG now shows enlarged prostate, upper tracts normal, next step:

(a) Redo Turp

(b) Trus bx

(c) CECT to r/o urothelial malignancy

(d) Start medication

Mention True and False respective to each statement (Q. No. 8 to 16)

8. Regarding T cell stimulation:

(a) MHC protein expressed on APC

(b) Type 1 and type 2 cytokines are counter-regulatory

(c) Stimulated T cells secrete cytokines

(d) During antigen priming, CD4+T cells develop into cells producing type 1 cytokines (e.g., Th 1 cells) or into cells producing type 2 cytokines

(e) Critical APC is dendritic cells

9. T cell activation:

(a) PLC → Activation of DAG and IP_3

(b) IP_3 activates → PKC

(c) DAG augment cytosolic Ca^{2+}

(d) Calcineurin buffers Ca^{2+} and calmodulin

(e) End result is the activation of a number of transcription factors that initiate gene expression

10. INK4 Cyclin D-CDK complex:

(a) The INK4 family of CDK inhibitors directly inhibits the assembly of cyclin D with CDK 4 and CDK 6
(b) Cyclin D expression is critical at the G_2M checkpoint
(c) Mutational inactivation of INK4 family members appears to be rare in prostate carcinoma
(d) By binding to cyclin D-CDK complexes, inhibit RB phosphorylation
(e) CIP/KIP family members bind most cyclin-CDK complexes

11. B-lymphocytes:

(a) Surface have Fc receptor
(b) Have 150 types of immunoglobulin in surfaces
(c) Immature cells express immunoglobulins in cytoplasm
(d) Plasma cells have complement receptors
(e) B cell express C3R

12. Immune tolerance:

(a) Lymphocytes are derived from bone marrow
(b) The primary lymphoid organs are the thymus, which is responsible for the selection and education of T cells
(c) Secondary or peripheral lymphoid tissue includes the spleen, lymph nodes
(d) The MHC describes a region of genes located on chromosome 3
(e) Important mechanism mediating tolerance to self proteins is deletion of self reactive B cells and T cells

13. Complement mediated:

(a) Alternate pathway is antibody independent
(b) The union of C3b with C6–C9 generates the membrane attack complex (MAC)
(c) C4 is most critical in complement pathway
(d) MAC attack lipid bilayer
(e) MAC kills via hypotonic lysis

14. Antibiotics:

(a) β-lactamase–inhibits cell wall synthesis
(b) Aminoglycoside inhibit protein synthesis
(c) Quinolones inhibits DNA synthesis
(d) TMPSMX inhibits folate synthesis
(e) Vancomycin inhibits cell wall synthesis

15. DNA fingerprinting:

(a) 99.9% of human DNA sequences are the same in every person
(b) Used in parental testing
(c) Most desirable method of collecting a reference sample is the use of a buccal swab
(d) DNA profiling uses repetitive sequences that are highly variable called variable number tandem repeats
(e) Samples can also be collected from stored sperms

16. Regarding T-cell stimulation:

(a) For the induction of most T cell–mediated immune responses, the critical APC is the dendritic cell
(b) Never directly recognizes allografts
(c) MHC is expressed over APC
(d) Secretes cytokine
(e) Interstitial dendritic cells are activated by TNF-α to become phagocytic cells and ingest pieces of foreign material and tissue debris

17. Which of the following is a CXC chemokine?

(a) MIG (b) Eotaxin
(c) RANTES (d) SLC

18. Immunosuppression cytokines:

(a) IL 1 (b) IL 10
(c) IL 12 (d) IL 14

19. Embryonal carcinoma express:

(a) CD 30 and CD 117
(b) CD 30 and keratin
(c) CD 30 and PLAP
(d) Keratin and PLAP

20. Biomaterials not used for engineering of genitourinary tissues:

(a) Polyglycolic acid

(b) Polylactic acid
(c) Poly(lactic-co-glycolic acid)
(d) Polypropylene

21. Apoptosis all are true *except*:

(a) Defense mechanism against malignancy
(b) BCL2 family cell cycle arrest
(c) Capsaicin – initiator
(d) Time – 60 sec

22. All are true *except*:

(a) CD-8- Receptor for MHC class 1
(b) CD 19 is pan B cell marker
(c) HIV receptor – CD 4
(d) CD3 part of T cell receptor

23. Not an advantage of adult stem cell over embryonal stem cell:

(a) Can be taken from multiple sites
(b) Ethical issues
(c) Pluripotent
(d) Less chances of differentiation into malignancy

24. Perineal pain with tender prostate PSA is 7.5:

(a) Repeat PSA
(b) TURP
(c) Analgesic and antibiotics
(d) TRUS guided biopsy

25. Pan Tcell marker:

(a) CD2 (b) CD3
(c) CD1 (d) CD10

26. Tyrosine kinase inhibitor action is:

(a) Compete with ATP, phosphorylating activity
(b) Alters cytoskeleton
(c) Produces proteins
(d) Generates free radicals

27. Stem cells can be retrieved from all *except*:

(a) Inner cell mass (b) Cord blood
(c) Bone marrow (d) Cardiac myocytes

28. Point mutation diagnosed by:

(a) FISH
(b) RFLP
(c) Karyotype
(d) Southern blot

29. Which of the following is false about molecular biology?

(a) Splicing: The removal of introns (spliced out) and the connection of exons (spliced together) in mRNA
(b) Telomere: An essential structural molecule of chromosome consisting of repetitive noncoding DNA and associated telomere specific binding proteins that cap and stabilise the chromosome
(c) Transcription synthesis of RNA on DNA template
(d) Transfection: Synthesis of proteins from mRNA template

30. The characteristics of synthetic biomaterials used in the reconstruction of genitourinary tract include:

(a) Rapidly biodegradable
(b) Greater surface area to volume ratio
(c) Not affected by pore size
(d) Inhibiting tissue fibrous ingrowth

31. Which of the following is abnormal in process of wound healing?

(a) Calcification
(b) Epithelialization
(c) Angiogenesis
(d) Neovascularisation

32. IFN-β is secreted by:

(a) Fibroblasts (b) Leucocytes
(c) Lymphocytes (d) Platelets

33. Calcium is stored in:

(a) Golgi (b) ER
(c) Caveolae (d) Mitochondria

34. Which of the following conditions have been linked to single gene mutation?

(a) Polycystic kidneys
(b) Vesicoureteric reflux
(c) Hypospadias
(d) Ureteric duplication

35. Pan B cell marker:

(a) CD 11 (b) CD 22
(c) CD 31 (d) CD 19

36. Which of the following is a critical contributor to the G1S checkpoint?

(a) GSTPl (b) TP 53
(c) Beta Catenin (d) CDC 25 B

37. Which of the following is an inhibitor of prostatic epithelial cell proliferation?

(a) Fibroblast growth factor – 1
(b) Vascular endothelial growth factor (VEGF)
(c) Transforming growth factor – beta
(d) Insulin like growth factor (IGF)

38. Labile energy source is:

(a) Fat
(b) Glucose
(c) Fructose
(d) Muscle protein
(e) Glycogen

ANSWERS

1.	A	10.	TFTFT	19.	B	28.	A	37.	C
2.	C	11.	TFTFT	20.	D	29.	D	38.	ABC
3.	A	12.	TTTFT	21.	D	30.	B		
4.	C	13.	TFFTT	22.	A	31.	A		
5.	C	14.	TTTTT	23.	C	32.	A		
6.	C	15.	TTTTT	24.	C	33.	B		
7.	C	16.	TFTTT	25.	B	34.	A		
8.	TTTTT	17.	B	26.	A	35.	D		
9.	TTTTT	18.	B	27.	D	36.	B		

CHAPTER 5

Reproductive and Sexual Function

1. **Which of the following hormones plays a central role in regulation of sertoli cell function?**
   (a) LH, FSH (b) FSH, estradiol
   (c) Prolactin (d) FSH, testosterone
2. **Which of the following contributes the majority of fluid from male ejaculate?**
   (a) Epididymis (b) Ejaculatory ducts
   (c) Prostate (d) Seminal vesicles
3. **The steroid peak during a human male's life occurs at:**
   (a) 2 months (b) 6 to 9 months
   (c) 10 to 15 years (d) 25 to 30 years
4. **Mitochondria are contained in which of the following sperm region?**
   (a) Tail (b) Head
   (c) Acrosome (d) Midpiece
5. **Which fetal hormone stimulates the development of the wolffian ducts?**
   (a) Estradiol (b) DHT
   (c) Estrone (d) Testosterone
6. **The majority of testosterone in plasma is bound to:**
   (a) Sex hormone binding globin (SHG)
   (b) Insulin
   (c) Prostaglandins
   (d) Cholesterol
7. **Which of the following should be the first line of investigation for a 30-year-old male with erectile dysfunction?**
   (a) Sildenafil citrate test
   (b) Cavernosometry
   (c) Intravenous injection of papaverine
   (d) Arterial (penile) color Doppler study
8. **Normal capacity of seminal vesicle:**
   (a) 3 to 4 ml (b) 10 to 15 ml
   (c) 20 to 25 ml (d) 5 to 10 ml
9. **On semen analysis, normal viscosity is:**
   (a) 4 mm threading (b) 7 mm threading
   (c) 14 mm threading (d) 20 mm threading
10. **In humans, sperm binds to which specific receptor?**
   (a) AD3 (b) ZP3
   (c) PI4 (d) PK2
11. **The ROS (reactive oxygen species) level for healthy donors with normal standard semen parameters is:**
   (a) 4×10^4 cpm/20 million sperm/ml
   (b) 8×10^4 cpm/10 million sperm/ml
   (c) 16×10^5 cpm/40 million sperm/ml
   (d) 1.5×10^4 cpm/20 million sperm/ml
12. **All of the following increase SHBG levels *except*:**
   (a) Cirrhosis (b) Anticonvulsants
   (c) Acromegaly (d) Estrogen
13. **All *except* one are absolute indications for vasography:**
   (a) Azoospermia
   (b) Complete spermatogenesis with many mature spermatids on testis biopsy
   (c) At least one palpable vas
   (d) Severe oligospermia with normal testis biopsy

14. Which brain area has been reported to control nocturnal penile erection?
(a) Midbrain raphe
(b) Substantia nigra
(c) Nucleus paragigantocellularis
(d) Lateral pre-optic area

15. Most common side effect observed with PDE 5 inhibitor therapy is:
(a) Headache
(b) Dyspepsia
(c) Flushing
(d) Visual disturbances

16. The most common side effect of MUSE is:
(a) Hypotension
(b) Dizziness
(c) Local urogenital pain
(d) Bleeding

17. Priapism is a full or partial erection that continues more than:
(a) 2 hours (b) 4 hours
(c) 6 hours (d) 8 hours

18. Phenylephrine is the preferred sympathomimetic used in the treatment of ischemic priapism because of its:
(a) $\alpha 1$= selective activity
(b) $\alpha 1$= and $\alpha 2$ activity
(c) $\beta 1$- selective activity
(d) $\beta 2$- selective activity

19. Which one of the following is deep dorsal vein shunt?
(a) Sacher (b) Al-Ghorab
(c) Ebbehoj (d) Barry

20. Behavioral therapy 'squeeze' technique was developed by:
(a) Masters and Johnson
(b) James Semans
(c) Rosen
(d) Hartmann

21. Half life of Dapoxetine:
(a) 1.5 hours (b) 26 hours
(c) 7 hours (d) 30 minutes

22. All of the following are three-piece inflatable penile prosthesis type *except:*
(a) AMS 700 CX (b) AMS 700 LGX
(c) AMS 700 CXR (d) AMS Ambicor

23. The no-scalpel technique for vasectomy reduces the rate of:
(a) Hematoma
(b) Vasectomy failures
(c) Recanalization
(d) Chronic orchialgia

24. Vasectomy was first described by:
(a) Sir Ashley Cooper (b) Johnson
(c) Giguere (d) Chapple

25. Most common cause of obstructive azoospermia:
(a) Klinefelter's syndrome
(b) Granuloma
(c) Vasectomy
(d) Trauma to testis

26. Which of the following is TRUE regarding outcomes for varicocele ligation?
(a) An average increase in motility by 20%
(b) Improved semen parameters in about two thirds of patients
(c) Spontaneous fertilization rate of 75%
(d) No improvement in semen parameters in azoospermic patients

27. The entire spermatogenic process in humans requires how many days?
(a) 32 (b) 64
(c) 128 (d) 256

28. Thirty years old with ED for 6 months duration. PDI was prescribed but symptoms does not improve:
(a) Psychogenic cause to be ruled out
(b) Continue PDI

(c) Evaluate organic cause failure
(d) Can be due to wrong dosage schedule

29. Testicular biopsy taken from:
(a) Medial upper pole (b) Medial lower pole
(c) Posterior inferiorly (d) Lateral inferiorly

30. Not indication of varicocelectomy:
(a) Large symptomatic
(b) Infertile couple with normal female fertility
(c) Small varicocele detected on USG
(d) Small testes < 2SD

31. Infertile couples with normal female parameters and male has low volume ejaculate, azoospermia and negative fructose. Next step is:
(a) TRUS to rule out ejaculatory duct obstruction
(b) Physical examination including palpating vas
(c) Endocrine workup
(d) Chromosomal analysis

32. Young male has right UDT and present with 10 cm abdominal mass and 6 cm pelvic mass:
(a) RPLND
(b) Biopsy of mass followed by chemotherapy
(c) RPLND followed by RT
(d) Excision of the mass

33. NSGCT with 10 cm LN mass with 10 times raised tumor markers, post chemotherapy 5 times raised tumor markers and 5 cm/LN mass:
(a) Salvage chemotherapy
(b) RPLND
(c) Excision of the mass
(d) Observation

34. Intramural MUSE most common side effect:
(a) Pain (b) Bleeding
(c) Priapism (d) Infection

Mention True and False respective to each statement (Q. No. 35 to 81)

35. Varicocele:
(a) Most common correctable surgical cause is infertility
(b) Gonadotropins usually decreased
(c) Motility is most commonly improved
(d) Nutcracker phenomenon causes decreased pressure in left venous system
(e) Right sided vein drains in IVC

36. Peyronie's disease:
(a) Vitamin E is proven treatment
(b) PABA is strongly recommended treatment
(c) Place of ESWL has been adequately determined
(d) Colchicine recommended due to effect on purine metabolism
(e) Tamoxifen is recommended due to effect on tubulin

37. Regarding spermatozoa:
(a) Length–60 nm
(b) Acrosome cap is contained in nucleus
(c) Axoneme has 5+2 arrangement
(d) PH 30 is important protein for fusion with oocyte
(e) Uterus transit time–>6 hours

38. Which statement is true?
(a) Inhibin B produced by human
(b) Inhibin B inhibits FSH
(c) FSH promote sertoli cells for spermatogenesis
(d) LH act on leydig cells for testosterone
(e) Inhibin B–is so named because it is a heterodimer composed of α and β subunits

39. Alprostadil:
(a) 90% metabolised in lung
(b) Priapism is rare
(c) Associated with pain in <5%
(d) Require refrigeration
(e) Increased cGMP to cause relaxation of penile muscle

40. Male infertility:
(a) Hormone abnormalities causes < 3% of infertility

(b) Increase FSH suggestive of disorder of spermatogenesis
(c) Prolactinoma is best diagnosed by MRI
(d) Antisperm antibodies are detected in approximately 10% of males presenting with infertility
(e) CBAVD is associated with 6% of cases of obstructive azoospermia

41. Testis:
(a) Volume (5-10) ml
(b) Interstitial tissue (20–30)%
(c) Seminiferous tubules open in rete tests
(d) The combined length of tubule is 250 meters
(e) Does not have somatic innervation

42. Regarding NO:
(a) Derived from lysine
(b) Arises from endothelium (EDRF)
(c) N-monomethyl-L arginine is a competitive inhibitor of NO synthetase
(d) NO stimulates guanyl cyclase
(e) All three NOS isoforms have been identified in the corpus cavernosum

43. Sildenafil:
(a) Oral intake leads to spontaneous erection
(b) Can lead to visual defects
(c) Half life 3-5 hours
(d) Beneficial in patients with pulmonary hypertension
(e) Contraindicated in patients taking nitrates

44. Varicocele:
(a) 5-7% of infertile population has varicocele
(b) Most common correctable surgical cause of male infertility
(c) Nutcracker phenomenon is for right side varicocele
(d) Motility is most effective finding in semen analysis
(e) Repair of subclinical varicocele does not improve fertility rates

45. Priapism:
(a) One of the cause can be RCC
(b) Ischemic priapism > 4 hours in duration irrespective of etiology implies a compartment syndrome
(c) A distal caverno glandular shunt should be the first choice
(d) The initial management of nonischemic priapism should be observation
(e) 1000 μg every 5-10 min until detumescence

46. Sildenafil:
(a) Heavy meal ingestion before sildenafil is contraindicated
(b) Standard dose 25–50 mg
(c) Sildenafil is the only PDE-5 inhibitor with a cardiac conduction precaution
(d) Nitrates are absolute contraindication
(e) Backache and myalgia are common side effects

47. Causes of asthenospermia:
(a) Genital tract infection
(b) Prolonged absenteeism
(c) Frequent ejaculation
(d) Structural defects
(e) Partial ejaculatory duct obstruction

48. Infertility:
(a) Normal pregnancy rate is 20–25%/month
(b) Peak fertility rate in female is at 26–30 years
(c) Male solely responsible for 40% of infertility cases
(d) Of infertile couples without treatment, 25% to 35% will conceive at some time by intercourse alone
(e) This baseline pregnancy rate of 1% to 3% per month must be kept in mind while evaluating the results of therapy

49. Seminal fluid:
(a) The human spermatozoon is approximately 60 μm in length
(b) The sperm mitochondria contain the enzymes required for the production of ATP, the primary energy source for the cell

(c) The head piece of the spermatozoon consist of mitochondria
(d) Acrosome, contains the enzymes required for penetration before fertilization
(e) Disulfide bonds, are thought to provide the sperm tail with the rigidity necessary for progressive motility

50. Sildenafil:
(a) PDE-5 inhibitors
(b) It can cause visual disturbances
(c) Precaution with antiarrhythmics
(d) Standard dose 25–50 mg
(e) The maximal recommended dosing frequency is once per day in most patients

51. Erectile dysfunction:
(a) Patients with MI within 8 weeks are stratified under high cardiac risk
(b) Heavy meal should be avoided before sildenafil
(c) Sildenafil does not cause exercise intolerance even in patient with IHD
(d) Patients at low risk may safely engage in sexual activity or receive treatment for ED
(e) Nitrate are absolutely contraindicated with 5-PDE

52. Asthenospermia can be due to:
(a) Longer abstinence
(b) Smoking can cause decrease in sperm density
(c) Frequent ejaculation
(d) Partial obstruction
(e) GI infection

53. Male infertility:
(a) LH leads to testosterone secretion from leydig cells
(b) FSH is produced from sertoli cells
(c) Inhibin A is predominantly produced in human
(d) Inhibin B decreases both FSH and LH
(e) Only inhibin not FSH is indicator of failure of spermatogenesis

54. Infertility:
(a) Fertile couple–pregnancy rate 20-25%
(b) Solely male factor contributing to infertility–40%
(c) Baseline pregnancy rate is 1% to 3% per month in infertile couples
(d) Of infertile couples without treatment, 25% to 35% will conceive at some time by intercourse alone
(e) Hormone abnormalities are present in 10% to 13% of infertile patients

55. Priapism:
(a) RCC may cause it
(b) AUA defines it as painful erection of more than 4 hours
(c) Maximum dose of phenylephrine is 2 mg
(d) Intracavernosal phenylephrine is repeated every two minutes with dose of 200–500 mg
(e) A distal caverno glandular (corporo-glandular) shunt should be the first choice

56. Erection:
(a) Parasympathetic causes NO release
(b) NO causes increase in cGMP in cavernosal smooth muscles and vascular cells
(c) cGMP causes release of intracellular Ca^{2++}
(d) PDE inhibitors–prevent degradation of CGMP
(e) Erection thus involves sinusoidal relaxation, arterial compression and venous dilatation

57. Sperm:
(a) 60 μm
(b) Acrosome is a part of nucleus
(c) PH 30 is an important fusion protein
(d) Axoneme has 5 + 2 arrangement
(e) Sperm is viable in uterus for more than 6 hours

58. About infertility:
(a) Sperm remain viable for 5 days
(b) Eggs remain viable for 1 day following ovulation

(c) In cystic fibrosis defect is in spermatogenesis
(d) Microdeletions of sections of the long arm of the Y chromosome have been identified in approximately 13% of azoospermic men
(e) In Kartagener's syndrome extra 'X' chromosome is hallmark

59. Regarding phosphodiesterase:
(a) PDE6 is present in corpora cavernosa tissue
(b) PDE5 is present in photoreceptor cells
(c) Inhibits cGMP activity by PDE5
(d) PDE inhibitor is successful in treatment of ED
(e) Low cytosolic calcium favors smooth muscle relaxation

60. Regarding priapism:
(a) Priapism >4 hours in duration irrespective of etiology implies a compartment syndrome
(b) Sickle cell disease accounts for 23% of adult cases of priapism
(c) Cavernosal blood gas and doppler cannot differentiate between high and low flow
(d) In high flow initial treatment is aspiration and evacuation
(e) In ischemic type, proximal shunt is preferred as initial management

61. Regarding varicocele:
(a) Most common surgically correctable cause of infertility
(b) Most improvement is seen in motility after surgical correction
(c) Nutcracker phenomena causes less pressure in left gonadal vein
(d) Right gonadal vein open into IVC
(e) Sperm count <20 million/ml has higher chances of infertility

62. Testosterone surge:
(a) Adult levels are achieved at 2 months
(b) Testosterone surge occur at 1 week after birth
(c) Development of wolffian duct is inducted by testosterone
(d) Development of prostate inducted by DHT
(e) Leydig cell is responsible for testosterone production

63. Carcinoma penis:
(a) For T_2 bilateral modified LND is done even in node (-ve) patient
(b) T_1 node (-ve) can be observed
(c) Sentinel node always seen in femoral canal
(d) Inguinal lymphadenectomy should be bilateral even for patients presenting with unilateral adenopathy at initial presentation of the primary tumor
(e) If superficial LN + ve then pelvic LN dissection done

64. Patient who develops 3 cm left testicular tumor, underwent left radical orchidectomy, histopathology showed 10% embryonal components, NSGCT, T2N0MO, management is:
(a) Left spermatic cord excision and modified RPLND
(b) Bilateral spermatic cord excision and bilateral RPLND
(c) Cisplatin based chemotherapy
(d) Radiotherapy for pelvic and abdominal lymph node
(e) Observation

65. Varicocele:
(a) Most common cause for secondary infertility
(b) Following surgical correction–Motility improves most
(c) Larger the varicocele better the results
(d) Bilateral varicocele should be always treated
(e) Subclinical varicocele does not need any operative intervention

66. In epididymal obstruction:
(a) Sperm quality is better in caput than cauda
(b) Post-gonococcal epididymitis, is rare today because of effective antibiotic therapy
(c) A preoperative sign of epididymal obstruction is palpable fullness of the epididymis more than 4 to 5 years after vasectomy

(d) Vasectomy is certainly one of the most common known causes of epididymal obstruction
(e) Sperm should be cryopreserved at the time of surgery

67. True regarding medical treatment of Peyronie's disease:
(a) Vit E is effective
(b) Potassium aminobenzoate side effects make it untouchable
(c) Extracorporeal shockwave therapy has been proposed as a treatment
(d) Radiotherapy should be avoided
(e) Tamoxifen stimulate the release of TGF

68. Tunica albuginea of penis:
(a) It is a single layered structure covering bilateral corpora cavernosa
(b) It is a double layered structure covering bilateral cavernosa and single layer over corpora spongiosum
(c) The most vulnerable area for prosthesis extrusion is between the 5 and 7 o'clock position
(d) Composed of collagen, smooth muscle and elastin
(e) It extends till glans

69. High flow priapism:
(a) The corpora cavernosa are not usually fully rigid or painful
(b) 1st line of treatment is aspiration and injection of phenylephrine
(c) It can't be diagnosed by USG doppler and blood gas analysis
(d) Nonischemic priapism, also termed arterial or high-flow priapism
(e) Penile or perineal trauma is most frequently associated

70. Sperm:
(a) Size is 60 μm
(b) Acrosome is in the nucleus
(c) Arrangement of tubules is 5 + 2
(d) The outer dense fibers, rich in disulfide bonds, are thought to provide the sperm tail with the rigidity necessary for progressive motility
(e) The sperm mitochondria contain the enzymes required for oxidative metabolism and for the production of ATP

71. Spermatogenesis:
(a) Gonadotropins are primary initiator
(b) One cycle takes 4 weeks
(c) Primary spermatocyte to secondary spermatocyte is spermatogenesis
(d) Sperm motility is maximum at caput of epididymis
(e) Sperm storage is maximum in caput of epididymis

72. Regarding priapism:
(a) Cavernous gas study shows acidosis within 4 hours in non-ischemic priapism
(b) Non-ischemic priapism after perineal trauma may be delayed on onset
(c) May be seen in newborn
(d) In old age, most commonly due to pharmacotherapeutic agent
(e) Priapism is associated with hematologic disease, most notably sickle cell disease

73. Regarding blood testis barrier/spermatogenesis:
(a) Sertoli cells divide into basal and adluminal component
(b) During meiosis, cell migrate to basal compartment
(c) Formation of primary into secondary spermatocyte is called as spermatogenesis
(d) Only the combination of FSH and testosterone supports a qualitatively and quantitatively fully normal level of sperm production
(e) Germ cells are required for blood testis barrier

74. Regarding blood testis barrier:
(a) Function importance of blood testis barrier is established

(b) Haploid cells are identified as self by immune system
(c) Spermatogenesis takes 64 days
(d) Motility is maximum in proximal corpus
(e) Vas deferens mobility governed by sympathetic stimulation

75. Varicocele:
(a) Following injury of testicular artery–50% chances of ischemic atrophy
(b) 30% incidence of varicocele in secondary infertility
(c) Maximum improvement in semen occur in morphology
(d) Testicular artery 0.5–1.5 mm
(e) Least chances of recurrence–Retroperitoneal varicocelectomy

76. Erectile dysfunction:
(a) Papaverine increases both cAMP and cGMP
(b) Prostaglandins increases cAMP only
(c) Sildenafil most common side effect in nasal congestion
(d) Sildenafil is contraindicated in HTN
(e) Alprostadil used in ED refers to PGE1

77. Regarding blood testis barrier:
(a) Sertoli cells divide into basal and albuminal component
(b) During meiosis, cell migrate to basal component
(c) Formation of secondary spermatocyte is called as spermatogenesis
(d) Germ cells are required for blood testis barrier
(e) Body does not recognize haploid cells as self

78. Regarding blood testis barrier:
(a) Functional importance of blood testis barrier is established
(b) Spermatogenesis takes 4 weeks
(c) Motility is maximum in proximal corpus
(d) Vas deferens motility is governed by sympathetic stimulation
(e) LH initiates spermatogenesis

79. Varicocele:
(a) Least chances of recurrence in retroperitoneal lymphadenopathy
(b) In minimal varicocele maximum improvement in quality of semen after surgery
(c) After varicocelectomy morphology improved but not motility
(d) 15% incidence in adolescent age group
(e) 70% incidence in primary infertility

80. Varicocele:
(a) Following injury of testicular artery–50% chances of ischemic atrophy
(b) Clinical varicocele is absolute indication of surgery
(c) 30% incidence of varicocele in secondary infertility
(d) Maximum improvement in semen analysis is in subclinical varicocele
(e) Testicular artery size is 0.5 mm to 1.5 mm

81. Erectile dysfunction:
(a) Papaverine increases both cAMP and cGMP
(b) Prostaglandins increases cAMP only
(c) Sildenafil most common side effect is nasal congestion
(d) Sildenafil is contraindicated in HTN
(e) Apomorphine is D1and D2 antagonist

Which of the Following Statement is Correct?

82. After ligation of testicular artery in varicocele surgery testicular supply derives from:
(a) Vasal artery
(b) Cremasteric artery
(c) Internal pudendal artery
(d) Internal spermatic artery
(e) Testicular artery

83. False about testosterone:
(a) Leydig cells make testosterone that induces development of the internal genitalia
(b) Converted to DHT by 5 α reductase

(c) Aromatase converts to estradiol in fatty tissue
(d) Testosterone feedback occurs mainly at the hypothalamus
(e) Normal testosterone production in men is approximately 5 g/day

84. Three years infertility, azoospermia, normal hormone levels and normal volume of ejaculate, cause may be:
(a) Unilateral absence of vas
(b) Bilateral absence of vas
(c) Bilateral obstruction of EJD
(d) Primary testicular failure
(e) Secondary testicular failure

85. Prosthesis erection:
(a) Short in size
(b) Glans tumescence is absent
(c) Preserve orgasm
(d) Minocycline/rifampicin coating decreases infection rate
(e) Reimplantation as soon as possible after removal of prosthesis for infection

86. Diagnosis criteria PME:
(a) Lack of ejaculatory control
(b) ED
(c) Long latency
(d) Sexual dissatisfaction
(e) Short latency time (intravaginal)

87. Which of the following dyscrasias causes priapism?
(a) Aplastic anemia
(b) Sickle cell anemia
(c) Thalassemia
(d) Leukemia
(e) Hereditary spherocytosis

88. Drugs used in retrograde ejaculation:
(a) Ephedrine (b) Imipramine
(c) Prostacycline (d) Darifenacin
(e) Oxybutanine

89. Causes of retrograde ejaculation:
(a) DM (b) RPLND
(c) TURP (d) MS
(e) Transverse myelitis

90. Neurotransmitter in penile erection:
(a) Acetylcholine (b) NO
(c) Dopamine (d) Methionine
(e) Adrenaline

91. All of the following are spermatotoxin *except*:
(a) Colchicine
(b) Calcium channel blockers
(c) Cimetidine
(d) Cefixitin
(e) Cannabis

92. Surgery in obese patients increases risk of:
(a) Mortality
(b) Heart attack
(c) Wound infection
(d) Peripheral nerve injury
(e) UTI

93. Vas deferens:
(a) Greatest muscle/lumen ratio in all hollow viscera of body
(b) Derived embryologically from the mesonephric (wolffian) duct
(c) Length 15-25 cm
(d) It is supplied by vesiculo deferential artery
(e) Function is to convert testosterone to DHT

94. Drugs in erectile dysfunction:
(a) Papaverine (b) Prostaglandin
(c) Phenylephrine (d) Phentolamine
(e) Phosphodiesterase stimulators

95. Priapism due to sickle disease in a 10 years male for 24 hours–treatment options:
(a) Packed cell administration
(b) Irrigation with heparinized saline
(c) Intracavernosal infection
(d) Shunt procedures
(e) Observation

96. Hydrocelectomy–most common complication:
(a) Chronic scrotal pain
(b) Hematoma
(c) Infection
(d) Testicular atrophy
(e) Recurrence

97. Primary testicular failure:
(a) Low testosterone
(b) Increased FSH
(c) Increased LH
(d) Normal testosterone
(e) Hypospermatogenesis

98. Which of the following is reduced in DIC?
(a) Platelets
(b) Fibrinogen
(c) FDP
(d) Prothrombin index
(e) Capillary fragility

99. Acid phosphatase is secreted by:
(a) RBC
(b) WBC
(c) Prostatic acinar cells
(d) Reticuloendothelial cells
(e) Osteoclast

100. Hyperuricemia with hyperuricosuria is seen in:
(a) Cancer chemotherapy
(b) Fanconi syndrome
(c) Tumor lysis syndrome
(d) Acute renal failure
(e) Uric acid stone

101. Highest source of androgen in men:
(a) Testis (b) Adrenal
(c) Prostate (d) Ejaculatory duct
(e) Vas deferens

102. Serum testosterone binds with:
(a) SHBG (b) Albumin
(c) α-methylglobulin (d) DHT
(e) CBG

103. Management of priapism all *except*:
(a) Intracavernosal papaverine
(b) Vacuum device
(c) Cavernosal aspiration and washing
(d) Winter's shunt
(e) Grayhack shunt

104. Blood testis barrier all *except*:
(a) Sertoli cell junction
(b) Germ cell not necessary
(c) Formed before spermatogenesis
(d) May be damaged by testicular tumor

105. Men after drinking alcohol not able to perform sex with wife and normal NPT:
(a) Masturbation
(b) Psychogenic ED with psychogenic counselling
(c) With sildenafil
(d) With organic counselling

106. Men with no issue for 4 years of marriage. Investigations revealed–Fructose–nil, no sperms on HPE, 0.5 ml volume:
(a) Palpation of vas (b) TRUS
(c) Testicular biopsy (d) MRI

107. For measurement of free testosterone, gold standard is:
(a) Testosterone assay
(b) Analog assay
(c) Biometric test
(d) Equilibrium dialysis

108. Regarding seminal vesicle false is:
(a) Store sperms
(b) Medial to vas
(c) Normally not palpable on DRE
(d) Controls by sympathetic stimulation

109. Cohort study all are true *except*:
(a) Beneficial for rare disease
(b) A cohort is a group of people who share a common characteristic or experience within a defined period
(c) Longitudinal study
(d) It is an analysis of risk factors and follows a group of people who do not have the disease

110. Odds ratio:
(a) Ab/cd (b) Ac/bd
(c) Ad/bc (d) Bc/ad

111. All are true *except*:
(a) LH and FSH from neurohypophysis
(b) Lactotrophs and corticotropes from adenohypophysis
(c) Neurohypophysis is ventral outpouching of hypothalamus
(d) Axis controlled by blood levels of hormone

112. All are true *except:*
(a) Most values lie in confident interval
(b) P value better predictor than confidence interval
(c) Level 1A evidence – case control studies
(d) Not significant implies not effective

113. NSGCT, post orchidectomy normal markers, CT shows 5 cm residual mass next step:
(a) VIP
(b) Resection of residual mass
(c) RPLND
(d) Modified RPLND with mass resection

114. Pivot study:
(a) BPH (b) Ca prostate
(c) Prostatitis (d) OAB

115. Editor Chief of Journal of Urology:
(a) William D Steers (b) Kevin T McVary
(c) Nitin Kekre (d) NP Gupta

116. Infertile couple, husband having Gd II varicocele and wife having PCOD management:
(a) Microscopic varicocelectomy
(b) IVF
(c) Embolization of varicocele
(d) Hormonal supplement to wife for ovulation

117. Not included in metabolic syndrome:
(a) Glucose intolerance
(b) HTN
(c) Sleep apnea
(d) Obesity

118. Intraurethral MUSE most common side effect is:
(a) Penile pain (b) Fibrosis
(c) Hypotension (d) Priapism

119. Twenty-five years old male has recent onset ED. Till 3 months back erection was normal. No history of trauma or illness. Management is:
(a) PDE-5 inhibitors
(b) Papaverine with color doppler
(c) FSH, LH and testosterone levels
(d) PDE-5 inhibitors with color Doppler

120. Highest pH in:
(a) 1 mol NaOH (b) Distill water
(c) Urine of normal man (d) Human blood

121. Most common micro-deletion causing azoospermia occurs in:
(a) Chromosome 17 (b) Y chromosome
(c) Chromosome 19 (d) X chromosome

122. What is the finding expected in azoospermia patient with AZFb and AZFc complete deletion?
(a) Total germinal aplasia/agenesis
(b) Immature/immotile spermatozoa
(c) Obstructive azoospermia
(d) Highly viscous semen

123. Blood testis barrier includes all *except*:
(a) Sertoli cells
(b) Myoid cells
(c) Endothelial cells
(d) Lymphatic cells

124. Azoospermia in all *except*:
(a) Varicocele
(b) Anti-sperm antibodies
(c) Torsion
(d) CBAVD

125. Which anti-hypertensive causes erectile dysfunction?
(a) α-blocker (b) β-blocker
(c) CCB (d) ACE inhibitor

126. Platelet receptor required for adhesion and plug formation:
(a) GP IIb/IIIa (b) Adenosine
(c) Fibrinogen (d) VWF

127. Which test is not required in the absence of vas?
(a) Testis FNAC
(b) Physical examination
(c) Sperm density
(d) Semen volume

128. APTT is not increased in:
(a) VIII (b) IX
(c) XI (d) V

129. In Pedigree analysis–affected male represented by:
(a) Solid square (b) Empty square
(c) Solid circle (d) Empty circle

130. Sperm enzymes are stored in:
(a) Head (b) Acrosome
(c) Middle pole (d) Tail

131. Mode of action of sildenafil:
(a) PDE 5 inhibitor
(b) Inhibits cyclic GMP
(c) Inhibits cyclic AMP
(d) PDE 5 stimulator

132. Test which should be mandatory before diagnosis of erectile function:
(a) NPTR
(b) Dynamic infusion cavernosometry and cavernosography
(c) Duplex USG
(d) CT angiography

133. Cavernous blood PO_2 30 mm Hg, pCO_2 60 mm Hg, pH 7.25, 4 hours delay in presentation: next to be done is:
(a) Aspiration and irrigation of the corpora cavernosa with adrenergic sympathomimetic agent
(b) Proximal shunt
(c) Observation
(d) Distal shunt

134. Phenylephrine is used in ischemic priapism because it is:
(a) α_1 selective (b) $\alpha_1\beta_1$ selective
(c) $\alpha_1\beta_2$ selective (d) α_2 selective

135. Best sperm quality after chronic obstruction is found in:
(a) Caput epididymis
(b) Corpus epididymis
(c) Cauda epididymis
(d) Same in above three

136. After non-obstructive azoospermia sperm extracted from:
(a) PESA (b) TESA
(c) MESA (d) TESE

137. Most common disadvantages of non-microsurgical varicocelectomy:
(a) Hydrocele (b) Recurrence
(c) Bleeding (d) Lymphocele

138. More than one testicular artery found in inguinal dissection in:
(a) 20% (b) 30%
(c) 50% (d) 10%

139. IIEF score is used in:
(a) Erectile dysfunction
(b) Sexual desire
(c) Intercourse satisfaction
(d) Ejaculation latency time

140. In human body nitric oxide is synthesized from:
(a) Arginine (b) Cystine
(c) Ammonia (d) Urea

141. Combined defects in sperm density, motility and morphology are most frequently caused by:
(a) Prostatitis (b) Varicocele
(c) Mumps (d) Filariasis

142. In fracture penis which is incorrect?
(a) Immediate surgical exploration and repair
(b) Cavernosometry is routine investigation
(c) In conservative management 10% develop chordee
(d) Diagnosis made reliably by history and physical examination alone

143. All *except* one are causes of low volume ejaculate:
(a) An ejaculation
(b) Vasoepididymal obstruction
(c) Hypogonadism
(d) Retrograde ejaculation

144. Seminal plasma mostly contains:
(a) Glucose (b) Fructose
(c) Maltose (d) Sucrose

145. Which of the following PDE is important for penile erection?
(a) PDE-2 (b) PDE-4
(c) PDE-3 (d) PDE-5

146. Priapism mostly commonly seen in:
(a) Leukemia
(b) Sickle cell anemia
(c) Peyronies disease
(d) Parkinson's disease

147. In micro-deletion of Y chromosome further treatment is:
(a) Hormonal manipulation
(b) ICSI
(c) Vaso-epidydomostomy
(d) Vasovasostomy

148. Regarding testicular biopsy in infertility, all are true *except*:
(a) Helps to plan treatment in azoospermia
(b) Bouin's solution is a fixative
(c) Can be used for sperm retrieval
(d) Should be done during varicocele surgery

149. Eggplant deformity is characteristic of:
(a) Posterior hypospadias
(b) Fracture penis
(c) Filariasis
(d) Peyronies disease

150. Seminal vesicles contributes .....% of semen volume.
(a) 40% (b) 30%
(c) 70% (d) 80%

151. Hematospermia is commonly due to:
(a) Trauma
(b) Malignancy of seminal vesicles
(c) Tuberculosis of prostate, seminal vesicles
(d) Non-specific inflammation of prostate, seminal vesicles

152. False about phenylephrine used in the treatment of priapism:
(a) Drug of choice for intracorporeal injection
(b) It is a non-selective α agonist which acts on α receptors
(c) Doesn't have β mediated chronotropic, or ionotropic effects
(d) Is diluted to 200 μgms per ml and given 0.5 ml to 1 ml

153. Following is not used for the treatment of peyronies disease:
(a) Carnitine
(b) Intralesional verapamil
(c) Extracorporeal shockwave therapy
(d) Radiation therapy

154. Half life of dapoxetine:
(a) 45 minutes (b) 1.5 hours
(c) 2 hours (d) 4 hours

155. An ejaculation can be caused by the following *except*:
(a) Androgen deficiency
(b) Sympathetic degeneration
(c) Bladder neck surgery
(d) Alpha adrenergic agonists

156. With which of the following is priapism most commonly associated?
(a) Sickle cell disease
(b) Advanced malignancy
(c) Coagulopathies
(d) Pulmonary diseases

157. Cause of post varicocelectomy hydrocele:
(a) Lymphatic obstruction
(b) Venous obstruction
(c) Increased intratesticular venous pressure
(d) Arterial obstruction

158. Testosterone is converted to DHT by:
(a) 5α reductase
(b) Lactate dehydrogenase
(c) Pyruvate kinase
(d) ALA

159. Absence or malformation of seminal vesicles is marked by:
(a) Citrate (b) Fructose
(c) Zinc (d) Glucose

160. Erectile dysfunction most common drug used:
(a) PDE inhibitor (b) Testosterone
(c) Papaverine (d) Phentolamine

161. Priapism most commonly seen in:
(a) Sickle cell anemia
(b) Coagulopathies
(c) Advance malignancy
(d) Lymphoma

162. Seminal fluid maximally formed by:
(a) Prostate (b) Seminal vesicle
(c) Testis (d) Vas deferens

163. Spermatogenesis in human require:
(a) 34 days (b) 44 days
(c) 54 days (d) 64 days

164. Sterility after vasectomy:
(a) 4-6 weeks (b) 8-10 weeks
(c) 12-16 weeks (d) 18-20 weeks

165. Most common complication of vasectomy:
(a) Hematoma (b) Infection
(c) Hydrocele (d) Sperm granuloma

166. Which of the following is the marker of testicular failure?
(a) Increased FSH
(b) Bilateral absence of vas
(c) Subnormal testicular volume
(d) Azoospermia

167. ADAM scoring is done for:
(a) Priapism
(b) Adult hypogonadism
(c) Degree of ED
(d) Peyronies disease

168. In azoospermia, percent of Y-chromosomal deletion:
(a) <5% (b) 5-10%
(c) 10-15% (d) 20-25%

169. Preferred technique for non-obstructive azoospermia is:
(a) Microsurgical epididymal sperm aspiration
(b) Percutaneous epididymal sperm aspiration
(c) Testicular sperm aspiration
(d) Testicular sperm extraction

170. Most common cause of impotence is:
(a) Psychogenic
(b) Organic
(c) Mixed psychogenic and organic
(d) Endocrine

171. Normal sperm count according to WHO criteria:
(a) 40 million/ml (b) 20 million/ml
(c) 60 million/ml (d) 80 million/ml

172. Drug which is used for the treatment of retrograde ejaculation?
(a) Ephedrine
(b) Pseudoephedrine
(c) Imipramine
(d) All of the above

173. True about varicocele is:
(a) Prevalence in general population on physical examination is 15-18%
(b) Incidence of secondary infertility in varicocele is 35-55%
(c) Incidence of male infertility in varicocele is 20-30%
(d) Large varicocele, less detrimental than small

174. Regarding infertility in varicocele patients:
(a) Incidence higher in primary infertility
(b) Incidence higher in secondary infertility
(c) Not associated with infertility
(d) Most affected factor is sperm viability

175. Most common improved parameter after varicocelectomy:
(a) Motility (b) Morphology
(c) Density (d) Vitality

176. Improvement in fertility after varicocelectomy occurs:
(a) Within 1 month (b) Within 1 year
(c) After 1 year (d) After 5 years

177. Impotence is defined as:
(a) Inability to maintain and sustain erection
(b) Inability to ejaculate
(c) Premature ejaculation
(d) Azoospermia

178. Priapism, most common cause:
(a) Sickle cell anemia
(b) Advanced malignancy
(c) Lymphoma
(d) Penile cancer

179. Blood testis barrier formed by all *except:*
(a) Sertoli cell junctions

(b) Myoid cells
(c) Endothelial cells
(d) Basal cells

180. Fructose secreted by:
(a) Seminal vesicles (b) Vas deferens
(c) Testis (d) Prostate

181. Torsion of tests, most common age group:
(a) Puberty (b) 20-25 years
(c) 40-50 years (d) 30-40 years

182. Sperm enzymes are stored in:
(a) Head (b) Acrosome
(c) Middle pole (d) Tail
(e) Head and tail

183. Most important in testosterone regulation is:
(a) FSH (b) LH
(c) Inhibin (d) Estradiol
(e) MIS

184. A 35 years old patient presented to infertility clinic, on genital examination testis is normal, semen analysis shows azoospermia, on hormonal evaluation FSH levels are normal. Next step in the evaluation includes:
(a) Vasography (b) TRUS
(c) Testis biopsy (d) CFTR testing

185. Preferred technique for non-obstructive azoospermia:
(a) MESA (b) PESA
(c) TESA (d) TESE

186. Complete absence of semen in ejaculate is called as:
(a) Azoospermia (b) Asthenospermia
(c) Aspermia (d) Teratospermia

187. A patient presented with low volume, azoospermic, acidic, fructose-negative semen that does not coagulate, diagnosis is:
(a) Chromosomal abnormalities
(b) Testicular atrophy
(c) Klinefelter's syndrome
(d) Ejaculatory duct obstruction

188. Absence vas is commonly associated with:
(a) Absent testis
(b) Renal agenesis
(c) Cryptorchidism
(d) Horseshoe kidney

189. Absolute contraindication for the use of PDE inhibitors:
(a) History of coronary artery disease
(b) History of hypertension
(c) Present congestive heart failure
(d) Present use of nitrates

190. Frontline investigation for vascular erectile dysfunction:
(a) Duplex USG
(b) Combined intracavernous injection and stimulation
(c) Dynamic infusion cavernosography
(d) Pudendal artery angiography

191. Priapism in pediatric age is most commonly caused by:
(a) Trauma
(b) Sickle cell disease
(c) Antihypertensive drugs
(d) Idiopathic

192. Egg plant deformity is seen in:
(a) Peyronies disease
(b) Fracture penis
(c) Rupture of urethra
(d) Priapism

193. After microsurgical inguinal dissection for varicocele, remaining veins is:
(a) Pampiniform (b) Cremasteric
(c) Vasal (d) Testicular

194. Retrograde ejaculation commonly seen with:
(a) Tamsulosin (b) Terazocine
(c) Doxazocine (d) Prazocine

195. Which of the following is a feature of mullerian inhibiting substance?
(a) Causes regression of mesonephric duct

(b) Causes regression of paramesonephric duct
(c) Converts testosterone to dihydrotestosterone
(d) Stimulates the second phase of testicular descent

196. The somatic innervation of the penis is by the:
(a) Cavernosal nerve
(b) Pudendal nerve
(c) Obturator nerve
(d) Hypogastric nerve

197. The absence of fructose in the semen suggests:
(a) Sertoli cell only syndrome
(b) Bilateral vasal obstruction
(c) Ejaculatory duct obstruction
(d) Testicular atrophy

198. All are features of Zoom's balanitis *except:*
(a) Also called plasma cell balanitis
(b) Occurs in uncircumcised men
(c) It is sexually transmitted
(d) Circumcision offers cure in the majority of cases

199. Apomorphine used for erectile dysfunction works as an:
(a) Dopaminergic antagonist
(b) Adrenergic antagonist
(c) PDE 5 inhibitor
(d) Dopaminergic agonist

200. Supersonic transporter deformity after prosthetic penile implant is due to:
(a) Poor glans support
(b) Oversize cylinder
(c) Cylinder erosion
(d) Cavernosal infection

201. Last portion of seminal fluid includes:
(a) Seminal vesicle (b) Prostate
(c) Cooper gland (d) Testis
(e) Epididymis

202. Congenital short urethra all is true *except*:
(a) Correct fusion of all elements of the penis
(b) During erection urethra and corpus spongiosum are not long or compliant enough to match compliance of other ventral tissue layers
(c) Type V anomaly
(d) Chordee without hypospadias
(e) Meatus is the tip of glans

203. WHO 2010 criteria for semen analysis includes all *except*:
(a) Vitality (live spermatozoa, %) >60%
(b) Semen volume >1.5 ml
(c) Total mortality >30%
(d) Semen volume/ml >15 million

204. Tail stump syndrome:
(a) Fibrous dysplasia of cyclidine
(b) Middle piece absent
(c) Flagella anomalies
(d) Acrosomal defect

205. Globozoospermia:
(a) Acrosomal defect
(b) Mid piece defect
(c) Kartagener syndrome
(d) Tail defect

206. Following are not PDE 5 inhibitors:
(a) Dutasteride
(b) Finasteride
(c) Tadalafil
(d) Sildenafil
(e) Zaprinast

207. Antidepressant not helpful in PME:
(a) Escitalopram (b) Venlafaxine
(c) Mirtazapine (d) Paroxetine
(e) Imipramine

ANSWERS

1.	D	26.	B	51.	FTTTT	76.	TTFFT	101.	A
2.	D	27.	B	52.	TTFTT	77.	TFFFT	102.	ABE
3.	A	28.	C	53.	TTFFF	78.	FFFTF	103.	ACDE
4.	D	29.	A	54.	TFTTF	79.	FFFTF	104.	C
5.	D	30.	C	55.	TTFFT	80.	FFFFT	105.	B
6.	A	31.	B	56.	TTFTT	81.	TTFFF	106.	A
7.	A	32.	B	57.	TTTFF	82.	AB	107.	D
8.	A	33.	A	58.	TTTTT	83.	ABCDE	108.	A
9.	A	34.	A	59.	FFTTT	84.	A	109.	A
10.	B	35.	TFTFT	60.	TTFFF	85.	ABCDE	110.	C
11.	D	36.	FFFFF	61.	TTFTT	86.	ABDE	111.	A
12.	C	37.	TTFTF	62.	FFTTT	87.	BD	112.	C
13.	D	38.	TTTTT	63.	TTFTT	88.	AB	113.	B
14.	D	39.	TTFTF	64.	TFTFF	89.	ABCDE	114.	B
15.	A	40.	TTTTT	65.	TTTFT	90.	AB	115.	A
16.	C	41.	FTTTT	66.	FTTTT	91.	ABD	116.	D
17.	B	42.	FTTTT	67.	FTTTT	92.	BCDE	117.	C
18.	A	43.	FTTTT	68.	FTTTF	93.	ABDE	118.	A
19.	D	44.	FTFTT	69.	TFFTT	94.	ABD	119.	D
20.	A	45.	TTTTF	70.	TTFTT	95.	CD	120.	A
21.	A	46.	TTFTF	71.	TFFTT	96.	B	121.	B
22.	D	47.	TTFTT	72.	FTTTT	97.	ABC	122.	A
23.	A	48.	TTFTT	73.	TFFTF	98.	AB	123.	D
24.	A	49.	TTFTT	74.	FFTFF	99.	ACDE	124.	C
25.	C	50.	TTTTT	75.	FFFTF	100.	ABCDE	125.	C

126. A	143. C	160. A	177. A	194. A
127. A	144. B	161. A	178. A	195. B
128. D	145. D	162. B	179. D	196. B
129. A	146. B	163. D	180. A	197. C
130. A	147. B	164. C	181. A	198. B
131. D	148. D	165. A	182. A	199. D
132. C	149. B	166. A	183. B	200. A
133. A	150. D	167. B	184. C	201. A
134. A	151. D	168. C	185. D	202. D
135. C	152. B	169. D	186. C	203. B
136. D	153. D	170. C	187. C	204. C
137. A	154. B	171. B	188. B	205. A
138. C	155. D	172. A	189. D	206. AB
139. A	156. A	173. A	190. B	207. A
140. A	157. A	174. B	191. B	
141. B	158. A	175. A	192. B	
142. B	159. B	176. B	193. D	

CHAPTER 6

Male Genitalia

1. **Which of the following genitourinary carcinoma has an isochromosome of 12 P identified in it?**
   (a) Testis (b) Prostate
   (c) Renal (d) Bladder
2. **Which of the following is not a contraindication for testosterone therapy in males?**
   (a) Angina pectoris (b) Breast cancer
   (c) Polycythemia (d) Gynecomastia
3. **All of the following are true about carcinoma penis *except:***
   (a) Can be associated with bad hygiene
   (b) More than 50% patients present with lymphadenopathy
   (c) Erythroplasia of queyrat is a precancerous condition
   (d) Circumcision if done any time before puberty provides 100% protection against Ca penis
4. **Without violating Gerota's fascia, the perinephric fluid collections can track in which direction?**
   (a) Superior (b) Medial
   (c) Inferior (d) Lateral
5. **Testicular biopsy specimen should be placed in:**
   (a) Zenker's
   (b) Bouin's
   (c) Buffered glutaraldehyde
   (d) All of the above
6. **Schiller-Duval body present in:**
   (a) Choriocarcinoma
   (b) Yolk sac tumor
   (c) Embryonal carcinoma
   (d) Seminoma
7. **The most common presentation of testicular cancer is:**
   (a) Painless testicular mass
   (b) Hemorrhage
   (c) Symptoms related to metastatic disease
   (d) Back pain
8. **Most common para testicular tumor:**
   (a) Cystadenoma
   (b) Mesothelioma
   (c) Sarcoma
   (d) Adenomatoid tumor
9. **What is the major difference between Bowen's disease and erythroplasia of Queyrat?**
   (a) Loss of rete pegs (b) Location
   (c) Keratin staining (d) Treatment options
10. **Which of the following agent used in combination therapy for penile cancer has been associated with significant pulmonary toxicity?**
    (a) Cisplatin (b) Paclitaxel
    (c) Methotrexate (d) Bleomycin
11. **The reported local recurrence rate after partial or total penectomy is:**
    (a) 0 to 8% (b) 10 to 20%
    (c) 20 to 25% (d) 35 to 45%
12. **Most common presenting symptoms of urethral cancer:**
    (a) Palpable urethral mass
    (b) Obstructive voiding symptoms
    (c) Urethral bleeding
    (d) Asymptomatic
13. **What artery is the major blood supply to the seminal vesicle?**
    (a) Hypogastric
    (b) Inferior vesical
    (c) Internal iliac
    (d) Vesiculo deferential artery

14. Most common cause of priapism in children:
(a) Sickle cell disease (b) Leukemias
(c) Drug induced (d) Trauma

15. Most common cause of premature ejaculation:
(a) Post surgical (b) Neurogenic
(c) Psychogenic (d) Drug induced

16. Urethral stricture commonly seen in straddle injury at:
(a) Penile urethral stricture
(b) Bulbo-membranous junction
(c) Posterior urethra
(d) Pan anterior urethral stricture

17. Within the age group 10 and 35 years, the incidence of carcinoma of the testis in males with intra-abdominal testes is:
(a) Equal to that in the general population
(b) Five times greater than that in the general population
(c) Ten times greater than that in the general population
(d) Twenty times greater than that in the general population

18. Incidence of single artery entering testis is:
(a) 20-30% (b) 30-40%
(c) 40-50% (d) 50-60%

19. Peak of testosterone occurs in the blood at all ages *except:*
(a) 12 and 18 weeks of gestation
(b) At 2 weeks of birth
(c) At 2 months of age
(d) At second decade

20. Which one of the following statement regarding blood testis barrier is correct?
(a) Spermatogonia and young spermatocytes are outside the blood-testis barrier in the adluminal compartment
(b) Mature spermatocytes and spermatids are sequestered above the barrier in the basal compartment
(c) The presence of germ cells is not necessary for the development of the barrier
(d) Testicular insult, such as biopsy, torsion, or trauma, will induce antisperm antibodies if the insult occurs before puberty

21. True about seminal vesicle are all *except:*
(a) 4 to 5 cm in length
(b) Blood supply from vesiculo deferential artery
(c) Does not store sperms
(d) Drain in inguinal lymph node

22. After 3 months of inguinal hernioplasty, men loses sensation over root of penis, nerve damaged is:
(a) Ilioinguinal (b) Genitofemoral
(c) Femoral (d) Iliohypogastric

23. True about embryonal NSGCT:
(a) CD 30 positive and CD 117 negative
(b) CD 30 negative and CD 117 negative
(c) CD 30 positive and CD 117 positive
(d) CD 30 negative and CD 117 positive

24. Percentage of NSGCT without raised tumor markers:
(a) 5% (b) 2%
(c) 10% (d) 20%

25. True about epididymis:
(a) Stores 100 million sperms
(b) Immotile sperms are seen in cauda
(c) DHT is the main extract
(d) Is temperature independent

26. Single most important factor for prognosis in NSGCT:
(a) RPLN (b) Size
(c) Type (d) Tumor markers

27. Most common proximal urethral carcinoma in females:
(a) Squamous cell carcinoma
(b) Adenocarcinoma
(c) Small cell carcinoma
(d) Transitional cell carcinoma

28. Difference between T1a and T1b carcinoma penis is all *except:*
(a) Beyond subepithelial tissues
(b) Lymphatic invasion
(c) Undifferentiated
(d) Vascular invasion

29. Cisterna chyli lies posterior to:

(a) Aorta
(b) IVC
(c) Left renal hilum
(d) Right crus of diaphragm

30. Measurement of free testosterone:

(a) Equilibrium dialysis
(b) Radioimmunoassay
(c) Non-radioactive immunoassay kits
(d) Automated platform assays that use chemiluminescent detection

Mention True and False respective to each statement (Q. No. 31 to 89)

31. Stricture urethra:

(a) Most significant complication is extravasation
(b) Gonococcal urethritis causes stricture in bulbar urethra
(c) USG has no role in detecting length and depth of spongiofibrosis
(d) Uroflowmetry is diagnostic
(e) In RGU, the length of the stricture can be underestimated

32. Urethral anatomy:

(a) Cuboidal epithelium is absent
(b) 8 mm is the narrowest part
(c) Glands of Littre open along the dorsal surface
(d) Cowper glands opens at bulbar region
(e) Glands of Littre is more numerous distally and less proximally

33. Testicular tumour:

(a) Poor risk patients should receive 4 cycles of BEP
(b) Most significant toxicity is pulmonary fibrosis
(c) VIP is 3rd line drug
(d) Salvage chemotherapy means autologous BMT and HDCT
(e) Bleomycin toxicity can be minimized by reduction in the forced inspiratory oxygen

34. Regarding tumour marker for testis:

(a) AFP is not raised in seminoma
(b) Beta HCG is raised in 5-10% cases of pure seminoma
(c) LDH is most sensitive for seminoma
(d) AFP is raised in upto 50-70% of NSGCT
(e) 40-45% of NSGCT have normal markers

35. Penile anatomy:

(a) Corpus spongiosum dual blood supply
(b) Blood is supplied to the skin of the penis by the left and right superficial external pudendal vessels
(c) The blood supply to the scrotal wall and ventral penile skin is based on the posterior scrotal artery
(d) The tunica albuginea of the corpus spongiosum is thinner than the tunica albuginea of the corpora cavernosa
(e) The deep drainage system consists of the crural and cavernosal veins

36. Penile carcinoma:

(a) 5 cm size inguinal LN–Adjuvant chemotherapy has better result
(b) In verrucous tumor superficial LN dissection is must
(c) High grade vascular invasive tumor–modified LN dissection is must
(d) Penile tumor involving urethra–partial amputation is not done
(e) Small lesion of T_1 grade 2 can be managed with organ preservation

37. Urethral anatomy:

(a) Spongiosum has dual blood supply
(b) Cuboidal epithelium not seen
(c) Narrowest diameter in urethra–8 mm
(d) Cowper glands opens into bulbar urethra
(e) Paired glands of Littre opens on both sides of external urethral meatus

38. Regarding carcinoma penis:

(a) Cigarette smoking is a common risk factor
(b) > 3 cm condyloma acuminata can be treated with local excision
(c) Holmium laser used for T1 lesion
(d) CECT always done when there is palpable inguinal LN

(e) Sentinel LN is located superomedial to the junction of the saphenous and femoral veins

39. Regarding management of carcinoma penis:

(a) Deep inguinal LN is deep to fascia lata
(b) T2 lesion with non palpable LN–bilateral modified inguinal lymphadenectomy is to be done
(c) Presence of vascular invasion as a prognostic indicator of inguinal lymph node metastasis
(d) When palpable inguinal LNs present then pelvic lymphadenectomy always to be done
(e) Squamous cell carcinoma is characteristically radioresistant

40. Testicular tumor:

(a) If history of scrotal violation is present than hemiscrotum always done along with radical orchiectomy
(b) PET-CT scan always done for finding various metastatic sites
(c) PET-CT to be done for decision making if retroperitoneal LN > 3 cm
(d) Increase β HCG excludes pure seminoma
(e) Doubling time for testicular tumor is 2 years

41. Testicular tumor:

(a) Seminoma is the 2nd most common testicular tumor in adults
(b) Increased AFP rules out pure seminoma
(c) S2 of HCG is 1000-10,000 mlU/ml
(d) Seminoma is radioresistant
(e) Localized seminoma is the most common presentation of GCT

42. A 24 years old diagnosed with NSGCT received 3 cycles of chemotherapy and now presents with 3 cm retroperitoneal LN, management is:

(a) When markers are increased, RPLND to be done
(b) If RPLND is required then it should be nerve sparing
(c) Stage IIIc good risk is given 4 cycles of BEP
(d) If markers are normal than nothing is to be done
(e) In seminomatous patients there is role of PET scan

43. Testicular blood supply:

(a) Blood supply goes posteriorly and inferiorly
(b) Anterior side of testis has fewer vessels
(c) Medial side of testis has fewer vessels
(d) The testicular veins form several highly anastomotic channels that surround the testicular artery as the pampiniform plexus
(e) Neural cross-communication may explain how pathologic processes in one testis may affect the function of the contralateral testis

44. Penile anatomy:

(a) It has 3 cylindrical structures
(b) Tunica albuginea protects erectile tissue
(c) Ejaculation is by ischiocavernosus
(d) Septum is not complete in between
(e) Onuf's nucleus is the somatomotor nucleus for penile erection

45. Testicular physiology:

(a) Inhibin B selectively suppresses FSH secretion in gonadotropes
(b) LH stimulates testosterone by leydig cells
(c) FSH stimulates Sertoli cells for spermatogenesis
(d) FSH and inhibin are predictors of infertility in humans
(e) Activins is negatively regulated by the binding protein follistatin

46. Which statement regarding ureter is true?

(a) Epithelial lining thickened in lower ureter
(b) Adventitia encompasses the blood vessels and lymphatics that travel along the ureter
(c) Ureteral peristalsis does not require outside autonomic input
(d) During ureteroscopy, perforation is most common in upper part
(e) For ureteric orifice dilation pressure required is 15 atm

47. Regarding staging of testicular tumor:

(a) Lymphovascular invasion without extending to tunica albuginea is T2
(b) Stage I marker raised following orchidectomy in NSGCT- RPLND to be done

(c) Contralateral biopsy is done at the time of orchiectomy
(d) Surveillance is option for T1
(e) Tumor invades in rete testes, surveillance cannot be done

48. Stricture urethra:
(a) OIU has good results in stricture less than 5 cm
(b) Uroflowmetry is good indicator for stricture
(c) End to end anastomosis has better prognosis in inflammatory rather than trauma
(d) Posterior urethral "strictures" are not included in the common definition of urethral stricture
(e) The depth and density of the scar in the spongy tissue can be deduced from the physical examination

49. Penile tumor:
(a) Sentinel LN is superficial superomedial
(b) Superficial LN are formed in superficial layer of superficial fascia
(c) In Ta high grade tumor minimal is superficial inguinal LND
(d) For inguinal node of 5 cm chemotherapy should be done before surgery
(e) T_1 tumor can be managed by CO_2 laser

50. Urethral stricture:
(a) Endoscopic alignment following trauma reduces need for surgery
(b) Transpubic approach gives extra 3-4 cm
(c) Inflammatory strictures urethrotomy is better than traumatic strictures
(d) RGU delineated exact length of stricture
(e) BMG is used for proximal bulbar stricture

51. Testis anatomy:
(a) Size 4.0-5.4 cm
(b) Volume 15-25 ml
(c) Tunica vasculosa is outermost layer
(d) Three layers of capsule
(e) Tunica vasculosa contain smooth muscle

52. Vascular anatomy of testis:
(a) Testicular artery courses post-inferiorly after penetrating tunica albuginea
(b) Medial midsection – vessels are less
(c) Lateral midsection – vessels are less
(d) Anterior midsection – vessels are less
(e) Inferior midsection – vessels are less

53. Anterior abdominal wall anatomy:
(a) Inferior epigastric artery is branch of external iliac artery
(b) Superior epigastric artery is a branch of inferior mammary artery
(c) Branches of superior epigastric artery passes through falciform ligament
(d) Intercostal branches does not supply rectus
(e) The rectus abdominis arises from the pubis medial to the pubic tubercle and inserts on the xiphoid process and adjacent costal cartilages

54. Penile anatomy:
(a) Has three cylindrical structures
(b) Incomplete septa is present between corpora cavernosa
(c) Bulbospongiosum causes rigid erection
(d) Ischiocavernosum causes ejaculation
(e) The corpus spongiosum has a dual blood supply

55. Stricture urethra:
(a) Dilation is treatment of choice for short penile stricture
(b) OIU is treatment of choice for < 2.5 cm bulbomembranous stricture
(c) Most dependable technique of anterior urethral reconstruction is the complete excision of the area of fibrosis, with a primary reanastomosis of normal urethra
(d) Holmium: YAG laser has been attempted for treatment with mixed results
(e) BMG gives best result in proximal bulbar stricture

56. Carcinoma penis:
(a) T_2 with node negative–surveillance appropriate
(b) Lymph node >4.5 cm give chemotherapy
(c) Superficial LN is in superficial layer of superficial fascia

(d) Sentinel LN is superomedial in groin
(e) Patients with small lesions of stage T1 grade 2 can be candidates for organ preservation

57. Carcinoma testis:
(a) NSGCT stage 1 after orchidectomy with increase tumor marker RPLND is done
(b) T_1 → Lympovascular invasion with tunica albuginea
(c) Seminoma stage 1 surveillance can be done
(d) Invasion to rete testes→surveillance is contraindicated
(e) Contralateral biopsy should be done to rule out CIS

58. Regarding penile artery:
(a) Common penile artery is the end branch of internal pudendal artery
(b) Dorsal artery of penis is below the buck's fascia
(c) Internal pudendal artery arises from anterior branch of internal iliac artery
(d) Dorsal artery runs between the dorsal vein and the dorsal penile nerve
(e) The three branches of penile artery are dorsal, bulbourethral and circumflex artery

59. Regarding testicular tumor:
(a) Increase in AFP indicates NSGCT
(b) Yolk sac is most common tumor of infant
(c) 10% of seminoma has increase in HCG
(d) AFP is raised in pure seminoma and choriocarcinoma
(e) Low stage seminoma can be treated with observation, radiotherapy or chemotherapy

60. Regarding testicular tumor:
(a) Orchidectomy done with transinguinal approach
(b) Orchidopexy decreases chances of carcinogenesis
(c) Teratoma contains all germ cell lines at same time
(d) Modified RPLND has advantage of ejaculation
(e) Spermatocytic seminoma never presents with metastasis

61. Regarding membranous urethral stricture:
(a) Dissection of Buck's fascia is done to increase compliance
(b) Infrapubectomy helps in repair without chordee
(c) Detachment of perineal body is done to shorten the course of urethra
(d) Progressive abdominal approach is used
(e) Closer the stricture to membranous urethra, longer it can be and still be reconstructed with anastomotic techniques

62. Urethral distraction injury:
(a) Is injury at membranous urethra
(b) In children usually do not extend to prostatic fossa
(c) In adult prostatic urethra usually involved
(d) Most common cause is straddle injury
(e) Accompany about 10% of pelvic fracture injuries

63. Testicular tumor:
(a) AFP elevation will indicate NSGCT
(b) HCG elevation will indicate NSGCT
(c) Stage III NSGCT–Hemiscrotectomy is done for scrotal violation along with orchidectomy
(d) Stage III, good risk NSGCT, 4- cycle B.E.P. given
(e) Increased tumor markers after orchidectomy, chemotherapy is given

64. In seminoma, post chemotherapy, scan there is a mass in retroperitoneum:
(a) Radiotherapy
(b) Bilateral RPLND is done
(c) FNAC is not accurate for diagnosis
(d) If mass is less than 3 cm, observation can be considered
(e) PET scan to evaluate regarding residual mass

65. P53 gene:
(a) Penile tumor has not been associated with it
(b) Associated with superficial low grade bladder tumor
(c) Acts on G_2M phase

(d) Close to 50% of all tumors have TP53 mutations
(e) P53 is on chromosome 17p

66. Alprostadil:
(a) Alprostadil refers to the exogenous form, PGE_1
(b) Doses of 10 to 20 µg, alprostadil produced full erections in 70% to 80% of patients with ED
(c) The most frequent side effects were pain at the injection site or during erection
(d) Priapism is rare
(e) Requires refrigeration

67. Penile erection:
(a) Nitric oxide increases c GMP
(b) PDE_6 is present in corpora cavernosa muscles
(c) PDE_5 is present in photoreceptor cells
(d) Inhibition of PDE by various agents proved useful in erectile dysfunction
(e) Innervation of penis is both autonomic and somatic

68. Regarding nervous and arterial supply of penis:
(a) Skin supplied by external pudendal artery
(b) The dorsal artery generally travels along the dorsum of the penis between the deep dorsal vein medially and the dorsal nerves laterally
(c) Pudendal nerves supply somatic motor and sensory innervation to the penis
(d) Cavernosal nerve is only sympathetic
(e) The internal pudendal artery becomes the common penile artery after giving off a branch to the perineum

69. Regarding testicular tumor:
(a) Yolk sac is the most common tumor in infant
(b) Spermatocytic tumor usually presents with metastasis
(c) Teratoma has various cell line at various stages of development
(d) In choriocarcinoma AFP is raised
(e) AFP is not raised in SGCT

70. Testicular physiology:
(a) LH stimulates testosterone production by Leydig cells in the interstitium
(b) Blood testis barrier is by Sertoli-Sertoli cell junction
(c) 60 – 70% volume of testis is formed by interstitial cell
(d) In male gonocytes mitosis occur at 7-9 years to life
(e) Testosterone is important for progressive spermatogenesis

71. Regarding stricture urethra:
(a) Endoscopic alignment following trauma decreases need for further surgery
(b) Transpubic approach provide extra length of 3-4 cm
(c) In inflammatory stricture results are better than in trauma
(d) RGU can tell exact length of stricture
(e) VIU – better results in inflammatory stricture

72. NSGCT:
(a) Yolk sac tumor, most common testicular tumor in infant
(b) Most of the teratoma deposits contain embryonal cell carcinoma
(c) 10% to 15% of patients with NSGCTs can be expected to have normal marker levels even at advanced stages of disease
(d) Most common site of late recurrence is retroperitoneum
(e) Choriocarcinoma may occur as a palpable nodule; the size depends on the extent of local hemorrhage

73. Anatomy of abdominal musculature:
(a) External oblique attaches to anterior border of thoracolumbar fascia
(b) Internal oblique originates from lower rib
(c) Psoas major originates from T10-L3
(d) Latissimus dorsi originates from medial border of thoracolumbar fascia
(e) Middle layer of thoracolumbar fascia separates sacrospinalis from quadratus lumborum

74. Regarding abdominal vasculature:
(a) Right gonadal vessel courses anterior to IVC
(b) Right iliac artery courses anterior to junction of common iliac vein
(c) Ureter courses posterior to ovarian artery
(d) Celiac trunk first branch of abdominal aorta
(e) Overlying the 2nd lumbar vertebrae, the paired renal arteries arises

75. Regarding carcinoma penis:
(a) Pearly penile papules caused by HPV 16
(b) Bowenoid papulosis is invasive disease
(c) Patient presenting with low grade T2 lymphadenectomy done
(d) Nuclear accumulation of p53 is an independent predictor of lymph node metastasis
(e) The presence and the extent of metastasis to the inguinal region are the most important prognostic factors

76. Regarding carcinoma penis:
(a) Bowenoid papulosis is in situ carcinoma with malignant potential
(b) Condyloma acuminata is malignant
(c) Sexually active male with verrucous carcinoma–radiotherapy best
(d) Verrucous carcinoma–locally destructive
(e) Pearly penile plaques is benign lesion

77. Regarding seminal vesicles:
(a) Volume 4-5 ml
(b) Produces fructose content of seminal plasma
(c) Seminal vesicles absent with absent vas
(d) Do not store sperm
(e) Contribute largest to ejaculate

78. Carcinoma testis:
(a) Elevated AFP means NSGCT
(b) hCG rise in 50% of seminoma
(c) Elevated tumor marker after radical orchidectomy for NSGCT–RPLND
(d) Scrotal ulceration in stage III hemiscrotectomy with radical orchidectomy
(e) Choriocarcinoma has near 100% increase in hCG

79. Anatomy of testes:
(a) Volume 5-10 ml
(b) Does not have somatic nerve supply
(c) Both ends of seminiferous ducts open into rete testes
(d) 25-40 ductules form into appendices
(e) Testicular biopsy is done from upper pole

80. Testicular tumor:
(a) β HCG increased in 70-90% of NSGCT
(b) β HCG increased in 5-10% of seminomas
(c) GCT doubling time is 10-30 days
(d) Negative tumor marker postoperatively – reliably rules out residual tumor
(e) Rx of stage I seminoma–RPLND

81. Regarding testicular tumor:
(a) Teratoma found in 1/3rd cases of residual tumors
(b) Teratoma can involve local vital structure by compression
(c) Radiotherapy and chemotherapy are effective options for stage I seminomas
(d) Contrast enhanced CT scan can evaluate viable cells in residual tumor
(e) Lymphomas are most common testicular tumor after 50 years of age

82. Testicular tumor:
(a) The usual presentation of a testicular tumor is a painful swelling of one gonad
(b) 3-14% incidence in cryptorchidism testis
(c) 5-10% incidence in opposite normal testis
(d) If epididymis is infiltrated, external iliac LN will be involved
(e) Most common bilateral testicular tumor is seminomas

83. Urethral injury:
(a) If urethra disrupted on RGU, endoscopic alignment should be tried first
(b) Non-infective hematoma should be drained

(c) Endoscopic alignment decreases difficulty in subsequent repair of urethroplasty
(d) Stabilized pelvic butterfly # should be fixed to assure transpubic approach
(e) RGU shows the exact length of stricture

84. Testicular tumor:
(a) β HCG increased in 70% to 90% of NSGCT
(b) β HCG increased in 5% to 10% of seminoma
(c) AFP is increased in 5% to10% of seminoma
(d) Negative tumor marker postoperatively reliably excludes residual tumor
(e) RPLND is the option for seminoma stage 1

85. Testicular tumor:
(a) Teratoma is found in one third cases of post chemotherapy residual tissue
(b) Teratoma can involve local vital structures by compression
(c) Radiotherapy and chemotherapy are effective against malignant teratoma
(d) CECT scan can rule out viable cells in retroperitoneum
(e) Immature teratoma consists of undifferentiated primitive tissues from each of the three germ cell layers

86. Testicular tumor:
(a) Doubling time is 1 year
(b) 3% to 14% incidence in cryptorchidism testis
(c) 3% to 10% incidence in the normal testis with contralateral cryptorchidism testis
(d) Tunica albuginea is a natural barrier to expansile local growth
(e) The slower growth rate of seminomas may be inferred from the observation that treatment failures may become evident after 2 to 10 years

87. Penile carcinoma:
(a) Four cm size LN–Adjuvant chemotherapy has better result
(b) If clinically LN is not present, no role of CT scan
(c) If verrucous carcinoma present–superficial LND should be done
(d) If high grade, invasive tumor without LN enlargement is present–superficial LND should be done
(e) In tumor arising from corpora partial penectomy is not considered

88. Urethral injury:
(a) If urethra disrupted on RGP, endoscopic alignment should be done within 7 days of injury
(b) Noninfected hematoma should be drained
(c) Endoscopic alignment decreases the difficulty in performing subsequent urethroplasty
(d) Stabilised pubic butterfly fracture should be fixed to assure transpubic approach
(e) Gentle attempts of Foley's can be attempted

89. Regarding urethral injury:
(a) RGU shows the correct length of stricture
(b) In bulbomembranous urethral disruption, primary realignment should be done
(c) Result of OIU is better in inflammatory than traumatic stricture
(d) End to end urethroplasty results are better in inflammatory than traumatic stricture
(e) If dye leakage is intraperitoneal it is indication for surgery

Which of the following statement is correct?

90. Teratomas of the testis are generally associated with:
(a) Normal tumor markers
(b) Elevated alfa fetoprotein
(c) Elevated beta HCG
(d) Elevated alfa fetoprotein and beta HCG

91. Penis blood supply true is:
(a) Penile skin is supplied by terminal branch of external pudendal artery
(b) Penile skin is supplied by terminal branch of internal pudendal artery

(c) Corpora cavernosa is supplied by dorsal and bulbar artery
(d) Corpora spongiosa is supplied by dorsal and bulbar artery
(e) Deep dorsal vein drains in prostatic venous plexus

92. **Testicular lymphatic drainage:**
(a) Right testis 1st echelon–Interaortocaval
(b) Right testis 1st echelon–Paracaval
(c) Left testis 1st echelon–Para-aortic and pretestis
(d) Left testis 1st echelon–Interaortocaval
(e) Right testis 1st echelon–Para-aortic

93. **Pelvic fracture with blood at meatus and unable to pass urine, all can be done *except:***
(a) SPC
(b) Endoscopic alignment
(c) RGU
(d) End to end anastomosis immediately
(e) Gentle attempt of catheter

94. **NSGCT stage II C, 3 × 3 cm is:**
(a) 3 cycles of BEP
(b) If increase tumor markers–salvage chemotherapy
(c) Surgical resection of residual masses after chemotherapy if visible residual masses and serum levels of tumor markers are normal
(d) Same management as of stage 3 NSGCT
(e) Role of PET scan for detection of post-chemotherapy residual masses

95. **Graft used in anterior urethral stricture commonly is:**
(a) Skin graft
(b) Bladder mucosal graft
(c) Bowel mucosal graft
(d) Saphenous vein graft
(e) Buccal mucosal graft

96. **Tumor marker in carcinoma testis is increased in:**
(a) Seminoma – 10%
(b) Choriocarcinoma – 100%
(c) Teratocarcinoma – 60%
(d) Embryonal carcinoma – 60%
(e) Teratoma – 25%

97. **Regarding GCT true is:**
(a) Yolk sac tumor is most common variant in adults
(b) Anaplastic seminoma is aggressive and lethal
(c) Embryonal body seen in immature teratoma
(d) Syncytiotrophoblast and cytotrophoblast seen in yolk sac tumor
(e) Increased β-hCG seen in choriocarcinoma

98. **VIU complication:**
(a) Extravasation (b) Bleeding
(c) Impotence (d) Hyponatremia
(e) Recurrence

99. **Young male, underwent right orchidectomy and chemotherapy for NSGCT – sperm analysis revealed count of 8 million sperm/ml, appropriate statement is:**
(a) Subfertility
(b) Subfertile because of increased β hCG
(c) Invalid sperm concentration because orchidectomy causes reduced in spermatogenesis
(d) May become normal after 2 years
(e) Count will not become normal as chemotherapy causes irreversible damage

100. **NSGCT with 30% embryonal cell component – invasion to rete testis with normal serum marker and chest X-ray, best option that ensures fertility and adequate tumor control:**
(a) Laparoscopic RPLND
(b) Modified RPLND
(c) Bilateral RPLND
(d) 2 cycle of chemotherapy
(e) Observation

101. **Narrowest portion of urethra:**
(a) External meatus
(b) Prostatic urethra

(c) Bulbomembranous urethra
(d) Bladder neck
(e) Penile urethra

102. Most important prognostic factor in carcinoma penis:
(a) Tumor size
(b) Well differentiated
(c) LN metastasis
(d) Urethral involvement
(e) Involved of glans

103. Chemotherapy in advanced carcinoma penis:
(a) Cisplatin (b) Bleomycin
(c) Adriamycin (d) Docitaxel
(e) Mitomycin C

104. Primary lymphatic drainage of left testis:
(a) Paraaortic (b) Interaortocaval
(c) Preaortic (d) Renal hilum
(e) Paracaval

105. Stage I testicular tumor, surveillance is contraindicated in:
(a) Vascular emboli
(b) Previous FNAC
(c) 5 cm tumor
(d) Cord involvement
(e) Embryonic component > 50%

106. Bulbourethral gland true is all *except*:
(a) Arises from urethral bud
(b) Between two layers of urogenital diaphragm
(c) Common site of infection
(d) Opens in prostatic urethra
(e) Before ejaculation small secretion from these glands are released

107. Denervation of kidney and ureter – true is:
(a) Pain sensation in response to inflammation and swelling is stopped
(b) No effect on renal autoregulation
(c) No effect at all
(d) Peristalsis affected
(e) Pain sensation is normal but autoregulation is affected

108. Carcinoma penis, MMS is not done in:
(a) Lesion >1 cm
(b) < 5 mm on glans
(c) CIS
(d) Lesion >3 cm with corpus cavernosum and corpus spongiosum involvement
(e) < 1 cm superficially invasive tumors

109. Modified LN dissection which is not done?
(a) Saphenovenous dissection
(b) Sartorious flap to cover the vessels
(c) LN dissection lateral to femoral artery
(d) Deep inguinal LN dissection upto inguinal ligament
(e) Shorter skin incision

110. Testicular tumor – true is:
(a) Yolk sac – most common variety in children
(b) Chemotherapy is treatment of choice for advance stage
(c) Overall 5 years survival – 50-60%
(d) In dysgenetic testis most common is– gonadoblastoma
(e) Adenocarcinoma – most common tumor of epididymis

111. In testicular tumor AFP not secreted by:
(a) Pure seminoma
(b) Pure choriocarcinoma
(c) Yolk sac tumor
(d) Teratoma
(e) Embryonal carcinoma

112. Alphafetoprotein half life:
(a) 5-7 days (b) 2-3 days
(c) 3-4 days (d) < 3 days
(e) 1.5 days

113. Alphafetoprotein not increased in:
(a) Teratoma
(b) Pure seminoma
(c) Pure choriocarcinoma
(d) Pure embryonal carcinoma
(e) Yolk sac tumor

114. Mohr's technique is contraindicated in:
(a) Recurrence of superficial lesion following conservative treatment
(b) Lesion of 2 cm involving subepithelial connective tissue
(c) Lesion of 1 cm involving corpus
(d) High grade tumor
(e) CIS

115. Catalona's modification of radical lymphadenectomy:
(a) Lateral dissection beyond femoral artery
(b) Lymph node removal below inguinal ligament
(c) Saphenous vein preserved
(d) Sartorious is transposed
(e) Smaller skin incision

116. Seminoma – surveillance not an option if:
(a) Vascular invasion
(b) >6 cm
(c) Young patients
(d) Increased β hCG
(e) Normal β hCG

117. 2 cm bulbomembranous stricture–treatment option:
(a) Optic internal urethrotomy
(b) End to end anastomosis
(c) Dilatation
(d) Preputial flap
(e) Buccal mucosa graft

118. Penile fracture:
(a) Most common cause is intercourse
(b) Site – transverse laceration at proximal shaft
(c) Urethral injury always seen
(d) Surgery is not a preferred option
(e) Pelvic fracture associated with penile fracture

119. Urethra narrowest at:
(a) External meatus
(b) Prostatic urethra
(c) Membranous urethra
(d) Bulbomembranous urethra
(e) Penile urethra

120. Most common differential diagnosis of testicular tumor:
(a) Hematocele (b) Spermatocele
(c) Torsion (d) Hydrocele
(e) Pyocele

121. Seminoma:
(a) Most common testicular tumor
(b) Most common site of spread is epididymis
(c) Most common cause is cryptorchidism
(d) Radioresistant
(e) Most common bilateral testicular tumor

122. CIS in testicular tumor:
(a) If one testis has GCT, biopsy always of contralateral testis
(b) Biopsy reliably diagnose CIS
(c) Cryopreservation of sperm is essential
(d) CIS–best treatment option is observation
(e) Develop from fetal gonocytes

123. BEP in testicular tumor:
(a) Strands for busulphan, etoposide, cisplatin
(b) Agranulocytosis is earliest side effect
(c) Alopecia is due to etoposide
(d) 4 cycles given at an interval of 3 weeks in poor risk
(e) Bleomycin is given on day 2, 9 and 16

124. Stratified squamous epithelium is seen in:
(a) Membraneous urethra
(b) Bulbar urethra
(c) Prostatic urethra
(d) Penile urethra
(e) Fossa navicularis

125. Most common site of stricture in PFUDD:
(a) Departure of the membranous urethra from the bulbospongiosus

(b) Prostatic urethra
(c) Penile urethra
(d) Bladder neck

126. Most common site of recurrence after RPLND:
(a) Paraaortic (b) Paracaval
(c) Interaortocaval (d) Common illiac

127. Stage and treatment of penile tumor with corpora cavernosa involvement and hard mobile 1 cm LN is:
(a) T2N1M0–bilateral superficial inguinal LND
(b) T2N1M0–bilateral superficial + deep inguinal LND
(c) T1N1M0–observation
(d) T21N1M0–bilateral superficial inguinal LND

128. Iliohypogastric nerve travels along:
(a) Between external oblique and internal oblique
(b) Between internal oblique and transverse abdominis
(c) Between transverse abdominis and transverse facialis
(d) Between transverse facialis and external oblique

129. Extravasation of urethral injury occurs at all *except:*
(a) Buttocks
(b) Perineum
(c) Scrotum
(d) Anterior abdominal wall

130. Distal carcinoma penis involving cavernosa with right 1 cm hard mobile lymph node. Stage and management:
(a) T2 N1 M0, bilateral superficial with right deep dissection
(b) Tl N1 M0, bilateral superficial with right deep dissection
(c) T2 N1 M0, bilateral superficial dissection
(d) T1 N1 M0, bilateral superficial dissection

131. Carcinoma urethra of size 1 cm, 2 cm proximal to navicular fossa. No lymph node involved:
(a) Partial penectomy
(b) Partial penectomy with bilateral inguinal dissection
(c) Partial penectomy with bilateral ilioinguinal dissection
(d) Radical penectomy

132. Patient has to undergo post orchidectomy treatment for lymph nodes for NSGCT. Surgeon will counsel for RPLND rather than chemotherapy for all reasons *except*:
(a) Most common site for metastasis is retroperitoneum
(b) Most accurate staging by RPLND
(c) Difficult to treat recurrence by RPLND
(d) Retroperitoneum not treated than fatal

133. Cowper gland location:
(a) Bulbar urethra
(b) Membranous urethra
(c) Superficial inguinal pouch
(d) Deep inguinal pouch

134. 1st branch of pudendal artery supplies which part of penis?
(a) Bulbar
(b) Cavernosal
(c) Dorsal
(d) Circumflex-cavernosal

135. Urethral trauma in emergency is best diagnosed by:
(a) RGU
(b) Conventional cystogram
(c) CT cystogram
(d) DRE

136. Graft not used in urethral reconstruction:
(a) Partial thickness skin
(b) Bladder epithelium
(c) Buccal mucosa
(d) Rectal mucosa

137. Pyramidalis supplied by:
(a) T11 (b) T12
(c) L1 (d) L2

138. Which statement is not true regarding round ligament?
(a) It passes medially through the broad ligament to fix the ovary to the lateral wall of the uterus
(b) Passes laterally, in the leaves of the broad ligament
(c) Exit through to inguinal canal and attach to the labial fat pad
(d) The superior gubernaculum becomes ligament of ovary

139. Salvage chemotherapy for NSGCT:
(a) MVAC (b) BEP
(c) VIP (d) GC

140. Premalignant condition in carcinoma penis:
(a) Penile plaques
(b) BXO
(c) Hirsute papillomas
(d) Coronal papillae

141. Stage III NSGCT good risk patient chemotherapy of choice:
(a) Two cycle BEP
(b) Three cycle BEP
(c) Autologous bone marrow transplant
(d) Four cycle BEP

142. Most common cancer in female urethra:
(a) Adenocarcinoma
(b) Squamous cell carcinoma
(c) Transitional cell carcinoma
(d) Adenosarcoma

143. Phases of imbibitions and inosculation takes:
(a) 24 and 48 hours respectively
(b) 48 and 24 hours respectively
(c) 24 hours each
(d) 48 hours each

144. Not a pre-malignant lesion of carcinoma penis:
(a) BXO
(b) Pearly penile papules
(c) Cutaneous horn
(d) Keratotic balanitis

145. Most important factor for prognosis in carcinoma penis:
(a) Age (b) Tumor size
(c) LN status (d) Metastasis

146. Testicular tumor causing precocious puberty in males:
(a) Leydig cell tumor (b) Seminoma
(c) Teratoma (d) Yolk sac tumor

147. Most common sign of carcinoma pelvis metastasis:
(a) Preputial swelling
(b) Priapism
(c) Discharge
(d) Tenderness

148. Adjuvant treatment done with post-chemotherapy RPLND:
(a) Hepatectomy (b) Splenectomy
(c) Nephrectomy (d) Pancreatectomy

149. Most important predictor of penile cancers survival:
(a) Grade (b) Stage
(c) Lymph node (d) Age

150. The most common paratesticular tumor is:
(a) Rhabdomyosarcoma
(b) Fibrosarcoma
(c) Sex cord tumor
(d) Adenocarcinoma

151. Surveillance in NSGCT, is not an indication:
(a) Absence of yolk sac
(b) Embryonal >40%
(c) Teratoma >50%
(d) T2

152. Seminoma with stage T2C, post-chemotherapy–4 cm discrete retroperitoneal mass, what is to be done?
(a) Bilateral RPLND
(b) Observation
(c) Get PET scan
(d) Removal of mass and bilateral RPLND

153. Most common site of recurrence for NSGCT:
(a) Lung (b) Retroperitoneal
(c) Liver (d) Bone

154. Spermatocytic seminoma, which should be done?
(a) Inguinal orchidetomy only
(b) Inguinal orchidectomy with radiotherapy to retroperitoneum
(c) Inguinal orchidectomy with two drug chemotherapy
(d) Inguinal orchidectomy with four drug chemotherapy

155. Stage I seminoma, all are treatment options *except*:
(a) Bilateral RPLND
(b) Single drug chemotherapy
(c) Radiotherapy
(d) Observation

156. True about periurethral gland *except*:
(a) Present in dorsolateral surface
(b) Skene gland are largest and most proximal to these glands
(c) Small diverticulum distally known as Lacuna Morgagni
(d) Drains into distal urethra

157. True about Leydig cell tumors, all *except*:
(a) Reinke's crystals
(b) Association with cryptorchidism
(c) Radical inguinal orchiectomy is the initial treatment of choice
(d) Not a GCT

158. In fracture pelvis percentage of patients who will have urethral injury is:
(a) 5% (b) 10%
(c) 15% (d) 20%

159. Weakest point of tunica albugenia:
(a) Ventral layer at 5 and 7 O'clock
(b) Dorsal at 1 and 11 O'clock
(c) Central at 2 and 4 O'clock
(d) Lateral at 8 and 10 O'clock

160. Which is incorrect regarding testicular CIS?
(a) CIS incidence 0.1%
(b) Tumor markers are not there for it
(c) Arises from fetal gonocytes
(d) CIS is evenly distributed

161. In NSGCT which is not associated with poor risk?
(a) Vascular invasion
(b) Embryonal carcinoma >40%
(c) Teratoma >50%
(d) T2 stage

162. Most common testicular tumor in infancy:
(a) Yolk sac tumor (b) Teratoma
(c) Seminoma (d) Leydig cell tumor

163. In stricture urethra onlay flap is most successful at:
(a) Bulbur urethra
(b) Penile urethra
(c) Prostatic urethra
(d) Membranous urethra

164. Regarding testicular sparing surgery, all are true *except*:
(a) For < 2 cm tumors
(b) Indicated in localized GCT in solitary testes
(c) Testicular cooling is mandatory
(d) Frozen section analysis of margins is imperative

165. Tumor markers for testicular carcinomas staged as:
(a) S1 S2 S3 S4 (b) S0 S1 S2 S3
(c) S0 S1 S2 (d) S1 S2 S3

166. In erythroplasia of queyrat all are treatment options *except*:
(a) Careful surveillance
(b) 5 FU cream
(c) Laser ablation with Nd:YAG
(d) Partial amputation

167. Costovertebral ligament insertion is from inferior margin 12th rib to:
(a) L_1 (b) L_2
(c) $L_1 L_2$ (d) $L_1 L_2 L_3$

168. Incorrect about inguinal nodes:
(a) Scrotum, perineal, penis drains into inguinal lymph nodes
(b) Divided into superficial and deep group of lymph nodes
(c) Both lie under fascia lata
(d) Glans drain into both groups of lymph nodes

169. True about scrotal skin all *except*:
(a) It is pigmented
(b) Rich in fat
(c) Lymphatics don't cross median raphe
(d) Contains sebaceous glands

170. Manifestation of ruptured posterior urethra are all *except*:
(a) Fracture pelvis
(b) Inability to pass urine
(c) Blood at meatus
(d) Sleeve like swelling of penis

171. Which of the following is most important determinant of carcinoma penis?
(a) Lymph node metastasis
(b) Depth of tumor
(c) Laterality of tumor
(d) Urethral involvement

172. Most common tumor of seminal vesicle is:
(a) Squamous cell carcinoma
(b) Adenocarcinoma
(c) Transitional cell carcinoma
(d) Adenosarcoma

173. Straddle injury to anterior urethra, the treatment is:
(a) Primary realignment
(b) Suprapubic cystostomy with delayed repair
(c) Catheterisation
(d) Immediate repair

174. In Stage I seminoma which of the treatment is not done?
(a) Surveillance (b) RPLND
(c) Chemotherapy (d) Radiotherapy

175. Most common tumor marker in seminoma is:
(a) βHCG
(b) PLAP
(c) LDH
(d) CA 19-9

176. Gain of the short arm of chromosome 12, most commonly as an isochromosome 12p, i(12p) is associated with:
(a) RCC
(b) Carcinoma prostate
(c) GCT
(d) Carcinoma bladder

177. The Tyson glands are located at:
(a) Frenulum of penis
(b) Perineal membrane
(c) Vagina
(d) Periurethral area

178. Only germ cell testicular tumor, that does not have a CIS stage:
(a) Embryonal carcinoma
(b) Spermatocytic seminoma
(c) Choriocarcinoma
(d) Classical seminoma

179. Orthoplasty is done for:
(a) Chordee release
(b) Undescended testes
(c) Torsion testes
(d) Urethral diverticulum

180. False about spermatocytic seminoma:
(a) Contributes < 1% of testicular tumors
(b) Arises from germ cell intraepithelial neoplasia
(c) Commonly seen in the 6th decade
(d) Usually benign and orchidectomy is the treatment of choice

181. Urethral injuries seen in:
(a) 5% of pelvic# in males
(b) 10% of pelvic# in males
(c) 30% of pelvic# in males
(d) 40% of pelvic# in males

182. Half life of HCG and AFP respectively:
(a) 24 to 36 hours, 3 to 7 days
(b) 24 to 36 hours, 2 to 3 days
(c) 5 to 6 hours, 3 to 5 days
(d) 2 to 3 hours, 3 to 7 days

183. Cremasteric artery is a branch of:
(a) Internal pudendal
(b) Obturator
(c) Inferior epigastric
(d) External iliac

184. Inner most covering of testis:
(a) Tunica albugenia
(b) Tunica vasculosa
(c) Tunica vaginalis
(c) Cremasteric fascia

185. The primary lymphatic drainage from the right testicle is to the:
(a) Interaortocaval group
(b) Pre-aortic group
(c) Para-aortic group
(d) Pre-aortic group and para-aortic groups

186. Treatment for stage I seminoma of the testis is:
(a) Orchiectomy alone
(b) Orchiectomy and chemotherapy
(c) Orchiectomy and radiotherapy
(d) Orchiectomy and retroperitoneal lymphadectomy

187. Which of the following substitute is commonly used in urethral stricture surgery?
(a) Bladder mucosal graft
(b) Buccal mucosal graft
(c) Scrotal skin grafts
(d) Vaginal mucosal tissue

188. Which of the following is the MOST radiosensitive tumor?
(a) Seminoma
(b) Cholangiocarcinoma
(c) Mucoepidermoid carcinoma parotid
(d) Breast carcinoma

189. Schiller-Duval bodies are found in:
(a) Spermatocytic seminoma
(b) Choriocarcinoma
(c) Yolk sac tumor
(d) Teratoma

190. Carcinoma in situ of the testis is a preinvasive precursor of all testicular germ cell tumors *except*:
(a) Anaplastic seminoma
(b) Spermatocytic seminoma
(c) Choriocarcinoma
(d) Yolk sac tumor

191. Reinke's crystals are a pathognomonic histologic feature of which of the following malignancy?
(a) Sertoli cell tumor
(b) Leydig cell tumor
(c) Juvenile granulosa tumor
(d) Gonadoblastoma

192. The following should be performed for the immediate assessment of a patient with pelvic fracture and suspected urethral injury:
(a) Ascending urethrogram with water soluble contrast
(b) Upper tract imaging
(c) Spinal CT scan
(d) Digital rectal examination

193. Erythroplasia of Queyrat is:
(a) Premalignant condition
(b) Red velvety well marginated lesion of glans
(c) Painless condition
(d) Atypical hyperplastic cells replace normal mucosa

194. The lumbo dorsal fascia is laterally contiguous with:
(a) External oblique aponeurosis
(b) Internal oblique muscle
(c) Transversus abdominal muscle aponeurosis
(d) Quadratus lumborum

195. Most common site of EGCT:
(a) Mediastinum
(b) Retroperitoneum
(c) Substantia nigra
(d) Pineal body

196. Which of following is most common site of late relapse of teratoma?
(a) Retroperitoneum (b) Mediastinum
(c) Lung (d) Brain

197. Testicular blood supply, all *except*:
(a) Internal spermatic artery
(b) External spermatic artery
(c) Cremasteric artery
(d) Pudendal artery

198. Blood supply of external genitalia and perineum of female is mainly by:
(a) External pudendal artery
(b) Internal pudendal artery
(c) Femoral artery
(d) Profunda femoris artery

199. Reinke's crystal characteristic of:
(a) Teratoma
(b) Sertoli cell carcinoma
(c) Gonadoblastoma
(d) Leydig cell carcinoma

200. Bulbar urethra is located in corpus spongiosum:
(a) Anteriorly
(b) Ventrally
(c) Dorsally
(d) Medially

201. Vas deferens develops from:
(a) Mesonephric duct
(b) Mullerian duct
(c) UGS
(d) Ureteric bud

202. Lymphatic flow of retroperitoneum is:
(a) Caudal and Left → Right
(b) Caudal and Right → Left
(c) Cephalad and Left → Right
(d) Cephalad and Right → Left

203. Gerotas fascia not fused at:
(a) Superiorly (b) Medially
(c) Laterally (d) Inferiorly

204. Which of the following is the most common cause of urethral stricture?
(a) Chlamydia (b) Trichomonas
(c) Gonococcal (d) Klebsiella

205. Stage-II seminoma, 5 years survival rate is:
(a) 100% (b) 90%
(c) 80% (d) 70%

206. Incidence of GCTs that are extragonadal in origin:
(a) 20-30% (b) 10-20%
(c) 5-10% (d) 3-5%

207. All *except* one can be ligated:
(a) Superior mesenteric artery
(b) Inferior mesenteric artery
(c) Left renal vein
(d) Inferior mesenteric vein

208. First branch of abdominal aorta:
(a) Inferior phrenic artery
(b) Celiac trunk
(c) SMA
(d) IMA

209. Testis sparing surgery, all are true *except:*
(a) Done when tumor < 2 cms
(b) Localised GCT in solitary testis
(c) Cooling the tests is mandatory
(d) Frozen section of tumor margin is imperative

210. Length of female urethra:
(a) 2 cm
(b) 3 cm
(c) 4 cm
(d) 5 cm

211. Most common site of recurrence after RPLND:
(a) Paraaortic
(b) Paracaval
(c) Interaortocaval
(d) Common illiac

212. Lymphatic drainage of prepuce:
(a) Bilateral superficial inguinal lymph node
(b) Internal iliac lymph node
(c) Bilateral deep inguinal lymph node
(d) External iliac lymph node

213. Bilateral inguinal dissection is indicated in which one of the following patient with carcinoma penis?
(a) Invasive primary with negative nodes
(b) Palpable nodes which disappear after treatment of primary
(c) Superficial primary with palpable lymph nodes
(d) Palpable nodes which disappear after antibiotic therapy

214. Stage of the testicular tumor, T2N3M0S1 is:
(a) I (b) II B
(c) III A (d) II C

215. Carcinoma penis with metastasis to 2 or fewer inguinal lymph nodes. 5-year survival after inguinal lymph node dissection is:
(a) 11% (b) 33%
(c) 55% (d) 77%

216. Clinical support for a bilateral procedure even if the contralateral nodal region was normal to palpation is based on the finding of contralateral metastases in:
(a) 10%
(b) 20%
(c) 30%
(d) 50%

217. Risk of metastasis in carcinoma penis depends on all *except:*
(a) DNA ploidy
(b) Vascular invasion
(c) Grade and depth
(d) Stage of disease (primary tumor)

218. Which is mandatory before the therapy for carcinoma penis?
(a) Biopsy (b) Antibiotics
(c) Circumcision (d) Dorsal slit

219. Lymph node involvement in carcinoma penis confirmed by:
(a) Excision (b) FNAC
(c) USG (d) MRI

220. The arterial supply to vas deferens is:
(a) Vesiculo deferential artery, a branch of the superior vesicle artery
(b) Vesiculo deferential artery, a branch of the inferior vesicle artery
(c) Internal pudendal artery
(d) Middle rectal artery

221. Length of vas:
(a) 20-30 cm (b) 30-40 cm
(c) 40-50 cm (d) 50-60 cm

222. Boundaries of retroperitoneal fossa are all *except:*
(a) Inferiorly–extraperitoneal pelvic structures
(b) Laterally–transversus abdominis musculature
(c) Posteriorly–sacrospinalis and quadratus lumborum
(d) Superiorly–pleura

223. Most common site of extragonadal GCT:
(a) Mediastinum
(b) Retroperitoneal
(c) Sacrococcygeal
(d) Pineal body

224. In carcinoma testis secondary tumor is more common with:
(a) More common after chemotherapy
(b) More common after radiotherapy
(c) More common after both CT and RT
(d) No association

225. Verumontanum is present at:
(a) Proximal half of prostatic urethra
(b) Distal half of prostatic urethra
(c) Proximal to external sphincter
(d) Distal to external sphincter

226. Most radiosensitive:
(a) Seminoma
(b) Yolk sac tumor

(c) Embryonal cell carcinoma
(d) Teratoma

227. Which is germ cell tumor?
(a) Anaplastic seminoma
(b) Adamantinoma
(c) Carcinoma rete testis
(d) Leydig cell tumor

228. Most common site of recurrence in GCT:
(a) Retroperitoneum (b) Mediastinum
(c) Pineal body (d) Liver

229. Most common tumor of seminal vesicles:
(a) Adenocarcinoma
(b) Metastasis
(c) Squamous cell carcinoma
(d) Transitional cell carcinoma

230. Cremasteric fascia arises from:
(a) Internal oblique
(b) External oblique
(c) Transversalis fascia
(d) Transverse abdominis

231. After urethral injury blood and urine can accumulate at all *except:*
(a) Scrotum and penis
(b) Anterior abdominal wall upto clavicle
(c) Perineum
(d) Leg

232. Single incision of choice for illioinguinal dissection for carcinoma penis:
(a) Ventral (b) S. shaped
(c) Oblique (d) Transverse

233. Most common complication after modified inguinal lymphadenectomy in carcinoma penis:
(a) Wound infection
(b) Seroma
(c) Lymphorrhea
(d) Skin necrosis

234. Investigations done for testicular tumor are all *except:*
(a) Aortography (b) CECT
(c) PET scan (d) Tumor markers

235. Percentage of urethral injury associated with pelvic fracture:
(a) 5% (b) 10%
(c) 15% (d) 20%

236. Regarding leydig cell tumor, all are true *except:*
(a) Radical inguinal orchidectomy is the initial treatment of choice
(b) 10% are benign
(c) Manifest as androgenital syndrome
(d) Reinke's crystals seen

237. Treatment of spermatocytic seminoma:
(a) High inguinal orchidectomy with retroperitoneal radiation
(b) High inguinal orchidectomy (HIO)
(c) HIO + 2 cycles of chemotherapy
(d) HIO + 4 cycles of chemotherapy

238. For treatment of Stage 1 seminoma after high inguinal orchidectomy, all are done *except:*
(a) Surveillance
(b) Single agent chemotherapy
(c) Modified RPLND
(d) Retroperitoneal radiotherapy

239. Tumor marker stages in use:
(a) S0, S1, S2 (b) S0, S1, S2, S3
(c) S1, S2, S3 (d) S0, S1, S2, S3, S4

240. High risk factors for metastasis in NSGCT are all *except:*
(a) Embryonal carcinoma (>40%)
(b) Teratoma (>50%)
(c) T2 Stage
(d) Vascular invasion

241. Most common testicular tumor in infants:
(a) Yolk sac tumor
(b) Teratoma
(c) Seminoma
(d) Embryonal cell carcinoma

242. True statement among following:
(a) Littre's glands open dorsally in urethra
(b) Littre's glands located more in proximal urethra

(c) Cowper's glands open in membranous urethra
(d) Diverticulum of Littre's called as cave of morgagni

243. Somatic innervation to the testis is provided by:
(a) Ilioinguinal nerve
(b) Genital branch of genitofemoral nerve
(c) Perineal branch of pudendal nerve
(d) None of the above

244. After ilioinguinal node dissection the area covered by:
(a) Adductor longus (b) Sartorius
(c) Posterior thigh flap (d) Gracilis

245. Distal urethral carcinoma in males best managed by:
(a) Partial penectomy
(b) Urethroscopic resection
(c) Radiotherapy
(d) Resection by laser

246. Most common histology of posterior urethral carcinoma in females:
(a) Squamous cell carcinoma
(b) Transitional cell carcinoma
(c) Adenocarcinoma
(d) Verrucous carcinoma

247. Management of inguinal region in a patient with carcinoma penis, T1G1 tumor and clinically negative nodes:
(a) Ilioinguinal node dissection
(b) Modified inguinal node dissection
(c) SLNB
(d) Observation

248. Verrucous carcinoma of penis caused by which HPV types?
(a) 6, 11 (b) 16, 18
(c) 31, 33 (d) 40, 45

249. The membranous urethra is lined by:
(a) Columnar epithelium
(b) Transitional epithelium
(c) Squamous epithelium
(d) Cuboidal epithelium

250. The artery of vas deferens is a branch of:
(a) Inferior vesicle artery
(b) Internal pudendal artery
(c) Middle rectal artery
(d) Superior vesicle artery

251. Which of the following structures does not enter the inguinal canal through the deep inguinal ring?
(a) Genitofemoral nerve
(b) Vas deferens
(c) Testicular artery
(d) Ilioinguinal nerve

252. The cowper's glands open at:
(a) Fossa navicularis
(b) Penile urethra
(c) Membranous urethra
(d) Bulbar urethra

253. Most urachal carcinomas are:
(a) Squamous carcinoma
(b) Sarcoma
(c) Transitional cell carcinoma
(d) Adenocarcinoma

254. Which is the most common type of testicular tumor found in children?
(a) Seminoma
(b) Lymphoma
(c) Yolk sac tumor
(d) Teratocarcinoma

255. The most frequently detected type of human papilloma virus in carcinoma penis is:
(a) Type 6 (b) Type 11
(c) Type 16 (d) Type 18

256. Most frequently detected HPV type in primary carcinomas:
(a) 6 (b) 16
(c) 19 (d) 44
(e) 45

257. Doubling time of testicular tumor is:
(a) <10 days (b) 10-30 days
(c) 30-150 days (d) 150-300 days
(e) 1-2 years

258. Following statement regarding penile anatomy is correct:

(a) Buck's fascia surrounds the corpora cavernosa and excludes the spongiosum
(b) There is communication between the vascular channels of the two cavernosa
(c) The common penile artery divides into two terminal branches
(d) Perforating branches of the cavernosal artery and circumflex arteries supply the penile skin

259. What is the normal testosterone production?

(a) 500 microgram/day
(b) 500 milligrams/day
(c) 1 gram/day
(d) 5 grams/day

260. The epididymis consists of:

(a) A single tightly coiled tubule 3–4 metres long
(b) A set of 12 radially arranged tubules joining the vas
(c) Single tube in the head and multiple tubules in the body and tail
(d) Multiple parallel tubes from rete testis to the origin of vas

261. Which of the following is a normal parameter in semen analysis according to 1999 WHO criteria?

(a) pH 7.50 – 7.65
(b) Count 1×10^7 per ML or more
(c) More than 30% with normal morphology
(d) More than 80% viable sperms

262. The most common cause of penile fracture is:

(a) Sexual intercourse
(b) Masturbation
(c) Road traffic accident
(d) Instrumentation of erect penis

263. Which of the following is correct regarding bladder rupture?

(a) Following blunt trauma, about 25% of bladder ruptures have concomitant pelvic fractures
(b) Gross hematuria with pelvic fracture is an absolute indication for immediate cystography
(c) Emergency exploration and closure is indicated in all extraperitoneal ruptures
(d) Following bladder closure, suprapubic cystostomy drainage is mandatory

264. Which of the following is true regarding seminal fluid?

(a) Spermatozoa represents 30% of the total ejaculate
(b) Major contribution of the volume of seminal plasma comes from the epididymis
(c) Average volume of normal human ejaculate is 7 ml
(d) Littre's glands and Cowper gland also contribute to seminal volume

265. Which of the following is correct regarding prosthetic insertion for erectile dysfunction?

(a) The glans penis does not increase in size with prosthetic erection
(b) With AMS LGX cylinders, no additional length can be obtained with device inflation
(c) Genesis is a two piece inflatable device
(d) Prosthetic insertion is the ideal treatment for situational erectile dysfunction

266. Which of the following is correct regarding Peyronie's disease?

(a) Spontaneous improvement is virtually unknown
(b) The calcific plaque is easily demonstrated using ultrasound examination
(c) Diminished plaque size and penile curvature is documented with colchicine
(d) Patients in the acute phase are ideal surgical candidates

267. In testosterone deficiency syndrome:

(a) Low serum testosterone is diagnostic
(b) Tiredness, dysphoria and hypoactive sexual desire are the most prominent symptoms

(c) Testosterone gel does not reproduce circadian rhythm
(d) Treatment should be initiated only if testosterone levels are diagnostic

268. What percentage of germ cell tumours are extragonadal in origin?
(a) 10% (b) 30%
(c) 45% (d) 60%

269. Which of the following is correct regarding testicular tumor metastasis?
(a) Non-seminomatous tumours are more sensitive than seminoma to chemotherapy
(b) False negative rates of CT to stage retroperitoneum is about 5%
(c) HCG more than 50,000 IU/l is a poor prognostic factor in seminoma
(d) The primary landing zone is different for left and right sided testicular tumors

270. Which of the following is a risk factor for penile cancer?
(a) HPV infection
(b) Neonatal circumcision
(c) Using latex condoms
(d) Sexual abstinence

271. Which of the following is a gold standard for anterior urethral strictures?
(a) Staged repair
(b) Onlay flap repair
(c) Excision and primary anastomosis
(d) Free graft onlay repair

272. The following instrument is used for a "no scalpel" vasectomy:
(a) Fine tipped forceps
(b) Castroviejo scissors
(c) Special mosquito clamp
(d) Snowden needle holder

273. Male with T2 penile tumor-partial penectomy done. Right inguinal lymph node FNAC s/o malignancy. Now treatment:
(a) Bilateral deep inguinal lymph node dissection
(b) Rt deep inguinal LN dissection
(c) Rt superficial inguinal LN dissection
(d) Pelvic lymph node dissection

274. Ta penile preputial tumor (noncircumcised) following not to be done in female partner:
(a) Imiquimod therapy
(b) Cervical biopsy
(c) Observation alone
(d) HPV vaccination
(e) Pap smear

275. Patient elected for right RPLND. The limit of left side of the dissection would be:
(a) Lateral border of aorta
(b) Medial border of aorta
(c) Mid aorta
(d) Right renal vein
(e) Left ureter medial border

276. Marker for testicular tumor:
(a) β-human classical gonadotropin
(b) PLAP
(c) LDH
(d) β-hCG
(e) AFP

277. Peyronies disease A/E:
(a) Need surgery (b) Pain on erection
(c) Infertility (d) Meatal stenosis
(e) Plaque associated

278. Which of the blood dyscrasis causes priapism?
(a) Thalassemia
(b) Sickle cell disease
(c) Leukemia
(d) Aplastic anemia
(e) Spherocytosis

279. Grafts used in anterior urethral stricture common:
(a) Bowel (b) Skin
(c) Bladder (d) Vein
(e) Buccal mucosa

280. About vasectomy true are:
(a) It does not protect against HIV and STD

(b) It is usually reversible
(c) It cause decrease libido
(d) It causes decreased erection and reduced ejaculate
(e) Barrier contraceptives should be used for 3 months

281. Testicular carcinoma markers true is/are:
(a) If AFP increased in SGCT, it is NSGCT
(b) Not used preoperatively
(c) AFP increases post chemoradiation
(d) AFP increase in 25-30% of NSGCT
(e) Post chemonormal level indicate cure

282. The most common complication of internal urethrotomy is:
(a) Bleeding
(b) Fournier's gangrene
(c) Stricture recurrence
(d) Priapism

283. The mediastinal NSGCTs differ in several ways from those originating in the testis or retroperitoneum, *except:*
(a) More sensitive to chemotherapy
(b) Carries poor prognosis
(c) Associated with serum alfa-fetoprotein (AFP) elevation
(d) Associated with hematological malignancies

284. The spermatocytic seminoma is characterized by all features given below, *except:*
(a) The peak incidence is in 6th decade
(b) Arises from intratubular germ cell neoplasia
(c) It is a benign tumor
(d) Always cured with orchiectomy

285. A 30 years old male was investigated for primary infertility. Testicular biopsy showed intratubular germ cell neoplasia on one side. What is the preferred treatment option for him?
(a) Radiotherapy
(b) Radical orchiectomy of that side
(c) Chemotherapy
(d) Wait and watch policy

286. Choose one of the investigations that is useful in evaluation of treatment responses and recurrence of the disease in retroperitoneal fibrosis.
(a) CECT
(b) MRI
(c) Gallium-67SPECT
(d) F-18 FDG PET

287. A 30 years old man presented with a moderately swollen penis associated with pain and diagnosed to have fracture penis. What is the next line of treatment?
(a) Conservative treatment
(b) Catheterisation
(c) Exploration and surgical repair
(d) Suprapubic urinary diversion

ANSWERS

1.	A	26.	A	51.	TTFTF	76.	FFFTT	101.	A
2.	A	27.	A	52.	TTTFF	77.	TTTTT	102.	C
3.	D	28.	C	53.	TFTFT	78.	TFFTF	103.	AB
4.	C	29.	A	54.	TTFFT	79.	FTFTT	104.	AB
5.	D	30.	A	55.	FTTTT	80.	FTTFF	105.	ABDE
6.	B	31.	FTFFT	56.	FTTTT	81.	TTTFT	106.	BCE
7.	A	32.	FFTTT	57.	FTTTF	82.	FTTTT	107.	ABC
8.	D	33.	TTFFT	58.	TTTTF	83.	TFTFF	108.	D
9.	B	34.	TTFTF	59.	TTTFT	84.	FTFFF	109.	AC
10.	D	35.	TTTTT	60.	TFTTT	85.	TTFFT	110.	BDE
11.	A	36.	FFTTT	61.	TTTTT	86.	FTTTT	111.	ABE
12.	C	37.	TTFTF	62.	TFFTT	87.	FTFTF	112.	A
13.	D	38.	TTFFT	63.	TFTFT	88.	FFTFT	113.	BCD
14.	A	39.	TTTTT	64.	FFTTT	89.	FTFFT	114.	ACD
15.	C	40.	FFFFF	65.	FFFTT	90.	D	115.	CDE
16.	B	41.	FFFFT	66.	TTTTT	91.	ADE	116.	ABD
17.	D	42.	FFFFT	67.	TFFTT	92.	AC	117.	AB
18.	D	43.	TFTTT	68.	TTTFT	93.	ABCE	118.	AB
19.	B	44.	TTFTT	69.	TFTFT	94.	ABCD	119.	A
20.	C	45.	TTTTT	70.	TTFTT	95.	ABDE	120.	ABCD
21.	D	46.	TTTTT	71.	TTFFF	96.	ABE	121.	ABCE
22.	A	47.	TFFTT	72.	TTTTF	97.	BDE	122.	BCDE
23.	D	48.	TFFTT	73.	FFFTT	98.	ABCE	123.	BCDE
24.	C	49.	TTFTF	74.	TTTFT	99.	D	124.	E
25.	C	50.	TTFFT	75.	FFTTT	100.	BDE	125.	A

126. A	160. A	194. C	228. A	262. A
127. A	161. C	195. A	229. A	263. B
128. B	162. A	196. A	230. A	264. D
129. A	163. A	197. D	231. D	265. A
130. A	164. C	198. B	232. C	266. B
131. A	165. B	199. D	233. B	267. B
132. C	166. A	200. C	234. A	268. A
133. B	167. D	201. A	235. B	269. D
134. A	168. C	202. D	236. B	270. A
135. A	169. B	203. D	237. B	271. A
136. D	170. D	204. C	238. C	272. B
137. B	171. A	205. C	239. B	273. BCD
138. D	172. B	206. D	240. B	274. AB
139. C	173. A	207. A	241. A	275. A
140. B	174. B	208. A	242. A	276. BCDE
141. B	175. B	209. C	243. D	277. ACD
142. B	176. C	210. C	244. B	278. ABC
143. D	177. A	211. A	245. A	279. ABCE
144. B	178. B	212. A	246. A	280. E
145. C	179. A	213. A	247. D	281. A
146. A	180. B	214. C	248. A	282. C
147. B	181. B	215. D	249. B	283. A
148. C	182. A	216. D	250. D	284. B
149. C	183. C	217. A	251. D	285. B
150. D	184. B	218. A	252. D	286. A
151. C	185. A	219. A	253. D	287. C
152. C	186. C	220. A	254. A	
153. B	187. B	221. B	255. C	
154. A	188. A	222. D	256. B	
155. A	189. C	223. A	257. B	
156. B	190. B	224. C	258. B	
157. B	191. B	225. C	259. D	
158. B	192. A	226. A	260. A	
159. A	193. A	227. A	261. C	

CHAPTER 7

Renal Physiology and Pathophysiology

1. **The usual intravenous solution for urine volume replacement after renal transplantation is:**
   (a) 0.45% saline (b) 0.9% saline
   (c) 0.25% saline (d) 0.20% saline

2. **The most common form of treatment for adults with end stage renal disease is:**
   (a) Kidney transplantation
   (b) Hemodialysis
   (c) Chronic ambulatory peritoneal dialysis
   (d) Medical management

3. **The regional arterial resistance of the kidney vessels is reduced by:**
   (a) Dopamine (b) Dobutamine
   (c) Noradrenaline (d) Isoprenaline

4. **Which of the following is not recommended in septic shock?**
   (a) Steroids
   (b) Activated protein C
   (c) Rituximab
   (d) Normal saline

5. **A young man develops gross hematuria 3 days after upper respiratory tract infection, the likely renal pathology is:**
   (a) IgA nephropathy
   (b) Minimal change disease
   (c) Membranous glomerulonephritis
   (d) Acute glomerulonephritis

6. **Recurrent gross hematuria is seen in:**
   (a) Alport's syndrome
   (b) IgA nephropathy
   (c) Focal segmental glomerulonephritis
   (d) Diabetes mellitus

7. **Crescent formation is characteristic of the following glomerular disease:**
   (a) Minimal change disease
   (b) Rapidly progressive glomerulonephritis
   (c) Focal and segmental glomerulonephritis
   (d) Rapidly nonprogressive glomerulonephritis

8. **Which of the following is the most significant sequel of renal papillary necrosis?**
   (a) Abscess formation (b) Obstruction
   (c) Stone (d) Calcification

9. **Indications for pretransplant native nephrectomy include all of the following *except:***
   (a) ADPKD
   (b) Recurrent hematuria
   (c) Chronic pyelonephritis
   (d) Small contracted kidney

10. **Most common type of rejection seen in post renal transplant recipients:**
    (a) Hyperacute
    (b) Acute
    (c) Chronic
    (d) All with equal frequency

11. **First branch of aorta:**
    (a) Inferior phrenic artery
    (b) SMA
    (c) IMA
    (d) Celiac trunk

12. Boundary of retroperitoneum are all *except:*

(a) Sacrospinalis and quadratus lumborum muscles
(b) Transversus abdominis muscle
(c) Diaphragm
(d) Rectus muscle

13. Which statement regarding lumodorsal fascia is not correct?

(a) The lumbodorsal fascia originates from the spinous processes of the lumbar vertebrae
(b) The posterior layer provides the posterior covering for the sacrospinalis muscle as well as the origin for the latissimus dorsi muscle
(c) As it progresses upward, it separates into three layers: posterior, middle and anterior
(d) The anterior layer of the lumbodorsal fascia forms the anterior margin of the retroperitoneum

14. Lymphatic flow in retroperitoneum is in direction:

(a) Cranially and left to right
(b) Cranially and right to left
(c) Caudally and left to right
(d) Caudally and right to left

15. Which statement regarding dromedary hump is not correct?

(a) Focal renal parenchymal bulge along the kidney's lateral contour
(b) This is of pathologic significance
(c) It is more common on the left than the right
(d) It is believed to be caused by downward pressure from the spleen or liver

16. Orientation of the kidney is in what direction?

(a) Upper poles are situated more medially and posteriorly than the lower poles
(b) Upper poles are situated more laterally and posteriorly than the lower poles
(c) Upper poles are situated more medially and anteriorly than the lower poles
(d) Upper poles are situated more medially and anteriorly than the lower poles

17. Permanent renal failure in adults is commonly defined as an irreversible glomerular filtration rate of less than:

(a) 5 ml/min (b) 10 ml/min
(c) 20 ml/min (d) 25 ml/min

18. In rupture of penile urethra extravasation will not spread to:

(a) Scrotum
(b) Deep to dartos fascia
(c) Flank
(d) Buttock

19. Relative to uterine vessel, ureter is:

(a) Anteriorly (b) Posteriorly
(c) Medially (d) Laterally

20. First human renal allograft was performed by:

(a) Voronoy (b) Carrel
(c) Austin (d) Collins

21. All *except* show, significant probability of disease recurrence and the risk of secondary graft failure:

(a) Focal segmental glomerulosclerosis
(b) Hemolytic-uremic syndrome
(c) Primary oxalosis
(d) Renal amyloidosis

22. Which factor contributes to the profound diuresis and natriuresis in BUO?

(a) Aldosterone (b) Renin
(c) Angiotensin (d) ANP

23. Aquaporin 2 is present at:

(a) Proximal tubule (b) LOH
(c) Distal tubule (d) Collecting duct

24. Greatest risk of ischemic renal injury is to:

(a) S1 portion of proximal tubule
(b) S3 portion of proximal tubule
(c) Medullary thick ascending limb
(d) Medullary thick descending limb

25. Which statement is not correct?
(a) Leydig cells of the testis are the major source of the testicular androgens
(b) Man undergoing bilateral simple orchiectomy is functionally castrate within 1 to 2 hours of surgery
(c) Only 2% of the total serum testosterone is unbound (free testosterone) in the plasma
(d) Testosterone is the major form of androgen found within the prostate gland

26. Which statement is not true regarding HDN of pregnancy?
(a) The left kidney becomes hydronephrotic more commonly than the right
(b) USG findings are hydroureteronephrosis extending to the pelvic brim
(c) MRU has been advocated as a noninvasive, nonradiating method of assessing those with hydronephrosis of pregnancy
(d) The majority of patients with symptomatic hydronephrosis of pregnancy can be managed with conservative measures

27. The Banff classification is accepted as the standard schema for diagnosing:
(a) Renal failure
(b) Transplant rejection
(c) Prostate cancer
(d) BPH

28. Kockerisation is done for mobilisation of which part of duodenum?
(a) First (b) Second
(c) Third (d) Fourth

29. True about blood testicular barrier is all *except:*
(a) Functional after puberty
(b) Both mechanical and functional component present
(c) For antisperm antibodies to form trauma occurs before puberty
(d) More appropriately termed the "blood—seminiferous tubule barrier"

30. CKD staging for children applied after:
(a) < 1 year of age (b) < 2 years of age
(c) > 1 year of age (d) > 2 years of age

31. Nesbitt procedure for Peyronie's disease is:
(a) Tunica albugenia is excised
(b) Penile shortening does not occur with this procedure
(c) Dorsal nerve of penis is retracted
(d) It is the method of choice for straightening congenital curvature of the penis

32. All are used in intermittent priapism *except:*
(a) Duloxetine (b) Baclofen
(c) PDEI 5 inhibitors (d) GnRH agonist

33. Most important to prevent reflux in intramural ureter is:
(a) Active urethral compression
(b) Mucosal coaptation
(c) Detrusor backing
(d) Pressure of valves

Mention True and False respective to each statement (Q. No. 34 to 86)

34. Regarding ATN:
(a) Most common predisposing factor in ischemia
(b) Forced alkaline diuresis is indicated to minimize nephrotoxicity
(c) Penicillin may cause ATN
(d) The S3 portion of the proximal tubule sustains the most severe injury
(e) The oliguric phase begins less than 24 hours after the inciting incident and may last for 1 to 3 weeks

35. Cyclosporine:
(a) Fungal polypeptide
(b) No nephrotoxicity
(c) Calcineurin inhibitor
(d) IL-2 production decreased
(e) Inhibits C-MYC and RAS

36. Regarding renal vasculature:

(a) Posterior segment is most consistent
(b) Anomalous vessel is most common from aorta
(c) Anomalous vessel is most common from renal artery
(d) Afferent arterioles arise from interlobular artery
(e) Arcuate artery is at the edge of cortico-medullary junction

37. Regarding renal vasculature:

(a) Anomalous renal vessel upto 35%
(b) Most common variation is supernumerary renal arteries
(c) Pyramid and major calyx are equal in number
(d) Renal papillae constitute the first gross structure of the renal collecting system
(e) There are 7 to 9 papillae per kidney

38. Anatomy of abdominal wall:

(a) Colle's fascia laterally attach to ischopubic rami
(b) Colle's fascia forms anterior margin of perineal membrane
(c) External oblique inserts into medial lip of iliac crest
(d) Internal oblique arises from lower eight ribs
(e) Iliopsoas inserts into lesser trochanter of femur

39. Ureter blood supply anatomy:

(a) Pelvic ureter–blood supply from lateral side
(b) Endoscopic dilation pressure–20-25 atm
(c) Stent always required after endoscopic balloon dilation
(d) Avulsion commonly occurs at distal 2/3rd of ureter
(e) Iatrogenic injury of ureter commonly at relation to ovarian vessels

40. Physiology of renal blood flow:

(a) Constriction of efferent arteriole causes–RBF and GFR
(b) Constriction of afferent arteriole causes–RBF and GFR
(c) Constriction of the afferent arteriole results in a decrease of PGC and GFR
(d) Endothelin is the most potent vaso-constrictor yet identified
(e) Filtration fraction–20%

41. Stimuli affecting the release of antidiuretic hormone:

(a) Hypo-osmolarity
(b) Ethanol
(c) Phenytoin
(d) Pregnancy
(e) Hypovolemia

42. Regarding diuresis:

(a) Classification of diuretics depends upon effect on Na^+ excretion
(b) Kaliuretic effect of loop diuretic can be blunted by K^+ sparing diuretics
(c) Acetazolamide is carbonic anhydrase inhibitor
(d) K^+ sparing diuretic acts on DCT
(e) Both loop diuretics and thiazide causes contraction of ECF volume

43. RVH:

(a) Renal atherosclerosis causes 20% of RVH
(b) Renal atherosclerosis involves distal arteriole
(c) Typical string of bead appearance seen in intimal fibroplasia
(d) Medial hyperplasia is most common among fibroplasia
(e) Intimal fibroplasia–Most common in elderly female

44. Testis anatomy:

(a) 4 cm – 5 cm in length
(b) Vol 25–35 ml
(c) 3 layers of testicular capsule
(d) Albuginea outermost layer
(e) Vasculosa has smooth muscles

45. Cyclosporine:
(a) It is a fungal cyclic protein
(b) It inhibits calcineurin
(c) Does not cause nephropathy
(d) Does not inhibit IL-2
(e) It inhibit, T cell mediated H-ras and myc release of IL-1

46. Renal physiology K^+:
(a) It is secreted by principal cell of medullary collecting duct
(b) Blockade of the Na channel by the diuretic amiloride leads to reduced Na reabsorption as well as K secretion
(c) K^+ excretion is not dependent of Na^+ concentration in tubules
(d) The cornerstone of medical therapy in PAL is mineralocorticoid receptor antagonist (i.e., spironolactone)
(e) Any condition that leads to increased aldosterone production, can lead to reduced potassium excretion

47. HCO_3 metabolism:
(a) Intracellular H_2O, under the influence of carbonic anhydrase, is combined with CO_2 to produce H^+ and HCO_3
(b) 60% is reabsorbed in PCT
(c) 20% is absorbed in thick ascending LOH
(d) Bicarbonate is not transported across PCT cells; its reabsorption is dependent upon H^+ secretion by the Na^+/H^+ antiporter
(e) There is no upper limit to bicarbonate reabsorption; in states of volume depletion

48. Fraction excretion of sodium >1 is seen with:
(a) ATN
(b) Obstruction
(c) Hepatorenal syndrome
(d) Rhabdomyolysis
(e) Multisystem organ failure

49. Renal anatomy:
(a) Gerota is enclosed from all sides
(b) Anterior to posterior→renal vein, artery and pelvis
(c) In lower pole fusion isthmus is at the level of L4
(d) Extension of cortex in between renal pyramid is column of bertin
(e) Renal pyramid ends at papilla

50. Aorta:
(a) Bifurcates at L4
(b) First branch is celiac artery
(c) Adrenal artery arises between celiac and superior mesenteric artery
(d) Four pairs of lumbar arteries are present
(e) Inferior mesenteric artery arises from right side

51. Urinary Na^+ in hyponatremia:
(a) SIADH > 20 mEq/l
(b) Cirrhosis < 20 mEq/l
(c) Nephrotic > 20 mEq/l
(d) Primary polydipsia > 20 mEq/l
(e) Undetectable in renal failure with euvolemia

52. HCO_3 reabsorption:
(a) More than 4300 mEq/l is filtered/day
(b) 80% absorbed in PCT
(c) 10 – 20% absorbed in DCT
(d) CO_2 combines with H_2O to form HCO_3 under carbonic anhydrase type 1
(e) There is no upper limit to bicarbonate reabsorption

53. Respiratory acidosis:
(a) Chronic respiratory acidosis compensated by renal mechanism
(b) Chemosensitive area is hypothalamus
(c) pH is low (acidemia) and pCO_2 is high
(d) PO_2 is more important than PCO_2 for regulation of ventilation
(e) Decrease ventilation → Decrease pH

54. A.V. fistula:
(a) Congenital more common in female
(b) Approximately 70% of fistulas occurring after needle biopsy of the kidney close spontaneously within 6 months
(c) Most congenital or cirsoid fistulas have been managed with nephrectomy
(d) Most commonly due to trauma
(e) Hemodynamic changes leads to bruit

55. Anomalous renal vasculature:
(a) Incidence up to 35%
(b) More common in arteries
(c) More common on left side
(d) Anomalous artery arises more commonly from arota
(e) Anomalous artery arises more commonly from renal artery

56. Regarding renal physiology:
(a) Glucose reabsorbed by PCT
(b) Sodium reabsorption along the TAHL, in the absence of water reabsorption
(c) Mg^{2+} maximum absorbed from PCT
(d) Aldosterone increases potassium secretion from S1-PCT
(e) 90% of filtered HCO_3^- is absorbed in PCT

57. Regarding renal physiology:
(a) 10% to 15% of Ca^{2+} absorption occurs in DCT
(b) About 15% of the filtered calcium is reabsorbed in the TALH
(c) Thiazide causes Ca^{2+} reabsorption in DCT
(d) Calcium reabsorption in the DCT is independent of Na^+ reabsorption
(e) Most calcium reabsorption occurs in the late S1 segment and early S2 segment of the PCT

58. Reading anatomy of ureter:
(a) Right longer than left by 1 cm
(b) Vas deferens crosses ureter anteriorly
(c) Ovarian artery crosses ureter anteriorly
(d) Ureter passes over the common iliac artery
(e) Fish look sign in lower ureter is seen in ureterocele

59. True about anatomy of retroperitoneum:
(a) Gerota covers kidney, adrenal, ureter and gonadal vessels
(b) In renal ectopia, adrenals are at normal location
(c) Renal vein crosses aorta anteriorly above superior mesenteric artery
(d) Left renal vein crosses anteriorly to aorta
(e) Right renal artery crosses anteriorly to IVC

60. Lymphatic drainage:
(a) Cisterna chyli arises at L1 vertebra behind aorta
(b) Drainage of right testis goes first to common iliac LN
(c) Drainage of left testis goes first to paraaortic LN
(d) Drainage of lymphatics goes from cephalad to caudad
(e) Drainage of testicular lymphatics goes from right to left

61. About Vitamin D:
(a) 25 (OH) cholecalciferol is given in cirrhosis
(b) 1.25 (OH) cholecalciferol is given in renal disease
(c) Vitamin D_3 is produced in skin
(d) Calcitrol is not given in renal failure
(e) 25 (OH) cholecalciferol is formed in liver

62. Renal damage can be prevented during surgery by:
(a) Local hypothermia is the most effective and commonly employed method for protecting the kidney from ischemic damage
(b) The optimum temperature for hypothermic in situ renal preservation is 30°C

(c) Mannitol is most effective when it is given 45 minutes before arterial occlusion
(d) Clamping of the renal artery with short periods of recirculation is less damaging than continuous arterial occlusion
(e) Manual renal compression to control intraoperative hemorrhage is less deleterious than simple arterial occlusion

63. Renal artery thrombosis:
(a) Unilateral chronic occlusion can present as oligouric renal failure
(b) Polycythemia vera can be etiological agent
(c) Acute arterial occlusion is more common on the right
(d) Renal arterial thrombosis commonly involves the proximal or middle third of the main renal artery
(e) Renovascular reconstruction is generally indicated when renal artery thrombosis or embolism occurs bilaterally or in a solitary kidney

64. Renal artery aneurysm:
(a) Saccular aneurysms generally occur at the bifurcation of the renal artery
(b) Fusiform aneurysms is the most common variant
(c) Fusiform are typically found in young hypertensive patients with stenosing fibrous renal arterial disease
(d) Dissecting aneurysm results from a tear in the internal elastic membrane of the renal artery
(e) The fusiform aneurysm is actually a poststenotic dilatation and can involve either the main renal artery or its branches

65. Renal anatomy:
(a) In column of Bertin, cortex is in between pyramid
(b) Renal papilla open into minor calyx
(c) Renal papilla joins into major calyx
(d) Gerota envelops all around the kidney
(e) Upper poles are situated more medially and posteriorly than the lower pole

66. Regarding venous anatomy:
(a) Right testicular vein drains into IVC above renal vein
(b) Left renal vein is longer
(c) Left testicular vein drain inferiorly in renal vein
(d) Common iliac veins lie medial and posterior to the iliac arteries
(e) Left renal vein crosses anterior to the aorta

67. Regarding abdominal aorta:
(a) Divides at L_4
(b) 1st branch celiac axis
(c) Five to 6 lumbar branches
(d) The final posterior branch from the aorta is the middle sacral artery
(e) The aorta enters the abdomen at the level of the 12th thoracic vertebrae

68. Criteria for dialysis:
(a) Serum $K^+ > 5$ mmol/l with no arrhythmias
(b) Hyperkalemia ($[K^+] > 6.5$ mmol/l)
(c) pH < 7.4
(d) Severe dysnatremia ([Na] > 160 or <115 mmol/l)
(e) Uremic pericarditis

69. Anion gap:
(a) Normal anion gap (9–14)
(b) Increase in ketoacidosis
(c) Normal in RTA
(d) Normal in ureterosigmoidostomy
(e) The predominant unmeasured anions include albumin and phosphate

70. Ureter:
(a) 3 layers of muscles
(b) Thickness increases in lower part

(c) When the bladder is distended the openings of the ureters are about 5 cm apart
(d) Avulsion common in proximal part
(e) Blood supply in abdominal ureter comes from medial side

71. Renal transplantation:

(a) Hyperacute rejection because of T cell
(b) OKT_3 effective in accelerated rejection
(c) Accelerated rejection can occur at any time within 1 month
(d) Cyclosporin–Calcineurin inhibitor decreases IL_2
(e) Mycophenolate mofetil–specific inhibitor of purine pathway

72. Cadaveric renal transplant:

(a) Hypothermia is contraindicated
(b) Primary brain tumor with no extracranial metastasis can be a potential donor
(c) Paracetamol intoxication can donate any organ
(d) Basal cell carcinoma (superficial and treated) can be a donor
(e) Can be done in patient who died of lung cancer

73. Bladder physiology:

(a) Predominantly contraction by M_2
(b) Maximum concentration of M_3 receptors
(c) Tolterodine–M_2 receptor selective
(d) Oxybutanin antichlolinergic effect is caused by its metabolite
(e) Tricyclic antidepressants have anticholinergic effect

74. Regarding metabolic derangement of CRF:

(a) Hypercalcemia with hypophosphatemia
(b) Hypomagnesemia
(c) Hypercalcemia
(d) Hypernatremia
(e) Metabolic alkalosis

75. Ureter:

(a) Arterial branches to the abdominal ureter approach from a medial direction
(b) True physical restriction of ureter is at PUJO
(c) Arterial vessels course longitudinally within the periureteral adventitia
(d) During ureteroscopy performation most common in upper part
(e) In ureteric orifice dilatation is done till 15–20 atm pressure

76. Regarding HCO_3:

(a) Daily excretion 4300 mEq/l
(b) 80%-90% absorbed by PCT
(c) 10%-20% absorbed by loop of Henle
(d) HCO_3 combines with H^+ to form H_2CO_3 which dissociates to CO_3 in membrane bound CA-II
(e) The TALH also reabsorbs filtered bicarbonate, mainly through H^+ secretion through the Na^+/H^+ exchanger

77. Anatomy of ureter:

(a) Arterial supply to pelvic ureter arises laterally
(b) Avulsion most common in distal third during ureteroscopy
(c) Iatrogenic injury most common behind ovarian artery
(d) True physical constrictor is at the crossing of iliac vessels
(e) The outermost layer is the adventitia

78. Regarding anatomy of anterior abdominal wall:

(a) Superior epigastric artery is a branch of internal mammary artery
(b) Inferior epigastric artery is a branch of external iliac artery
(c) Intercostal artery does not supply rectus
(d) Superior epigastric artery gives branches to falciform ligament
(e) Arcuate line is a horizontal line that demarcates the lower limit of the posterior layer of the rectus sheath

79. Which statement is true?

(a) Camper's fascia is superficial fibrofatty layer
(b) Colles' fascia is continuous with Scarpa's fascia
(c) Scarpa's fascia is continuous with dartos fascia
(d) Inguinal ligament forms boundary of femoral triangle
(e) Cloquet's node is lateral to femoral vein

80. Regarding Na^+ excretion:

(a) PCT absorbs 20–40%
(b) LOH absorbs 25–40%
(c) Glucose reabsorption is driven by passive Na^+ reabsorption
(d) In collecting duct aldosterone acts on intercalated cells for Na^+ absorption
(e) In medullary CD is impermeable to water in basal state

81. K^+ excretion:

(a) Net secretion of potassium in the CCT
(b) K^+ excretion is not dependent on Na^+ concentration in CD
(c) Amiloride stimulates apical channels and abolishes K^+ secretion
(d) K^+ wasting occur in Mg^{2+} deficiency
(e) In CCD condition that causes decreased luminal flow rates, or increased aldosterone production, can lead to reduced potassium excretion

82. Regarding respiratory acidosis:

(a) PO_2 is more important than PCO_2 for ventilation
(b) Chemoreceptors for CO_2 are present in hypothalamus
(c) pH decreases with hypoventilation
(d) $PaCO_2$ is elevated above the upper limit of the reference range
(e) In chronic respiratory acidosis compensation is by renal mechanism

83. Hyponatremia with urinary Na^+ excretion:

(a) In SIADH urinary $Na^+ > 20$
(b) In RTA urinary $Na^+ > 20$
(c) In nephrotic syndrome urinary $Na^+ > 20$
(d) In cirrhosis urinary $Na^+ < 20$
(e) Renal failure urinary $Na^+ < 20$

84. Regarding renal pathology:

(a) Inulin is best measure for GFR
(b) Molecular weight of creatinine is 50-D
(c) Creatinine is produced by enzymatic conversion
(d) Cephalosporin falsely increases the creatinine
(e) As GFR falls, tubular secretion of creatinine increases and PCr may not change noticeably until there has been a significant drop in GFR

85. Pregnancy and renal physiology:

(a) In pregnancy if creatinine is > 0.8 mg–needs further evaluation
(b) Transient increase in GFR and effective plasma flow
(c) Renal length increases by 1 cm
(d) GFR increases by 10%
(e) Hydroureter occurs due to progesterone

86. Cyclosporine:

(a) Fungal peptide
(b) Calcineurin inhibitor
(c) Never nephrotoxic
(d) Suppresses the expression of K-ras
(e) Decrease IL2 secretion

Which of the following statement is correct?

87. FE Na >1 is seen with:

(a) Prerenal failure
(b) ATN
(c) AGN
(d) Obstruction
(e) Sepsis

88. GFR true is:

(a) Depends on muscle mass
(b) Cock-Craft is inaccurate method of calculating creatinine clearance
(c) In liver cirrhosis GFR is overestimated
(d) Creatinine clearance may overestimate GFR as renal function slowly declines
(e) Best measure is inulin clearance

89. Renin angiotensin system:

(a) Renin secreted by kidney
(b) Renin stimulation by stimulation of α-adrenergic nerves
(c) Renin stimulation by agents that increase adenylate cyclase activity
(d) Angiotensinogen is produced in lung
(e) ACE produced by lung

90. Treatment of coagulopathy in CRF:

(a) Dialysis
(b) Cryoprecipitate
(b) Transfusion
(d) Desmopressin
(e) Conjugated estrogen

91. Physically important constriction of ureter:

(a) VUJ
(b) UPJ
(c) Crossing of iliac vessels
(d) Crossing of gonadal vessels
(e) Crossing of broad ligament

92. CRF diet avoided:

(a) Banana
(b) Orange
(c) Iodized salt
(d) Melons
(e) Milk

93. Which of the following can be ligated without serious consequences?

(a) Gonadal artery
(b) Anterior division of internal iliac artery
(c) IMA
(d) Middle suprarenal
(e) Brachial artery

94. Artery arising from aorta at lower border of L1:

(a) Celiac artery
(b) SMA
(c) IMA
(d) Main renal only
(e) Middle suprarenal

95. Objective assessment supporting diagnosis of CKD:

(a) Poor appetite
(b) Anemia
(c) Hypertension
(d) IHD
(e) Small kidney on USG

96. CKD patients done is:

(a) Adequate hydration
(b) Severe protein restriction
(c) BP monitoring
(d) Oral hematinics
(e) Immunization of hepatitis B

97. In renal transplant donor function after donating kidney becomes:

(a) 80%
(b) 70%
(c) 60%
(d) 50%
(e) 90%

98. Immunosuppression in renal transplant–not used:

(a) FK-506
(b) OKT-3
(c) Cyclosporine
(d) Azathioprine
(e) Mitomycin

99. Indications of urgent hemodialysis:

(a) Potassium >5.6
(b) S. creatinine 4.5 mg/dl with pericarditis
(c) S. creatinine 4.5 with pH 7.25
(d) S. creatinine >5.5 with mental obtundation
(e) S. creatinine >6.5 with generalized anasarca in absence of dyspnea and tachycardia

100. Which of the following is formed in kidney?

(a) 25 OH D3 → 1,25 OH D3
(b) 1,25 OH D3 → 25 OH D3
(c) 25 OH D3 → 24,25 OH D3
(d) 24,25 OH D3 → 25 OH D3
(e) 1,25 OHD3 → 24,25 OH D3

101. In selective angioembolization in renal trauma causing AV fistula – agents used:

(a) Gelfoam
(b) Detachable balloon
(c) Steel coil
(d) Autologous blood products
(e) Ethanol

102. Posterior relation of kidney:

(a) Latissimus dorsi
(b) Quadratus lumborum
(c) Serratus posterior inferior
(d) Psoas major
(e) Diaphragm

103. Association of RAS:

(a) Takayasu's
(b) Neurofibromatosis
(c) Turner's
(d) Pheochromocytoma
(e) MCDK

104. Following inhibits renin:

(a) Captopril (b) Enalapril
(c) Methyldopa (d) Clonidine
(e) Propranolol

105. Potentially nephrotoxic:

(a) Mannitol (b) Acetylcysteine
(c) Ampicillin (d) Urografin 76%
(e) Cefuroxime

106. Hematoma of kidney within gerota can extend:

(a) Inferiorly upto bony pelvis
(b) Medially
(c) Superiorly
(d) Laterally
(e) In the scrotum along the spermatic cord

107. Renal vein thrombosis all *except*:

(a) Associated with nephritic syndrome
(b) Dehydration precipitate it in children
(c) Patient can be asymptomatic
(d) Associated with increased antithrombin III and fibrinogen levels
(e) Anticoagulation is treatment

108. Loop diuretics are all *except*:

(a) Furosemide (b) Bumetanide
(c) Ethacynic acid (d) Triamterine
(e) Thiazide

109. All are renin inhibitors *except*:

(a) Beta blocker (b) Enalapril
(c) Captopril (d) Clonidine
(e) Methyldopa

110. In transplantation renal artery anastomosis to:

(a) Internal iliac artery
(b) External iliac artery
(c) Superior vesical artery
(d) Aorta
(e) Native renal artery

111. Cyclosporin all *except:*

(a) Inhibit activation of IL2
(b) Inhibit lymphokines production
(c) Ketoconazole reduces levels
(d) Cyclosporine increases digoxin toxicity
(e) Oral cyclosporine is not refrigerated

112. Side effects of cyclosporine all *except*:

(a) Hypertension
(b) Nephrotoxicity
(c) Weight gain
(d) Neutropenia/lymphocytopenia
(e) Hypercholesterolemia

113. Association of RAS is seen in:

(a) Neurofibromatosis
(b) Takayasu
(c) Turner's syndrome
(d) Pheochromocytoma
(e) Kawasaki syndrome

114. RVT all *except*:

(a) Associated with nephritic syndrome
(b) Dehydration
(c) Patient can be asymptomatic
(d) There is a role of anticoagulants in treatment
(e) Surgery is mainstay treatment

115. Regarding cyclosporine true is:

(a) Metabolized through cytochrome 450
(b) Given with ketoconazole increases its serum concentration
(c) Drug of choice in acute rejection
(d) Nephrotoxicity
(e) Contraindicated in cadaveric transplant

116. PTA with stenting is indicated in:

(a) Osteal narrowing
(b) Partial intimal injury
(c) Not amenable to angiography
(d) Renal artery stenosis with CKD
(e) Restenosis after PTA

117. Anemia in CRF – true is:

(a) Reduced erythropoietin
(b) Reduced RBC survival
(c) Increased hemolysis during hemodialysis
(d) Bone marrow depression by toxins
(e) Functional iron deficiency

118. Indications of renal artery stenting:

(a) Hilar stenosis
(b) Osteal stenosis
(c) Stenosis with severe hypertension
(d) Stenosis with CKD
(e) Renal artery dissection

119. Mortality in renal failure:

(a) 10% (b) 20%
(c) 30% (d) 40%
(e) 50%

120. Side effects of cisplatin:

(a) Pulmonary fibrosis
(b) Alopecia
(c) Bone marrow suppression
(d) Renal insufficiency
(e) Neuropathy

121. Epididymal arterial supply:

(a) Through superior epididymal artery
(b) Through inferior epididymal artery
(c) Cremasteric artery
(d) Through branches of superior vesical artery
(e) All of the above

122. Drug dose need not be altered in renal insufficiency:

(a) Cloxacillin (b) Streptomycin
(c) Amikacin (d) Cephalexin
(e) Aztreonam

123. Bilateral smooth small kidneys:

(a) Congenital hypoplasia
(b) Generalised arteriosclerosis
(c) Chronic glomerulonephritis
(d) Reflux nephropathy
(e) MCKD

124. Narrowing of ureter at all *except:*

(a) PUJ
(b) VUJ
(c) Illiac vessel crossing
(d) Sacral promontory crossing
(e) Gonadal vessel crossing

125. Kidney produces:

(a) PTH (b) Insulin
(c) Rennin (d) 1,25 DHCC
(e) Erythropoietin

126. Artery arises from aorta between celiac axis and renal artery:

(a) SMA (b) Adrenal
(c) Inferior phrenic (d) IMA
(e) Gonadal

127. Renin secretion stimulated by:

(a) Increased cAMP
(b) Increased intracellular calcium
(c) Reduced perfusion pressure
(d) Adrenergic antagonist
(e) Reduced sodium in DCT

128. Renal artery stenosis associated with:

(a) Takayasu
(b) Neurofibromatosis
(c) Turner's syndrome
(d) Pheochromocytoma
(e) Middle aortic syndrome

129. Hormone secreted by kidney acting on cell surface receptor:

(a) ADH (b) Aldosterone
(c) Calcitonin (d) Vitamin D
(e) PTH

130. In pre-renal failure urine: plasma creatinine ratio >30:1, most likely explanation will be:

(a) Urea absorbed from tubules
(b) Dehydration
(c) Decreased renal plasma flow
(d) Creatinine is not absorbed from renal tubules
(e) Release of ADH

131. Glutaraldehyde – true:

(a) Toxic and strong irritant
(b) Carcinogenic
(c) Pungent, colorless oily liquid
(d) Used in electron microscopy as preservative
(e) Used for industrial water treatment

132. Compound papilla:

(a) Formed by fusion of pyramids
(b) Associated with reflux and back pressure changes
(c) Restricted only at poles
(d) Associated with scarring
(e) Prevent reflux by collapsing of collecting duct

133. In cadaveric kidney, which donor is not a contraindication?

(a) Astrocytoma
(b) Superficial skin tumor
(c) Carcinoma colon
(d) Carcinoma–lung
(e) Intraductal carcinoma of breast

134. Selective renal artery angiography done:

(a) As a primary investigation in suspected renal mass in solitary kidney
(b) In determinant solid renal mass on CT
(c) To differentiate between solid and cystic
(d) Bleeding following PCNL
(e) In evaluation of renal artery stenosis

135. Ureteral narrowing seen at:

(a) UPJ
(b) Crossing of gonadal vessels
(c) Crossing of iliac vessel
(d) Sacral promontory
(e) Ureteric orifice

136. Cyclosporine toxicity all are true *except*:

(a) Graft tenderness
(b) No history of fever
(c) Normal urine output
(d) Slow increase in creatinine

137. GFR most significant determinant:

(a) Transglomerular pressure
(b) Renal plasma flow
(c) Glomerular permeability
(d) Oncotic pressure

138. Recurrent TCC after renal transplant:

(a) Thiopeta (b) BCG
(c) Mitomycin (d) Fulguration

139. Kidney longitudinal axis is due to:

(a) Psoas
(b) Quadratus lumborum
(c) Erector spinae
(d) Diaphragm

140. Renal artery aneurysm surgery all are true *except:*

(a) Calcified – 1.5 cm
(b) Noncalcified 3.5 cm
(c) Aneurysmal dissection
(d) Associated with hypertension

141. Fetal lobulation:

(a) Normal variant
(b) Disappear by 5 years
(c) Disappear by puberty
(d) Disappear by 30 years of age

142. All are true regarding angiotensin *except*:

(a) AT2 receptor causes renal ischemia
(b) AT1 receptor causes aldosteronism
(c) PG blunts the effect of afferent arteriole
(d) Effect more pronounced on efferent

143. Warm ischemia time for kidney:

(a) 15 min (b) 20 min
(c) 30 min (d) 45 min

144. Twenty two years old girl with pain in left flank, USG suggestive of HDN and ureter not visualised, DTPA 18 ml/min. Management is:

(a) Pyeloplasty (b) Nephrectomy
(c) MRU (d) CTU

145. Pretransplant nephrectomy indication:

(a) Autosomal-recessive polycystic kidney disease
(b) Medically refractory hypertension
(c) Chronically infected kidneys
(d) Suspected renal or urothelial cancer

146. Which is correct regarding urinary obstruction?

(a) FE_{Na} is greater in BUO
(b) Increase FE_K in UUO
(c) Urine pH is greater in UUO
(d) Post obstructive diuresis more in UUO

147. Smallest vein in kidney is:

(a) Lobular (b) Interlobar
(c) Arcuate (d) Segmental

148. Dose modification not required at GFR 50 ml/min:

(a) Ceftriaxone (b) Cefoperazone
(c) Linezolid (d) Cefixime

149. Least complication occurs if damaged is:

(a) SMA (b) IMA
(c) Celiac plexus (d) Renal artery

150. BUN increases in all *except*:

(a) Dehydration
(b) Shock
(c) Congestive heart failure
(d) Liver failure

151. Most common presentation of stone in transplanted kidney:

(a) Decrease urine output
(b) Pain from loin to tip of penis
(c) Pain from groin to loin
(d) Dietal crisis

152. Time of bilateral pretransplant nephrectomy:

(a) Simultaneously (b) 6 weeks before
(c) 6 months before (d) Any time

153. CKD stage of kidney damage with moderate decrease in GFR?

(a) 2 (b) 3
(c) 4 (d) 5

154. In cockcroft gault formula constant value used in females is:

(a) 0.75 (b) 0.85
(c) 1.05 (d) 1.15

155. Most susceptible segment in renal ischemia:

(a) JG apparatus
(b) Ascending thick LOH
(c) S3 segment of PCT
(d) S3 segment of DCT

156. Creatinine clearance is not the perfect way to measure GPR due to all *except*:

(a) As GFR falls, tubular secretion of creatinine increases and PCr may not change noticeably until significant drop in GFR
(b) Creatinine production may decrease with liver cirrhosis
(c) Variable rate throughout day
(d) Affected by rhabdomyolysis

157. Patient with serum creatinine 2.7 mg/dl requires renal angiography, best way to protect renal function is:

(a) Saline diuresis
(b) Mannitol infusion
(c) Furosemide before study
(d) Dopamine throughout the study

158. Most effective agent for preserving residual renal function in CRF:

(a) Alpha blockers
(b) Dihydropyridine CCB
(c) ACE inhibitors
(d) Beta blockers

159. FE_{Na} in prerenal ARF is:

(a) $<1\%$ (b) $>1\%$
(c) $>10\%$ (d) $<10\%$

160. Immunosuppressive drug that can replace cyclosporine:

(a) Tacrolimus (b) Steroids
(c) AZT (d) Mycophenolate

161. First successful renal transplantation done in:

(a) 1952 (b) 1954
(c) 1956 (d) 1958

162. Major cell types in collecting ducts are:

(a) Intercalated and principal cell
(b) Intercalated cells
(c) Principal cells
(d) Macula densa

163. All are true regarding phosphate *except*:

(a) About 85% to 90% of filtered phosphate is reabsorbed, primarily in the PCT
(b) High luminal pH favors calcium phosphate complexion
(c) PTH enhances phosphate excretion
(d) Approximately 60% of the phosphate in the diet is absorbed by the intestine

164. Each of the following is a major determinant used to calculate total body osmolarity of body fluids *except*:

(a) Plasma Na^+ (b) Plasma K^+
(c) Plasma glucose (d) BUN

165. Main site of renal HCO_3^- reabsorption is:

(a) PCT (b) LOH
(c) DCT (d) CD

166. Renal artery dilation occurs with:

(a) CO (b) ANP
(c) NE (d) ET

167. Most common aneurysm of renal artery:

(a) Intrarenal (b) Fusiform
(c) Saccular (d) Dissecting

168. ACE inhibitors are useful in:

(a) Unilateral RAS with normal contralateral kidney
(b) Bilateral RAS
(c) RAS in solitary kidney
(d) RAS in transplant kidney

169. Lap. Donor nephrectomy: order of ligation:
(a) Ureter, vein, artery
(b) Ureter, artery, vein
(c) Vein, artery, ureter
(d) Artery, vein, ureter

170. Most accurate marker of GFR is:
(a) Serum creatinine
(b) BUN
(c) Cystatin
(d) Urinary creatinine

171. Which is incorrect for PCT?
(a) Absorb 75% of the filtrate
(b) 100% of glucose
(c) 80% of water
(d) Glutamine to ammonia for acidification

172. Oliguric ARF, which of the following is present, *except*?
(a) Anemia (b) Uremia
(c) Hypercalcemia (d) Acidosis

173. Renal artery stenosis is present in all *except*:
(a) Takayasu's
(b) PAN
(c) Fibromuscular dysplasia
(d) Atherosclerosis

174. Poor risk factor in atherosclerosis, all *except*:
(a) Hyperhomocysteinemia
(b) Decreased fibrinogen levels
(c) Decreased HDL levels
(d) Increased waist-hip ratio

175. GFR best measured by:
(a) MAG-3 (b) DTPA
(c) DMSA (d) Gallium scan

176. Treatment option in hyperkalemia, all *except*:
(a) IV $NaHCO_3$
(b) Ion exchange resin orally
(c) Oral coconut water
(d) 25% dextrose infusion

177. Minimum MAP below which filtration ceases:
(a) 20 mm Hg (b) 30 mm Hg
(c) 40 mm Hg (d) 50 mm Hg

178. Most significant determinant of GFR is:
(a) Renal plasma flow
(b) Glomerular permeability
(c) Oncotic pressure
(d) Transglomerular (hydraulic) pressure

179. Sympathetic nerve supply of ureter:
(a) $T_{10} - L_2$ (b) $T_{11} - L_2$
(c) $T_{11} - L_1$ (d) $T_{10} - T_{11}$

180. Ureteral constriction is not present at:
(a) PUJ
(b) UVJ
(c) Crossing of iliac vessel
(d) Crossing at vas deferens/uterine vessels

181. Psoas major incorrect is:
(a) Originates from 12th rib to 5th lumbar vertebra
(b) Flexion of hip
(c) Inserts into greater trochanter
(d) Joins iliacus

182. Which of the following is not a branch of celiac trunk?
(a) Common hepatic
(b) Left gastric
(c) Splenic
(d) Superior mesenteric artery

183. Uromodulin secreted by:
(a) S_3 segment of LH
(b) DCT
(c) Thin ascending loop
(d) Thick ascending loop

184. Incorrect about water reabsorption in PCT:
(a) Passive process
(b) Water absorptions occur by transcellular pathways through aquaporin-2 channels
(c) Paracellular movement of water reabsorption occurs across the tight junctions between cells

(d) Water absorptions occur by transcellular pathways through aquaporin-1 channels

185. Principal cells present in:
(a) DCT
(b) Cortical collecting tubules
(c) Medullary collecting tubules
(d) Loop of Henle

186. Which of the following is a vasoconstrictor for kidney?
(a) ANP (b) NO
(c) Serotonin (d) CO

187. Which of the following is not a vasoconstrictor?
(a) Endothelin (b) Angiotensin II
(c) NO (d) Nor adrenaline

188. MDRD formula for creatinine clearance doesn't include:
(a) Age (b) Sex
(c) Race (d) Weight

189. Corkcroft Gault formula doesn't include:
(a) Plasma creatinine
(b) Urinary creatinine
(c) Age
(d) Weight

190. Low fractional excretion of sodium is seen in all *except*:
(a) Prerenal azotemia
(b) Acute tubular necrosis
(c) Glomerulonephritis
(d) Hepatorenal syndrome

191. IgA nephropathy – deposits along:
(a) Mesangial cells
(b) Mesangiocapillary
(c) Basement membrane
(d) Capillary

192. Cyclosporine toxicity – most important is:
(a) Nephrotoxicity
(b) Secondary malignancy
(c) DM
(d) Hypertension

193. Which of the following is false regarding creatinine clearance?
(a) More accurate than inulin clearance
(b) Plasma creatinine is most widely used marker of GFR
(c) Production rate varies from individual to individual
(d) Advantage of being easy to perform (no intravenous infusion), is cheap, and is readily available

194. Among these most common cause of renal transplantation is:
(a) Chronic glomerulonephritis
(b) Malignant nephrosclerosis
(c) Polycystic kidney
(d) Chronic pyelonephritis

195. Creatinine clearance correlates with:
(a) GFR
(b) Tubular reabsorption
(c) Renal plasma flow
(d) Tubular function

196. In ischemic injury which portion sustain the most common injury:
(a) TAL of Henle
(b) Cortical collecting duct
(c) Juxtaglomerular apparatus
(d) Proximal tubule

197. Kidney length in vertical direction is:
(a) 8 – 10 cm (b) 10 – 12 cm
(c) 6 – 8 cm (d) 12 – 14 cm

198. Medial aspect of kidney is rotated anteriorly by:
(a) 0 degree (b) 10 degree
(c) 30 degree (d) 40 degree

199. Renal column of Bertin is the extension of:
(a) Cortex (b) Medulla
(c) Pyramid (d) Papilla

200. Ureteral peristalsis arises from:
(a) Renal calyx (b) Renal pelvis
(c) UVJ (d) Upper ureter

201. Afferent arteriole arises from:
(a) Interlobular (b) Arcuate
(c) Interlobar (d) Vasa recta

202. First and most consistent branch of renal artery is:
(a) Posterior branch (b) Anterior branch
(c) Inter lobar (d) Vasa recta

203. The following statements are correct *except*:
(a) Macula densa is located in ascending limb of loop of Henle
(b) Afferent arterioles contain juxtaglomerular cells
(c) The conversion of angiotensin I to angiotensin II occurs in the liver
(d) 70% of filtered K is absorbed in PCT

204. Erythropoietin is produced by:
(a) Glomerular tufts
(b) Renal interstitial fibroblasts
(c) Juxtaglomerular cells
(d) Macula densa

205. Gerota's fascia opens:
(a) Superiorly
(b) Inferiorly
(c) Medially
(d) Laterally

206. Renal arteries arises at the level of:
(a) T12 (b) L1
(c) L2 (d) L3

207. The segment of kidney most variable in origin of its blood supply:
(a) Apical (b) Middle
(c) Lower (d) Posterior

208. Intra operatively ureter can be identified as it enters the pelvis:
(a) At the superior border of sacrum
(b) At the crossing of uterine artery
(c) Over the common iliac artery where internal iliac artery arises
(d) At the aortic bifurcation

209. Which of the following best describes the function of thin descending loop of nephron?
(a) Impermeable to water, slightly permeable to Na, Cl
(b) Permeable to water, impermeable to Na, Cl
(c) Impermeable to water, highly permeable to Na, Cl
(d) Impermeable to water and Na, Cl

210. False about angiotensinogen:
(a) It is a 452 amino acid protein
(b) Functions as serine protease inhibitor similar to alfa-1 antitrypsin
(c) Liver is the primary site of storage where it is synthesised
(d) Estrogen and glucocorticoids increases the angiotensinogen levels in the blood

211. Stage of CKD when GFR is 26 ml/1.73 m/min:
(a) Stage 2 (b) Stage 3
(c) Stage 4 (d) Stage 5

212. False about acute interstitial nephritis (AIN):
(a) Clinical picture although variable usually involves abnormal urinary sediment
(b) Renal biopsy is not usually required for the confirmation of diagnosis
(c) Most common cause of granuloma formation is sarcoidosis
(d) Nephrotic range proteinuria is frequently seen in AIN due to NSAIDS

213. In the treatment of hyperkalemia which of the following doesn't alter the serum K^+ levels:
(a) Insulin + glucose
(b) Sodium bicarbonate
(c) Calcium gluconate
(d) Nebulised albuterol

214. Which of the following disease doesn't recur after renal transplantation?
(a) FSGS (b) HUS
(c) ADPKD (d) Primary oxaluria

215. False about medial fibroplasia:
(a) Most common fibroplasia constituting 30 to 40% of fibrous lesions
(b) Occurs in women between 25 and 50 years of age
(c) Often involves both renal arteries
(d) None of the above

216. Following immunosuppressant causes diabetes:
(a) Mycophenolate mofetil
(b) Cyclosporine
(c) Sirolimus
(d) Azathioprine

217. Postoperative IV fluid of choice after renal transplantation:
(a) 0.25% NaCl (b) 0.45% NaCl
(c) 0.9% NaCl (d) 3% NaCl

218. After transplantation the minimum duration after which couple is advised to plan for pregnancy:
(a) 3 months (b) 6 months
(c) 12 months (d) 24 months

219. Drug which increases the levels of cyclosporine in the blood:
(a) Rifampicin (b) Phenobarbitone
(c) Ketoconazole (d) Phenytoin

220. Regarding fertility after transplantation all of the following true *except*:
(a) After successful kidney transplantation, levels of FSH, LH, testosterone usually becomes normal and spermatogenesis improves
(b) Among male recipients who have fathered children, there has been increase in congenital abnormalities in the offspring
(c) Impregnation be delayed atleast 1 year after transplantation
(d) Successful renal transplantation usually restores fertility in premenopausal women

221. False about renal artery stenosis after renal transplantation:
(a) It can be due to atheroma or faulty suture technique
(b) Can present with impaired renal function
(c) Finding of bruit over the kidney graft is a reliable sign of diagnosis
(d) Percutaneous transluminal angioplasty is the initial treatment of choice

222. False regarding the outcome following revascularisation of atherosclerotic renal artery disease:
(a) Outcome is similar irrespective of preoperative serum creatinine levels
(b) Outcome is good when there is deterioration in the renal function where angiotensin receptor blockers are used to control HTN
(c) Preoperative kidney size >9 cm good outcome
(d) Bilateral renal artery stenosis good outcome

223. True physical constriction of ureter is seen at:
(a) UPJ
(b) UVJ
(c) At the crossing of gonadal vessels
(d) Where ureter crosses iliac vessels

224. Mechanism of absorption of HCO_3- in PCT:
(a) Active diffusion
(b) Action of carbonic anhydrase
(c) Passive diffusion
(d) No absorption in PCT

225. An average of how many glomeruli are found in each kidney?
(a) 4 millions
(b) 2 millions
(c) 8 millions
(d) 1 million

226. The vas deferens is lined by:
(a) Pseudostratified columnar epithelium
(b) Stratified columnar epithelium
(c) Stratified squamous epithelium
(d) Transitional ciliated epithelium

227. The normal ratio of intramural length to ureter diameter is:
(a) 5:1 (b) 3:1
(c) 6:1 (d) 1:1

228. Which is not correct regarding renal blood flow?
(a) It is about 1200 ml/min
(b) It is about 20% of the cardiac output
(c) It is about 4 ml/gm/min
(d) Renal medulla receives 60% of blood

229. The gold standard in identifying the kidney causing renovascular hypertension is:
(a) Differential renal vein renin estimation
(b) Captopril DTPA renal dynamic scan
(c) Isotope renogram
(d) MR angiogram

230. The most serious toxicity of cyclosporine therapy is:
(a) Ototoxicity
(b) Pulmonary fibrosis
(c) Nephrotoxicity
(d) Hepatotoxicity

231. The major site of synthesis angiotensinogen is:
(a) Liver
(b) Kidney
(c) Vascular endothelium
(d) Lungs

232. Girlie's disease is:
(a) Intimal fibroplasias
(b) Perimedial fibroplasias
(c) Fibromuscular hyperplasia
(d) Medial fibroplasias

233. Post obstructive diuresis is due to all *except*:
(a) Retained salt and water
(b) Retained urea and nitrogenous products
(c) Impaired concentrating ability
(d) Impaired glucose tolerance

234. Dromedary hump is:
(a) Found commonly on right kidney
(b) One of the fetal lobulation in left kidney
(c) A normal variant secondary to downward pressure from spleen or liver
(d) Needs surgical intervention when found

235. Which of the following statements regarding anatomical position of kidneys is false?
(a) Lower poles of both kidneys lie farther from midline than upper pole
(b) Lower poles of kidneys are pushed slightly more anterior than upper pole
(c) Medial aspect of each kidneys is rotated anteriorly at an angle of about 90 degree from the true coronal plane
(d) None of the above

236. False statement regarding renal artery stenosis after renal transplantation:
(a) Usually diagnosed because of hypertension
(b) Atheroma, faulty suture technique and immunological mechanisms are proposed as etiological factors
(c) Bruit over the transplant kidney is a reliable sign of renal artery stenosis
(d) Percutaneous transluminal angioplasty is the treatment of choice

237. The true physical restriction of ureteral lumen occurs at:
(a) Ureteropelvic junction
(b) Ureterovesical junction
(c) At the level of sacroiliac joint
(d) Where ureter crosses the iliac vessels

238. 38-year-old man with hypertension, Serum creatinine >2.4, RBC cast, 3+ protein, 10-20 RBC/HPF:
(a) MRI (b) Renal biopsy
(c) RGP (d) CT scan

239. Post transplant most common recurrence seen in:
(a) Membranoproliferative glomerulonephritis
(b) Focal segmental glomerulosclerosis
(c) Chronic GN
(d) Membranous GN

240. HCO_3^- maximum absorbed by:
(a) PCT (b) DCT
(c) LOH (d) CD

241. First successful renal transplant was done in:
(a) 1954 (b) 1944
(c) 1962 (d) 1965

242. Hyperacute rejection due to:
(a) Preformed antibodies against HLA-1
(b) ABO mismatch
(c) Alloantibodies
(d) Anti lymphocytes

243. Gonadal vessels in relation to ureter:
(a) Anterior
(b) Posterior
(c) Lateral
(d) Not immediately related

244. A 60-year-old male with cardiac pacemaker with creatinine 3 mg % with acute pyelonephritis, which of the following investigation is most appropriate?
(a) MRI
(b) Non-contrast CT
(c) USG
(d) Radioisotope scanning

245. First segmental branch of renal artery is:
(a) Apical (b) Anterior
(c) Posterior (d) Medial

246. The structures seen at renal hilum from anterior to posterior:
(a) Renal artery, renal pelvis, renal vein
(b) Renal vein, renal artery, renal pelvis
(c) Renal pelvis, renal vein, renal artery
(d) Renal pelvis, renal artery, renal vein

247. False about post infection glomerulonephritis in children is:
(a) Group A beta hemolytic streptococci is the most common causative organism
(b) Complete regression occurs in only 10% of cases
(c) Recovery is possible in patients on dialysis
(d) C3 comes down to normal level within 2 months

248. Stimulation for renin release are all *except:*
(a) Renal ischemia
(b) Low sodium delivery
(c) Beta agonist
(d) Agents decreasing adenylyl cyclase activity

249. Angiotensin II causes all *except:*
(a) Epinephrine release
(b) Vasoconstriction
(c) Release of aldosterone
(d) Development of tubulointerstitial fibrosis, tubular atrophy and apoptosis

250. All of the following are indications of dialysis *except:*
(a) Pulmonary edema with evidence of water retention
(b) Potassium > 6.5 within ECG changes
(c) pH < 7.1 with bicarbonate < 10
(d) Convulsion and disorientation

251. Gerotas fascia is deficient at:
(a) Inferiorly (b) Medially
(c) Laterally (d) Superiorly

252. Vasa recta are formed by:
(a) Interlobular arteries
(b) Efferent arterioles

(c) Afferent arterioles
(d) Arcuate arteries

253. All are true about right renal artery, *except:*
(a) It is at higher level than the left renal artery
(b) It lies posterior to right renal vein
(c) It lies anterior to pancreas
(d) It is a branch of abdominal aorta

254. All are true about renal collecting system, *except:*
(a) Upper pole is situated more medially and posteriorly
(b) Medial aspect of kidney is more posterior
(c) There are usually three major calyces
(d) Renal pyramids fuse during development, thus forming compound papillae

255. Fluid of choice for post-obstructive diuresis:
(a) 5% dextrose (b) NS and RL
(c) NS (d) RL

256. Which parameter is decreased with BUO in post obstructive phase?
(a) FE_{Na} (b) FE_k
(c) ANP (d) Acidification

257. Drugs acting on RAAS pathway:
(a) Brimonidine (b) Cilnidipine
(c) Metoprolol (d) Quinapril
(e) Aliskiren

258. ARF may be precipitated in nephron-sparing surgery in all *except:*
(a) Solitary kidney
(b) Tumor size < 5 cm
(c) > 50% parenchymal excision
(d) Ischemia > 60 minutes

259. All the following drugs cause interstitial nephritis *except* one:
(a) Methicillin (b) NSAIDS
(c) Isoniazid (d) Rifampicin

260. Mechanism of action of cisplatin toxicity in PCT:
(a) Reactive oxygen species
(b) Lipid peroxidation
(c) Mitochondrial change
(d) Increase in SH group

261. Treatment of cisplatin toxicity, all *except:*
(a) Fluid restriction
(b) Free radical scavengers
(c) Ion chelation
(d) Glutathione depletion

262. Drug safe in renal failure:
(a) Cephalexin (b) Cloxacillin
(c) Gentamycin (d) Imipenem

263. Renal axis changed in all *except:*
(a) Renal abscess
(b) Adrenal tumor
(c) Retroperitoneal tumor
(d) Renal duplication

264. Weight of the kidney in proportion to the adult weight is:
(a) 0.4% (b) 0.5%
(c) 0.2% (d) 0.3%

265. Narrowest part of nephron:
(a) PCT (b) DCT
(c) LH (d) CD

266. Position of epididymis to testis:
(a) Posterolateral (b) Posteromedial
(c) Anterolateral (d) Anteromedial

267. Renal artery stenosis is seen in all *except:*
(a) Atherosclerosis
(b) Fibromuscular dysplasia
(c) Middle aortic syndrome
(d) All of the above

268. True about left renal vein is:
(a) Crossed anteriorly by SMA
(b) Joined by the portal vein

(c) IMV drains into left renal vein
(d) Located behind left renal artery

269. Regarding microalbuminuria – true is:
(a) Predictor of nephropathy in DM type I
(b) Irreversible
(c) Seen only in DM
(d) Detected by chemical test

270. Erythropoietin is used for:
(a) Total bone marrow aplasia
(b) Pure red cell aplasia
(c) Anemia of chronic renal disease
(d) Polycythemia

271. In ARF all are true *except:*
(a) Hypouricemia
(b) Hyponatremia
(c) Hyperkalemia
(d) Hypermagnesemia
(e) Hypocalciuria

272. In ARF due to ATN all can occur *except:*
(a) Urinary sodium >40
(b) $FE_{Na} > 1$
(c) Renal failure index > 1
(d) Urine osmolarity >500
(e) Urine : plasma creatinine ratio <20

273. ANP all are true *except:*
(a) Secreted by cardiac myocytes
(b) Causes systemic hemodynamic and renal changes
(c) Increased GFR
(d) Causes diuresis and natriuresis
(e) Reduces vascular permeability

274. FSGS all *except:*
(a) Most common cause of nephritic syndrome in children
(b) Poor response to steroids
(c) Biopsy diagnostic
(d) 50% recurrence in transplant
(e) Multifactorial

275. Indications of renal replacement in CRF all *except:*
(a) Uremic pericarditis
(b) Uremic encephalopathy
(c) Sodium < 115
(d) Uremic myopathy/neuropathy
(e) pH < 8.1

276. As in relation to ureter, uterine vessels are:
(a) Anterior (b) Posterior
(c) Medial (d) Lateral
(e) Not related

277. Secretion of potassium from collecting duct depends on all *except:*
(a) Luminal flow (b) Luminal sodium
(c) Serum potassium (d) Calcitonin level
(e) Aldosterone

278. In 38 years adult male on MHD which vaccinations are indicated:
(a) Hepatitis-A (b) Pneumococcus
(c) Typhoid (d) Varicella
(e) HPV

279. Tyson glands location:
(a) External urethral meatus
(b) Internal urethral meatus
(c) Balanopreputial sulcus
(d) Membranous urethra

280. Best investigation to measure for GFR:
(a) Inulin (b) Tc 99 DTPA
(c) Sr creatinine (d) IVP

281. Kidney size is decreased in all *except:*
(a) CGN
(b) Renal artery stenosis
(c) MCDK
(d) Hypoplasia

282. Which of the following disease commonly recurred after renal transplantation?
(a) ADPKD

(b) Alport syndrome
(c) Primary oxalosis
(d) Renal dysplasia

283. Nitric oxide precursor:
(a) Arginine
(b) Citrulline
(c) N_2O
(d) Arachidonic acid

284. Subcapsular hemorrhage with associated hypertension seen in:
(a) ASK-UPMARK kidney
(b) LUMP kidney
(c) 'S' shape kidney
(d) PAGE kidney

285. Hypothermia provides complete renal protection from arterial occlusion for:
(a) 1 hour (b) 2 hours
(c) 3 hours (d) 4 hours

286. Which segment of kidney is largest?
(a) Apical
(b) Anterior
(c) Basilar
(d) Posterior

287. The renal blood flow is:
(a) 5% of cardiac output
(b) 10% of cardiac output
(c) 20% of cardiac output
(d) 30% of cardiac output

288. What is the most common new tumor in recipients after transplantation?
(a) Renal
(b) Lung
(c) Lymphoproliferative
(d) Skin

289. Which of the following immunosuppressive agents is associated with diabetes?
(a) Mycophenolate mofetil
(b) Sirolimus
(c) Tacrolimus
(d) Azathioprine

290. String of heads appearance on angiography is seen in:
(a) Intimal fibroplasia
(b) Medial fibroplasia
(c) Perimedial fibroplasia
(d) Fibromuscular hyperplasia

291. Angiotensinogen is secreted in the:
(a) Macula densa
(b) Juxtaglomerular cells
(c) Liver
(d) Lungs

292. Blood supply of ureter in pelvis comes from:
(a) Posteriorly (b) Laterally
(c) Anteriorly (d) Posteromedially
(e) Medially

293. Renal axis is altered in all *except*:
(a) Adrenal tumor
(b) Retroperitoneal tumor
(c) Renal abscess
(d) Duplex system
(e) Horseshoe kidney

294. Artery that can be safely ligated:
(a) Inferior mesenteric artery
(b) Middle colic artery
(c) Bilateral internal iliac
(d) External iliac
(e) Superior mesenteric artery

295. Anterior relation of ureter:
(a) Inferior vesical artery
(b) Superior vesical artery
(c) Vas deferens
(d) Uterine artery
(e) Middle rectal artery

296. Calcineurin inhibitors are:
(a) Azathioprine (b) Tacrolimus
(c) Sirolimus (d) Everolimus
(e) Rapamycin

297. Uric acid secreted by:
(a) PCT
(b) DCT
(c) Cortical collecting duct
(d) Outer medullary collecting duct
(e) Inner medullary collecting duct

298. Hormone produced by kidney are all *except*:
(a) Erythropoietin
(b) Renin
(c) 1, 25-OH vitamin D
(d) Calcitriol
(e) Vasopressin

299. Dialysis indication are all *except*:
(a) pH < 7.1
(b) >10 S. creatinine
(c) Volume overload with pulmonary edema
(d) Pericarditis
(e) Hyperkalemia with ECG changes

300. First renal transplant in India was done by:
(a) AP Pandey
(b) Mohan Rao
(c) Peter Morris
(d) HS Bhatt

301. Mortality in ATN:
(a) 1%
(b) 15%
(c) 50%
(d) >15%

302. Rituximab:
(a) Monoclonal antibody to CD 20
(b) Monoclonal antibody to CD10
(c) Inhibits calcineurin and interleukin-2 production
(d) Inhibit purine synthesis

303. Indication for dialysis all *except:*
(a) Pericarditis
(b) Potassium 4.5-5.5
(c) Encephalopathy
(d) Output <200 ml/12 hours

304. Which of the following is correct regarding retroperitoneal vasculature?
(a) Right gonadal artery crosses posterior to the inferior vena cava
(b) Common iliac arteries lie anterior to the common iliac veins
(c) Left renal artery lies anterior to the renal vein
(d) Renal arteries are the first paired branches of abdominal aorta

305. In the kidneys:
(a) Renal medulla and renal pyramid are synonymous terms
(b) Apex of the pyramid is called renal sinus
(c) Columns of Bertin are extensions of medulla towards the capsule
(d) Left kidney is shorter and wider than the right kidney

306. Which of the following regarding the intra-renal vasculature is correct?
(a) The first and most constant branch is the lateral segmental branch
(b) The segmental arteries divide into arcuate arteries
(c) Afferent arteries to the glomeruli are branches of interlobular arteries
(d) The arcuate arteries are perpendicular to the edge of the corticomedullary junction

307. True about renal vasculature:
(a) Right renal vein runs anterior to IVC
(b) Right gonadal vein drain into Right renal vein
(c) Right renal artery is longer than left renal artery
(d) Left renal vein is longer than Right renal vein
(e) Left renal vein runs anterior to aorta

308. In transplant main renal artery can be anastomosed to:
(a) Deep femoral artery
(b) External iliac artery
(c) Internal iliac artery
(d) Inferior epigastric artery
(e) Common iliac artery

309. Absolute C/I for renal transplantation:

(a) Flow cytometric cross reaction B cells
(b) HIV seropositivity
(c) CDC positive of T and B cell
(d) CDC positive for B cell

310. Following drugs are not sulfonamide diuretics:

(a) Ethacrynic acid
(b) Loop diuretics
(c) Torsemide
(d) Furosemide
(e) Bumetanide

311. In unobstructed ureter DJ stenting will cause:

(a) Decrease renal pelvic pressure
(b) Atrophy of ureteric mucosa
(c) Atrophy of ureteric smooth muscle
(d) Decrease ureteric contractions
(e) Increase ureteric contraction

312. RAS true:

(a) FMO young patients
(b) Common in male
(c) Atheromatous plaque extending to origin is most common
(d) Sever in arteriosclerosis in arterioles in RAS/ischemic kidney
(e) Ischemic kidney contracted

313. MDRD includes all *except*:

(a) Age
(b) Gender
(c) Ethnicity
(d) Creatinine
(e) Mass (body weight)

314. Contrast induced nephropathy (CIN):

(a) Ventricular EF <40% is not a risk factor
(b) 25% increase in creatinine from baseline within 3 days in absence of other factors
(c) Higher contrast volume is risk factor
(d) Tubular damage + ischemia is mechanism
(e) N-acetyl cystine protects by scavenging free redical

315. Which part of the loop of Henle is critical to the formation of the interstitial concentration gradient?

(a) Thin descending loop of Henle in outer zone
(b) Thin descending loop of Henle in inner zone
(c) Thin ascending loop of Henle
(d) Thick ascending loop of Henle

316. A woman aged 40 years presented with secondary hypertension due to bilateral renal artery stenosis. The angiogram showed 'string of beads' appearance. What is the likely diagnosis and treatment?

(a) Intimal fibroplasia and stenting
(b) Medial fibroplasia and conservative treatment
(c) Perimedial fibroplasia and intervention
(d) Fibromuscular hyperplasia and intervention

ANSWERS

1.	A	31.	D	61.	TTTFT	91.	ABC	121.	E
2.	B	32.	A	62.	TFFFF	92.	ABCDE	122.	AE
3.	A	33.	C	63.	FTFTT	93.	ACD	123.	ABCDE
4.	C	34.	TTFTT	64.	TFTFT	94.	BE	124.	ABC
5.	A	35.	TFTTF	65.	TTFFT	95.	ABCE	125.	ACDE
6.	B	36.	TFFTT	66.	FTTTT	96.	ABCDE	126.	AB
7.	B	37.	TTFTT	67.	TFFTT	97.	A	127.	ACE
8.	B	38.	TFFFT	68.	FTFTT	98.	E	128.	ABE
9.	D	39.	TFTFT	69.	TTTTT	99.	BD	129.	ABDE
10.	C	40.	FFTTT	70.	TTTTT	100.	A	130.	BCE
11.	A	41.	FFFTT	71.	FFTTT	101.	D	131.	ACDE
12.	D	42.	TTTTT	72.	TTTTT	102.	BDE	132.	ABCD
13.	D	43.	FFFTF	73.	FFFTT	103.	AB	133.	CDE
14.	B	44.	TTTFF	74.	FFTFF	104.	ABE	134.	DE
15.	B	45.	TTFFF	75.	TFTTT	105.	ACE	135.	ACE
16.	A	46.	FTFTT	76.	FTTFT	106.	A	136.	A
17.	B	47.	TFTTT	77.	TFTTT	107.	D	137.	A
18.	D	48.	TTFFF	78.	TTFTT	108.	DE	138.	B
19.	B	49.	FTTTT	79.	FTTTF	109.	DE	139.	A
20.	A	50.	TFTTF	80.	FTTFT	110.	ABDE	140.	A
21.	D	51.	TTFTF	81.	TFFTT	111.	C	141.	A
22.	D	52.	FTFFT	82.	FTTTT	112.	D	142.	A
23.	D	53.	TFTFT	83.	TTFTF	113.	AB	143.	C
24.	B	54.	FFTTT	84.	TFTTT	114.	E	144.	A
25.	D	55.	TTTFT	85.	TTTFT	115.	ABD	145.	A
26.	A	56.	TTFFT	86.	TTFFT	116.	ADE	146.	A
27.	A	57.	TTTTF	87.	ABE	117.	ABCDE	147.	B
28.	B	58.	FTTTF	88.	ADE	118.	ABCD	148.	D
29.	C	59.	TTFTF	89.	ABCE	119.	E	149.	B
30.	D	60.	TFTFT	90.	BCDE	120.	CDE	150.	D

151.	A	185.	B	219.	C	253.	A	287.	C
152.	B	186.	A	220.	B	254.	B	288.	C
153.	B	187.	C	221.	C	255.	C	289.	C
154.	B	188.	D	222.	A	256.	D	290.	B
155.	C	189.	B	223.	B	257.	BCDE	291.	C
156.	C	190.	B	224.	B	258.	B	292.	B
157.	A	191.	A	225.	B	259.	C	293.	C
158.	C	192.	C	226.	A	260.	A	294.	A
159.	A	193.	A	227.	A	261.	B	295.	D
160.	A	194.	A	228.	D	262.	B	296.	B
161.	B	195.	A	229.	A	263.	A	297.	E
162.	A	196.	D	230.	C	264.	C	298.	E
163.	D	197.	B	231.	A	265.	C	299.	B
164.	D	198.	C	232.	B	266.	A	300.	B
165.	A	199.	D	233.	D	267.	D	301.	C
166.	A	200.	A	234.	C	268.	A	302.	A
167.	C	201.	A	235.	B	269.	D	303.	B
168.	A	202.	A	236.	A	270.	C	304.	C
169.	B	203.	C	237.	B	271.	A	305.	A
170.	C	204.	B	238.	B	272.	D	306.	C
171.	A	205.	D	239.	B	273.	E	307.	CDE
172.	C	206.	C	240.	A	274.	A	308.	BCE
173.	B	207.	A	241.	A	275.	E	309.	C
174.	B	208.	C	242.	A	276.	A	310.	A
175.	A	209.	B	243.	A	277.	D	311.	E
176.	C	210.	C	244.	C	278.	B	312.	CE
177.	C	211.	C	245.	C	279.	C	313.	E
178.	D	212.	B	246.	B	280.	A	314.	BCDE
179.	A	213.	C	247.	B	281.	C	315.	C
180.	D	214.	C	248.	D	282.	C	316.	D
181.	C	215.	A	249.	A	283.	A		
182.	D	216.	B	250.	D	284.	D		
183.	D	217.	B	251.	A	285.	C		
184.	B	218.	C	252.	B	286.	B		

CHAPTER 8

Upper Urinary Tract Obstruction and Trauma

1. **First person to describe endoscopic stent placement to relieve ureteral obstruction:**
   (a) Albarran (b) Watterson
   (c) Zimskind (d) Denstedt

2. **The most common genitourinary organ injured from external trauma is:**
   (a) Kidney (b) Ureter
   (c) Bladder (d) Prostate

3. **Dismembered pyeloplasty is not suitable in:**
   (a) High ureteral insertion
   (b) Dependent ureteral insertion
   (c) Accessory or aberrant lower pole vessels
   (d) Lengthy or multiple proximal ureteral strictures

4. **In retroperitoneal fibrosis, all are true *except:***
   (a) Most common in 40-60 years of age
   (b) Predominant in males
   (c) Predominant in females
   (d) Fibrotic mass generally centered at L4-L5

5. **In a patient with a pre-existing ureteropelvic junction (UPJ) obstruction, gross hematuria following trauma is usually due to:**
   (a) Coexisting renal lithiasis
   (b) Renal contusion
   (c) Laceration through the thinned renal cortex
   (d) Rupture of renal pelvis

6. **Most common cause of retroperitoneal fibrosis:**
   (a) Idiopathic (b) Drugs
   (c) Post surgical (d) Neoplastic

7. **In pelvic lipomatosis:**
   (a) Lower urinary tract symptoms are uncommon
   (b) Constipation is uncommon
   (c) Pain is common
   (d) Hypertension occurs in upto 50% of patients

8. **Which of the following studies best for diagnosis of PUJO in a 10 years old boy with creatinine of 1.5?**
   (a) NCCT kidney
   (b) DMSA renogram
   (c) Diuretic DTPA scan
   (d) Duplex ultrasonography of the kidneys

9. **Which of the following studies best predicts whether renal functional recovery will occur after reconstruction of an obstructed kidney?**
   (a) Diuretic MAG 3 scan
   (b) Diuretic DTPA scan
   (c) DMSA renogram
   (d) Duplex ultrasonography of the kidneys

10. **How much of ureteral defect can be bridged with Boari flap?**
    (a) 10-12 cm (b) 12-15 cm
    (c) 15-18 cm (d) 8-10 cm

11. **Which surgery is most commonly associated with ureteral injury?**
    (a) Hysterectomy
    (b) Colorectal surgery
    (c) Transabdominal urethropexy
    (d) Abdominal vascular surgery

12. **Which statement is not true regarding endometriosis?**
    (a) Endometriosis of the urinary tract is predominantly found in the bladder
    (b) Eighty percent of ureteral endometriosis is intrinsic and primarily involves the distal ureter
    (c) The left side is more often affected
    (d) Significant portion of patients with ureteral endometriosis do not have genitourinary symptoms

13. **Who coined the term endopyelotomy?**
    (a) Ramsay (b) Badlani
    (c) Lingeman (d) Perminger

14. **Contraindications to a percutaneous endopyelotomy includes all *except:***
    (a) >2 cm of obstruction
    (b) Active infection
    (c) Uncorrected coagulopathy
    (d) Presence of crossing vessel

15. **During endopyelotomy incision should be made in which direction to avoid injury to crossing vessel?**
    (a) Anteriorly (b) Posteriorly
    (c) Laterally (d) Medially

16. **Aberrant or accessory lower pole vessels when found in association with the UPJ obstruction, which is the best pyeloplasty option?**
    (a) Dismembered pyeloplasty
    (b) Foley YV plasty
    (c) Culp-DeWeerd Spiral Flap
    (d) Scardino-Prince Vertical Flap

17. **Which pyeloplasty was originally designed for repair of PUJO with high insertion of ureter?**
    (a) Dismembered pyeloplasty
    (b) Foley YV plasty
    (c) Culp-DeWeerd Spiral Flap
    (d) Scardino-Prince Vertical Flap

18. **Which drug is not associated with RPF?**
    (a) Methyldopa (b) Hydralazine
    (c) Blockers (d) ACE inhibitors

19. **Renal trauma with >1 cm parenchymal depth of renal cortex without collecting system rupture or urinary extravasation:**
    (a) Grade 1 (b) Grade 2
    (c) Grade 3 (d) Grade 4

20. **DM patient with Serum creatinine of 6.5 with bilateral HDN in AUR, management is:**
    (a) Catheterisation with electrolyte monitoring
    (b) Bilateral DJ stenting
    (c) Bilateral PCN
    (d) Dialysis

21. **DM patient with Serum creatinine of 2.5 with bilateral upper ureteric stone, management is:**
    (a) Bilateral DJ stenting with right uretero-lithotomy later
    (b) Right URS with left DJ stenting
    (c) Bilateral PCN with left URSL later
    (d) Right DJ stenting with left URSL later

22. **Young girl following trauma with hemodynamic stable CT reveals no contrast in left kidney:**
    (a) Observation
    (b) Explore and salvage
    (c) Nephrectomy
    (d) DTPA scan

23. **4 years girl suspected of having PUJ obstruction next best step:**
    (a) IVP
    (b) MCU
    (c) CT urography
    (d) Diuretic renography

Mention True and False respective to each statement (Q. No. 24 to 55)

24. **PUJO:**
    (a) Most common abnormality is contralateral PUJO

(b) Dismembered pyeloplasty discovered by Anderson hynes
(c) Foley VY plasty when crossing vessels are present
(d) Presence of crossing vessel decreases the success rate of endopyelotomy
(e) In doubtful cases IVU is done

25. Regarding lower genitourinary tract:
(a) Sacrospinous ligament divides greater and lesser sciatic foramen
(b) Injury to obturator nerve causes weakness of abduction of thigh
(c) Colles' fascia attaches to posterior edge of urogenital diaphragm
(d) Colles' fascia attaches to ischiopubic rami
(e) Colles' fascia is continuous with the dartos fascia of the penis and scrotum

26. UPJO:
(a) Endopyelotomy is best for antigravity, small pelvis, short segment
(b) For crossing vessel–VY plasty is best
(c) On IVP if ureter is delineated then obstruction is ruled out
(d) The Culp-DeWeerd spiral flap is generally best suited for box shape pelvis
(e) The scardino prince has vertical flap

27. Ureterocalicostomy:
(a) When the UPJ is associated with horseshoe kidney, Ureterocalicostomy may be useful to provide completely dependent drainage
(b) Parenchyma overlying the lower pole calyx must be resected rather than simply incised
(c) Indwelling nephrostomy tube should be considered
(d) The renal capsule is closed over the cut surface of the parenchyma
(e) Anastomosis should be covered with perinephric fat

28. Retrocaval ureter:
(a) M : F – 6:1
(b) Ureter with an S-shaped, fish hook, or shepherd's crook appearance is classified as type 1
(c) Supracardinal vein forms IVC
(d) IVC transection and end to end anastomosis is treatment of choice
(e) Minimal symptoms can be managed conservatively

29. Regarding genitourinary anatomy:
(a) Aorta divides at L4
(b) IMA arises at right side
(c) Horseshoe kidney ascent is blocked by SMA
(d) Middle adrenal artery arises below SMA
(e) Lumbar arteries are in 6-8 pairs

30. Endometriosis:
(a) Peak age is 16-20 years
(b) Premenopausal woman commonly affected
(c) Ureter is involved more commonly than bladder
(d) Hematuria is always present in ureteric involvement
(e) If renal function is normal and there is no hydronephrosis with no functional obstruction, hormone therapy may be prescribed

31. Ovarian vein syndrome:
(a) Pain during pregnancy
(b) Right ovarian vein drain into IVC
(c) Only involve right side
(d) Majority response to conservative therapy
(e) Some author believe it's a myth

32. Ureterocalicostomy:
(a) Kidney should be mobilized
(b) Omental wrap is done over the ureter
(c) Extensive mobilization of ureter
(d) Lower pole amputation
(e) Capsule should not be closed near the anastomosis

33. Urinary obstruction in adult:

(a) Foley V.Y. plasty is appropriate for PUJ with crossing vessels
(b) Ureterocalicostomy is a recommended as salvage procedure for failed pyeloplasty
(c) Crossing vessels does not influence success of surgery
(d) Superior and posterior puncture during percutaneous endopyelotomy prevent torque
(e) Transureteroureterostomy is contra-indicated in RPF

34. Regarding retrocaval ureter:

(a) Standard repair is pyelopyelostomy
(b) Persistent anterior cardinal vein leads to retrocaval ureter
(c) In lower pole fusion of kidney, isthmus get stucked at superior mesenteric artery
(d) Normally developed IVC results from persistence of the right subcardinal vein suprarenally and the right supracardinal infrarenally
(e) Asymptomatic retrocaval ureter doesn't require any treatment

35. 28 years old male with serum creatinine > 3.0 mg/ml with recurrent nephrolithiasis and 5 cm lower ureteric stricture with small capacity bladder, treatment is:

(a) Ureterocalicostomy with excision of structure
(b) Boari flap
(c) Ileal ureter
(d) Transureteroureterostomy
(e) Auto transplant

36. Retrocaval ureter:

(a) Supracardinal vein persisted as IVC
(b) Diuretic renography is used to confirm the presence of obstruction
(c) Ureterolysis is treatment of choice
(d) Most of them are observed during childhood
(e) Exclusively on right side

37. Retrocaval ureter:

(a) Posterior cardinal vein is responsible for anomaly
(b) IVC resection and end to end anastomosis is treatment of choice
(c) Asymptomatic patient with retrocaval ureter should also be treated
(d) Type I is S shaped
(e) Point of maximal obstruction in type I is lateral to the lateral margin of the IVC

38. RPF:

(a) Male to female ratio is 5 : 1
(b) Age 40–60 years
(c) Extends from renal hilum to bifurcation of great vessels
(d) 70% of the cases, the disease is idiopathic
(e) Medial deviations at L_3–L_4

39. Ovarian vein syndrome:

(a) Pain during pregnancy
(b) Described only on right side
(c) Some author has convincing evidence–that it is a myth
(d) Treatment is ureterolysis and ovarian vein resection
(e) Mostly treated by conservative measures

40. Regarding endometriosis:

(a) Ureteric involvement is more common than bladder
(b) Most common in premenopausal
(c) 80% of ureteric involvement is intrinsic
(d) Involvement of ureter always causes hematuria
(e) Patients with ureteral endometriosis can have asymptomatic obstruction of the kidney with a loss of renal function

41. Steps of ureterocalicostomy:

(a) Kidney should be mobilised down
(b) Avoid extensive mobilisation of ureter
(c) Closure of renal parenchyma around ureter
(d) Lower pole amputation
(e) Omental wrap of ureter

42. Unilateral ureteric obstruction:
(a) First phase < ↑ renal blood flow (RBF) ↑ ureteral pressure (UP)
(b) 2nd phase < ↓ RBF ↑ UP
(c) 3rd phase < ↓ RBF
(d) First phase 12 hours
(e) Last phase by arteriolar constriction

43. Bilateral ureteric obstruction:
(a) It is triphasic
(b) Post obstructive diuresis is well marked
(c) Post obstruction ↑FE_{Na}, ↑FE_K
(d) Concentrating ability after relief of obstruction remains intact
(e) Blood flow from inner to outer cortex

44. Whitaker test:
(a) < 15 suggestive of obstruction
(b) It is an invasive test
(c) Bladder drainage is must
(d) 10 ml/min is fill rate
(e) Sensitivity and specificity of only 79% and 50%

45. Gun shot injury with hematoma:
(a) Blunt injury with gross hematuria warrants exploration
(b) CT is more useful than USG
(c) Renal artery avulsion can be diagnosed on CT and is an indication for nephrectomy
(d) Penetrating injury usually managed non-operatively
(e) All patients with blunt trauma and gross hematuria should undergo imaging by CT scan

46. 20 years old male with HDN and dull aching pain:
(a) IVU–Investigation of choice
(b) If in an IVP, ureter is visualised it rules out PUJO
(c) If on RGP, narrowing at PUJ and dilation above → makes diagnosis of PUJO
(d) Provocative IVP → 0.3 – 0.5 mg/kg furosemide used
(e) DTPA scan is must in all cases

47. Unilateral ureteric obstruction:
(a) 1st phase last more than 2 hours
(b) 1st phase characterize by arteriolar constriction
(c) In 3rd phase RBF and ureteral pressure decreased
(d) In 1st phase RBF and ureteral pressure increased
(e) In 2nd phase RBF decreased and ureteral pressure increased

48. Bilateral ureteric obstruction:
(a) Triphasic
(b) After release decrease K^+ excretion
(c) Na^+ overload
(d) Does not cause diuresis
(e) In first phase there is modest dilatation of RBF as compare to UUO

49. Endometriosis:
(a) Prevalent in premenopausal women
(b) Extrinsic > intrinsic
(c) Upper urinary tract should be imaged in all patients with endometriosis
(d) Ureter involvement > bladder involvement
(e) Cyclical hematuria always in ureteral involvement

50. Retrocaval ureter:
(a) Normally developed IVC results from persistence of the right supracardinal vein suprarenally and the right subcardinal infrarenally
(b) Type I crosses at the level of the L3
(c) Male to female = 6 : 1
(d) IVC transection and reanastomosis is treatment of choice
(e) In asymptomatic patient with minimal caliectasis observation is best

51. Regarding pyeloplasty:
(a) Laparoscopic fenger pyeloplasty is recommended for large intrarenal pelvis with PUJ obstruction
(b) Foley V-Y pyeloplasty is for large PUJ with aberrant vessels
(c) Last to be removed in pyeloplasty is drain
(d) If after removal of stent fever occurs–urgent PCN should be done
(e) Continuous suture is not preferable as it causes ureteric ischemia and stenosis

52. Regarding technical point of ureterocalicostomy:
(a) Lower pole amputation
(b) Omental wrapping
(c) Proximal ureter is spatulated medially
(d) Suturing of kidney parenchyma around the ureter
(e) Mobilisation of kidney

53. Radionuclide renography:
(a) DTPA is solely excreted by GFR
(b) Excretion rate of DTPA is 50%
(c) Renal plasma flow can be calculated by MAG3
(d) MAG is solely secreted by tubular secretion
(e) MAG3 is more useful in patients with renal insufficiency, but DTPA is more economical

54. Regarding idiopathic RPF:
(a) More common in males
(b) Extends lateral to psoas
(c) From renal hilum to bifurcation of aorta
(d) Medial deviation at $L_{3,4}$
(e) Common in 4th to 6th decades

55. About retrocaval ureter:
(a) IVC formed by supracardinal vein
(b) Male : female = 6 : 1
(c) Type II is more common
(d) Surgery is always required
(e) Treatment of choice–division of IVC and reanastomoses

Which of the following statement is correct?

56. Biofilm true is:
(a) Shield bacteria from environmental challenges
(b) Biofilm EPS, is also referred to as slime
(c) Increase protection include the slower growth rate of the bacteria with associated physiologic changes
(d) Biofilms may form on living or non-living surfaces
(e) Protects the bacteria from neutrophils

57. PUJ obstruction:
(a) F-15 DTPA (b) F+20 DTPA
(c) MAG 3 (d) DMSA
(e) None of the above

58. PUJ obstruction:
(a) Not associated with VUR
(b) Foley's V-Y plasty–done in high ureter insertion
(c) On USG can differentiate between MCDK and PUJO
(d) In PUJO kidneys with <15% differential function–nonsalvageable in adults
(e) Endopyelotomy–success rate >90% if not crossing vessel

59. PUV true:
(a) "Keyhole" sign of a dilated bladder above a dilated prostatic urethra
(b) Type I most common
(c) Type III valves have a worse prognosis
(d) Pulmonary hypoplasia is the most common cause of mortality
(e) Immediate catheterization

60. Retrocaval ureter:
(a) Present in the sixth decade of life
(b) Left-sided circumcaval ureter has been reported
(c) Type I crosses at the level of the L3 and type II crosses at the level of UPJ

(d) Definitive diagnosis can be made noninvasively using 3DCT imaging
(e) A spatulated ureteroureterostomy is performed only if patient is symptomatic

61. Hemorrhagic kidney:
(a) Perirenal hematoma in etiology
(b) Decreased renal perfusion on angiogram
(c) Excess secretion of renin
(d) Kidney usually maintains reniform shape
(e) Hypertension is a common finding

62. Serum alkaline phosphatase raised in all *except*:
(a) Primary hypothyroidism
(b) Primary hyperparathyroidism
(c) Bony metastasis
(d) Liver metastasis
(e) Cholestasis

63. Gillenwater study on dog w.r.t. release of UUO:
(a) 100% recovery of GFR after 7 days of UUO
(b) 70% recovery of GFR after 14 days of UUO
(c) 50% recovery of GFR after 14 days of UUO
(d) 30% recovery of GFR after 4 days of UUO
(e) Complete renal loss after 6 weeks

64. Idiopathic RPF diagnosis is helpful by following:
(a) Hypertension
(b) Hematuria
(c) Backache
(d) Increased serum creatinine
(e) Feeling of inability to empty bladder completely

65. Anomalies associated with PUJ obstruction:
(a) Contralateral PUJO (b) MSK
(c) MCDK (d) ADPKD
(e) Ectopic ureter

66. In a patient with shock, minimal parameters accessed are:
(a) Pulse oxymetry (b) ECG
(c) CVP (d) BP monitoring
(e) Urine output

67. Management of patient with S. creatinine 4.2 mg/dl and suspected PUJO:
(a) IVU
(b) MR urography
(c) NCCT
(d) DTPA
(e) PCN and if fall in creatinine, confirm with DTPA scan

68. Ca-cervix stage IIA – SCC treatment options:
(a) Radical hysterectomy
(b) Radiation
(c) Radiation + chemotherapy
(d) Pelvic exenteration
(e) Observation

69. Precursors for hepatic gluconeogenesis during starvation:
(a) Glycerol fatty acids (b) Amino acids
(c) Lactate (d) Citrate
(e) Maltose

70. Zinc is a co-factor in:
(a) Glutamate dehydrogenase
(b) Glutathione peroxidase
(c) Alkaline phosphatase
(d) Carbonic anhydrase
(e) Superoxide dismutase

71. Acid phosphatase is secreted by:
(a) RBC
(b) WBC
(c) Prostatic acinar cells
(d) Reticuloendothelial cells
(e) Osteoclast

72. Which of the following is reduced in DIC?
(a) Platelets (b) Fibrinogen
(c) FDP (d) Prothrombin index
(e) Capillary fragility

73. Creatinine is produced:
(a) Muscle (b) Heart
(c) Kidney (d) Liver
(e) Lung

74. Renal physiology all are true *except*:
(a) Only sympathetic control
(b) Renal blood supply 600 ml/min
(c) O_2 supply/blood supply per gram tissue mass more than brain
(d) Directly measure by RAH
(e) Cortex less blood than medulla

75. HASTE in ureteric obstruction:
(a) MR urography (b) DTPA
(c) CECT (d) Doppler USG
(e) X-ray KUB

76. In Page kidney seen:
(a) Unilateral hypersecretion of renin
(b) Hypertension
(c) Seen with blunt trauma abdomen
(d) Perirenal hematoma is common etiology
(e) RVT is usually seen

77. Earliest manifestation of septicemia:
(a) Respiratory alkalosis
(b) Respiratory acidosis
(c) Metabolic alkalosis
(d) Metabolic acidosis
(e) Hypoventilation

78. RPF which is not characteristic?
(a) Anteriorly deviated aorta
(b) Medially deviated ureter
(c) Hydronephrosis
(d) Poor/reduced renal function
(e) Plaques extending from aortic bifurcation into renal hilum

79. Ureteric injury:
(a) Most common cause is gynecological surgery
(b) Simple hysterectomy > radical hysterectomy
(c) If diagnosed after 3 weeks PCN followed by delayed repair
(d) Ligation of ureter should be treated with removal of ligature if detected immediately
(e) Minor ureteral perforation can be treated with ureteral stenting

80. Preferred calyx for endopyelotomy:
(a) Superior–posterior
(b) Middle–posterior
(c) Inferior–posterior
(d) Middle–anterior
(e) Inferior–anterior

81. Post-radiotherapy ureteric stricture:
(a) Within 5 months of treatment
(b) If not symptomatic in 1 year no follow-up is required
(c) Majority of cases is asymptomatic – causes silent CRF
(d) Prior pelvic surgery increases risk
(e) Stricture length varies with dose

82. Retroperitoneal fibrosis:
(a) Pain present in only 5%
(b) CT to confirm the diagnosis
(c) Medial deviation of ureter
(d) Tamoxifen is contraindicated
(e) Ormond in 1928 described RPF

83. In unilateral acute ureteral obstruction initially:
(a) Increased renal blood flow and increased pressure
(b) Normal blood flow and increased pressure
(c) Decreased blood flow and increased pressure
(d) Decreased blood flow and decreased pressure
(e) Increased blood flow and decreased pressure

84. Blunt renal trauma:
(a) CECT scan is the single most important investigation
(b) Hematuria proportionate to renal injury
(c) Previous anomalies make kidney liable to injury
(d) Exploration is done in all cases
(e) Late complication can be hypertension

85. Most preferred route for endopyelotomy:
(a) Upper pole posterior
(b) Middle pole posterior
(c) Lower pole anterior
(d) Renal pelvis
(e) Lower pole posterior

86. Which nerve is affected in psoas hitch?
(a) Genitofemoral nerve (b) Sciatic nerve
(c) Femoral nerve (d) Obturator nerve

87. Blunt trauma abdomen in a twelve years old female is hemodynamically stable, CECT-RK-normal, LK–no perfusion no function after 1 hour, renal function is normal next step:
(a) Observation (b) Heparin
(c) Angio stenting (d) Surgery

88. Grade III renal trauma on CT, vitals are stable with one episode of hematuria:
(a) Immediate exploration and repair
(b) Embolization
(c) Observation and surgery when needed
(d) Cystoscopy with DJ stenting

89. Retroperitoneal fibrosis:
(a) Most commonly in 6th decade
(b) Ureter deviated medially at L3-L4
(c) Most common malignancy involved is lymphoma
(d) Male to female ratio is 6:1

90. Both extrinsic and intrinsic obstruction of ureter seen in:
(a) Endometriosis
(b) Pelvic lipomatosis
(c) Retrocaval ureter
(d) Testicular vein thrombophlebitis

91. Not a drug for RPF:
(a) Amphetamines (b) Phenacetine
(c) Phenytoin (d) Hydralazine

92. Female patient with retroperitoneal mass encasing ureter and great vessels with bilateral HDN. Pelvic examination and local examination is normal:
(a) Idiopathic RPF
(b) Pelvic malignancy
(c) Retrocaval ureter
(d) Ovarian vein thrombophlebitis

93. Five cm post-surgery ureteric stricture. History of recurrent nephrolithiasis with hypertension, 65% renal function on DTPA, Serum creatinine 2.5 mg%, bladder capacity <300 ml. Treatment option is:
(a) Transureteroureterostomy
(b) Ileal transplant
(c) Autotransplant
(d) Nephrectomy

94. Stab injury in mid ureteric transection, repair is by:
(a) Transureteroureterostomy
(b) Ureteroureterostomy
(c) Boari flap
(d) Psoas hitch

95. Earliest grade which reflux upto PUJ?
(a) II (b) III
(c) IV (d) V

96. Investigation of choice in renal trauma:
(a) USG (b) IVP
(c) CT scan (d) X-Ray KUB

97. Most common type of renal injury is:
(a) Renal parenchymal (b) Renal pelvis
(c) Renal vein (d) Renal artery

98. The model in which renal subcapsular hematoma produces renin induced hypertension is called:
(a) Page kidney
(b) Ask Upmark kidney
(c) Bosniak's 3 cysts
(d) Goldblatt kidney

99. The landmark used during emergency exploration of a patient with suspected left renal trauma and retroperitoneal hematoma:

(a) Left ureter
(b) Interior mesenteric vein
(c) Splenorenal ligament
(d) Tail of pancreas

100. Retroperitoneal fibrosis is idiopathic in:

(a) 30% (b) 50%
(c) 70% (d) 90%

101. Which of the following procedure has highest failure rate in the treatment of UPJ obstruction?

(a) Ballon dilatation
(b) Antegrade incision of UPJ
(c) Retrograde laser ureterotomy
(d) Retrograde ureteroscopic incision of UPJ

102. True about retrocaval ureter:

(a) It is due to persistence of anterior cardinal vein in the retroperitoneum
(b) "S" shape deformity on retrograde pyelography is diagnostic
(c) Definitive diagnosis can be made by IVU
(d) Surgery is not indicated in all the cases

103. True about JJ stents:

(a) Increases ureter peristalsis
(b) Decreases the intrarenal pressure
(c) Increases the intrarenal pressure
(d) It provides better drainage than nephrostomy

104. Not an absolute indication of renal exploration after trauma:

(a) Hemodynamic instability with shock
(b) Expanding, pulsatile renal hematoma
(c) Suspected renal pedicle avulsion
(d) Non viable tissue

105. Grade of injury when ureter transection is <50% following trauma:

(a) Grade 1 (b) Grade 2
(c) Grade 3 (d) Grade 4

106. The most important complication of long standing pelvic lipomatosis is:

(a) Cystitis glandularis
(b) Carcinoma in situ
(c) Adenocarcinoma
(d) Squamous cell carcinoma

107. Which of the following protein is known to mediate the inflammatory response in retroperitoneal fibrosis?

(a) Ceroid (b) Calcineurin
(c) Calcitonin (d) Retinoid

108. Retroperitoneal fibrosis caused by all *except*:

(a) Methysergide (b) β-blockers
(c) Phenacetin (d) Tamoxifen

109. Most common site of endometriosis in genitourinary tract:

(a) Bladder (b) Kidney
(c) Ureter (d) Prostate

110. Which one of the following is not a contraindication for dismembered pyeloplasty?

(a) High insertion ureter
(b) Small inaccessible intrarenal pelvis
(c) Multiple proximal ureteric stricture
(d) Long proximal ureteric stricture

111. All of the following is relative contraindication for transureteroureterostomy *except*:

(a) Chronic pyelonephritis
(b) Urothelial malignancy
(c) Nephrolithiasis
(d) Insufficient length of donor ureter

112. Indication of urgent nephrostomy:

(a) Anuria with calculus in solitary kidney
(b) Febrile patient with hydronephrosis
(c) Pregnant lady with recurrent colic
(d) Palpable kidney with PUJ obstruction in children

113. Drugs causing retroperitoneal fibrosis all *except:*
(a) Phenoxybenzamine (b) Amphetamine
(c) Methyldopa (d) Methysergide

114. Tear drop bladder is found in all of the following *except:*
(a) Pelvic lipomatosis
(b) Perivesical hematoma
(c) Iliopsoas hypertrophy
(d) Intraperitoneal rupture of bladder

115. Retrocaval ureter occur as a result of defect in the formation of:
(a) Ureter
(b) IVC
(c) SVC
(d) Both ureter and IVC

116. Contraindication for transureteroureterostomy is:
(a) Large soft tissue loss
(b) Urolithiasis
(c) GUTB
(d) Obstructed megaureter

117. Which is not an indication of contrast study in blunt renal trauma?
(a) Gross hematuria
(b) Microscopic hematuria
(c) Hypotension
(d) Associated organ injury

118. Exploration in blunt renal trauma, absolute indication:
(a) Persistent hemodynamic instability
(b) Urinary extravasation
(c) Gross hematuria
(d) Abdominal distention

119. Procedure done in hydronephrosis:
(a) Anderson-Hyne's pyeloplasty
(b) Hyne's Mikculiz pyeloplasty
(c) Colonoplasty
(d) Gastroplasty

120. True about UPJ is all *except:*
(a) VUR associated with UPJO in 7-18%
(b) UPJO associated with VUR in 0.7-3.2%
(c) On MCU-contrast not filling the pelvis with dilated ureter suggestive of UPJO
(d) Contrast not draining from pelvis but rapid emptying of ureter on postvoid film of MCU suggestive of UPJO
(e) UPJO and VUR should not be treated simultaneously

121. Ureterocystoplasty all are true *except:*
(a) Is a type of augmentation cystoplasty
(b) Unilateral severe HDUN can be considered for ureterocystoplasty
(c) Preservation of ureteral sheath is of no importance
(d) Ureter opened longitudinally throughout its length
(e) Bladder is opened in sagittal plane

122. A 7 years old child with stenosis at PUJ undergone open pyeloplasty. After 1 year he developed stricture at the same site. Now he is best managed by:
(a) Endopyelotomy
(b) Laparoscopic pyeloplasty
(c) Open pyeloplasty
(d) Nephrectomy

123. One cm bulbar urethral stricture after trauma best managed by:
(a) Anastomotic urethroplasty
(b) VIU
(c) Laser incision of the stricture
(d) Gradual dilatation

124. Most common cause of surgical ureteric injury:
(a) Open abdominal hysterectomy
(b) Laparoscopic hysterectomy
(c) LSCS
(d) Vaginal hysterectomy

125. In retroperitoneal fibrosis the best diagnostic information is currently given by:
(a) MRI
(b) Gallium scintigraphy
(c) IVP and cavography
(d) Computer tomography

126. Imaging of choice in suspected renal injury is:
(a) MR urography
(b) Isotope renogram
(c) Contrast enhanced CT
(d) Intravenous urography

127. All of the following cause distinct narrowing in ureteric course *except*:
(a) Ureteropelvic junction
(b) At the iliac vessel crossing
(c) At the gonadal vessel crossing
(d) Ureterovesical junction

128. Which nerve is most likely to be injured during the psoas hitch procedure?
(a) Femoral nerve
(b) Obturator nerve
(c) Iliohypogastric nerve
(d) Genitofemoral nerve

129. Blunt trauma abdomen lady after hemodynamic stability investigation of choice:
(a) Contrast enhanced CT
(b) High contrast IVP
(c) Ultrasonography
(d) Doppler USG
(e) MRI

130. Retrocaval ureter true is:
(a) For treatment resection and uretero-ureteric anastomosis done
(b) Due to persistence of supracardinal vein
(c) Present in 3-4th decade
(d) Always on right even on bilateral IVC
(e) IVP fish hook deformity at obstructive level

131. Second week after bilateral ureteric obstruction all are true *except*:
(a) Tubular function improved
(b) Both glomerular and tubular function not improved
(c) Tubular acidification and concentration defect may persist
(d) GFR may be improving after 10 weeks
(e) FR function improved

132. About pelvic lipomatosis true is:
(a) Steroid treatment is highly successful
(b) Does not cause progressive azotemia
(c) High riding prostate can be seen
(d) Excision of mass is commonly performed procedure
(e) Classic pear shaped bladder with surrounding translucency seen on IVU

133. Ovarian vein syndrome true is:
(a) Periureteric phlegmon with periarthritis is etiology
(b) Antibiotic treatment results in resolution of ureteric obstruction
(c) Most common in pubertal females
(d) Only seen at right side
(e) A well documented postpartum condition

134. Renal resistive index true is:
(a) PSV-EDV/PSV
(b) PSV-EDV
(c) RI>0.7 associated with increased intrarenal resistance and ureteral obstruction
(d) Abnormal never occurs in unobstructed kidney
(e) EDV-PSV

135. How do you approach to the renal pelvis in open pyelolithotomy?
(a) Anterior
(b) Posterior
(c) Lateral
(d) Medial

136. Which of the following is mandatory following pyeloplasty?
(a) Stenting
(b) Nephrostomy
(c) External drain
(d) Nephropexy

ANSWERS

1.	C	29.	TFFFF	57.	AB	85.	B	113.	A
2.	A	30.	TTFFT	58.	BCD	86.	A	114.	D
3.	D	31.	FTFTT	59.	ABCDE	87.	A	115.	B
4.	C	32.	TTFTT	60.	BCDE	88.	C	116.	B
5.	B	33.	FTFTT	61.	ABDE	89.	D	117.	B
6.	A	34.	TFFTT	62.	B	90.	A	118.	A
7.	C	35.	FTFFF	63.	ABDE	91.	C	119.	A
8.	C	36.	TTFFF	64.	ACD	92.	A	120.	D
9.	C	37.	TFFTT	65.	AC	93.	C	121.	C
10.	B	38.	FTTTT	66.	ABCDE	94.	B	122.	B
11.	A	39.	FFTTT	67.	E	95.	B	123.	A
12.	B	40.	FTFFT	68.	BC	96.	C	124.	A
13.	B	41.	TTFTT	69.	ABC	97.	A	125.	D
14.	D	42.	TTTFT	70.	ABDE	98.	A	126.	C
15.	C	43.	FTTFT	71.	ACDE	99.	B	127.	C
16.	A	44.	FTTTT	72.	AB	100.	C	128.	D
17.	B	45.	FTTFT	73.	A	101.	A	129.	A
18.	D	46.	TFTTF	74.	BCE	102.	D	130.	ACE
19.	C	47.	FFTTT	75.	A	103.	C	131.	BD
20.	A	48.	FTTFF	76.	ABCD	104.	D	132.	CE
21.	C	49.	TTFFF	77.	A	105.	B	133.	ABE
22.	A	50.	FTFFT	78.	A	106.	A	134.	AC
23.	D	51.	FFTTT	79.	ACDE	107.	A	135.	B
24.	TTFTT	52.	TTFTT	80.	B	108.	D	136.	A
25.	TFTTT	53.	TFTTT	81.	CDE	109.	A		
26.	FFFFT	54.	TFFFT	82.	BC	110.	A		
27.	TTTTT	55.	FFFFF	83.	A	111.	D		
28.	FTTFT	56.	ABCDE	84.	ACE	112.	A		

CHAPTER 9

Urinary Urolithiasis and Endourology

1. **Most common complication of PCNL:**
   (a) Hemorrhage (b) Infection
   (c) Hemothorax (d) Pneumothorax

2. **Most important pathogenetic factor for uric acid stone formation is:**
   (a) Low urine pH (b) Low urine volume
   (c) Hyperuricosuria (d) Hypercalciuria

3. **Most common organism associated with infection stones:**
   (a) E coli (b) Pseudomonas
   (c) Proteus (d) Staphylococcus

4. **Risk of recurrence for first stone formers within the subsequent 10 years is:**
   (a) 10% (b) 30%
   (c) 50% (d) 75%

Mention True and False respective to each statement (Q. No. 5 to 36)

5. **Cystinuria:**
   (a) Autosomal dominant
   (b) Heterozygous form stones
   (c) Stone formation most common in young patients
   (d) pH of urine should be raised to 6.5 to 7.0
   (e) More resistant than calcium oxalate monohydrate for ESWL

6. **Lower ureteric stone 1cm size:**
   (a) Laser probe should be away from stone
   (b) Lithoclast used only with NS
   (c) Stone fragmentation and simultaneous fragment removals possible with laser
   (d) EHL—risk of ureteral perforation is maximum
   (e) Hol:YAG is best

7. **Regarding PCNL:**
   (a) Large stones may need for sandwich therapy
   (b) Pneumatic lithotripsy used for RIRS
   (c) Bleeding more common in superior calyceal puncture
   (d) Supracostal puncture should be in deep inspiration
   (e) Air in a posterior calyx filled with contrast agent has been described as "Mickey mouse ears"

8. **PCNL for staghorn:**
   (a) Bacteremia can be cause of hypotension
   (b) Bacteremia may be present in post-operatively even if pre-op culture is sterile
   (c) Secondary hemorrhage is usual cause of bleeding after 10 days
   (d) Untreated struvite staghorn calculi eventually destroy the kidney and pose a significant risk to the patient's life
   (e) Stone burden is the single most important factor in determining the appropriate treatment modality for a patient with renal calculi

9. **Regarding PTH:**
   (a) Primary hyperparathyroidism is the cause of nephrolithiasis in about 5% of cases
   (b) Stimulate osteoclast for demineralization of bone
   (c) Increase phosphate absorption in kidney
   (d) Increase calcium absorption in intestine
   (e) Periods of hypocalcemia, PTH synthesis and secretion are increased

10. **Vitamin D:**
   (a) 25-OH formed in liver
   (b) Calcitriol synthesis can occur in macrophages in granulomatous conditions
   (c) The major source of vitamin D–is dermal synthesis of the precursor compound cholecalciferol
   (d) Second hydroxylation occurs within the tubular cell
   (e) D3 supplemented in renal failure

11. **Sudden right flank pain in 20 years old:**
   (a) Ureteral stone can be the diagnosis
   (b) If hematuria present, can suggest RCC
   (c) Rupture of AML is most common
   (d) IVU is investigation of choice
   (e) USG is the best initial investigation

12. **Regarding uric acid renal stone:**
   (a) Easily detected by CT scan
   (b) Stone of 3 cm PCNL is treatment of choice
   (c) Stone 1 cm in pelvis–ESWL
   (d) Metabolic work up not necessary
   (e) Hyperuricosuria is defined by urinary uric acid exceeding 600 mg/day

13. **Regarding Ca^{++} metabolism:**
   (a) PTH increases Ca^{++} absorption at PCT
   (b) Vitamin D_3 increases Ca^{++} absorption at PCT
   (c) PTH stimulates calcitriol production by increasing 1α-hydroxylase levels
   (d) 1α-hydroxylase is found in tubular cells
   (e) Most calcium reabsorption occurs in the late S2 segment and early S3 segment of the PCT

14. **Citrate in urolithiasis:**
   (a) Pure hypocitraturia makes 10% of nephrolithiasis
   (b) Hypocitraturia is most correctable cause of calcium oxalate stones
   (c) Citrates promotes spontaneous nucleation of calcium stones
   (d) Promotes inhibitory effect of Tamm-Horsfall glycoprotein
   (e) Profound hypocitraturia, perhaps the most important factor in stone formation in RTA

15. **PCNL for stone disease:**
   (a) If on puncture dirty urine aspirated procedure is abandoned and only PCN placed
   (b) Supracostal approach is done in deep inspiration
   (c) Anterior calyces are more laterally located and posterior calyces are more medially located
   (d) The depth of needle penetration is monitored by keeping the C-arm in vertical position
   (e) Needle puncture directly into the fornix of a calyx is the safest route of percutaneous entry

16. **Ureteroscopy:**
   (a) Impacted stone in upper part of ureter is recovered by dormia basket
   (b) 6 mm ureteric perforation at the level of stone warrants ureterolithotomy
   (c) DJ stent should be routinely used to prevent ureteric orifice stenosis
   (d) Laser causes lesser chances of migration of stone
   (e) Use of UASs during flexible ureteroscopy shortens operating times, reduces renal pelvic pressures, and can limit endoscope damage

17. **RTA:**
   (a) Distal RTA–hyperkalemia
   (b) Uric acid stone are most commonly seen in RTA 1
   (c) The hallmark is a hyperchloremic metabolic acidosis with a high urinary pH (>5.5) in the presence of persistently low serum HCO_3
   (d) Type 1 (distal) is of particular significance to urologists
   (e) Type 4 RTA is associated with chronic renal damage, usually seen in patients with interstitial renal disease and diabetic nephropathy

18. Regarding renal stone:
(a) Hydroxy apatite → RTA 1
(b) Hydroxy apatite → Hyperparathyroidism
(c) Metabolic evaluation deferred by 6 months of surgery
(d) PTH must be determined in recurrent stone formers
(e) Primary hyperoxaluria is due to increased GI absorption

19. Calcium metabolism:
(a) PTH acts on PCT
(b) Ca^{2+} absorption in thick ascending LOH is dependent on PTH
(c) About 15% of the filtered calcium is reabsorbed in the TALH
(d) Calcium reabsorption is regulated in DCT region by the actions of PTH
(e) The DCT accounts for 10% to 15% of Ca^{++} reabsorption

20. Regarding PCNL:
(a) Bulls eye sign when needle hub is aligned with shaft in the direction of 'X-ray'
(b) To assess the needle depth C arm is rotated to 30°
(c) Puncture is made in deep inspiration
(d) Ideal puncture should pass through fornix
(e) Most common complication is pelvic perforation

21. Staghorn calculus–post PCNL–hypotension and clear urine:
(a) Send blood for culture
(b) IV fluids and vasopressin
(c) Champ nephrostomy and angioembolisation
(d) Upgrade to higher antibiotics
(e) More than 6% patient require transfusion following bleeding following PCNL

22. Patient undergoing PCNL for struvite stone:
(a) Sterile urine can be seen with bacteremia
(b) NCCT–100% sensitive for residual fragments
(c) Superior calyceal puncture–more chances of bleeding
(d) Ureteric catheterization is first step
(e) Anterior calyceal puncture causes less bleeding

23. Regarding nephrolithiasis:
(a) Citrate binds with Ca^{+2}
(b) Urate stones occurs in alkaline urine
(c) Hol: YAG should not be used in cystine stone
(d) Distal RTA – Hyperkalemia, hypochloremia with metabolic acidosis
(e) Crystals precipitated in an alkaline urine are calcium phosphate and triple-phosphate

24. Regarding extracorporeal lithotripsy:
(a) EHL is associated with maximum chances of subcapsular hematoma
(b) EHL is better than electromagnetic with regard to power
(c) If F_1 is larger it is associated with lesser pain
(d) F_1 should be at stone
(e) Piezoelectric has insufficient power to break stone effectively

25. Urolithiasis:
(a) Morbidly obese with small stone burden, retrograde ureteroscopy with lithotripsy should be done
(b) 1 cm upper ureteric calculus–flexible URS is an option
(c) 1.7 cm lower calyceal stone–flexible URS is an option
(d) 1.7 cm lower calyceal stone–PCNL is treatment of choice
(e) Calyceal diverticulum stone–ESWL treatment of choice

26. Regarding intracorporeal lithotripsy:
(a) Laser fiber should be placed away from urothelium
(b) EHL probe should be on the stone
(c) NS only to be used in EHL
(d) Ballistic is safest with lowest perforation
(e) Calcium oxalate monohydrate is hardest to break

27. Urolithiasis and ESWL:
(a) Upper ureteric 1 cm stone ESWL treatment of choice
(b) Urine culture should be sterile
(c) 2 cm inferior calyceal stone ESWL should be used
(d) Piezoelectric lithotripter produces plane shockwaves with directly converging shock fronts
(e) 1.5 cm UPJ stone with grossly hydronephrosis → ESWL is an option

28. Intracorporeal lithotripsy:
(a) EHL has narrow safety margin
(b) Ultrasonic lithotripsy is the efficient combination of stone fragmentation and simultaneous fragment removal
(c) Pneumatic and ultrasonic can combine in single instrument
(d) Ultrasonic used for soft infected staghorn stone
(e) KTP laser is best laser for intracorporeal lithotripsy

29. True about anatomy of PCN:
(a) Right kidney posteriorly covered by diaphragm
(b) Puncture best done in deep inspiration
(c) Bleeding is more in superior than inferior calyceal puncture
(d) Lung injury increases if puncture is at 10th intercostal space
(e) Puncture is done with C-arm rotated in 30 degree axis

30. Regarding lithotripsy:
(a) EHL probe is placed over stone
(b) Holmium laser to fragment all stones regardless of composition
(c) Only NS used with lithoclast
(d) Stone migration maximum with pneumatic
(e) Perforation maximum with pneumatic

31. Post PCNL presenting with hypotension and clear urine:
(a) Clamp nephrostomy immediate angio-embolization
(b) Higher antibiotics
(c) Vasopressor and fluid therapy
(d) Blood culture and blood to be arranged
(e) Explore the patient

32. Hypocitraturia:
(a) Isolated defect in 1% of calcium renal stones
(b) Promotes inhibitory effect of Tamm-Horsfall protein
(c) Promotes Ca^{2+} nucleation
(d) Women tend to have higher urinary citrate measurements than men
(e) In RTA most important metabolic defect is hypocitraturia

33. After PCN:
(a) Hypotension without significant blood loss can be due to bacteremia
(b) Bacteremia can occur with sterile urine culture
(c) Massive hematuria after 10 days–secondary hemorrhage
(d) Upper post calyceal puncture most often associated with bleeding
(e) Upper calyceal puncture done during deep expiration

34. Which statement is not true?
(a) Stent placed routinely after ureteroscopy to prevent ureteric orifice stenosis
(b) In large impacted stone it's safe to use dormia basket under fluoroscopy
(c) EHL is the most effective intracorporeal lithotripsy
(d) If 6 mm ureteric perforation occurs at the level of stone during ureteroscopy, conversion to open should be considered
(e) Vision in flexible is better than rigid

35. Regarding intracorporeal lithotripsy:
(a) EHL is the most powerful source of energy
(b) During lithotripsy ureteric probe should be in contact with stone

(c) Laser probe should be 0.5 mm away from stone
(d) Up migration of stone is less by laser
(e) Laser is better than ultrasonic for hard stone

36. Regarding intracorporeal lithotripsy:
(a) For soft, diverticular stone ultrasonic is better
(b) Perforation of upper ureter is more common than lower ureter stone
(c) Flexible ureteroscopy is used for mid ureteral stone
(d) For upmigrated stone flexible ureteroscopy is best
(e) KTP absorbed by H_2O and not by Hb

Which of the following statement is correct?

37. Secondary cause of RTA:
(a) Hyperparathyroidism
(b) Obstructive uropathy
(c) ATN
(d) AGN
(e) Idiopathic hypocalciuria

38. Most appropriate for laparoscopic ureterolithotomy:
(a) 12 mm long stone impacted at lower ureter with functioning kidney
(b) 22 mm long stone impacted with non-functioning kidney
(c) 4 mm at lower ureter
(d) 18 mm in upper ureter
(e) 22 mm long stone impacted in mid ureteral with functioning kidney

39. 10 weeks primigravida with right ureteric colic, investigation done:
(a) Routine urinalysis (b) USG
(c) X-ray KUB (d) CT
(e) MRI

40. Which are most resistant to ESWL?
(a) Cystine
(b) Uric acid
(c) Struvite
(d) Calcium oxalate monohydrate
(e) Calcium oxalate dihydrate

41. Renal colic in female with second trimester of pregnancy – treatment option:
(a) Analgesics (b) URS
(c) Stenting (d) PCN
(e) Antegrade removal

42. Renal hypercalciuria:
(a) Increased intestinal absorption
(b) Occurs due to defective tubular absorption
(c) Increased PTH
(d) High fasting urinary calcium levels
(e) Serum Ca is normal

43. Hypocitraturia:
(a) < 320 mg/day in urine
(b) Associated with chronic diarrhea
(c) Atkin's diet is prescribed to patient
(d) Associated with stone formation
(e) Renal tubular acidosis

44. Contraindication of ESWL are all *except*:
(a) Pregnancy
(b) UTI
(c) Bleeding diathesis
(d) Very obese patients
(e) History of pancreatitis

45. Most common complication of PCNL:
(a) Bleeding (b) Pleural effusion
(c) Colonic perforation (d) Fever
(e) Urinary leak

46. Which of the following factor help in decision making ESWL/PCNL?
(a) Stone size
(b) Composition
(c) Hydronephrosis
(d) Calyceal anatomy
(e) Congenital anomaly

47. **Drug used in renal colic:**
(a) Indomethacin (b) Bethanechol
(c) Aceclofenac (d) Ephedrine
(e) Vasopressin

48. **AVF/pseudoaneurysm incidence after PNL:**
(a) 0.5% (b) 2%
(c) 5% (d) 10%
(e) 20%

49. **Following are responsible for recurrent stone formation after removal of staghorn calculus:**
(a) Retained fragment
(b) Decreased magnesuria
(c) Increase calciuria
(d) Increase oxaluria
(e) RTA with recurrent stone

50. **Which stone is undetectable on stone protocol CT scan?**
(a) Uric acid
(b) Cystine
(c) Indinavir
(d) Dihydroxy adenine

51. **10% hemiacidrin is used to dissolve struvite stone – it causes:**
(a) Hyperkalemia
(b) Hypermagnesemia
(c) Hyperammonia
(d) Hyperoxalemia
(e) Hyperphosphatemia

52. **True regarding uric acid calculus:**
(a) Most important factor is low urinary pH
(b) Low pH is commonly caused by altered ammonium metabolism due to insulin resistance
(c) Low pH is a risk factor for uric acid and calcium oxalate
(d) Thiazide diuretics is the treatment of choice
(e) Enhancement in CT >1000 HU

53. **Lower calyx 2.5 cm stone treatment option:**
(a) ESWL
(b) PCNL
(c) Nephrectomy
(d) Pyelolithotomy
(e) Observation

54. **Randall plaque forms in the basement membrane of:**
(a) Proximal convoluted tubule
(b) Thick limb of loop of Henle
(c) Thin limb of loop of Henle
(d) Distal convoluted tubule

55. **Radiolucent stones are:**
(a) Oxalate
(b) Phosphate
(c) Cystine
(d) Uric acid

56. **Investigations for acute ureteric colic:**
(a) Hemogram (b) Urinalysis
(c) IVU (d) NCCT
(e) CECT

57. **Treatment option for 2 cm (obstructing) stone at L4 transverse process:**
(a) Push back and PCNL
(b) Flexible ureteroscopy with laser
(c) ESWL
(d) Lap surgery
(e) Open surgery

58. **In acute abdomen, commonly done useful investigations:**
(a) USG (b) NCCT
(c) CECT (d) PET
(e) ECHO

59. **Urinary stone disease usually not diagnosed by:**
(a) IVU (b) USG
(c) MRI (d) PET
(e) NCCT

60. **Which of the following is present in struvite stone in excess to ammonium and magnesium?**
(a) Calcium (b) Carbonate
(c) Phosphate (d) Sulphate
(e) Uric acid

61. Best imaging for ureteric colic:
(a) USG (b) NCCT
(c) X-ray KUB (d) Doppler
(e) IVU

62. Advise to prevent recurrence of stone disease:
(a) Adequate fluid intake for urine output of around 2 litres
(b) Weight reduction
(c) Daily thiazide
(d) Restrict salt intake
(e) Stop calcium intake

63. Nephrocalcinosis associated with:
(a) RTA
(b) MSK
(c) Hyperparathyroidism
(d) Alport syndrome
(e) Bartter's syndrome

64. Pain in ureteric colic due to:
(a) Scratching of mucosa simulate nociceptors
(b) Visceral-type pain to the sympathetic distribution of the kidney and ureter
(c) Muscle spasm are typically produced over the distributions of the subcostal, iliohypogastric, ilioinguinal, and/or genitofemoral nerves
(d) Distension in renal collecting system
(e) All of the above

65. ESWL – difficulty in fragmentation:
(a) Calcium phosphate
(b) Cystine
(c) Triple phosphate
(d) Brushite
(e) Calcium oxalate dihydrate

66. Young female with left ureteric colic on evaluation 4 mm calculus at L2-L3 with no PCS dilatation – management:
(a) Pain relief and expectant management
(b) ESWL
(c) URS
(d) DJ stenting
(e) PCN

67. Following vitamin deficiency causes stone:
(a) Vitamin A (b) Vitamin E
(c) Vitamin D (d) Vitamin B_{12}
(e) Pyridoxine

68. Urease producing organisms are:
(a) Staphylococcus (b) Klebsiella
(c) E. coli (d) Citrobacter
(e) Streptococci

69. Common complication of ureterenoscopy is:
(a) Mucosal injury
(b) Ureteral perforation
(c) Stricture
(d) Bleeding
(e) Avulsion

70. Alkaline therapy used in following stone:
(a) Cystine
(b) Uric acid
(c) Calcium oxalate stone
(d) Calcium phosphate
(e) Struvite

71. Proximal RTA all *except*:
(a) Hyperkalemia
(b) Nephrocalcinosis
(c) Normal urinary pH
(d) Abnormal vitamin D metabolism
(e) Hypophosphatemia

72. Radiolucent stone:
(a) Uric acid (b) Cystine
(c) Struvite (d) Calcium oxalate
(e) Calcium phosphate

73. Radio-opaque are:
(a) Uric acid (b) Xanthine
(c) Cysteine (d) Adenine
(e) Calcium oxalate monohydrate

74. Stone in acidic urine are:
(a) Uric acid

(b) Cysteine
(c) Calcium oxalate monohydrate
(d) Calcium phosphate
(e) Struvite

75. Nephrocalcinosis is seen in:
(a) RTA
(b) Hyperparathyroidism
(c) Sarcoidosis
(d) MSK
(e) Chronic glomerulonephritis

76. Selective angiography indicated in:
(a) In evaluation of renal artery stenosis
(b) Gross hematuria after PCNL
(c) Hemodynamic instability after renal biopsy
(d) Graft failure after renal transplantation
(e) Gross hematuria in bladder malignancy

77. Optimal pH for prevention of crystallization of uric acid stone:
(a) 5.5-6 (b) 6-6.5
(c) 6.5-7 (d) 7-7.5
(e) 7.5-8

78. Regarding lithotripsy:
(a) Holmium laser has maximum chance of ureteral wall perforation
(b) Holmium YAG – thin flexible fiber
(c) Ultrasonic lithotripter best for fragmentation and simultaneous removal of stone
(d) Pneumatic lithotripter maximum chances of retrograde propulsion
(e) EHL is least costly, has smaller probes and good probe flexibility

79. Struvite stone beside magnesium and ammonium composed of:
(a) Carbonate (b) Sulfate
(c) Phosphate (d) Urate
(e) Calcium oxalate

80. Safe investigation in pregnancy for ureteric calculus:
(a) USG (b) IVP
(c) CT (d) MRI
(e) Renal scintiscan

81. Radiolucent calculus:
(a) Xanthine (b) Uric acid
(c) $CaPO_4$ (d) Cystine
(e) Calcium oxalate

82. Hyperuricemia with hyperuricosuria is seen in:
(a) Cancer chemotherapy
(b) Loop diuretics
(c) High dose HOCM
(d) Xanthinuria
(e) Ethambutol

83. Intracorporeal lithotripsy–true:
(a) Ultrasonic is best for URS
(b) Hol:YAG cannot be used with flexible fiber
(c) Hol:YAG may produce cyanide with uric acid stone
(d) EHL probe is essential on underwater spark plug
(e) Retrograde propulsion is maximum with pneumatic lithotripter

84. Photoacoustic laser:
(a) Holmium (b) Nd;YAG
(c) Freddy (d) Diode

85. Laser fiber (µm) most commonly used for ureteric calculus:
(a) 200 (b) 365
(c) 500 (d) 1000

86. Safest site for PCNL:
(a) Infundibulum (b) Calyceal neck
(c) Papillae (d) Fornix

87. Endemic stones all are true *except*:
(a) Always recur after treatment
(b) Cereal based diet
(c) Peak age – 3 years
(d) Ammonium citrate with calcium oxalate

88. Reabsorptive hypercalciuria:
(a) Serum calcium is elevated
(b) PTH is stimulated
(c) Fasting urine calcium is suppressed
(d) Intestinal calcium absorption is elevated

89. **Corpora amylacea:**
(a) Always associated with infection
(b) Not premalignant
(c) Formed by prostatic secretions around epithelial cells
(d) Proteinaceous material

90. **Twenty-eight weeks pregnant woman with 8 mm upper ureteric stone:**
(a) URS (b) PCNL
(c) ESWL (d) Conservative

91. **Six years old with staghorn calculous:**
(a) PCNL
(b) Open nephrolithotomy
(c) URS
(d) ESWL

92. **Lady with 3 cm ureteric stone at the level of L3 in solitary kidney with S creatinine of 2.2 mg/dl. After placing PCN renal function improved. Nephrostogram shows no dye beyond stone. Management is:**
(a) Nephrectomy
(b) PCNL
(c) URS with DJ stenting
(d) Stent with ESWL

93. **Drug not used in treatment of hypercalcemia:**
(a) Furosemide (b) Saline hydration
(c) Thiazide (d) Calcitonin

94. **In type IV RTA:**
(a) Hyperkalemia
(b) Hypokalemia
(c) Alkalosis
(d) Urine pH cannot be below 5.5

95. **Guidewire used in access is of:**
(a) 0.038 inch (b) 0.038 Fr
(c) 0.038 cm (d) 0.038 mm

96. **Most common type of RTA with stone:**
(a) Type 1 (b) Type 2
(c) Type 3 (d) Type 4

97. **Twenty-year-female patient has right HDN with parenchyma 1 cm. Bilateral staghorn calculus with deranged KFT, DTPA right – 70%, left – 30% plan is:**
(a) Right PCNL followed by left PCNL
(b) Right PCNL with left nephrectomy
(c) Left PCNL followed by right PCNL
(d) Bilateral renal diversion and then PCNL

98. **Twenty-year-female with bilateral staghorn calculus with normal renal function test, right HDN with DTPA 99% with parenchyma 1.5 cm. Left non HDN, treatment plan:**
(a) Right PCNL followed by left PCNL
(b) Right PCNL with left nephrectomy
(c) Left PCNL followed by right PCNL
(d) Bilateral simultaneous PCNL

99. **Young female with urosepsis, bilateral HDN, serum creatinine 6.0, serum K+ 6.8, BU 130, Na^+ 127; bilateral ureteric calculus with echogenic debris:**
(a) Bilateral PCN
(b) Right PCN with stent left side
(c) Dialysis
(d) Observation with antibiotics

100. **Patient underwent PCNL for renal stone, complete stone clearance. Post PCNL complete obstruction at PUJ present, what is the next step?**
(a) Pyelostomy
(b) Remove nephrostomy
(c) Internal stenting followed by pyeloplasty
(d) Nephrectomy

101. **Randall's plaque is composed of:**
(a) Calcium apatite
(b) Calcium phosphate
(c) Calcium silicate
(d) Calcium carbonate

102. Which of the following is not present in RTA?
(a) Inability to acidify urine
(b) Hypercitraturia
(c) Nephrocalcinosis
(d) Non-anion gap

103. Hyperparathyroidism, which cause is incorrect?
(a) Increase Ca^{2+} reabsorption in DCT
(b) Decrease phosphate reabsorption
(c) Calcitriol stimulates PTH synthesis
(d) Direct action on GI reabsorption of Ca^{2+}

104. Cause of endemic pediatric vesical calculus:
(a) Dietary deficiency of phosphate
(b) Dietary excess of calcium
(c) Dietary deficiency of calcium
(d) Dietary excess of phosphate

105. The following urinary abnormalities are seen in patients with Type I RTA *except*:
(a) Hypercalciuria
(b) Hypocitraturia
(c) Increased urinary pH
(d) Hyperuricosuria

106. The following statements are true about urinary stones *except*:
(a) Inflammatory bowel disease predisposes to oxalate stones
(b) Pyridoxine can be used to treat hyperoxaluria
(c) Calcium oxalate dihydrate stones are common with renal tubular acidosis
(d) Hypercalciuria is seen after prolonged immobilization

107. The urinary crystals that are formed in acidic urine include the following *except*:
(a) Whewellite (b) Uric acid
(c) Cystine (d) Struvite

108. Most common artery that is injured during PCNL is:
(a) Posterior segmental artery
(b) Anterior segmental artery
(c) Renal artery
(d) Splenic artery

109. In distal renal tubular acidosis the following statements are true *except*:
(a) Urine pH is below 5.0
(b) Stones are usually calcium phosphate
(c) Systemic acidosis is present
(d) Stones form in the collecting ducts

110. Hypomagnesemic urolithiasis caused by all *except:*
(a) Laxative abuse
(b) Inflammatory bowel disease
(c) Chronic thiazide therapy
(d) Chronic citrate therapy

111. False about cystinuria:
(a) It is caused by autosomal recessive error of transepithelial transport involving intestine and kidneys
(b) Crystallization occurs when excreted concentration is above 250 mg/l
(c) Relatively more radiopaque and diagnosed on plane X-ray
(d) Staghorn calculi or multiple, pus filled calyces are common

112. False about pregnancy associated hydronephrosis:
(a) Commonly starts from 1st trimester
(b) Usually resolves within 6 weeks following delivery
(c) Left side is more common than right side
(d) Ureter dilatation doesn't extend below pelvic brim

113. The wavelength of Hol-YAG laser:
(a) 1060 cm (b) 2100 cm
(c) 520 cm (d) 10600 cm

114. Incidence of primary bladder calculi is highest during:

(a) 1st decade (b) 2nd decade
(c) 3rd decade (d) 4th decade

115. Mineralogical name for calcium oxalate monohydrate:

(a) Whewellite (b) Weddellite
(c) Brushite (d) Whitlockite

116. Microscopic appearance of cystine calculi:

(a) Hexagonal
(b) Envelope shaped
(c) Hourglass
(d) Rectangular

117. Not a cause of acquired renal tubular acidosis:

(a) Obstructive uropathy
(b) Idiopathic hypercalciuria
(c) Cystinuria
(d) Recurrent pyelonephritis

118. Most common primary urethral calculi:

(a) Calcium oxalate
(b) Calcium phosphate
(c) Uric acid
(d) Magnesium ammonium phosphate

119. Infective calculi most commonly caused by:

(a) E coli (b) Pseudomonas
(c) Proteus (d) Staphylococcus

120. False about primary hyperoxaluria:

(a) Type 1 is most common and due to deficiency of alanine/glyoxylate aminotransferase enzyme
(b) Type 2 is due to deficiency of glyoxylate reductase/hydroxypyruvate reductase
(c) Urinary oxalate levels increased without increase in serum levels
(d) Without treatment death is common before 20 years of age

121. Most important pathogenetic mechanism of uric acid stones:

(a) Decreased urinary pH
(b) Low urine volume
(c) Hyperuricosuria
(d) Hypercalciuria

122. False regarding stones during pregnancy:

(a) Age adjusted incidence of stones is similar in multiparous and primipara women
(b) Incidence is similar in pregnancy and non-pregnancy states
(c) Incidence is more on left side than right side
(d) Ureteric stones twice common than renal stones

123. True about triangulation technique used during percutaneous access to upper collecting system:

(a) Ability to maintain both the mediolateral, cephalocaudal planes as in the 'eye-of-the needle' technique
(b) Ability to monitor the depth of the needle continuously
(c) Typically 21-gauge needle is used to maintain the angle of entry
(d) Can be used to place the needle at any location and angle

124. Stones in distal renal tubular acidosis are composed of:

(a) Calcium oxalate
(b) Calcium phosphate
(c) Struvite
(d) Mixed stones

125. Jackstone calculus is composed of:

(a) Calcium oxalate monohydrate
(b) Ammonium urate
(c) Struvite
(d) Cystine

126. The following stones can be disintegrated using ESWL *except*:

(a) Uric acid

(b) Calcium magnesium ammonium phosphate
(c) Calcium oxalate dehydrate
(d) Cystine

127. Uric acid calculi:
(a) Are radiolucent
(b) Occur in men only
(c) Commonly occur in urine with a pH of less than 5.5
(d) Are always associated with hyperuricemia

128. In a patient with an infected staghorn calculus, where the urine pH is 8, the most likely causative organism:
(a) Escherichia coli
(b) Proteus mirabilis
(c) Enterococcus faecalis
(d) Klebsiella

129. Medical management of struvite stone is all *except*:
(a) Acetohydroxamic acid
(b) Mercaptopropionyl glycine
(c) Fluorofamide
(d) Hydroxyurea

130. Most common stone in RTA:
(a) $CaPO_4$
(b) Calcium oxalate monohydrate
(c) Uric acid
(d) Calcium oxalate dihydrate

131. All of the following are seen in distal RTA *except*:
(a) Hyperkalemia
(b) Hyperchloremia
(c) Hypercalcemia
(d) Nephrocalcinosis

132. In alkaline urine which stone occurs?
(a) Uric acid
(b) Calcium oxalate monohydrate
(c) Cystine
(d) Calcium phosphate

133. Composition of matrix cast:
(a) Mucoprotein
(b) Tamm-Horsfall protein
(c) Albumin
(d) Globulin

134. Prostatic calculi composition:
(a) Corpora amylacea with inspissated material
(b) $CaPO_4$ with 20% matrix
(c) Calcium oxalate
(d) Triple phosphate

135. Which of the following investigations is most important in acute abdomen?
(a) Non-contrast CT
(b) Contrast enhanced CT
(c) X-ray abdomen supine and erect
(d) MRI

136. A 30-year-old female patient with recurrent colicky flank pain for 6 months showing no radiopaque shadow on X-ray KUB least likely is:
(a) Staghorn calculus
(b) Uric acid calculus
(c) Ureteric stricture
(d) PUJ obstruction

137. Uric acid is the part of which metabolic pathway?
(a) Purine
(b) Methionine
(c) Fructose
(d) Allantoin

138. What is the treatment of choice of renal stone, 10-30 mm in size?
(a) ESWL
(b) PCNL
(c) Open pyelolithotomy
(d) Laparoscopic pyelolithotomy

139. In a patient with acute ureteric colic, the investigation that will give the accurate result:

(a) X-ray KUB
(b) Non-contrast spiral CT
(c) IVU
(d) Contrast-enhanced CT

140. Which of the following stone is formed in short bowel syndrome?

(a) Cystine (b) Oxalate
(c) Xanthine (d) Phosphate

141. Which of the following enzyme defect is present in type-1 primary hyperoxaluria?

(a) Alanine glyoxalate aminotransferase
(b) D-glyoxylate DH
(c) L-glyoxalate DH
(d) N-glyoxalate DH

142. Hexagonal crystals are of:

(a) Phosphate (b) Cystine
(c) Matrix (d) Xanthine

143. FDA approved ESWL in year:

(a) 1978 (b) 1980
(c) 1982 (d) 1984

144. ESWL is contraindicated if the serum creatinine is more than:

(a) 1.2 mg/dl (b) 2 mg/dl
(c) 3 mg/dl (d) 5 mg/dl

145. All are urease producing organisms, *except:*

(a) Proteus
(b) E coli
(c) Pseudomonas
(d) Streptococcus hemolyticus

146. Contraindication for PCNL:

(a) Bleeding disorder
(b) Pelvic stone
(c) Calyceal stone
(d) Solitary kidney

147. In pregnancy and urolithiasis, true is:

(a) Mostly on left side
(b) Ureteric > renal stones
(c) Increased incidence in the first trimester
(d) Mostly operative intervention is required

148. Radiolucent stone is:

(a) Uric acid
(b) Calcium oxalate monohydrate
(c) Calcium oxalate dihydrate
(d) Calcium phosphate

149. Differential diagnosis of ureteric colic in pregnancy are all *except*:

(a) Renal rupture
(b) Acute appendicitis
(c) Ectopic pregnancy
(d) Acute pyelonephritis

150. Contributory factor for calculi formation in children:

(a) Genetic
(b) Anatomic abnormality
(c) Metabolic
(d) All of the above

151. Absorptive hypercalciuria type 1, all are true *except:*

(a) Normal fasting urine calcium
(b) Reduced intestinal absorption of sodium
(c) Normal serum calcium
(d) Upgradation of vitamin D receptor in intestine
(e) Renal phosphate wasting

152. Renal hypercalciuria all are true *except:*

(a) Increase renal tubular absorption of calcium
(b) Increased urinary calcium
(c) Normal serum calcium
(d) Increased intestinal absorption of calcium
(e) Associated with secondary hyperparathyroidism

153. Resorptive hypercalciuria all are true *except:*

(a) Most common associated with primary hyperparathyroidism

(b) Decreased bone resorption
(c) Increased renal production of vitamin D3
(d) Increased intestinal absorption of calcium
(e) Increased serum calcium

154. Contraindications of ESWL are all *except:*
(a) Uncorrectable coagulopathy
(b) Morbid obesity
(c) Severe spinal deformity
(d) Pregnancy
(e) Hypertension

155. Not a feature of holmium laser intracoporeal lithotripsy:
(a) Weak shockwaves
(b) Reduced incidence of stone retrograde propulsion
(c) Used for all stones irrespective of composition
(d) Photothermal reaction
(e) Fragmentation and suction can be done simultaneously

156. PNL for staghorn all are true *except:*
(a) General anesthesia ideal
(b) Supine position
(c) Posterior calyceal puncture ideal
(d) Ureteric catheter facilitates identification
(e) C-arm at 30 degree is preferred for puncture

157. Regarding Steinstrasse all are true *except:*
(a) Stream of stones
(b) 2-10% of ESWL incidence
(c) Increased incidence with increased stone size
(d) Increased incidence with pre-existing ureteric obstruction
(e) Surgery required in all cases

158. Complications of ureterorenoscopy are all *except:*
(a) Urethral stricture
(b) Ureteral avulsion
(c) Urosepsis
(d) Ureteral perforation
(e) Damage to scope

159. Obstruction of calculus most common location:
(a) UPJ
(b) UVJ
(c) Crossing of gonadal artery
(d) At the crossing of iliac vessels

160. First line investigation for a patient presenting with renal colic:
(a) USG
(b) IVP
(c) CT scan abdomen
(d) MR urogram

161. A 44 years old patient presented with right loin pain, fever with chills, on USG dilated collecting system, with internal echoes, next step in the management includes:
(a) Retrograde stenting
(b) PCN
(c) Broad spectrum antibiotics
(d) Observation

162. The main cause of hypercalcemia in hospitalized patients is:
(a) Hyperparathyroidism
(b) Malignancy
(c) Steroid usage
(d) Iatrogenic

163. Hyperparathyroidism causes which type of hypercalciuria?
(a) Type 1 absorptive
(b) Type 2 absorptive
(c) Resorptive
(d) Renal leak

164. All of the following stones formed in acidic urine *except:*
(a) Calcium oxalate
(b) Uric acid
(c) Cystine
(d) Phosphate

165. **Which of the following is not an indication of treatment of asymptomatic 4 mm calyceal stone?**
(a) Patient with solitary kidney
(b) Women considering pregnancy
(c) When the patient is a pilot
(d) Elderly patients

166. **Following stones difficult to fragment by ESWL *except:***
(a) Uric acid
(b) Calcium oxalate monohydrate
(c) Cystine
(d) Brushite

167. **Following lithotripsy has narrowest safety margin:**
(a) EHL (b) LASER
(c) Ballistic (d) Ultrasonic

168. **Organism producing urease are all *except:***
(a) Proteus (b) Serratia
(c) Klebsiella (d) E coli

169. **Urinary crystals that precipitate in acidic urine include all *except:***
(a) Uric acid
(b) Cystine
(c) Calcium oxalate
(d) Calcium phosphate

170. **What is the wavelength of a hol: YAG laser?**
(a) 532 nm (b) 2100 nm
(c) 980 nm (d) 1650 nm

171. **In distal renal tubular acidosis the following statements are true *except:***
(a) Urine pH is below 5.0
(b) Stones are usually calcium phosphate
(c) Metabolic acidosis may be present
(d) Stones form in the collecting ducts

172. **Endemic bladder calculi are mostly composed of:**
(a) Calcium phosphate
(b) Calcium oxalate
(c) Ammonium acid urate
(d) Triple phosphates

173. **Urgent nephrostomy is required in:**
(a) Pyonephrosis
(b) Recurrent renal colic in pregnancy
(c) Fever with hydronephrotic kidney
(d) Anemia with uremia
(e) PUJ obstruction with palpable kidney

174. **Resistant to ESWL are:**
(a) Uric acid
(b) Calcium oxalate dehydrate
(c) Calcium oxalate monohydrate
(d) Cystine
(e) None of the above

175. **Radiolucent stones are:**
(a) Uric acid (b) Cystine
(c) Calcium oxalate (d) Struvite
(e) Calcium phosphate

176. **Predisposing factor for uric acid stone are all *except*:**
(a) pH < 5.5
(b) Low urine volume
(c) Hyperuricemia
(d) pH > 5.5
(e) Diabetes mellitus

177. **First PCNL done by:**
(a) Fernstrom and Johannsen
(b) Marshall
(c) Goodman
(d) Arthur Smith
(e) Smoth and Boyce

178. **First percutaneous nephrostomy:**
(a) Goodwin (b) Clayman
(c) Johannson (d) Peter Gilling

179. **Not used for medical management of ureteric stone:**
(a) Nifedipine (b) Tamsulosin
(c) Phentolamine (d) Alfuzosin

180. **Which of the following is not an inhibitor of urinary stone formation?**
(a) Citrate
(b) Cystine
(c) Tamm-Horsfall protein
(d) Nephrocalcin

181. **Which of the following medication is not associated with stone formation?**
(a) Magnesium trisilicate
(b) Potassium citrate
(c) Ephedrine
(d) Guaifenesin

182. Envelope shaped crystals are seen in calculi with:
(a) Calcium oxalate (b) Brushite
(c) Struvite (d) Cystine

183. Febuxostat is useful in urinary stones related to:
(a) Hypercalcemia (b) Oxalosis
(c) Hyperuricemia (d) Cystinuria

184. Alken guide rod with ball tip is used for:
(a) Retrograde intrarenal surgery
(b) Percutaneous nephrolithotomy
(c) Rigid ureteroscopy
(d) Retroperitoneoscopy

185. Which of the following is used for medical expulsive therapy of urinary stones?
(a) Sympathomimetics
(b) Anticholinergics
(c) Alpha blockers
(d) Flavoxate

186. Highest perforation rates in ureteric stones is encountered with:
(a) Ballistic lithotripsy
(b) LASER lithotripsy
(c) Sonotrode
(d) Electrohydraulic lithotripsy

187. Female with turbid urine, pH-5.7, 50 pus cell/HPF, 10-12 RBC, WBC cast, following will not grow in urine culture:
(a) Pseudomonas
(b) E. coli
(c) Clostridium perfringens
(d) Klebsiella pneumoniae
(e) Proteus

188. Commonly seen in patients with calcium oxalate stones:
(a) Calcium restriction should be advised
(b) Uric acid stone and hyperuricosuria is a risk factor
(c) Patients commonly demonstrate increased intestinal calcium absorption
(d) Loop diuretics are associated with decreased urinary calcium excretion
(e) Associated with hypercalciuria

189. Second trimester of pregnancy stone detected. Treatment option are:
(a) Antegrade PCNL (b) Analgesic
(c) DJ stenting (d) URS
(e) PCN

190. In PCNL puncture is made through:
(a) Major calyx (b) Infundibulum
(c) Minor calyx (d) Fornix
(e) Pelvis

191. Metabolic evaluation for urinary lithiasis is indicated in:
(a) First time stone formers
(b) Renal insufficiency
(c) Osteoporosis
(d) Stone other than struvite, urate, cystine
(e) Solitary kidney

ANSWERS

1.	A	25.	TTFTF	49.	ABCDE	73.	CE	97.	A
2.	A	26.	TFFFF	50.	C	74.	ABC	98.	B
3.	C	27.	TTFTF	51.	BE	75.	ABCDE	99.	A
4.	C	28.	TTTFF	52.	ABC	76.	ABC	100.	C
5.	FFTTT	29.	TTTTT	53.	BD	77.	A	101.	A
6.	TFTTT	30.	FTFTF	54.	C	78.	BCDE	102.	B
7.	TFTTT	31.	FTTTF	55.	CD	79.	C	103.	A
8.	TTTTT	32.	FTFTT	56.	D	80.	AD	104.	D
9.	TTTFT	33.	TTTTF	57.	ABCDE	81.	A	105.	D
10.	TTTTT	34.	FFFFF	58.	AB	82.	A	106.	C
11.	TFFFT	35.	FTFTT	59.	D	83.	E	107.	D
12.	TTTFT	36.	FTTTF	60.	C	84.	A	108.	A
13.	FFTTT	37.	ABC	61.	AB	85.	B	109.	A
14.	TTFTT	38.	E	62.	ABD	86.	C	110.	D
15.	TTTTT	39.	AB	63.	ABCDE	87.	A	111.	C
16.	FFFTT	40.	A	64.	E	88.	C	112.	C
17.	FFTTT	41.	ACD	65.	BD	89.	C	113.	C
18.	TTFTF	42.	ABCDE	66.	A	90.	A	114.	A
19.	FFTTT	43.	ABDE	67.	ACDE	91.	A	115.	A
20.	TFTTF	44.	E	68.	AB	92.	B	116.	A
21.	TTFTF	45.	A	69.	ABCDE	93.	D	117.	C
22.	TTTTF	46.	ABCDE	70.	ABC	94.	A	118.	D
23.	TFFFT	47.	AC	71.	ABC	95.	A	119.	C
24.	FFTFT	48.	A	72.	A	96.	A	120.	C

121.	A	137.	A	153.	B	169.	D	185.	C
122.	C	138.	B	154.	E	170.	B	186.	A
123.	B	139.	B	155.	E	171.	A	187.	ADE
124.	B	140.	B	156.	B	172.	C	188.	BCE
125.	A	141.	A	157.	E	173.	A	189.	BCDE
126.	D	142.	B	158.	A	174.	D	190.	AD
127.	A	143.	D	159.	B	175.	A	191.	BCE
128.	B	144.	B	160.	A	176.	D		
129.	B	145.	B	161.	B	177.	A		
130.	A	146.	A	162.	B	178.	A		
131.	A	147.	B	163.	C	179.	C		
132.	D	148.	A	164.	D	180.	B		
133.	A	149.	A	165.	D	181.	B		
134.	A	150.	A	166.	A	182.	A		
135.	A	151.	A	167.	A	183.	C		
136.	A	152.	A	168.	D	184.	B		

CHAPTER 10

Neoplasms of Upper Urinary Tract

1. **The P53 tumor suppressor gene plays a critical role in:**
   (a) Apoptosis
   (b) Angiogenesis
   (c) DNA replication
   (d) Signal transduction

2. **Von Hippel-Lindau (VHL) disease predisposes patients to:**
   (a) Epididymal carcinoma
   (b) Clear cell carcinoma
   (c) Papillary renal cell carcinoma
   (d) Adrenocortical carcinoma

3. **Most common renal involvement seen in tuberous sclerosis include:**
   (a) RCC (b) Renal cysts
   (c) Angiomyolipoma (d) Oncocytoma

4. **Involvement of the IVC with RCC occurs in:**
   (a) 0 to 5% (b) 5% to 10%
   (c) 10% to 15% (d) 15% to 20%

5. **Sunitinib is used for:**
   (a) Metastatic renal cell carcinoma
   (b) Castration resistance prostate cancer
   (c) Hormone resistance prostate cancer
   (d) Adenocarcinoma of bladder

6. **Treatment of choice for 1 cm diverticular stone in kidney of a 30 years old male:**
   (a) ESWL (b) PCNL
   (c) RIRS (d) Nephrolithotomy

7. **Most common renal malignancy:**
   (a) Clear cell carcinoma
   (b) Medullary carcinoma
   (c) Papillary carcinoma
   (d) Sarcoma

8. **Radiolucent stone:**
   (a) Uric acid
   (b) Calcium monohydrate
   (c) Calcium dehydrate
   (d) Calcium oxalate

9. **Vessel that can cause troublesome bleeding during placement of pelvic laparoscopic ports:**
   (a) Superficial circumflex iliac
   (b) External pudendal
   (c) Superficial inferior epigastric
   (d) Superficial superior epigastric

10. **Primary hyperparathyroidism is the cause of nephrolithiasis in:**
    (a) 2% (b) 20%
    (c) 5% (d) 10%

11. **Most common malignancy-associated hypercalcemia is:**
    (a) Lung and breast
    (b) Renal cell carcinoma
    (c) Head and neck
    (d) Lymphoma and myeloma

12. **The most common type of stone associated with distal RTA is:**
    (a) Calcium phosphate
    (b) Calcium oxalate monohydrate
    (c) Calcium oxalate dihydrate
    (d) Uric acid

13. **Single most important test to delineate the nature renal mass is:**

(a) IVU (b) USG
(c) CECT (d) MRI

14. The risk of malignancy for category II renal cysts is:
(a) Nil (b) 0% to 5%
(c) 5% to 10% (d) 10% to 15%

15. Which is the most lethal tumor?
(a) RCC (b) Ca urinary bladder
(c) Ca prostate (d) Ca testis

16. Paraneoplastic syndromes are found in how many patients with RCC?
(a) 10% (b) 20%
(c) 30% (d) 40%

17. During PCNL most common site for venous bleed is from:
(a) Posterior calyx
(b) Posteromedial calyx
(c) Medial calyx
(d) Inferior calyx

18. Site for randall plaque is:
(a) Basement membrane of thin loop of Henle
(b) DCT
(c) PCT
(d) Collecting tubules

19. Patient has partial staghorn calculus with urine showing urease splitting organism, what should be avoided?
(a) Fluoroquinolones
(b) Orthophosphate
(c) Acetohydroxamic acid
(d) PCNL

20. Indication of repair in renal artery aneurysm are all *except:*
(a) Calcified 1.5 cm artery
(b) Female of child bearing age
(c) Uncalcified 3 cm artery
(d) Sypmtomatic

21. Diabetic 4 cm upper urinary tract tumor:
(a) Radical nephroureterectomy
(b) Pyelectomy
(c) Simple nephrectomy
(d) Endoscopic fulguration

Mention True and False respective to each statement (Q. No. 22 to 72)

22. AML:
(a) Benign tumor
(b) Arises from perivascular epithelial cells
(c) Almost always present in TS
(d) Wunderlich syndrome is seen in 10% cases
(e) Female: Male:: 10: 1

23. Regarding tumor of kidney:
(a) Chromophobe is better prognosis than clear cell RCC
(b) In oncocytoma prominent necrosis or hypervascularity is seen
(c) Oncocytoma has cart wheel appearance on angiography
(d) AML < 4 cm management is conservative
(e) AML–30 HU is diagnostic

24. Regarding RCC:
(a) Adrenal involvement–T3a
(b) IVC involvement better seen in CT than MRI
(c) N3–>5 cm
(d) Tumor grossly extends into vena cava below diaphragm–T3b
(e) Tumor > 7.0 cm and ≤ 10.0 cm and confined to the kidney– T2a

25. AV fistula:
(a) Most common type is acquired
(b) Congenital fistula occur equally in both sexes
(c) Congenital fistula constitute 22% to 25% of all renal arteriovenous fistulas
(d) Congenital fistula generally do not become manifest until adult life
(e) 70% of fistulas occurring after needle biopsy of the kidney close spontaneously within 18 months

26. Dorsal lumbotomy:
(a) Muscle cutting incision
(b) Done in supine position
(c) Can be done bilaterally without changing position
(d) Advantage in obese patients
(e) Incision of choice in upper polar RCC for open nephrectomy

27. Upper tract malignancy:
(a) CECT can differentiate between Ta and T_1
(b) CECT should be done to detect upper tract malignancy in patients with bladder cancer
(c) CECT can detect upper tract CIS
(d) CECT suspicious of mass with normal urine cytology excludes malignancy
(e) With CT urography the sensitivity for detecting upper tract malignant disease approaches 100%

28. Target therapy in RCC:
(a) Sunitinib is mTOR inhibitor and considered as 1st line drug in metastatic RCC
(b) Sorafenib is tyrosine kinase inhibitor used as adjuvant in locally advanced RCC
(c) Solitary metastasis in liver–resection is better than target therapy
(d) IFN better than target therapy in metastatic RCC
(e) Bevacizumab is an IgG1 monoclonal antibody recognizing and binding all VEGF isoforms

29. RCC:
(a) Chromophobic better prognosis them bellini duct RCC
(b) Oncocytoma arises from distal tubule
(c) Cart-wheel appearance can reliably differentiate RCC from oncocytoma
(d) Adrenal involvement in T3a
(e) LN > 5 cm is N3

30. RCC:
(a) Chest CT scan is mandatory
(b) CT better than MRI for detection of IVC thrombus
(c) PET–CT should be done in cases for multiple metastasis
(d) Enlarged hilar or RPLN 2 cm or more in diameter on CT almost always harbor malignant change
(e) In RCC with IVC thrombus venacavography is best reserved for patients with equivocal MRI findings

31. Regarding AML:
(a) 20 HU is diagnostic on CT
(b) 20% cases has tuberous sclerosis
(c) < 4 cm lesion can be put on surveillance
(d) It arises from distal collecting duct
(e) Cart-wheel appearance on angiography

32. Renal cyst:
(a) 30 years male with 3 cm incidental cyst-observation
(b) 8 cm cyst at renal hilum–Aspiration and sclerotherapy
(c) Lap unroofing is best for 8 cm lower pole cyst
(d) Solid enhancing cyst Bosniak III requires partial nephrectomy
(e) >5 cyst in both kidneys can be potential donor candidate for renal transplantation

33. Regarding simple renal cyst:
(a) Common age group 40–50 years
(b) Anechoic
(c) Well marginated
(d) Complete transmission of sound
(e) HU-0

34. Urolithiasis:
(a) Upto 70% of adults with distal renal tubular acidosis have kidney stones
(b) Cystinuria is manifested when concentrations exceed 250 mg/l
(c) Hydroxyapatite stone is in primary hyperparathyroidism
(d) 3% of all patients undergoing a full metabolic evaluation will demonstrate no abnormalities
(e) First-time stone formers have a 50% risk of recurrence within the subsequent 10 years

35. **Oncocytoma:**
   (a) Most common benign tumor
   (b) Granularity is due to mitochondria
   (c) If contralateral kidney is abnormal, 4 cm polar oncocytoma can be managed by partial nephrectomy
   (d) Cart-wheel appearance is seen on angiography
   (e) Most renal oncocytomas cannot be differentiated from malignant RCC by clinical or radiographic means

36. **RCC:**
   (a) Necrosis is bad prognosis
   (b) Sunitinib and sorafenib are useful in locally advanced RCC
   (c) IFN has been used for metastatic RCC
   (d) Target therapy has been found to be useful only in clear cell variant
   (e) Cytoreductive nephrectomy followed by systemic treatment should be considered in patients with synchronous metastatic disease

37. **Renal artery aneurysm:**
   (a) Incidence–0.09–0.3%
   (b) Saccular is least common
   (c) Fusiform common in young hypertensive
   (d) Intrarenal in 50%
   (e) Dissecting aneurysm is due to rupture in external elastic layer

38. **AML:**
   (a) Benign clonal neoplasm
   (b) Almost always occur in TS
   (c) Origin from perivascular epithelioid cell
   (d) Wunderlich syndrome most feared and significant complication
   (e) Female : Male = 10 : 1

39. **Forty years young male with fever, UTI and solid enhancing mass lesion:**
   (a) FNAC should be done
   (b) Clear cell carcinoma mostly associated with VHL
   (c) Proangiogenic factor mostly involve in RCC is VEGF
   (d) Best treatment of 7 cm RCC is laparoscopic RN
   (e) RCC < 3 cm can be safely observed in this patient

40. **Renal cystic disease:**
   (a) Acquired renal cytic disease depends upon duration of dialysis
   (b) Rovsing operation for deroofing causes reduction in HTN
   (c) When RCC occurs in ESRD patients the age at occurrence averages 5 years younger
   (d) The male-to-female ratio is significantly greater in ESRD patients with RCC than in the general population with RCC
   (e) The incidence of RCC in ESRD is 3 to 6 times that of the general population

41. **Renal oncocytoma:**
   (a) Most common benign tumor
   (b) Prominent necrosis or hypervascularity is common
   (c) Cart wheel appearance on angiography
   (d) Granularity is due to mitochondria
   (e) 4 cm polar lesion can be managed by partial nephrectomy

42. **AML:**
   (a) Four cm tumor with bleeding requires nephretomy
   (b) USG – Hypoechoic
   (c) CECT is diagnostic
   (d) 30% of AMLs are found in patients with tuberous sclerosis syndrome
   (e) Fat is must for diagnosis

43. **RCC:**
   (a) 3% of all adult malignant neoplasm
   (b) 50% present with triad of symptoms
   (c) Hypertension is one of the presentation
   (d) Hypercalcemia is due to bone metastasis
   (e) Clear cell forms 80%

44. RCC:
- (a) T1 is more than 8 cm
- (b) Spindle cell histology has good prognosis
- (c) Invasion of IVC is poor prognosis
- (d) Routine MRI can differentiate between caval thrombus and tumor
- (e) LN metastasis–5 years survival (0-30%)

45. RCC:
- (a) If LN involvement is present in children, lymphadenectomy should be done
- (b) Lymphadenectomy is controversial in adults
- (c) Lower pole 3 cm tumor adrenalectomy is required
- (d) Interferon beta derived from fibroblast
- (e) Interferon alpha derived from recombinant mammalian cells

46. RCC:
- (a) Interferon alpha response rate is 60%
- (b) Avigan is vaccine used in RCC
- (c) MDR1 gene for P-glycoprotein helps in influx of cytotoxic drugs
- (d) TIL is obtained ex-vivo
- (e) Adjunctive nephrectomy can cause regression of metastasis

47. Fuhrman's grade:
- (a) Depends on cell size
- (b) Depends on nucleoli character
- (c) Most RCC have pseudocapsule of compressed parenchyma and fibrous tissue
- (d) Doppler USG has better resolution than MRI for detecting thrombus
- (e) In large tumor renal vein can be ligated first for easy dissection of artery

48. Renal tumor:
- (a) Chromophobic RCC has better survival than bellini duct RCC
- (b) Cart-wheel appearance on angioplasty cannot differentiate between AML and RCC
- (c) Adrenal involvement is T3a
- (d) N3 involvement denotes as LN > 5 cm
- (e) Involvement of IVC by renal tumor below the diaphragm is considered as stage 3c

49. Benign renal tumor:
- (a) Less than 4 cm AML is managed conservatively
- (b) Oncocytoma arises from DCT
- (c) 20% of AML occurs in TS
- (d) 30 HU on CT is suggestive of AML
- (e) Simple cyst represents 70% of all asymptomatic renal masses

50. In medullary carcinoma of kidney:
- (a) It occurs with sickle cell disease
- (b) Present in 5th decade
- (c) Aggressive chemotherapy has a role in treatment
- (d) Histologically resemble papillary carcinoma
- (e) Highly infiltrative

51. In a 2 years old boy with right testicular NSGCT, pathology reveals 3 cm lesion, no vascular invasion, 10% embryonal cell component, clinical staging T1N0M0, options regarding further management is:
- (a) Radiotherapy
- (b) Chemotherapy
- (c) Observation
- (d) All of the above

52. VHL is characterized by:
- (a) Clear cell carcinoma
- (b) Retinal angioma
- (c) Hepatic hemangioma
- (d) Pancreatic islets cell tumor
- (e) Carcinoma prostate

53. Regarding angiomyolipoma:
- (a) Benign tumor
- (b) F:M = 10 : 1
- (c) Occurs in all cases of tuberous sclerosis
- (d) Ultrastructurally, AML is packed with numerous large mitochondria
- (e) Wunderlich's syndrome, has been found in up to 10% of patients and represents the most significant and feared complication

54. For RCC metastatic evaluation includes:
(a) KFT (b) LFT
(c) CT chest (d) CT abdomen
(e) Bone scan

55. RCC:
(a) MDR 1 increases aggressiveness of tumor
(b) Papillary hypovascular and better prognosis
(c) RCC develops in about 70% of patients with von Hippel-Lindau disease
(d) Paraneoplastic occurs in 20%
(e) Hypercalcemia is due to osteolytic resorption

56. RCC with IVC thrombus:
(a) Doppler can be better than CT for vena cava thrombus
(b) MRI can differentiate between tumor and bland thrombus
(c) If MRI is equivocal perform contrast inferior venacavography
(d) Multiplanar CT is as good as MRI in IVC thrombus
(e) In patients where MRI is contraindicated, transesophageal echo is performed

57. Renal cyst:
(a) Common in 40-50 years
(b) USG diagnosis
(c) Thick walled
(d) Well defined
(e) Anechoic

58. Oncocytoma:
(a) Most common benign tumor
(b) Cart-wheel appearance on angiography
(c) Granularity due to mitochondria
(d) Nuclear aneuploidy
(e) <3 cm with opposite kidney normal–partial nephrectomy

59. RCC:
(a) 3% of all adult malignancies
(b) Lymphadenectomy–therapeutic importance not proved
(c) < 3 cm lower pole tumor–adrenalectomy to be done
(d) Involved colon–partial resection with radical nephrectomy
(e) RCC is most lethal among bladder and prostate malignancies

60. Regarding RCC:
(a) Chromophobe adenoma has better prognosis than Bellini duct carcinoma
(b) Adrenal gland metastasis is T3a
(c) CT better than MRI to detect cranial extent of IVC infiltration
(d) Tumor infiltrating 6th segment of liver and colon with no other metastasis initially treated with immunotherapy for better outcome
(e) Single lung metastasis has best results

61. Simple renal cyst:
(a) CT attenuation 20-140 HU
(b) Smooth rim with no calcification
(c) Thick septa
(d) No blood vessels and do not communicate directly with nephrons
(e) No enhancement of IV contrast

62. Regarding benign renal tumor:
(a) Oncocytoma arises from distal collecting tubule
(b) Central stellate scar is found on CT
(c) AML <4 can be observed
(d) Spokewheel pattern on angiography is unreliable sign
(e) FNAC is compromised by difficulty distinguishing oncocytoma from the granular forms of conventional RCC or the eosinophilic variants of chromophobe or chromophilic RCC

63. Angiomyolipoma:
(a) TS seen in 50% patient with AML
(b) On USG–Hypoechoic
(c) Enhancement on CT is diagnostic
(d) Asymptomatic 3 cm tumor, observation can be attempted
(e) It is benign tumor

64. Oncocytoma:
(a) Most common benign tumor of kidney
(b) Cart-wheel appearance on angiography
(c) Granularity due to mitochondria
(d) If < 4 cm with (N) contralateral kidney–partial nephrectomy can be done
(e) HMB–45 is positive

65. Renal cyst:
(a) 8 cm cyst–symptomatic, painful near hilum – Rx aspiration and sclerotherapy
(b) Represent 70% of asymptomatic renal masses
(c) 3 cm asymptomatic → observation
(d) Found in more than 50% of patients older than 50 years
(e) 8 cm lower pole cyst→laparoscopic deroofing is best

66. RCC:
(a) Paraneoplastic syndrome–20%
(b) RCC develops in about 50% of patients with von Hippel-Lindau disease
(c) Chromophilic RCC has better prognosis than chromophobic RCC
(d) Belleni duct carcinoma most commonly seen in 5th–7th decade
(e) Belleni duct carcinoma seen only in patients with SCA

67. Ureteric tumor:
(a) In low grade tumor endoscopic management can be done
(b) If endoscopy +ve and cytology –ve observation can be done
(c) If cytology +ve, endoscopy –ve and IVP is –ve nephroureterectomy should be done
(d) T_3 tumor should be treated with adjuvant chemotherapy
(e) Most common site of urothelial tumor is upper ureter

68. Regarding angiomyolipoma (AML):
(a) Tuberous sclerosis (TS) is seen in upto 50% cases of AML
(b) On USG it is hypoechoic
(c) Enhancement on CT is diagnostic
(d) If 6 cm AML bleeds, nephrectomy should be considered
(e) AML is usually bilateral in TS patients

69. Regarding oncocytoma:
(a) Most common benign tumor
(b) Cart-wheel appearance on angiography
(c) Granularity due to mitochondria
(d) If less than 4 cm with compromised contralateral kidney–partial nephrectomy can be considered
(e) The central stellate scar observed on CT scan

70. Renal cyst:
(a) Eight cm cyst near hilum and is symptomatic–treatment is aspiration and sclerosis
(b) Eight cm lower pole cyst–treatment is marsupialisation
(c) Five cm asymptomatic cyst–treatment is observation
(d) Five cm cyst in bilateral kidney–patient can be potential donor
(e) Eight cm upper pole cyst–treatment is laparoscopic deroofing

71. Regarding RCC:
(a) Paraneoplastic syndrome is present in 20% of patients
(b) RCC develops in about 50% of patients with VHL disease
(c) Papillary have good prognosis and is hypovascular
(d) In metastatic tumor MDR-2 mutation is seen
(e) Bellini duct carcinoma is present most commonly in 5th to 7th decade

72. Regarding ureteric tumor:
(a) In low grade tumor endoscopic management can be done
(b) If endoscopy is positive and cytology is negative–surgery should be done
(c) If cytology is positive and endoscopy and IVU is negative nephroureterectomy should be done

(d) In T3 tumor adjuvant chemotherapy will yield good result
(e) The risk of tumor recurrence in a remaining ureteral stump is 33% to 75%

Which of the following statement is correct?

73. Sunitinib-mechanism of action is:
(a) Inhibitor of VEGFR2
(b) Humanized monoclonal antibody against VEGF-A
(c) Inhibitor of PDGFR
(d) Inhibitor of *c-KIT*
(e) Inhibitor of fms-like tyrosine kinase-3

74. AML – most useful and reliable investigation:
(a) CT
(b) Radionuclide scan
(c) USG
(d) MRI
(e) X-ray KUB

75. Renal biopsy is laparoscopically contraindicated in:
(a) Renal failure
(b) Anticoagulation
(c) Solitary kidney
(d) Uncontrolled hypertension
(e) Morbid obesity

76. Which renal tumor involve renal vein / IVC?
(a) Oncocytoma
(b) Clear cell RCC
(c) AML
(d) Papillary RCC
(e) Upper tract TCC involving kidney

77. PNET of kidney:
(a) Derived from neural crest
(b) Associated with Ewing's sarcoma family
(c) Immunotherapy is the primary treatment
(d) Minimal enhancement in CT scan is characteristic
(e) HPE homer wright rosettes seen

78. Paraneoplastic syndrome of RCC – all *except*:
(a) Anemia (b) Polycythemia
(c) Hypertension (d) Hyperkalemia
(e) Hypercalcemia

79. Hormonal treatment for RCC:
(a) Medroxyprogesterone acetate
(b) Stanazol
(c) Ethyl estradiol
(d) Tamoxifen
(e) Megestrol acetate

80. Following partial nephrectomy for 3 cm RCC after 12 months follow up, investigations required:
(a) LFT and RFT
(b) USG abdomen
(c) CECT
(d) History and clinical examination
(e) X-ray chest

81. Prognostic factor for renal cell carcinoma is:
(a) Lymph node staging
(b) DNA ploidy
(c) IVC involvement
(d) Histological subtype
(e) Nuclear grade

82. Reninoma:
(a) Type of hemangiopericytoma
(b) Associated with factor VIII immuno-histopathological staining
(c) Hypokalemia common
(d) Hyperkalemia common
(e) Antiandrogen is treatment

83. Renal cyst and RCC coexists in:
(a) ADPKD (b) TS
(c) VHL (d) ARCD
(e) Medullary sponge kidney

84. Anticancer hormone:
(a) Tamoxifen (b) Bicalutamide
(c) Goserelin (d) Sunitinib
(e) Methotrexate

85. 48-year-old male, right RCC with single lung metastasis, FNAB clear cell carcinoma, treatment option:

(a) Cytoreductive nephrectomy
(b) Metastasectomy
(c) Targeted molecular therapy
(d) Chemotherapy
(e) Radiotherapy

86. Upper urinary tract TCC most common site:

(a) Upper pole calyx (b) Lower pole calyx
(c) Lower ureter (d) Upper ureter
(e) Renal pelvis

87. 90-year-old female patient, DM with CAD with good performance status, 3 cm left RCC, rational treatment:

(a) Nephron sparing surgery
(b) Radical nephrectomy
(c) Microwave therapy
(d) Observation
(e) Cryoablation

88. Which of the following drugs is the front line choice for metastatic renal cell cancer with poor risk factors?

(a) Sunitinib
(b) Pazopanib
(c) Axitinib
(d) Temsirolimus

89. Radiological findings of RCC:

(a) Heterogeneous mass
(b) Enhancement
(c) Calcification
(d) Change in renal outline
(e) Increase density

90. Routine screening for renal cell carcinoma is not justified in:

(a) Patients in end stage renal disease
(b) Patients with tuberous sclerosis
(c) Patients with autosomal dominant polycystic kidney disease
(d) Patients with known VHL syndrome

91. 4 cm RCC – treatment option in 60-year-old male:

(a) Partial nephrectomy
(b) Radical nephrectomy
(c) Immunotherapy
(d) Chemotherapy
(e) Radiotherapy

92. Hereditary RCC in VHL:

(a) Young age
(b) Multifocal and unilateral
(c) Multicentric and bilateral
(d) Papillary
(e) Retinal angiomas

93. Incidence of AML in tuberous sclerosis:

(a) 10% (b) 30%
(c) 40% (d) 50%
(e) 75%

94. 70-year-old diabetic, ejection fraction 40%, known CAD, 2.5 cm homogenous solid, right renal mass – treatment option:

(a) Radical nephrectomy
(b) Lap cryoablation
(c) Observation with 6 monthly ultrasound
(d) NSS
(e) Lap radical nephrectomy

95. Radiological features of malignant renal mass:

(a) Calcification
(b) Contrast enhancement
(c) Heterogeneous enhancing lesion
(d) Increase density
(e) Change in contour of kidney

96. Best prognosis for renal cell carcinoma is in:

(a) Chromophobe cells (b) Clear cell
(c) Spindle cell (d) Diploid
(e) Aneuploidy

97. Localised renal pelvis transitional cell carcinoma – treatment options are:

(a) Radical nephrectomy
(b) Radical nephroureterectomy

(c) Chemotherapy
(d) Immunotherapy
(e) Endoscopic treatment

98. Regarding renal cell carcinoma which is not correct?
(a) Suprahepatic IVC thrombus– treatment of choice is chemotherapy
(b) LN dissection prolongs survival
(c) Surgery best for organ confined disease
(d) Most common cause of death in VHL is RCC
(e) Renal oncocytoma – good prognosis

99. Immunotherapy in metastatic RCC – all *except*:
(a) Response rate for IL2 is 15%
(b) Remission occurs and last for >2 years
(c) Best given IV
(d) Results better with medroxyprogesterone
(e) Most effective in single lung metastasis

100. Characteristics of simple renal cortical cyst:
(a) No enhancement
(b) Smooth sharp margin
(c) Mixed density
(d) No internal echoes
(e) Thorough transmission of wave

101. Causes of hypertension in RCC:
(a) Partial renal artery obstruction
(b) Increased renin
(c) Increased cortisol
(d) Hyperkalemia
(e) Increased ICT due to brain metastasis

102. Cytoreductive therapy for RCC with multiple lung metastasis, Hb 10.0, serum calcium 10.2 after correction, diagnosis of metastatic disease 11 months after nephrectomy and LDH levels twice of normal and karnofsky 80%. It will be classified as grade:
(a) Very poor (b) Poor
(c) Intermediate (d) High

103. Female with bilateral AML with past history of seizures with bilateral flank pain is associated with which chromosomes and mode of inheritance:
(a) AD 16,9 (b) AD 16,4
(c) AR 16,9 (d) AR 16,4

104. Best prognosis for RCC:
(a) PNET (b) Carcinoid
(c) Sarcoma (d) Adult Wilms

105. All are true *except*:
(a) VHL–pheochromocytoma
(b) VHL–clear cell RCC
(c) MEN 2 with RET–pheochromocytoma
(d) Wilms–13p11

106. Fetal hepatotoxicity:
(a) Sunitinib (b) Sorafenib
(c) Temsirolimus (d) Pazopinib

107. A 72 years old man incidentally detected to have right small solid renal mass (size: 2.8 cm) on routine ultrasound examination of abdomen, what is your line of management?
(a) FNAC of the mass
(b) Radiofrequency ablation
(c) Active surveillance
(d) Partial nephrectomy

108. Anatrophic kidney dissection, sequence of steps:
(a) Ice slush - clamp - surgery - declamp
(b) Ice slush - surgery
(c) Clamp - ice slush - surgery - declamp
(d) Surgery - clamp - ice slush

109. Lady with seizure and angiomyolipoma is associated with:
(a) Autosomal dominant 4 and 16
(b) AR 4 and 16
(c) AD 9 and 16
(d) AR 9 and 16

110. Most commonly associated with angiomyolipoma:
(a) Tuberous sclerosis

(b) VHL
(c) Neurofibromatosis
(d) Birt Hogg Dube syndrome

111. Liquid nitrogen cryotherapy used in:
(a) Renal carcinoma
(b) Bladder carcinoma
(c) Testicular carcinoma
(d) Ureteric carcinoma

112. Good prognosis for renal carcinoma:
(a) Ca-9
(b) TP 53 staining is positive
(c) Thrombocytopenia
(d) Bone metastasis

113. Diabetic patient with low grade carcinoma renal pelvis. Management is:
(a) Radical nephroureterectomy
(b) Partial nephrectomy
(c) Ureteroscopic resection of tumor
(d) Percutaneous resection

114. VHL is associated with which RCC:
(a) Clear cell (b) Papillary
(c) Chromophobe (d) Sarcomatoid

115. RCC with single metastasis, best prognosis with:
(a) Pulmonary (b) Liver
(c) Spine (d) Brain

116. ECOG score — light physical activity without assistance is scored as:
(a) 0 (b) 1
(c) 2 (d) 3

117. Surgery is curative in RCC in all *except*:
(a) T3b N0M0 (b) T2N1M0
(c) T1N0M0 (d) T2N0M0

118. 3.5 cm upper polar mass best treatment:
(a) Partial upper polar nephrectomy
(b) Retroperitoneal radical nephrectomy
(c) Transperitoneal radical nephrectomy
(d) Partial upper polar nephrectomy with ipsilateral adrenalectomy

119. Loss of heterozygosity on chromosome 16q is associated with which malignancy?
(a) RCC
(b) WT
(c) Angiomyolipoma
(d) Leydig cell tumor

120. Most common site of carcinoma ureter (TCC):
(a) Proximal 1/3rd (b) Distal 1/3rd
(c) Mid 1/3rd (d) Renal pelvis

121. Chromophobe cell variant is a type of:
(a) RCC (b) Testicular tumor
(c) Oncocytoma (d) Wilms tumor

122. Most common benign renal mass:
(a) AML
(b) Renal cyst
(c) RCC
(d) Multiloculated cystic nephroma

123. All *except* one is seen in VHL:
(a) Epididymal cystadenoma
(b) Cyst of pancreas
(c) Oncocytoma
(d) Renal cyst

124. AML on USG is:
(a) Hypoechogenic
(b) Hyperechogenic
(c) Hyperechogenic with shadowing
(d) Isoechogenic

125. Lymphadenectomy in carcinoma of renal pelvis:
(a) Improves prognostication
(b) Improves survival
(c) Therapeutic
(d) Not to be done

126. Biopsy in RCC is not used because:
(a) Difficulty in differentiating between oncocytoma and eosinophilic RCC

(b) Needle track seeding
(c) Risk of infection
(d) Risk of bleeding

127. Most common sarcoma of kidney:
(a) Leiomyosarcoma
(b) Liposarcoma
(c) Rhabdomyosarcoma
(d) Osteosarcoma

128. Birt-Hogg-Dubé syndrome has all *except*:
(a) Chromophilic
(b) Oncocytoma
(c) Cutaneous fibrofolliculomas
(d) Spontaneous pneumothoraces

129. Right kidney: cytology positive, normal intravenous urography and retrograde pyelography, normal cystoscopy, and normal biopsy findings from the bladder and urethra:
(a) RGP
(b) RGP with ureteropyeloscopy
(c) IVP
(d) Repeat properly collected upper tract samples

130. Four cm central renal tumor with Serum creatinine 1 mg/dl, contralateral kidney normal in 55-year-old male, treatment of choice is:
(a) Open radical nephrectomy
(b) Partial nephrectomy
(c) Observation
(d) Lap radical nephrectomy

131. Patient with history of seizure, bilateral incidental 3 cm renal mass on CT with -20 HU, what is the diagnosis and treatment to be done?
(a) TS with AML with observation
(b) TS with AML with bilateral partial nephrectomy
(c) RCC with bilateral radical nephrectomy
(d) RCC with bilateral partial nephrectomy

132. 5 cm upper pole RCC in right kidney in patients with DM, 25% function of left kidney, what is to be done?
(a) Right partial nephrectomy
(b) Radical nephrectomy
(c) Observation if age is 80 years
(d) Cryosurgery if age is 80 years

133. Drug not used in metastatic RCC:
(a) Bevacizumab (b) Trastuzumab
(c) Sorafenib (d) Sunitinib

134. All are true about VHL *except*:
(a) Transmitted in AD fashion
(b) May have cyst in pancreas and epididymis
(c) Pheochromocytoma is the most common cause of death
(d) Mutated or absent VHL gene causes increased VEGF

135. Sunitinib is used in:
(a) Metastatic RCC
(b) Metastatic adrenocortical tumor
(c) Metastatic bladder malignancy
(d) Metastatic prostate malignancy

136. Sunitinib–Mechanism of action:
(a) Tyrosine kinase inhibitor
(b) IgG1 monoclonal antibody recognizing and binding all VEGF isoforms
(c) Inhibits Raf kinase
(d) Inhibits PDGF

137. The most common renal tumor in patients with sickle cell trait is:
(a) Renal medullary carcinoma
(b) Oncocytoma
(c) Angiomyolipoma
(d) Medullary renal tumor

138. VHL, chromosome involved is:
(a) 6 (b) 5
(c) 4 (d) 3

139. VHL mutated gene is:
(a) Tumor inhibitor
(b) Tumor promotor
(c) Tumor suppressor
(d) Tumor initiator

140. Incidence of renal neoplasm principally adenomas in patients receiving chronic hemodialysis is:
(a) Less than 1% (b) 10–20%
(c) 10% (d) 20–30%

141. USG not a very useful modality in which renal pathology?
(a) Renal tumor (b) Hydronephrosis
(c) Malrotations (d) Ureteric stone

142. Hyperechoic renal mass lesion with shadowing on USG is seen in:
(a) Oncocytoma
(b) Angiomyolipoma
(c) RCC
(d) Wilms' tumor

143. Best modality to diagnose a renal mass is:
(a) MRI gadolinium (b) Contrast CT
(c) USG (d) Angiography

144. All the following are tumor suppressor gene in humans *except*:
(a) RB gene (b) p53
(c) APC (d) erb-B2

145. Following is not a relative contraindication of retroperitoneal approach:
(a) Previous percutaneous renal surgery
(b) Previous open renal surgery
(c) History of radiotherapy
(d) History of xanthogranulomatous pyelonephritis

146. Which of the following is not a poor prognostic factor for metastatic RCC?
(a) Karnofsky performance core <80%
(b) Elevated lactate dehydrogenase (> 1.5 times upper limit of normal)
(c) Elevated corrected calcium (> 10 mg/dl)
(d) Prior nephrectomy status

147. True about recurrence after partial nephrectomy for RCC:
(a) Incidence is 30 to 50%
(b) Most commonly seen in tumor bed
(c) Commonly due to persistence of the tumor
(d) Thermal ablation is a treatment option

148. Following is true regarding the prenatal ultrasonography of renal cysts:
(a) In MCKD cyst are distributed peripherally
(b) In MCKD renal cysts are usually communicating
(c) A cyst in the upper pole of kidney is usually a dilated upper pole of duplex kidney
(d) Presence of central large cyst is characteristic of MCDK

149. Familial renal cell carcinoma has been associated with:
(a) Tuberous sclerosis
(b) Renal cystic disease
(c) Renal angiomyolipoma
(d) Von Hippel-Lindau disease

150. Wunderlich's syndrome is associated with:
(a) Oncocytoma
(b) Angiomyolipoma
(c) Metanephric adenoma
(d) Multilocular cystic nephroma

151. First and most constant branch of renal artery:
(a) Posterior (b) Anterior
(c) Apical (d) Basal

152. Most common type of renal sarcoma:
(a) Liposarcoma
(b) Leiomyosarcoma
(c) Angiosarcoma
(d) Fibrosarcoma

153. Most common site of RCC:
(a) PCT (b) DCT
(c) Glomeruli (d) CD

154. Most common site of renal metastasis:
(a) Liver (b) Lung
(c) Breast (d) Colon

155. For 15 cm RCC nephrectomy done, continuous low grade fever, most common cause:
(a) Deep seated wound infection
(b) Distal metastasis
(c) Foreign body
(d) Paraneoplastic syndrome

156. Poorest prognostic factor in RCC is:
(a) Lymph node involvement
(b) Perinephric fat involvement
(c) Thrombus in IVC
(d) Histological subtype

157. Biological agent used in metastatic renal cell carcinoma:
(a) Sunitinib (b) Leuprolide
(c) Bicalutamide (d) Finasteride

158. Which of the following is most fatal genitourinary malignancy?
(a) Prostate (b) Kidney
(c) Bladder (d) Penile

159. Which one of the following is found in VHL?
(a) Cerebellar hemangioblastoma
(b) Epididymis cystadenoma
(c) Endolymphatic tumor
(d) All of the above

160. Investigation of choice for IVC thrombosis in case of RCC:
(a) USG
(b) MRI
(c) CT scan
(d) Transesophageal ECHO

161. Spontaneous regression of metastasis after primary treatment is seen with:
(a) RCC (b) Lung cancer
(c) Gastric cancer (d) Colorectal cancer

162. The most common metastasis to spontaneously regress in RCC:
(a) Liver (b) Lung
(c) Bone (d) Adrenal

163. Renal biopsy is most commonly associated with:
(a) Hematuria (b) Flank pain
(c) Hypotension (d) Tachycardia

164. Regarding renal malignancy all are true *except:*
(a) > 15 HU enhancement of solitary lesions suggestive of malignancy
(b) 20 HU enhancement suggestive of oncocytoma
(c) Solid masses with <–20 HU–indicative of fat are diagnostic of AMLs
(d) MRI is the investigation of choice for RCC with IVC thrombus

165. Regarding VHL all are true *except:*
(a) Autosomal dominant inheritance
(b) Cysts seen in epididymis and pancreas
(c) Chromosome 3 mutation
(d) Associated with increase in VEGF

166. Simple renal cyst all are true *except:*
(a) Most common benign tumor of kidney
(b) 70% of asymptomatic masses
(c) M: F ratio 1:2
(d) 50% incidence in age >50 years
(e) Solitary mostly

167. Renal oncocytoma all are true *except:*
(a) 3-7% of all solid renal tumors
(b) Benign
(c) Truly encapsulated
(d) Cannot be differentiated from RCC
(e) Histopathology shows large mitochondria

168. Stauffer's syndrome all are true *except:*
(a) Seen in renal cell carcinoma
(b) 3-20% incidence
(c) Alkaline phosphatase increased in 50%
(d) PT increase in 67%
(e) Bilirubin increase in 20-30%

169. RCC with thrombus in venous system all are true *except:*
(a) Level determined by distal extent
(b) Level determined by proximal extent
(c) Cardiopulmonary bypass required for thrombus extending into right atrium
(d) Deep hypothermic circulatory arrest can be maintained for 40 min
(e) Venovenous bypass can be an alternative for supradiaphragmatic thrombus not extending into right atrium

170. Complications of partial nephrectomy in RCC all are true *except:*
(a) Hemorrhage
(b) Renal insufficiency
(c) Urinary fistula
(d) Pneumothorax
(e) Infections

171. Clear cell RCC is most commonly seen in:
(a) VHL syndrome
(b) HPRCC
(c) Acquired renal cystic disease
(d) Birt-Hogg-Dube syndrome

172. Balkan nephropathy commonly causes:
(a) RCC
(b) Ureteral tumors
(c) Bladder carcinoma
(d) Prostate carcinoma

173. Risk factor for RCC includes all *except:*
(a) Smoking
(b) Obesity
(c) Hypertension
(d) Excessive coffee intake

174. Which variant of RCC has affinity for the ulex europaeus?
(a) Clear cell (b) Papillary
(c) Collecting duct (d) Belleni duct

175. RCC classic triad includes:
(a) Flank pain (b) Fever
(c) Hematuria (d) Lump

176. SSIGN score for clear cell RCC incorporates:
(a) TNM stage (b) Tumor size
(c) Nuclear grade (d) Histology

177. Pluck technique, should be reserved for:
(a) Renal cell carcinoma
(b) Prostate carcinoma
(c) Proximal, low-grade urothelial tumors
(d) Bladder carcinoma

178. Chromophobe cell carcinoma of the kidney is a distinct entity of renal cell carcinoma and is proposed to arise from:
(a) Mesenchymal derivatives
(b) Proximal tubular epithelium
(c) Glomerulus and/or loop of Henle
(d) Cortical portion of collecting duct

179. Von Hippel-Lindau disease predisposes patients to:
(a) Bilateral testicular tumors
(b) Bilateral clear cell renal tumors
(c) Bilateral papillary renal carcinoma
(d) Bilateral adrenocortical carcinoma

180. First laparoscopic nephrectomy was done by:
(a) Schussler (b) Clayman
(c) Figenshau (d) Gaur

181. To differentiate RCC from pseudotumor modality of choice is:
(a) DMSA (b) CT
(c) USG (d) MRI

182. Which of the following is true regarding oncocytoma of the kidney?
(a) They are derived from proximal renal tubules
(b) Frozen section clearly distinguishes oncocytoma from RCC
(c) Percutaneous biopsy is strictly contraindicated
(d) Radiologically it can be indistinguishable from RCC

183. Papillary RCC is associated with trisomy of:
(a) Chromosomes 2 and 13
(b) Chromosomes 7 and 17
(c) Chromosome 3
(d) Chromosomes 5 and 15

184. Which of the following is not an approved treatment modality for renal cell carcinoma?
(a) Cryoablation
(b) Radiofrequency ablation
(c) HIFU
(d) Laparoscopic partial nephrectomy

185. Which of the following is correct about unilateral renal agenesis?
(a) Ipsilateral gonad is frequently absent
(b) Ipsilateral ureter is absent in all cases
(c) Fifty percent of women have concomitant uterine anomaly
(d) Adrenal agenesis occurs in 10–17% of individuals

186. Postradical nephrectomy with high drain serosanguinous discharge on POD1 with fever, following evaluation should be done:
(a) Fluid and blood culture
(b) CECT abdomen and pelvis
(c) Serum and fluid creatinine
(d) Serum albumin and chyle in drain fluid
(e) Serum and fluid hemoglobin

187. Noninvasive papillary carcinoma bladder false is:
(a) Nuclei are elongated with inconspicuous nucleoli
(b) Mitoses are rare
(c) Umbrella cells are usually present in low grade
(d) Low grade associated with delicate branching pattern on histology
(e) Branching not seen

188. About Lesch-Nyhan syndrome true:
(a) Poor reflexes
(b) Extrapyramidal syndrome
(c) Mental retardation
(d) Hyperuricemia
(e) Bladder stone

189. Differential diagnosis of 46 years female with history of myomectomy 2 years back, now complaint of right sided abdominal pain for year, palpable mobile mass, non-tender soft abdomen, urine c/s 60000 cfu, mix flora.
(a) PID
(b) Torsion of ovary
(c) Chronic pyelonephritis
(d) Renal ptosis
(e) Stone

190. Thrombus in IVC and renal vein is associated with:
(a) Papillary RCC
(b) AML
(c) Nephritic syndrome
(d) Conventional RCC
(e) Transitional cell carcinoma invading kidney

191. About RCC staging (AJCC 2009) false is:
(a) Adrenal ipsilateral involvement is T3a
(b) CT sensitivity for IVC thrombosis is 96%
(c) Segmental renal vein involvement is T3b
(d) Renal sinus fat involvement without Gerota's invasion in T3a
(e) MRI and multiplanner CT for IVC thrombosis diagnosis are nearly equivalent

192. Regarding upper tract TCC true is:
(a) Perinephric fat involvement through renal parenchyma is T3
(b) Regional lymphadenectomy should be done along with nephroureterectomy
(c) Neoadjuvant chemotherapy should be given in all patients
(d) T2 is renal parenchymal involvement
(e) Stage is the most important prognostic factor

193. A 40 years lady with 12 cm lower pole renal mass with surrounding hematoma with Hb of 7 gm/dl, on NCCT –30 HU, next management is:
(a) Angioembolization
(b) Partial nephrectomy
(c) Radical nephrectomy
(d) Observation
(e) RFA

194. A 45 years old man presented with total painless hematuria of 2 weeks duration. Plain X-ray KUB and Ultrasound scanning revealed 2 cm complex cyst with mural calcification on right kidney. What is the next investigation of choice?
(a) CECT
(b) MRI
(c) PET-CT
(d) Nuclear scintigraphy

ANSWERS

1.	A	26.	FFTTF	51.	FTTTF	76.	B	101.	ABE
2.	B	27.	FTFFT	52.	TTTTF	77.	ABDE	102.	B
3.	C	28.	TFTFT	53.	TFFFT	78.	ABCE	103.	A
4.	B	29.	TTFFF	54.	TTFTF	79.	AE	104.	B
5.	A	30.	FFFFT	55.	TTFTT	80.	D	105.	D
6.	B	31.	TTTFF	56.	TTTTF	81.	ABCDE	106.	A
7.	D	32.	TFTTF	57.	TTFTT	82.	ABC	107.	A
8.	A	33.	TTTTT	58.	FFTTT	83.	BCD	108.	C
9.	C	34.	TTTTT	59.	TTFTT	84.	ABC	109.	A
10.	C	35.	FTTTT	60.	TFFFT	85.	ABC	110.	A
11.	A	36.	TFTTT	61.	FTFTT	86.	E	111.	A
12.	A	37.	TFTFF	62.	TTTTT	87.	D	112.	A
13.	C	38.	TFTTF	63.	TFFTT	88.	D	113.	D
14.	B	39.	FTTTF	64.	FTTTT	89.	ABCDE	114.	A
15.	A	40.	TFTTT	65.	FTTTT	90.	A	115.	A
16.	B	41.	FFTTT	66.	TTTFF	91.	AB	116.	B
17.	A	42.	TTTTF	67.	TFFTF	92.	ACDE	117.	A
18.	A	43.	TFTTT	68.	TFFTT	93.	B	118.	D
19.	B	44.	FFFTF	69.	FTTTT	94.	C	119.	B
20.	A	45.	TTFTT	70.	FFTFT	95.	ABCDE	120.	D
21.	A	46.	FFTFF	71.	TTTFF	96.	A	121.	A
22.	TTFTF	47.	FTTFT	72.	TTFTT	97.	BE	122.	B
23.	TFTTF	48.	TTFFF	73.	ACDE	98.	AB	123.	C
24.	FFFTT	49.	TFFFF	74.	A	99.	BD	124.	B
25.	TTTTT	50.	TFTFT	75.	B	100.	ABDE	125.	A

126.	A	141.	D	156.	A	171.	A	186.	AD
127.	B	142.	B	157.	A	172.	B	187.	BE
128.	A	143.	B	158.	B	173.	D	188.	CDE
129.	B	144.	D	159.	D	174.	C	189.	D
130.	B	145.	A	160.	B	175.	B	190.	CD
131.	A	146.	D	161.	A	176.	C	191.	AC
132.	A	147.	D	162.	B	177.	C	192.	ABE
133.	B	148.	C	163.	A	178.	D	193.	C
134.	C	149.	D	164.	B	179.	B	194.	A
135.	A	150.	B	165.	B	180.	B		
136.	C	151.	A	166.	D	181.	A		
137.	A	152.	B	167.	C	182.	D		
138.	D	153.	A	168.	C	183.	B		
139.	C	154.	B	169.	A	184.	C		
140.	C	155.	A	170.	D	185.	B		

CHAPTER 11

The Adrenals

1. Finasteride reduces prostate volume by:
(a) 10% (b) 20%
(c) 40% (d) 50%

2. Familial pheochromocytoma in VHL:
(a) Type 1 (b) Type 2A
(c) Type 2B (d) Type 2C

3. Lymphatic drainage of adrenal:
(a) Hilar in right
(b) Paracaval in left
(c) Paraaortic in left
(d) Paraduodenal in right

4. False about familial Wilms' tumor:
(a) 10% incidence
(b) 17, 19 chomosome
(c) Early onset
(d) Bilateral present

5. True about pheochromocytoma:
(a) Post operative ionotropic support depends upon the duration of surgery
(b) Intraoperative BP hikes depends upon the size of the tumor
(c) 6 cm tumor can be done laparoscopically
(d) Incidence of pheochromocytoma in VHL is 40%

Which of the following statement is correct ?

6. Pheochromocytoma-anesthetic agent used:
(a) Isoflurane (b) Guanethidine
(c) Halothane (d) Fentanyl
(e) Thiopental

7. Features of primary aldosteronism (Conn's) is:
(a) Hypertension (b) Hypernatremia
(c) Edema (d) Increased K^+
(e) Decreased pH

8. Adrenal anatomy false is:
(a) Right adrenal lies posterolateral to IVC
(b) Posterior surface of both adrenals in contact with posterior diaphragm
(c) Inferior phrenic artery is the main blood supply
(d) Covered by Gerota's fascia
(e) Adrenal medulla constitutes 90% of gland

9. MIBG used in:
(a) Carcinoid
(b) Islet cell tumor
(c) Pheochromocytoma
(d) Neuroblastoma
(e) Wilms' tumor

10. Conn's syndrome manifestation:
(a) Hypertension (b) Hyperkalemia
(c) Increased Na^+ (d) Edema
(e) Metabolic acidosis

11. Pheochromocytoma-anesthetic drugs used are:
(a) Thiopentone (b) Propofol
(c) Halothane (d) Ketamine
(e) Isoflurane

12. Pheochromocytoma is localized by:
(a) Iodine 131 MIBG scan
(b) CT (c) MRI
(d) DTPA (e) PET scan

13. Conn's syndrome (hyperaldosteronism):
(a) Edema (b) Hypertension
(c) Hyperkalemia (d) Hypernatremia
(e) Acidosis

14. Tumor arising from adrenal cortex:
(a) CAH
(b) Ganglioneuroma
(c) Pheochromocytoma
(d) Paragangliomas
(e) Neuroblastoma

15. Most direct way to demonstrate pituitary hypersecretion of ACTH is:
(a) 24-hour excretion of cortisol in the urine
(b) Concurrent measurement of both plasma ACTH and cortisol
(c) Measure ACTH level in the petrosal venous sinus and compare the level with the peripheral level
(d) Morning plasma aldosterone (ng/dl) to renin (ng/ml/hr) ratio (ARR)

16. Primary hyperaldosteronism what is to be done to ensure hypokalemia:
(a) Normal Na (b) Low Na
(c) Low K (d) Normal K

17. In primary hyperaldosteronism which is to be done to check hypokalemia?
(a) Low Na diet (b) Low K diet
(c) Normal Na diet (d) Normal K diet

18. Hypokalemia associated with:
(a) Meta Acidosis (b) Meta Alkalosis
(c) Resp Acidosis (d) Resp Alkalosis

19. Primary hyperaldosteronism all *except*:
(a) Hypokalemia (b) Low PRA
(c) High aldosterone (d) Hyperkalemia

20. Clonidine suppression test differentiate between:
(a) Paraganglioma and pheochromocytoma
(b) Functioning and non-functioning pheochromocytoma
(c) Pheochromocytoma and essential HTN
(d) Functional and non-functional myelolipoma

21. False about adrenal gland:
(a) Adrenal weight at birth is larger than in adult
(b) Measure up to 5 cm in length, 3 cm in width and 1 cm thick
(c) The fetal adrenal cortex increases rapidly during the first 6 weeks of life
(d) Healthy, non stressed adult, the glands weigh about 5 g each

22. Normotensive in pheochromocytoma:
(a) 5% (b) 10%
(c) 15% (d) 20%

23. All are present in Cushing's syndrome, *except:*
(a) Hyperkalemia
(b) Weight gain
(c) Metabolic alkalosis
(d) Stria

24. Rate limiting step in adrenal cortical steroid synthesis is:
(a) Pregnenolone
(b) 17 oxy ketosteroid
(c) 11 deoxy cortisone
(d) 21 deoxy cortisone

25. cGMP is degraded by:
(a) Phosphodiesterase (b) Pyruvate kinase
(c) Tyrosine kinase (d) NO

26. Shortest plasma half life:
(a) Cortisone (b) Cortisol
(c) Prednisolone (d) Aldosterone

27. Which of the following is not true for adrenals?
(a) Cortex maintain 3 layers
(b) Medulla contains chromaffin cells
(c) Adrenal absence is associated with renal agenesis
(d) Most of adrenal is cortex

28. Which one of the following is not present in MEN II?
(a) Pancreatic tumors
(b) Parathyroid adenoma
(c) Pheochromocytoma
(d) Medullary carcinoma thyroid

29. Sex steroids are secreted by which layer of adrenal cortex?
(a) Zona glomerulosa (b) Zona fasciculate
(c) Zona reticularis (d) Zona vasculosa

30. Most common cyst from which adrenocortical carcinoma arises:
(a) Endothelial (b) Epithelial
(c) Pseudocyst (d) Parasitic

31. Adrenal cortex is derived from:
(a) Endoderm (b) Mesoderm
(c) Ectoderm (d) Neural crest

32. About adrenal, one of the following statement is true:
(a) Pheochromocytomas are malignant in 90% of cases
(b) Pheochromocytoma may be found with VHL
(c) Twenty percent of patients with pheochromocytoma are normotensive
(d) Elevated levels of catecholamines in urine is seen in 10% of patients

33. The best treatment of adrenal adenoma resulting in Conn's syndrome is:
(a) Open adrenalectomy
(b) Laparoscopic adrenalectomy
(c) Partial adrenalectomy
(d) Bilateral adrenalectomy

34. Adrenals are supplied by:
(a) Inferior phrenic
(b) Branch from aorta
(c) Branch from ipsilateral renal artery
(d) All of the above

35. Adrenal medulla is innervated by:
(a) Pre-ganglionic sympathetic
(b) Post-ganglionic parasympathetic
(c) Pre-ganglionic cholinergic
(d) Post-ganglionic cholinergic

36. Best investigation for pheochromocytoma:
(a) CT (b) USG
(c) IVP (d) Angiography

37. Primary hyperaldosteronism all *except:*
(a) Hypokalemia (b) Hypertension
(c) Edema (d) Decrease in renin

38. Which is not the symptom of hyperaldosteronism?
(a) Hypokalemia
(b) Hypomagnesemia
(c) Hyponatremia
(d) Alkalosis

39. Pheochromocytoma all are true *except:*
(a) Incidence 0.1-0.6% in hypertensive patients
(b) Malignant in 50%
(c) Associated with NF in 1-2% cases
(d) 10% normotensive
(e) Is one of the common causes of hypertension

40. Adrenal cystic lesions all are true *except:*
(a) Incidental mostly
(b) Mostly unilateral
(c) 15% have calcification
(d) 45% lymphangiomatic
(e) Percutaneous drainage contraindicated

41. In pheochromocytoma '10% tumor' applies all *except:*
(a) Malignant (b) Adults
(c) Outside adrenal (d) Bilateral

42. The blood supply of the left adrenal gland is from:
(a) Aorta
(b) Aorta, left renal artery and inferior phrenic artery
(c) Left renal and inferior phrenic artery
(d) Aorta and left renal artery

43. The pattern of hypertension in a patient with pheochromocytoma is:
(a) Sustained
(b) Paroxysmal
(c) Sustained with superimposed paroxysms
(d) All of the above

44. Most common cause of Conn's syndrome is:

(a) Bilateral hyperplasia
(b) Adrenal adenoma
(c) Adrenal carcinoma
(d) Familial hyperaldosteronism

45. Investigations to diagnose s/o malignancy in incidental adrenal mass:

(a) Isointensity MRI (b) Histology
(c) Grade (d) Size
(e) Metabolic activity

46. Adrenal anatomy true are:

(a) Supplied by postganglionic fibers
(b) In renal agenesis, adrenal present but in orthotropic position
(c) All control all responses
(d) Glomerulosa layer outermost
(e) Left adrenal gland is more superiorly located than right

47. Non germ cell testicular tumor are:

(a) Sertoli cell
(b) Seminoma
(c) Leyding cell tumor
(d) YST
(e) Lymphoma

48. The antihypertensives of choice in primary aldosteronism are:

(a) Phenoxybenzamine and propranolol
(b) Prazosin and eplerenone
(c) Spironolactone and eplerenone
(d) Guanethidine and spironolactone

ANSWERS

1.	B	11.	AE	21.	C	31.	B	41.	B
2.	D	12.	ABC	22.	B	32.	B	42.	B
3.	C	13.	BD	23.	A	33.	B	43.	D
4.	A	14.	A	24.	A	34.	D	44.	B
5.	C	15.	C	25.	A	35.	A	45.	DE
6.	AE	16.	B	26.	D	36.	A	46.	BD
7.	AB	17.	A	27.	C	37.	C	47.	ACE
8.	ABCD	18.	D	28.	A	38.	C	48.	C
9.	ACD	19.	D	29.	C	39.	B		
10.	AC	20.	A	30.	C	40.	E		

CHAPTER 12

Urine Transport, Storage and Emptying

1. **Which of the following disorders may commonly lead to irritative voiding symptoms?**
   (a) Parkinson's disease
   (b) Renal cell carcinoma
   (c) Bladder diverticula
   (d) Prostate cancer
2. **Following cerebrovascular accident, involvement of which of the following is likely to lead to urinary incontinence?**
   (a) Internal capsule (b) Basal ganglia
   (c) Thalamus (d) Cerebellum
3. **Postganglionic sympathetic nerve fibres to the urinary bladder release:**
   (a) Acetylcholine
   (b) Epinephrine
   (c) Norepinephrine
   (d) Vasoactive intestinal polypeptide
4. **Botulinum toxin relaxes detrusor muscle tone by:**
   (a) Enhancing nitric oxide release
   (b) Blocking synaptosome associated membrane receptor (SNARE) proteins
   (c) Presynaptic neurovesical reuptake inhibition
   (d) Postsynaptic neurovesical antagonist
5. **The most common urodynamic abnormality in patients with voiding dysfunction, dysfunction secondary to Parkinson's disease is:**
   (a) Detrusor overactivity
   (b) Striated sphincter dyssynergia
   (c) Impaired sensation during filling
   (d) Impaired detrusor contractility
6. **Which of the following is the most common complication in absorbable stapled ileal pouches?**
   (a) Urine leak
   (b) Valve failure
   (c) Ureteral stricture
   (d) Ischemic pouch contraction
7. **Pouch stone development occurs most commonly with:**
   (a) T-pouch
   (b) Kock pouch
   (c) Penn pouch
   (d) Gastric ileus composite pouch
8. **Chronically elevated bladder filling pressures are detrimental to the upper tracts. The lowest pressure threshold most often reported to cause problems is:**
   (a) 20 cm H_2O (b) 30 cm H_2O
   (c) 40 cm H_2O (d) 50 cm H_2O
9. **Intrinsic smooth muscle pacemaker sites for ureter are located at:**
   (a) Major calyces
   (b) Minor calyces
   (c) Both major calyces and minor calyces
   (d) None of the above
10. **Peritoneum can be assessed transvaginally through the:**
    (a) Posterior fornix
    (b) Anterior fornix
    (c) Rectovaginal septum
    (d) Lateral fornices
11. **All are causes of "pear shaped" urinary bladder *except:***
    (a) Pelvic lipomatosis
    (b) Pelvic fibrosis
    (c) Iliopsoas hypertrophy
    (d) Retroperitoneal fibrosis

12. Most common cause of VVF in developing countries:
(a) Trauma (b) Obstructed labour
(c) Iatrogenic (d) Post surgical

13. Creating an antireflux mechanism is most difficult with anastomosis to the ......
(a) Stomach (b) Ileum
(c) Cecum (d) Sigmoid colon

14. Stress urinary incontinence:
(a) Is principally a disease of young females
(b) Is associated with urinary frequency and urgency
(c) May be corrected by surgically increasing the volume of the bladder
(d) Is a disease of aging produced by shortening of the urethra

15. True about apomorphine:
(a) Agonist of D1 and antagonist of D2 in brain
(b) Agonist of D1 and D2
(c) Antagonist of D1 and agonist of D2
(d) Antagonist of D1 and D2

16. When ileum used in augmentation cystoplasty?
(a) Contracture (b) Dehiscence
(c) Perforation (d) Stricture

17. Small contracted bladder with GFR 30:
(a) Stomach not used for augmentation because of HUS
(b) Stomach used because of least metabolic complications
(c) Ileum not used because poor contractibility
(d) Ileum used because renoprotective

18. Post radical prostatectomy has continuous incontinence:
(a) Sling has best overall performance rate
(b) AUS should only be used after 2 years
(c) Trial of injections durasphere before AUS
(d) Rule out anastomotic stricture before AUS

19. Young girl with continuous incontinence with normal intermittent voiding suggest:
(a) Ectopic ureter
(b) Ureterovaginal fistula
(c) Vesicovaginal fistula
(d) Urge incontinence

20. True about Lisch Gregor ureteric implantation:
(a) It's purely extravesical
(b) Combined extra and intravesical
(c) Intravesical
(d) Only done laparoscopically

Mention True and False respective to each statement (Q. No. 21 to 51)

21. Vaginal repair can be considered in VVF:
(a) High fistula
(b) Radiation associated
(c) Large vagina size
(d) Pliable tissue
(e) Fistula near ureteric orifice

22. Regarding anatomy of anterior abdominal wall:
(a) Superior epigastric artery is a branch of internal mammary artery
(b) Inferior epigastric artery is a branch of external iliac artery
(c) Intercostal artery does not supply rectus
(d) Superior epigastric artery gives branches to falciform ligament
(e) Arcuate line is a horizontal line that demarcates the lower limit of the posterior layer of the rectus sheath

23. Ureter:
(a) Arterial branches to the abdominal ureter approach from a medial direction
(b) True physical restriction of ureter is at PUJO
(c) Arterial vessels course longitudinally within the periureteral adventitia
(d) During ureteroscopy performation most common in upper part
(e) In ureteric orifice dilatation is done till 15-20 atm pressure

24. BCG:
(a) Attenuated mycobacterium bovis
(b) Increase fibronectin in urine is good prognosis
(c) TP 53 most frequent altered gene in bladder tumors
(d) BCG delays progression
(e) If two attempts of BCG fail, there is no further role of BCG therapy

25. In neurogenic bladder upper tract changes occur:
(a) >40 cm H_2O of DLPP
(b) <20 cm H_2O of DLPP
(c) DESD
(d) Hyperreflexic bladder
(e) Decrease compliance with hypocontractile bladder

26. Regarding artificial urinary sphincter:
(a) In men with post-prostatectomy incontinence, the bulbous urethra is route of implantation
(b) AUS cuff in children is placed at the bladder neck
(c) In the male patient with SUI who has not had previous radical prostatectomy, the cuff is placed around the bladder neck
(d) Swelling is the most likely cause of urinary retention in the immediate postoperative period
(e) Skin pathogens are the most commonly cultured organism with perioperative infections

27. Supratrigonal VVF:
(a) Martius flap cannot be used
(b) Peritoneal flap cannot be brought down by vaginal approach
(c) Most common in obstructed labor
(d) IVP should always be done
(e) Cannot be done by vaginal approach

28. Women with SUI with ALPP < 58 treatment options are:
(a) Biofeedback
(b) Pubovaginal sling
(c) Bladder neck suspension
(d) AUS
(e) Collagen injection

29. Orthotopic neobladder:
(a) Prostatic biopsy is taken during cystectomy, if orthotopic is planned
(b) Continuous CIC is required for always
(c) Hyperchloremic acidosis is more in orthotopic neobladder than in ileal conduit
(d) Ileal is the most commonly used segment
(e) The innervation of the striated urethral rhabdosphincter arises from the branches of the pudendal nerve

30. VVF supratrigonal:
(a) Obstructed labour is a cause
(b) IVP is not mandatory
(c) O'Connor repair is transabdominal approach
(d) Martius flap cannot be used
(e) In transvaginal repair peritoneal transposition is not done

31. Upper tract damage occurs in:
(a) DLPP > 40
(b) DLPP < 20
(c) DESD
(d) Overactive bladder
(e) AG number < 40 is suggestive of BOO

32. Following TAH, elderly female presents with total incontinence:
(a) VVF is most common cause
(b) Ureterovaginal fistula must be excluded
(c) Martius flap used for abdominal repair
(d) O'Connor flap is used in transvaginal repair
(e) Repair should be done after 8 months

33. Neural dysraphism:
(a) Myelomeningocele accounts for 90% of open neural tube defect
(b) Folate deficiency causes myelodysplasia
(c) Formation of spinal cord begins development at 18th day of gestation
(d) VUR is present in 3 to 5%
(e) VUR if not corrected can progress in 30–40%

34. Urodynamics with neurogenic bladder:
(a) DM–DESD
(b) Parkinson's disease–Normal compliance
(c) Suprasacral injury–Overactive bladder with DESD
(d) Autonomic reflexia below T_6
(e) Autonomic reflexia treatment is sublingual nifedipine with α blocker

35. Urethral pressure profile:
(a) UPP is measured along with whole length of urethra

(b) Maximum urethral closing pressure is the difference of urethral and intravesical pressure
(c) The urethral pressure is fluid pressure needed to just open a closed urethra
(d) Functional profile length is the length of the urethra along which the urethral pressure exceeds intravesical pressure in women
(e) Pressure transmission ratio: The increment in urethral pressure on stress as a percentage of the simultaneously recorded increment in intravesical pressure

36. Detrusor pressure:
(a) Pdet = Pves – Pabd
(b) Pdet can be measured directly
(c) Pdet > 30 cm indicates obstruction
(d) Pdet at Qmax if > 100–Indicates obstruction
(e) VLPP < 60 can cause ISD

37. Upper tract changes with obstruction occurs in:
(a) DLPP > 40
(b) DLPP< 20 mm Hg
(c) DESD
(d) Hypereflexia
(e) High complaint bladder

38. Vesicovaginal fistula:
(a) Repair mandatory after 3-6 months
(b) If discovered within 36-48 hours–immediate repair
(c) Management is individual based
(d) Radiation induced fistula repaired after 6-12 months
(e) Most common type of acquired fistula of the urinary tract

39. Regarding augmentation cystoplasty:
(a) Ileal cystoplasty is indicated for small capacity bladder
(b) In orthotropic bladder–Asymptomatic E. coli treatment is for 7-14 days
(c) Detubularization and reconfiguration should always be performed during augmentation cystoplasty
(d) The majority of bladder stones in this population of patients are struvite
(e) The main disadvantage of auto augmentation is a limited increase in bladder capacity

40. Continuous incontinence developing after radical abdominal hysterectomy:
(a) Most common cause is VVF
(b) Rule out ureterovaginal fistula
(c) O'Connor repair is transvaginal operation to treat VVF
(d) Martius flap is used in transabdominal surgery for VVF
(e) Ideally treated after 3-6 months

41. VVF:
(a) Most VVF in western world caused by malignancy
(b) In India most commonly caused by obstetrics causes
(c) All VVF can be repaired by transvaginal surgery
(d) Interposition of viable omentum is done
(e) In obstetric causes, VVF can be repaired within 4 weeks

42. Urethral support:
(a) Puborectal ligament
(b) Vesicopelvic ligament
(c) Uterosacral ligament
(d) Cardinal ligament
(e) Bulbourethral muscle

43. In Neurogenic bladder, upper tract changes occurs if:
(a) > 40 cm DLPP
(b) 40-20 cm DLPP
(c) < 20 cm of DLPP
(d) Underactive bladder
(e) DESE

44. Regarding urodynamic studies:
(a) Qmax < 10 ml/sec 70–80% have obstruction
(b) Qmax > 50 ml/sec–never obstruction
(c) AUA score of 30 will always require surgery
(d) If residual urine volume > 250 ml, requires surgery
(e) CMG is always done when nocturia > 4 times

45. 65 years female with stress urinary continence with ALPP of <38 cm, following are the Rx option:

(a) Biofeedback
(b) Collagen injection
(c) Artificial urinary sphincter
(d) Vaginal suspension procedures
(e) Pubourethral sling

46. Stress incontinence:
(a) Preceded with urgency
(b) Involuntary loss without detrusor contraction
(c) Can cause life threatening condition
(d) Post TURP 6-15% of patients will remain with overactive bladder
(e) CO_2 cystometry is better than liquid cystometry

47. Regarding pharmacology of bladder:
(a) M2 receptor causes contraction of bladder
(b) Tolterodine is M2 selective
(c) Side effect of oxybutynin is due to its active metabolite
(d) Intravesical pressure decreases as compliance decreases
(e) Compliance decreases due to increase in collagen

48. Regarding voiding:
(a) Initiated by onuf nucleus
(b) First step is increase in intravesical pressure
(c) Bladder distention causes increased sympathetic stimulation
(d) Lesion at pons causes DESD
(e) Micturition center is at pons

49. Regarding urodynamic studies:
(a) At Q max <10 ml/sec, 70% to 80% have obstruction
(b) Q max > 50 ml/sec, obstruction is never present
(c) Needle electrode is best for EMG
(d) If residual volume more than 250 ml is indication for surgery
(e) Cystoscopy is always done when nocturia is more than 4 times

50. 65-year-old male with SUI with ALPP <38 cm H_2O following are the treatment options:
(a) Biofeedback
(b) Collagen injection
(c) Artificial sphincter
(d) Suspension procedure (vaginal)
(e) Pubovaginal suburethral sling

51. Regarding incontinence:
(a) SUI is involuntary loss of urine
(b) Can cause life threatening condition
(c) CO_2 cystometry is better than liquid cystometry
(d) Urge incontinence is the voluntary loss of urine
(e) Postoperatively 6% to 15% have OAB

Which of the following statement is correct?

52. Metabolic abnormality in intestinal segment, true:
(a) Stomach–Hypochloremic, hypokalemic metabolic alkalosis
(b) Jejunum–Hypochloremia, hyperkalemic, hyponatremic metabolic acidosis
(c) Ileum–Hyperchloremia, hypokalemia, hypocalcemia metabolic acidosis
(d) Colon–Hyperchloremia, hypokalemia, hypocalcemia metabolic acidosis
(e) Stomach-Hypochloremic, hypokalemic metabolic acidosis

53. Non refluxing ureterovesical anastomosis is:
(a) Leadbetter and Clask (b) Goodwin
(c) Nesbit (d) Strickler
(e) Serosal tunnel

54. Anticholinergics with grade A recommendation that can be given in OAB:
(a) Atropine (b) Oxybutynin
(c) Probanthine (d) Darifenacin
(e) Tolterodine

55. Mixed incontinence includes:
(a) Overflow (b) Stress
(c) Continuous (d) Urge
(e) Postvoid

56. Orthotropic neobladder is contraindicated in females in:
(a) Trigone involvement with CIS
(b) Urethra involved

(c) Bladder neck involved
(d) T3
(e) Lymph node mass

57. 6 months after LSCS, lady presents with cyclical hematuria, causes (she is lactating):
(a) Endometriosis of bladder
(b) Youssef syndrome
(c) Choriocarcinoma
(d) Lactational amenorrhea
(e) Second pregnancy

58. Urinary diversion false:
(a) Mechanical bowel preparation done
(b) Refluxing causes more stenosis than non-refluxing
(c) Alkalosis causes osteomalacia
(d) Osteomalacia may be due to vitamin D resistance
(e) Alkaline phosphatase in osteomalacia may be normal or decreased

59. A 32-year-old female patient – LSCS done 6 months before, presented with cyclical hematuria during menstruation:
(a) Vesicouterine fistula
(b) Vesical endometriosis
(c) Endometroid tumor of bladder
(d) TCC bladder
(e) H. mole

60. Non-reflexing ureteroenteric anastomosis:
(a) Bricker (b) Wallace
(c) Pogano (d) Goodwin
(e) Strickler

61. Ureterosigmoidostomy complications:
(a) Acidosis (b) Alkalosis
(c) Hypokalemia (d) Hyperkalemia
(e) Hyperchloremia

62. In VVF repair, flap used:
(a) Omental flap (b) Martius flap
(c) Gabriel flap (d) Mathew flap
(e) Gracilis flap

63. DESD treatment is:
(a) Baclofen
(b) Dantrolene sodium
(c) Bethanechol
(d) Sphincterotomy
(e) SPC

64. One day old female with lower abdominal mass – USG showed mass between rectum and bladder:
(a) Sacrococcygeal teratoma
(b) Fluid filled vagina
(c) Hydrocolpos
(d) Prolapsed ureterocele
(e) Prolapse urethra

65. In DESD treatment which is not used?
(a) Sphincterotomy
(b) SPC
(c) Baclofen
(d) Dantrolene
(e) Diversion procedures

66. Non-reflux urinary diversion is:
(a) Wallace (b) Bricker
(c) Wipple (d) Strickler
(e) Goodwin

67. In VVF–which arterialized flap is used?
(a) Gracilis
(b) Martius
(c) Omental
(d) Rectus abdominis
(e) Bone flap

68. Most important factor for healing of VVF:
(a) Bladder relaxant to prevent spasm
(b) Proximal urinary diversion to keep bladder dry
(c) Continuous bladder drainage by catheter
(d) Absolute bed rest
(e) Antibiotics

69. Non-refluxing ureteroenteric anastomosis:
(a) Strickler
(b) Wallace
(c) Goodwin
(d) Nipple split valve
(e) Pogano

70. Urge incontinence – drugs used:
(a) Darifenacin
(b) Pseudoephedrine
(c) Propranolol

(d) Prazosin
(e) Trospium

71. **Post-prostatectomy incontinence – drugs used is:**
(a) Alpha blocker
(b) Beta blocker
(c) Alpha agonist and cholinergic drugs
(d) Beta agonist and cholinergic drugs
(e) Duloxetine

72. **Complex VVF is associated with:**
(a) DM
(b) Obstructed labour
(c) Supratrigonal
(d) Involving bladder neck
(e) Post irradiation

73. **Cyclical hematuria seen in:**
(a) VVF
(b) Uterovesical fistula
(c) Vesical endometriosis
(d) Pseudohermaphrodite
(e) True hermaphrodite

74. **Most common collagen accumulation in obstructive uropathy:**
(a) 1 (b) 2
(c) 3 (d) 4

75. **Which parameter significantly affects results of retropubic surgery for SUI?**
(a) Obesity
(b) Age
(c) Comorbidity
(d) Previous surgery

76. **Girl with normal voiding with continuous incontinence:**
(a) Ectopic ureter and IVU is done
(b) Vesicovaginal fistula and cystoscopy is done
(c) Dysfunctional voiding and urodynamic study is done
(d) Ureterovaginal fistula and ultrasound is done

77. **Autoaugmentation-Demucosation of intestine leads to:**
(a) Contraction of intestinal patch
(b) Tissue necrosis
(c) Mucosal regrowth
(d) Anatomotic patch

78. **Most common long-term complication of illeal conduit:**
(a) Nephrolithiasis
(b) Anastomotic stenosis
(c) Pyelonephritis
(d) Stomal stenosis

79. **Difference between male and female bladder neck:**
(a) Less adrenergic innervation
(b) Longitudinal muscles extend upto mid-urethra
(c) Thickened smooth muscle is circular
(d) Thickened striated muscle at meatus

80. **BPH with bilateral hydroureteronephrosis, serum creatinine of 6.5, PVR-600 ml, volume of prostate-35 ml, bladder palpable with night wetting. Immediate treatment is:**
(a) Catheterise with electrolyte monitoring
(b) TURP
(c) Dialysis
(d) Urodynamic study

81. **Posthysterectomy patient has normal voiding with continuous leakage:**
(a) Vesicovaginal fistula
(b) Youssef syndrome
(c) UTI
(d) Ureterovaginal fistula

82. **UNIPOINT:**
(a) Urinary (b) Prostatism
(c) Neurogenic (d) Infection

83. **GUTB with small contracted bladder. GFR 25 ml:**
(a) Stomach conduit for better contraction
(b) Stomach conduit better for no acidosis
(c) Ileum for low side effect
(d) Ileum for less nutritional loss

84. **Patient with palpable bladder with overflow incontinence. Bilateral HUN with serum creatinine of 6.0:**
(a) TURP
(b) PUC with electrolyte monitoring

(c) SPC
(d) Bilateral PCN

85. Not an anti-cholinergic:
(a) Propanthin (b) Tolteridine
(c) Solifenacin (d) Papozanib

86. Patient has undergone low anterior resection for carcinoma rectum with radiotherapy develops LUTS. DRE-enlarged prostate. Cause:
(a) BPH
(b) Neurogenic bladder
(c) Radiation cystitis
(d) Rectovesical fistula

87. Patient has undergone hysterectomy for fibroid. 5 days later after removal of catheter develops continuous leakage with normal voiding. Diagnosis is:
(a) VVF
(b) Ureterovaginal fistula
(c) Urethrovaginal fistula
(d) Ectopic ureter

88. Hinman syndrome:
(a) Non-neuropathic neuropathic bladder disorder
(b) Neuropathic bladder
(c) Megacystis
(d) Obstructive bladder with PUV

89. In Penn pouch which segment of bowel is used?
(a) Ileal (b) Jejunal
(c) Iliocecal (d) Sigmoid

90. After colonic diversion not seen is:
(a) Hyperkalemia
(b) Hypomagnesemia
(c) Hyperchloremia
(d) Hypocalcemia

91. VVF – abdominal approach is preferred to vaginal in all *except*:
(a) Obstetric VVF
(b) Small bladder
(c) Radiation VVF
(d) Large fistula

92. Drug with grade A evidence for stress incontinence is:
(a) Duloxetine
(b) Imipramine
(c) Ephedrine
(d) Methoxamine

93. Trapped prostate is:
(a) Sympathetic hyperactivity with enlarge prostate
(b) Bladder neck obstruction with enlarge prostate
(c) Enlarge prostate with stricture
(d) Bladder neck obstruction with stricture

94. To differentiate between hypermotility and ISD, test is:
(a) DLPP
(b) VLPP
(c) Q tip test
(d) Pressure transfer ratio

95. Calcium is stored in:
(a) Golgi (b) ER
(c) Caveolae (d) Mitochondria

96. Type of incontinence seen in urethral obstruction:
(a) Overflow
(b) Stress
(c) Urge
(d) No incontinence

97. All *except* one is used for periurethral injection:
(a) Autologous fat
(b) Silicone
(c) Teflon
(d) Autologous bone

98. Most common urodynamic abnormality seen in parkinsonism:
(a) Detrusor hyperreflexia with no dyssynergia
(b) Detrusor hyperreflexia with DESD
(c) Detrusor areflexia
(d) Detrusor hyperreflexia with pseudo dyssynergia

99. Type of bladder abnormality seen in DM are all *except*:
(a) Impaired bladder sensation
(b) Decreased cystometric capacity
(c) Decreased bladder contractility
(d) Increase in PVR

100. Detrusor instability and detrusor hyper-reflexia terms differ from each other as the latter has:
(a) Neurological lesion
(b) Bladder instability
(c) Urodynamically abnormal
(d) Increase tone in bladder

101. Drugs given in overactive bladder are all *except*:
(a) Tolterodine (b) Capsaicin
(c) Resiniferatoxin (d) Finasteride

102. Involuntary urine leakage occurs in all *except*:
(a) Stress incontinence
(b) ISD
(c) Urge incontinence
(d) None of the above

103. Continuous urinary leakage from:
(a) Ureterovaginal fistula
(b) Stress incontinence
(c) ISD
(d) Urge incontinence

104. Mitrofanoff was first used in:
(a) Mainz (b) Le bag
(c) Indiana (d) Penn pouch

105. Pelvic fracture extraperitoneal rupture of bladder investigation to be done in:
(a) CT cystogram (b) IVP
(c) X-ray pelvis (d) MRI

106. Patient with extraperitoneal rupture with pelvic fracture, treatment of choice:
(a) Suprapubic cystostomy
(b) Transurethral catheterization
(c) Exploration and bladder repair
(d) Exploration and bladder repair with fixation of pelvic fracture

107. Elderly treatment for depression with bladder pain syndrome, drug of choice:
(a) Amitriptyline (b) Nortriptyline
(c) Desipramine (d) Imipramine

108. Patient is having injury at cervical vertebral, which is more important complication?
(a) Reflux neurogenic bladder
(b) Atonic bladder
(c) Detrusor sphincter dysnergia
(d) Large hypoplastic bladder

109. CIC devised by:
(a) Lapides (b) Badlani
(c) Arthur Smith (d) Nitti

110. Bladder functional evaluation by:
(a) Urodynamic study
(b) MCU
(c) Cystoscopy
(d) IVU

111. Which of the following of mechanism of duloxetine?
(a) Combined norepinephrine and 5-HT reuptake inhibitor
(b) 5-HT reuptake inhibitor
(c) Norepinephrine reuptake inhibitor
(d) Combined epinephrine and 5-HT reuptake inhibitor

112. Solifenacin acts on:
(a) M_1 (b) M_2
(c) M_3 (d) M_4

113. Martius flap is not useful in:
(a) Bladder neck
(b) High posterior wall
(c) Trigone
(d) Urethra

114. Bladder neck reconstructions using anterior wall of bladder neck:
(a) Tanagho (b) Monti
(c) Leadbetter (d) Young and Dees

115. In the male patient with SUI who has not had previous radical prostatectomy, the cuff of AUSis placed at:
(a) Bladder neck
(b) Membranous urethra
(c) Prostatic urethra
(d) Bulbar urethra

116. Ureter increases in diameter and length following increase in intraluminal pressure:
(a) Peristalsis (b) Stress reaction
(c) Creep (d) Hysteresis

117. RMP of ureteral smooth muscle depends on:
(a) K^+ ion (b) Na^+ ion
(c) Ca^{++} ion (d) Cl^- ion

118. Phosphorylation of which substance is involved in the contractile process?
(a) Actin (b) Myosin
(c) Calmodulin (d) Actinomycin

119. Calcium binding protein during smooth muscle contraction:
(a) Calmodulin (b) Actin
(c) Myosin (d) Actinomycin

120. C-fiber induced micturition reflex can be measured by:
(a) Urodynamic study
(b) Pressure flow study
(c) Ice water urodynamic
(d) Uroflometry

121. Female urethral sphincter incorrect is:
(a) Striated sphincter covers distal 2/3rd of urethra
(b) Smooth muscle covers middle 1/3rd of urethra
(c) Mucosa and submucosa are involved in continence
(d) Decrease adrenergic innervation as compare to males

122. In a normal continent women, what is the least VLPP?
(a) < 60 (b) 60 – 80
(c) 80–100 (d) Does not exist

123. Compliance true is:
(a) Not a measurable quantity
(b) Always < 5 cm H_2O
(c) Does not change in BOO
(d) 12 ml/cm H_2O

124. Le Duc anastomosis which is not true?
(a) Is a refluxing anastomosis
(b) Involves both small and large bowel
(c) 5% incidence of stricture and a 2% incidence of leak
(d) The mucosa is not reapproximated over the top of the ureter but rather sutured to the side of it

125. Not true about Le Bag is:
(a) A 20 cm segment of ascending colon and a corresponding length of terminal ileum are isolated
(b) Two incised segments are sewn to one another forming the posterior plate of the reservoir
(c) This reservoir is folded and rotated 180 degrees into the pelvis
(d) Neobladder is closed posteriorly

126. Most common late complications of ileal conduit:
(a) Acute pyelonephritis
(b) Metabolic acidosis
(c) Stromal obstruction
(d) Bleeding

127. Baseline, or resting, ureteral pressure is approximately:
(a) < 5 cm H_2O (b) 5–10 cm H_2O
(c) 10–20 cm H_2O (d) 20–40 cm H_2O

128. Which layer of bladder continues with Waldeyer's sheath?
(a) Superficial layer (b) Deep layer
(c) Detrusor layer (d) All the layers

129. Micturitional Urethral Pressure profilometry is done to diagnose:
(a) Urethral hypermobility
(b) Intrinsic sphincter deficiency
(c) Bladder outlet obstruction
(d) Sphincter abnormality

130. The valsalva leak point pressure in a young healthy female is:
(a) Infinite (b) < 40 cm
(c) < 20 cm (d) < 10 cm

131. Following is not a feature of Hinman Syndrome:
(a) Incontinence
(b) Recurrent UTI
(c) Incomplete emptying
(d) Hematuria

132. According to AMID classification type 1 synthetic mesh:
(a) Pore size 30 to 50 mm
(b) Pore size 50 to 75 mm
(c) Submicronic pore size
(d) Pore size > 75 mm

133. For following reasons vaginal approach is preferred over abdominal for bladder neck closure *except*:
(a) Prior pelvic surgery
(b) Prior pelvic radiotherapy
(c) When martius flap is used
(d) In patients with inability to place in lithotomy position

134. False about Fowler Syndrome:
(a) Abdominal distention
(b) No sensation
(c) Increased bladder capacity > 1L
(d) Feeling of urgency

135. Most common cause of vesicoenteric fistula:
(a) Extensive local colonic malignancy
(b) Diverticulitis
(c) Crohn's disease
(d) Radiotherapy

136. Following is not a feature of Gouverneur's Syndrome:
(a) Frequency (b) Dysuria
(c) Hesitancy (d) Tenesmus

137. Spinning top deformity on voiding cystourethrogram is seen in:
(a) Posterior urethral valves
(b) Vesicoureteric reflux
(c) Detrusor and external sphincter dyssynergia
(d) Hinman's disease

138. Most common cause of vesicovaginal fistula is:
(a) Obstetric trauma and child birth
(b) Gynecological operations
(c) Carcinoma cervix
(d) Carcinoma urinary bladder

139. Gouverneur's syndrome is:
(a) Vesicovaginal fistula
(b) Ureterovaginal fistula
(c) Vesicoenteric fistula
(d) Urethrorectal fistula

140. Which of the following bowel substitute used in the urinary tract causes metabolic alkalosis?
(a) Jejunum (b) Ileum
(c) Stomach (d) Colon

141. Hinman's syndrome is characterized by the following *except*:
(a) Incontinence
(b) Poor emptying of bladder
(c) Recurrent urinary infections
(d) Hematuria

142. Iatrogenic vesicovaginal fistulae (VVF):
(a) Are more common in patients who have previously received radiotherapy to pelvis
(b) Usually present in the immediate postoperative period
(c) Commonly involve large defects
(d) Usually present with hematuria

143. Which of the following investigations is mandatory in patients with suspected VVF?
(a) Cystography
(b) Intravenous urography
(c) Retrograde ureteropyelography
(d) Pelvic CT scan

144. Vesicocolic fistula is caused most commonly by:
(a) Diverticulosis (b) Crohn's disease
(c) Tuberculosis (d) Malignancy

145. Clinically bladder is palpable and percussible at least with what volume?
(a) 50 ml (b) 150 ml
(c) 250 ml (d) 450 ml

146. In detrusor overactivity all are used *except*:
(a) Darifenacin (b) Trospium
(c) Bethanechol (d) Oxybutynin

147. Normal voiding pressure in female does not exceed:
(a) 60 mm of Hg (b) 50 mm of Hg
(c) 40 mm of Hg (d) 30 mm of Hg

148. 23-year-old lady, 3 weeks after LSCS developed continuous incontinence with regular urethral voiding cause:
(a) Infratrigonal vesicovaginal fistula
(b) Vesicouterine fistula
(c) Ureterovaginal fistula
(d) Supratrigonal vesicovaginal fistula

149. Post-abdominoperineal resection, patient presents with retention of urine–further management is:
(a) Trial of catheter removal after α blocker
(b) Urodynamics
(c) CIC
(d) TURP

150. Which nerve is affected in psoas hitch?
(a) Genitofemoral nerve
(b) Sciatic nerve
(c) Femoral nerve
(d) Obturator nerve

151. TVT is applied at:
(a) Bladder neck
(b) Mid urethra
(c) Distal urethra
(d) Any place around bladder outlet

152. Superficial layer of the trigone of bladder is formed by:
(a) Longitudinal muscle of ureter
(b) Detrusor
(c) Waldeyer's fascia
(d) Colles' fascia

153. Micturition center is in:
(a) Pons (b) Medulla
(c) Thalamus (d) Hypothalamus

154. Capacity of bladder is approximately:
(a) 300 ml (b) 400 ml
(c) 500 ml (d) 600 ml

155. Which of the following drugs is NOT used in the treatment of overflow incontinence?
(a) Baclofen (b) Distigmine
(c) Bethanecol (d) Duloxetine

156. Investigation for bladder function:
(a) USG
(b) IVP
(c) MCU
(d) Urodynamic study

157. Clean intermittent catheterization was introduced by:
(a) Lapides (b) Bosnick
(c) Badlani (d) Ramsay

158. Most important excitatory neurotransmitter for micturition in CNS:
(a) ACTH (b) Glutamate
(c) Serotonin (d) Dopamine
(e) Glycine

159. For contraction of bladder with most potent and most common muscarinic receptor respectively is:
(a) M2 and M3 (b) M3 and M2
(c) M1 and M2 (d) M2 and M4
(e) M2

160. The fine longitudinal smooth muscle fibers of ureter extending from ureteric orifices to internal urethral meatus:
(a) Mercier bar
(b) Bell muscle
(c) Verumontanum
(d) Internal sphincter

161. Deep layer of trigone is formed by:
(a) Longitudinal muscle of ureter
(b) Waldeyer's sheath
(c) Outer longitudinal muscle of bladder
(d) Inner circular muscle of bladder

162. Predominant muscurinic receptors mediating contraction of bladder:
(a) M1 (b) M2
(c) M3 (d) M4

163. Decreased compliance of the bladder seen in all *except:*
(a) Radical hysterectomy
(b) Tubercular cystitis
(c) BOO
(d) Intrasacral lesion

164. A 36 years old male came with recurrent voiding dysfunction. Cystoscopy, clinical examination are normal. There is no history of fever, trauma, probable diagnosis is:
(a) Bladder neck dysfunction
(b) Neurogenic bladder
(c) Ectopic ureter
(d) Fowler's syndrome

165. Vincent's Curtesy sign is seen in:
(a) Hypocontractile bladder

(b) Hypercontractile bladder
(c) Hinman syndrome
(d) Prune Belly syndrome

166. UMN/LMN lesions of bladder can be differentiated by:
(a) Bethanechol test
(b) Ice water test
(c) Potassium sensitivity test
(d) Cystoscopy

167. Normal voiding pressure in males:
(a) 10-20 cm H_2O (b) 20-40 cm H_2O
(c) 40-60 cm H_2O (d) 60-80 cm H_2O

168. CIC is first invented by:
(a) Lapides (b) Bradly
(c) Michell (d) Dmochowski

169. Malignancy in bladder diverticulum doesn't have stage:
(a) T1 (b) T2
(c) T3 (d) T4

170. Most common cause of VVF in developing countries:
(a) Surgical injury (b) Radiotherapy
(c) Malignancy (d) Obstetric trauma

171. After enterocystoplasty which of the following segment of bowel doesn't cause metabolic acidosis:
(a) Stomach (b) Ileum
(c) Jejunum (d) Sigmoid colon

172. Vincent's Courtesy sign is seen in:
(a) SUI (b) OAB
(c) VUR (d) VVF

173. Fowler's syndrome refers to:
(a) Idiopathic detrusor over activity
(b) Urinary retention in neurologically intact young women
(c) Post-operative retention
(d) Retention after spinal cord injury

174. Autonomic hyperreflexia is seen in lesions at:
(a) Cauda equina syndrome
(b) Diabetic autonomic neuropathy
(c) Spinal cord injury above T6-T8
(d) L4-L5 disc compression

175. A 24 years old female patient with 23 weeks pregnancy with LSCS came with dribbling of urine after 4 weeks, diagnosis is:
(a) Ureterovaginal fistula
(b) Supratrigonal vesicovaginal fistula
(c) Ureterovesical fistula
(d) Ectopic ureter
(e) Stress incontinence

176. Bourne test is done for:
(a) Vesicovaginal fistula
(b) Ureterovaginal fistula
(c) Colvesical fistula
(d) Vesicouterine fistula
(e) Urethrorectal fistula

177. External sphincter supply is by all *except*:
(a) L5 (b) S1
(c) S2 (d) S3
(e) S5

178. DLPP for bladder decompensation is:
(a) 10 (b) 20
(c) 30 (d) 40

179. Martius flap blood supply all *except:*
(a) Anterior labial vessels
(b) Posterior labial vessels
(c) Obturator artery
(d) External pudendal artery

180. PTFE most important side effects:
(a) Migration (b) Allergy
(c) Erosion (d) Infection

181. Which of the following is correct regarding ureteral smooth muscle?
(a) The resting membrane potential is –33 to –70 mV
(b) RMP is determined primarily by the distribution of sodium
(c) Increased permeability to sodium results in depolarization
(d) Repolarization is due to permeability of magnesium

182. According to McGuire, what is the intra-vesical pressure at which upper tract deterioration is known to occur?
(a) 10 cm H_2O (b) 20 cm H_2O
(c) 40 cm H_2O (d) 70 cm H_2O

183. Which of the following is a potassium channel opener?
(a) Midodrine (b) Capsaicin
(c) Pseudoephedrine (d) Pinacidil

184. Following procedure are not for SUI:
(a) Sacrocolpopexy
(b) Transvaginal tape
(c) Burch colposuspension
(d) Transobturator sling (tension free)
(e) MMK

185. Botulinum toxin is used in:
(a) Low compliance with VUR
(b) Detrusor sphincter dyssynergia
(c) Detrusor hyperreflexia
(d) Detrusor areflexia
(e) Detrusor asymmetry

186. Mirabegron is:
(a) Anticholinergic (b) Alpha agonist
(c) Alpha blocker (d) Beta agonist
(e) Beta antagonist

187. Which are not useful for treatment of OAB?
(a) Oxybutynin (b) Darifenacin
(c) Propantheline (d) Atropin
(e) Tolterodine

188. About nocturia true is:
(a) Nocturnal polyuria diminished with age
(b) Nocturnal polyuria–20-30% of 24 hours output
(c) Nocturia index <1 will always requires voiding at night
(d) Polyuria defined as > 2.8 l in 24 hours
(e) Slow wave sleep occurs in early phase

189. During bladder filling, intraluminal ureteral pressure:
(a) Increases, and the frequency of contractions increase
(b) Increases, and the frequency of contractions decrease
(c) Increases, and the frequency of contractions is unchanged
(d) Decreases once the frequency of contractions decrease

190. The common metabolic abnormality associated with incorporation of intestinal segments in the urinary tract is:
(a) Hypochloremic metabolic acidosis
(b) Hyperchloremic metabolic acidosis
(c) Hypokalemic metabolic alkalosis
(d) Hyperkalemic metabolic acidosis

191. Which of the following drugs is not instilled into the bladder immediately after transurethral resection of bladder tumor?
(a) BCG (b) Mitimycin
(c) Epirubicin (d) Thiotepa

192. The most common complication of vesicovaginal fistula repair is:
(a) Ureteral injury
(b) Rectal injury
(c) Recurrence of fistula
(d) Bladder neck incompetence

193. A 25 years old lady reported with acute urinary retention and lower abdominal discomfort. Catheterization yielded 1200 ml of urine. Neurological examination is normal. MRI of brain and spinal cord also normal. This lady has:
(a) Urethral stricture
(b) Fowler's syndrome
(c) Elseberg syndrome
(d) Psychogenic retention

194. The BOURNE test is useful in the diagnosis of:
(a) Vesicovaginal fistula
(b) Ureterovaginal fistula
(c) Colovesical fistula
(d) Vesicouterine fistula

ANSWERS

1.	A	34.	FTTFT	67.	ABCD	100.	A	133.	D	166.	B
2.	A	35.	TTFTT	68.	ACE	101.	D	134.	D	167.	B
3.	C	36.	TFFTT	69.	ACDE	102.	D	135.	B	168.	A
4.	B	37.	TFTTF	70.	AE	103.	A	136.	C	169.	B
5.	A	38.	FTTTT	71.	E	104.	D	137.	C	170.	D
6.	A	39.	TFTTT	72.	BCDE	105.	A	138.	B	171.	A
7.	B	40.	TTFFT	73.	BCE	106.	B	139.	C	172.	B
8.	C	41.	FTFTT	74.	C	107.	A	140.	C	173.	B
9.	B	42.	TTFFF	75.	D	108.	C	141.	D	174.	C
10.	A	43.	TFFFT	76.	A	109.	A	142.	B	175.	B
11.	D	44.	FFFFF	77.	A	110.	A	143.	B	176.	C
12.	B	45.	FTTTT	78.	C	111.	D	144.	A	177.	D
13.	B	46.	FTFTF	79.	A	112.	C	145.	B	178.	D
14.	D	47.	FFTFT	80.	A	113.	B	146.	C	179.	A
15.	B	48.	FFFFT	81.	D	114.	A	147.	D	180.	A
16.	A	49.	TFTFF	82.	B	115.	A	148.	C	181.	A
17.	B	50.	FTTTT	83.	B	116.	C	149.	A	182.	C
18.	D	51.	TFFFT	84.	B	117.	A	150.	A	183.	D
19.	A	52.	ABCD	85	A	118.	B	151.	B	184.	A
20.	A	53.	ABDE	86.	C	119.	A	152.	A	185.	BC
21.	FFTTF	54.	BDE	87.	B	120.	C	153.	A	186.	D
22.	TTFTT	55.	BD	88.	A	121.	B	154.	C	187.	D
23.	TFTTT	56.	C	89.	C	122.	D	155.	D	188.	BDE
24.	TFTTT	57.	B	90.	A	123.	D	156.	D	189.	A
25.	TFTTT	58.	BCE	91.	A	124.	A	157.	A	190.	A
26.	TTTTT	59.	A	92.	A	125.	D	158.	B	191.	A
27.	TFTTT	60.	CDE	93.	A	126.	A	159.	B	192.	C
28.	FTTTT	61.	BCE	94.	B	127.	A	160.	B	193.	B
29.	TFTTT	62.	ABE	95.	B	128.	B	161.	B	194.	C
30.	TFTTF	63.	ABD	96.	A	129.	C	162.	C		
31.	TFTTT	64.	ABCDE	97.	D	130.	A	163.	D		
32.	TTFFF	65.	BE	98.	D	131.	D	164.	B		
33.	TTTTT	66.	DE	99.	B	132.	D	165.	B		

CHAPTER 13

Bladder, Lower Genitourinary Calculi and Trauma

1. **The most common histologic bladder cancer cell type is:**
   (a) Squamous (b) Adeno
   (c) Urothelial (d) Small cell

2. **Which of the following is the most commonly mutated gene in high grade muscle invasive bladder cancer?**
   (a) Cyclin A (b) TP 53
   (c) HRA 5 (d) FGFR 3

3. **The conversion of normal urothelium to dysplasia is associated with chromosome 9 deletion in:**
   (a) 5% of cases (b) 25% of cases
   (c) 50% of cases (d) 75% of cases

4. **What are the chances for the smokers to have bladder cancer as compared to non-smokers?**
   (a) Two to six fold greater
   (b) 8 to 10 fold greater
   (c) 11 to 15 fold greater
   (d) Almost 20 times greater

5. **What is the bladder outlet obstruction index for a man with a voided volume of 310 mls, a Qmax of 13 mls/sec and a Pdet at Qmax of 90 cm H_2O_2?**
   (a) 86 (b) 70
   (c) 74 (d) 64

6. **Bicalutamide-mechanism of action:**
   (a) Androgen biosynthesis inhibitor
   (b) Androgen receptor antagonist
   (c) Androgen receptor agonist
   (d) Newer LHRH agonist

7. **After transurethral resection of the ejaculatory ducts, the patient develops retrograde ejaculation. What is the next step of management?**
   (a) Watchful waiting
   (b) Intrauterine insemination
   (c) ICSI
   (d) Pseudoephedrine trial

8. **Yohimbine acts as:**
   (a) Alpha1 agonist
   (b) Alpha1 antagonist
   (c) Alpha 2 agonist
   (d) Alpha 2 antagonist

9. **Primary genetic abnormality in low grade bladder cancer is associated with:**
   (a) Long arm of chromosome 9
   (b) Short arm of chromosome 9
   (c) Long arm of chromosome 13
   (d) Short arm of chromosome 13

10. **Which one of the following is not the ureterocolic anastomosis?**
    (a) Leadbetter-Clark (b) Strickler
    (c) Pagano (d) Le Duc

11. **Islands of benign-appearing urothelium situated in the lamina propria is termed as:**
    (a) Urothelial metaplasia
    (b) von Brunn's nests
    (c) Cystitis cystica
    (d) Cystitis glandularis

12. Most common group of lymph node involved in bladder cancer is:

(a) Perivesical (b) Obturator
(c) External iliac (d) Common iliac

13. Which statement regarding genetics of bladder tumor is not correct?

(a) 9q losses is associated with development of low grade superficial tumor
(b) High grade cancers are associated with p53 and chromosome 17 deletions
(c) Precise molecular analysis has been far from complete for chromosome 13 because most often entire chromosome is missing
(d) Abnormal expression of RB occur primarily in aggressive TCCs

14. Not true regarding smoking and urinary bladder carcinoma is:

(a) Higher number of p53 mutation occurs in smokers
(b) Risk correlates with number of cigarettes and duration of smoking
(c) Reduction of risk down to baseline occurs 5 years after cessation of smoking
(d) Cigarette smokers have up to a four-fold higher incidence of bladder cancer than do people who have never smoked

15. Predisposing factors for squamous cell carcinoma are all *except:*

(a) Chronic indwelling catheter
(b) Calculi
(c) S. hematobium
(d) Analgesic abuse

16. Most common long-term complication of extracorporeal ileal ureteral anastomosis is:

(a) Malignancy (b) Stenosis
(c) Pyelonephritis (d) Obstruction

Mention True and False respective to each statement (Q. No. 17 to 63)

17. Regarding TURBT:

(a) Coagulation current should be used at ureteric orifice
(b) The most significant complication of laser therapy is perforation of a hollow, viscous organ such as overlying bowel
(c) Proximal urethral biopsy is indicated for orthotopic neobladder
(d) If urethral margin +ve, orthotropic neobladder should not be done
(e) Best laser for TURBT is CO_2

18. Biomechanics:

(a) Laplace Law Tension = Pves × Radius/2-diameter
(b) The resting or contractile force developed at any given length depends on the direction in which the change in length is occurring and on the rate of length change
(c) Increase collagen causes increase contractility
(d) Female with low pressure and low contractility can have normal flow
(e) Cross striation seen in smooth muscles

19. Pharmacology of urinary bladder:

(a) The bladder ice-water urodynamic test has been suggested as a method to assess the C fiber-mediated micturition reflex
(b) Oxybutynin is M_3 selective
(c) M_3 receptors are believed to be the most important for contraction
(d) Capsaicin desensitize unmyelinated C fibers
(e) Normal bladder sensation is by unmyelinated C fibers

20. Non-invasive bladder tumor:

(a) Second look TURBT done only when muscle not found in first TURBT

(b) 2nd look done after 6-8 weeks of initial TURBT
(c) MMC given after 24 hours of TURBT
(d) Laser TURBT better than conventional TURBT
(e) In Ta low grade–BCG is best

21. Regarding BCG therapy:

(a) Binds to fibronectin on tumor urothelial cells
(b) Useful in residual papillary tumor
(c) T_1 recurrence rate is 5–10%
(d) T_1 progression rate is 40%
(e) Decreases CIS by 80%

22. Carcinoma urinary bladder:

(a) Tentacle invasion is most common mode of spread
(b) Most common lymph node involved is obturator node
(c) T_{3a} is involvement of outer half of muscle
(d) Involvement of muscular propria is considered as T2
(e) CIS is a flat, high-grade lesion confined to urothelium

23. TURBT:

(a) Bipolar cautery can be used with saline
(b) CO_2 laser can be used for TURBT
(c) Small tumors may be resected using the cold cup biopsy forceps alone
(d) BCG should be given after one week of TURBT
(e) Redo TURBT should be done after 6 weeks of initial TURBT

24. Regarding embryology:

(a) Bladder derived from vesicoureteral canal lined by ectoderm
(b) Collagen increases with age
(c) Bilateral MCDK patient can live up to puberty
(d) Trigone is derived from mesoderm
(e) Urothelium matures by 13 weeks to 16 weeks

25. Calcineurin:

(a) Serine protein phosphatase
(b) Elevated Ca^{2+} results in the activation of the enzyme
(c) The association of calmodulin with calcineurin alters the structure of catalytic subunit, leading to activation of its phosphatase activity
(d) Calcineurin dephosphorylates the NLS of NFAT, allowing the transcription factor to translocate into the nucleus
(e) Tacrolimus inhibits calcineurin and IL 2 production

26. Ca bladder/orthotopic neobladder:

(a) T_{3a}-Deep detrusor muscle is involved
(b) Orthotopic bladder has less metabolic complication than ileal conduit
(c) Ileum is best for neobladder formation
(d) Prostate urethral Bx should be done prior to orthotopic bladder construction
(e) Lifetime CIC is required in neobladder due to decrease bladder sensation

27. Superficial TCC:

(a) Mitomycin C is given within 24 hours of TURBT
(b) BCG is given 1 week after TURBT
(c) Quinolones can affect the validity of BCG
(d) BCG is given for both low and high risk groups
(e) High grade TCC with muscularis mucosa involvement, repeat TURBT after 4 weeks

28. Testicular trauma:

(a) 75% of testicular trauma is blunt trauma
(b) Contusion without rupture can lead to significant bleeding

(c) Degree of hematoma correlates well with severity of injury
(d) Testicular hematoma without rupture can be easily observed
(e) Absence of hematoma rules out testicular rupture

29. Bladder rupture:

(a) Extraperitoneal rupture usually associated with pelvic fracture
(b) All penetrating or intraperitoneal injuries resulting from external trauma should be managed by immediate operative repair
(c) < 30% associated with nonurological injury
(d) Dense, flame-shaped collection of contrast material in the pelvis is characteristic of extraperitoneal extravasation
(e) Microscopic hematuria with pelvic fracture is an absolute indication for cystography

30. Bladder with 3 cm tumor on lateral wall near ureteric orifice:

(a) Following TURBT BCG should be given within 1 week
(b) Mitomycin should be given weekly for 12 weeks
(c) Radical cystectomy should be offered as an option
(d) Partial cystectomy can be done
(e) Repeat TURBT after 16-20 weeks

31. Regarding urinary marker in carcinoma urinary bladder:

(a) BTA track is for complement 'H' protein
(b) Immunocyte not affected by benign condition
(c) Urovision checks chromosomal foci
(d) Urovision is useful in equivocal cytology
(e) NMP 22 has low sensitivity but high specificity

32. Patient with gunshot injury:

(a) Gross hematuria with blunt trauma, renal injury should be suspected
(b) Penetrating injury usually does not require operative intervention
(c) USG should be initial investigation of choice
(d) If renal avulsion occurs nephrectomy should be done
(e) Often small entrance wounds do not lead to massive destruction in body

33. Regarding urodynamics:

(a) Pressures greater than 90 cm H_2O suggest urethral hypermobility
(b) DLPP > 20 cm of H_2O cause upper tract damage
(c) Pdet = Pves – Pabd
(d) A VLPP of less than 60 cm H_2O indicates the presence of significant ISD
(e) The standard catheter for routine urodynamics should be a transurethral, double-lumen catheter

34. Urothelial tumor:

(a) Most common finding is filling defect on IVP
(b) CECT is investigation of choice for planning of conservative management
(c) Urine cytology (+) and endoscopy (–ve) →Surgical management indicated
(d) Urine cytology (–ve) and endoscopy (+ve) → Surgical management indicated
(e) Low grade tumor of renal pelvis with normal opposite kidney, conservative surgery can be done

35. TCC of urinary bladder:

(a) CT scan can distinguish T2 vs T3a
(b) The urothelium of the normal bladder is three to seven layers thick

(c) Lamina propria is a tunica muscularis mucosa containing scattered smooth muscle fibers
(d) Most common node involved is obturator
(e) Cystitis cystica is liquified von Brunn's nest

36. TCC of urinary bladder:
(a) Dysplasia denotes epithelial changes intermediate between normal urothelium and CIS
(b) Cystitis follicularis is a subepithelial nodule akin to lymphoid follicle
(c) Cystitis glandularis is precursor of adenocarcinoma
(d) In exstrophy most common malignancy is adenocarcinoma
(e) Urachal adenocarcinoma of bladder has better prognosis than adenocarcinoma elsewhere

37. Bladder malignancy:
(a) Squamous metaplasia in TCC is treated as conventional TCC
(b) Squamous changes develops in 80% of paraplegics
(c) Squamous cancers occur in patients 10 to 20 years younger than patients with TCC
(d) TCC of diverticulum–early stage migration
(e) Adenocarcinoma is associated with cystitis cystica

38. Chemotherapy in TCC:
(a) Acrolein is responsible for cyclophosphamide's carcinogenic effect
(b) Mesna increases carcinogenicity of cyclophosphamide
(c) Pelvic radiation increases risk of TCC by 2-4 folds
(d) Cigarette smokers have up to a four-fold higher incidence of bladder cancer
(e) Mitomycin C is intravesical chemotherapy of choice

39. TCC bladder–Treatment:
(a) BCG should be given after surgery once bleeding stops
(b) BCG should be given 1 week after surgery
(c) Persistent fever for more than 48 hours after BCG → ATT should not be given
(d) Lateral wall tumor – TURBT should be done under GA
(e) Small TURBT can be done with TURP

40. Regarding BCG:
(a) BCG-refractory is defined as recurrence or persistence of lesser degree, stage, or grade after an initial course
(b) BCG should be given for 6 weeks for TaG1
(c) Further courses of BCG or chemotherapy beyond two are not recommended routinely, as they will fail 80% of the time
(d) If the initial treatment was chemotherapy, a course of BCG should be undertaken
(e) UTI is contraindication to BCG therapy

41. CIS of bladder:
(a) Urine cytology is positive in 80–100%
(b) Muscle progression in 40–80% of cases
(c) Low grade tumor confined to urothelium
(d) Present in 25% of patients with high grade superficial tumors
(e) Endoscopically invisible

42. Investigation for TCC:
(a) Overnight urine is required for cytology
(b) Urine cytology is false +ve in inflammation
(c) NMP-22 can be used in follow up in place of cystoscopy in low grade tumor
(d) Flow cytometry has not been found to be more clinically valuable than conventional cytology
(e) Even in patients with high-grade tumors, urinary cytology may be falsely negative in 20%

43. Staging of TCC:

(a) Failure to detect microscopic nodal disease with MRI is similar to that with CT

(b) More than 1.0 cm node is metastatic

(c) Understaging and overstaging remain persistent problems with both CT and MRI, occurring in about 30%

(d) Correlation of CT findings with pathologic findings of the cystectomy specimen is 65% to 80%

(e) CT detects metastatic disease in regional lymph nodes in 50% to 85% of cases

44. Development of bladder:

(a) Urinary bladder develop from ectodermal lined urogenital sinus

(b) Trigone developed from endonephros

(c) Bladder compliance is thought to change during development

(d) The vesicourethral canal gives rise to the bladder and pelvic urethra

(e) Right and left common excretory ducts fuse in midline forming primitive trigone

45. Receptors of bladder:

(a) α_1 is more common than α_2 in causation of LUTS

(b) α receptor > β in bladder base

(c) β receptor > α in bladder body

(d) Female bladder has more adrenergic innervation

(e) $\beta_3 > \beta_2$ receptor in bladder body

46. Neurophysiology of bladder:

(a) Low compliance in sacral level injury

(b) Post ganglionic sympathetic fibers in bladder secretes norepinephrine

(c) Preganglionic sympathetic fibers in bladder secretes norepinephrine

(d) Micturition control at thoracic cord level

(e) The most common long-term expression of lower urinary tract dysfunction after CVA is phasic detrusor overactivity

47. Patient with known superficial bladder cancer of T_1 with bleeding:

(a) Emergency cystoscopy should be done

(b) Repeat TUR can demonstrate worse prognostic findings in up to 25% of specimens

(c) Second resection changed treatment in one third of cases

(d) BCG in preventing progression appears to be higher in patients if a restaging TURBT was performed before instillation of BCG

(e) ReTURBT is recommended 1 to 4 weeks after the initial resection

48. Regarding carcinoma urinary bladder:

(a) Progression of carcinoma not reduced with mitomycin C

(b) Progression is reduced in high grade but not in low grade with BCG

(c) BCG decreases progression over short-term but not in long-term

(d) BCG is most effective intravesical chemotherapy

(e) BCG is used to treat residual papillary lesion

49. Carcinoma urinary bladder: TURBT in T_1 high grade:

(a) More chances of perforation while doing resection in a diverticula

(b) Cold biopsy is better as it reduces incidence of cautery artifact

(c) Urine cytology is +ve in more than 90% of cases

(d) If there is no muscle in specimen indication for repeat biopsy

(e) Early cystectomy is preferred for T1high grade

50. Superficial bladder cancer:

(a) Low-grade Ta lesions recur at a rate of 50% to 70%

(b) High-grade T1 lesions recur in more than 80% of cases

(c) Most important risk factor for progression is grade, not stage

(d) Approximately 70% of bladder tumors are non-muscle invasive at presentation

(e) Among non-muscle invasive, 70% present as stage T1

51. Regarding cell cycle:

(a) Rb gene main regulator at G_1S checkpoint

(b) TP53 mediates both G_1S and G_2M arrest

(c) BAX is the most well studied pro-apoptotic BCL2 family member

(d) G_1 (for gap 1) is when the cell prepares to duplicate its DNA

(e) Cyclin D expression is critical at the G_2M checkpoint

52. Overactive bladder:

(a) Tolterodine is muscarinic antagonist

(b) Tolterodine causes less dryness of mouth than oxybutynin

(c) Hydrodistention is treatment of choice

(d) The frequency volume chart remains the principal method of evaluating frequency and nocturia in an objective way

(e) Incontinence follows urgency and is involuntary

53. Carcinoma bladder:

(a) Risk increases after pelvic radiotherapy

(b) Pelvic metastasis initially to obturator lymph node

(c) Diverticular disease involve musculature early

(d) In paraplegic SCC most common (80%)

(e) Acrolein metabolite of cyclophosphamide is carcinogenic

54. Urothelium:

(a) 2-3 cell layer thick with umbrella cells

(b) Scattered muscle cells in tunica muscularis layer

(c) von Brunn's nests are islands of benign-appearing urothelium situated in the lamina propria

(d) Cystitis cystical liquefied Von Brunn's nests

(e) Cystitis glandularis is similar to cystitis cystica except that the transitional cells have undergone glandular metaplasia

55. Carcinoma bladder:

(a) BCG best given after 2 weeks of TURBT

(b) Treatment of TB if fever >103°F after BCG therapy

(c) Granulomatous prostatits often asymptomatic

(d) 6 weeks of therapy followed by maintenance gives long remission interval for pTa and pT1 disease

(e) Quinolones in particular may affect the viability of BCG and should be avoided if possible during the course of BCG treatments

56. Regarding pharmacology of bladder:

(a) M_2 receptor causes contraction of bladder

(b) Tolterodine is M_2 selective

(c) Side effect of oxybutynin is due to its active metabolite

(d) TCA has anticholinergic effect

(e) Intravesical pressure decreases due to increase in collagen

57. **Bladder tumor:**
(a) Intravesical follicle is analogous with lymphoid cells anywhere in body
(b) Inverted papilloma is associated with TCC else wherein urinary bladder
(c) Cystitis glandularis is associated with adenocarcinoma of bladder
(d) Incidence of leukoplakia is more in patient of bladder calculus and chronic infection
(e) Cystitis cystica is von Brunn's nests in which urothelium has undergone eosinophilic liquefaction

58. **BCG:**
(a) Attenuated mycobacterium bovis
(b) Increase fibronectin in urine–good prognosis
(c) BCG prevents progression of disease
(d) If two attempt of BCG fails, third attempt of BCG should not be tried
(e) Treatment by BCG generally begun 2 to 4 hours after tumor resection

59. **Carcinoma bladder:**
(a) Low grade superficial tumor 5 years recurrence 30%
(b) ¼ of superficial high grade tumor progress to muscle invasion
(c) CIS has 80% response rate with BCG
(d) 50% of high grade lesion progress to muscle invasion
(e) High grade T1 tumor recur in 50% of cases

60. **Bladder tumor:**
(a) Intravesical folliculitis is analogous with lymphoid follicles elsewhere
(b) Inverted papilloma is associated with TCC elsewhere in urinary bladder
(c) Cystitis glandularis is precursor of adenocarcinoma
(d) Incidence of leukoplakia is more in patients with bladder stone and chronic infections
(e) Multicentric recurrent tumor should be treated with cystectomy

61. **BCG:**
(a) Attenuated mycobacterium bovis
(b) Increase fibronectin in urine is good prognosis
(c) TP 53 most frequent altered gene in bladder tumors
(d) BCG delays progression
(e) If two attempts of BCG fails there is no further role of BCG therapy

62. **Regarding TURBT:**
(a) Half of patients with muscle/invasive bladder cancer (10%) already have occult distant metastases
(b) 50% are nonmuscle invasive at presentation
(c) When repeat TURBT is done after original procedure, tumor recurrence is seen in upto 30% to 40% of cases
(d) If the bladder lesion is small, it may be amenable to cold-cup biopsy and fulguration
(e) Finer diameter loops project a more concentrated current and therefore cut more easily

63. **Regarding carcinoma urinary bladder:**
(a) Low grade Ta–recurrence rate is 30%
(b) T1 high grade tumor progress to muscle invasion in one fourth of cases
(c) BCG has good response on CIS
(d) 50% of high grade lesion are muscle invasive
(e) Sessile tumor has more chances to progress than papillary tumors

Which of the following statement is correct ?

64. **Which of the following inflammation/infection is NOT a risk factor for bladder cancer?**
(a) Gonorrhea
(b) Schistosomiasis
(c) Human papilloma virus
(d) BK virus

65. In an old patient 4th cycle of BCG was to be given. During therapy there is resistance at bulbar urethra, but catheter is negotiated. Initial hematuria occurred which resolves later. Next step:

(a) Give BCG therapy
(b) Course given after decreasing dose
(c) Give full course with prophylaxis of ATT
(d) Perineal compression given
(e) Abandon the procedure

66. TURBT of 2 × 2 cm of high grade growth involving lamina propria without detrusor involvement:

(a) TaG3
(b) Relook TURBT
(b) BCG in this setting may be helpful
(d) Prepare the patient for early cystectomy
(e) Intravesical mitomycin given

67. Common lymph node involved in carcinoma bladder:

(a) Internal iliac
(b) External iliac
(c) Obturator
(d) Para-aortic
(e) Inguinal

68. Which of the following is most common carcinoma occurring in urinary bladder?

(a) Adenocarcinoma
(b) SCC
(c) TCC
(d) Adenosarcoma
(e) Small cell carcinoma

69. All are contraindications of BCG *except*:

(a) Total incontinence
(b) Cirrhosis
(c) UTI
(d) Immunosuppression
(e) Stress incontinence

70. Chemotherapy in bladder carcinoma (intravesically):

(a) Mitomycin C
(b) Gemcitabine
(c) Doxorubicin
(d) Cisplatin
(e) Cyclophosphamide

71. CIS of bladder:

(a) BCG contraindicated
(b) Cytology 80-90% positive
(c) HPE–poorly differentiated TCC with involvement of muscularis propria
(d) Erythematous velvety appearance
(e) May be positive with severe symptoms of dysuria, frequency and urgency

72. Intravesical drugs which is used to prevent recurrence of bladder carcinoma:

(a) Interferon
(b) Cisplatin
(c) Cyclophosphamide
(d) Adriamycin
(e) Methotrexate

73. Most important risk factor for TCC progression:

(a) Grade of tumor
(b) LN involvement
(c) Invasion of muscularis propria
(d) Invasion of lamina propria
(e) Lymphovascular invasion

74. 45-year-old with 3 foci of 2 cm PUNLMP, treatment options:

(a) TURBT + BCG
(b) Laser coagulation
(c) Radical cystectomy
(d) Radical RT
(e) BCG + mitomycin

75. Contraindication of BCG:

(a) Gross hematuria

(b) UTI
(c) T1G3 tumor
(d) Muscle invasive tumor
(e) Total incontinence

76. For radical cystectomy indications are:
(a) Multiple recurrences
(b) Involvement of bladder neck + prostatic urethra
(c) Diffuse CIS
(d) Recurrence not responding to BCG
(e) Multiple superficial tumor

77. Intravesical chemotherapy – which agent is given?
(a) Mitomycin C (b) Adriamycin
(c) Cisplatin (d) Methotrexate
(e) Cyclophosphamide

78. In urothelial TCC – risk factor for recurrence:
(a) High grade
(b) Bladder neck TCC
(c) CIS
(d) Multifocality
(e) High stage

79. Intravesical BCG contraindicated in:
(a) Active UTI
(b) Hematuria
(c) CIS
(d) Immunosuppressed
(e) True incontinence

80. Complication of TURBT:
(a) Clot retention
(b) Perforation
(c) High risk of tumor seeding
(d) Obstruction of ureteric orifice can occur
(e) Urethral stricture

81. Intravesical therapeutic option in multiple superficial urinary bladder malignancy:
(a) Mitomycin
(b) Cisplatin
(c) Cyclophosphamide
(d) Methotrexate
(e) Adriamycin

82. In radical cystectomy structure removed:
(a) Bladder with terminal ureter
(b) Anterior vaginal wall
(c) Uterus
(d) Entire urethra in female
(e) Bulbar urethra + perineal skin

83. Male auxillary genital glands:
(a) Seminal vesicle
(b) Prostate
(c) Epididymis
(d) Bulbourethral gland
(e) Penis

84. Broad based high grade bladder tumor, muscle not identified in specimen next step:
(a) Intravesical BCG
(b) Intravesical mitomycin
(c) ReTURBT after 4 weeks
(d) CPE after 3 months

85. Bladder and urethra lymphatic supply is:
(a) Prepubic (b) Inguinal
(c) Internal iliac (d) Obturator

86. Which is not carcinogenic for urothelium?
(a) Hypoxanthine
(b) Smoking
(c) Balkan nephropathy
(d) Analgesics

87. Urothelial carcinoma with stage T1G3 with no muscle in biopsy. Next stage is:
(a) Repeat biopsy after 2 weeks
(b) BCG
(c) Mitomycin
(d) Repeat cystoscopy after 3 weeks

88. Lamina propria involved, in which stage?
(a) T1 (b) Ta
(c) Tcis (d) T2

89. **Fifty-year-old smoker with hematuria normal DRE, cytology and CECT negative, what is to be done?**
(a) Finasteride (b) TURP
(c) Cystoscopy (d) Observation

90. **CT regimen least toxic in carcinoma urinary bladder:**
(a) MVAC
(b) CVM
(c) Gemcitabine-Cisplatin
(d) PEB

91. **On TURBT posterior wall of urinary bladder has 2 cm diverticula with associated CIS. Tumor was high grade, no muscularis propria seen, muscularis mucosa involvement present, what is treatment?**
(a) Radical cystectomy
(b) Partial cystectomy
(c) Intravesical mitomycin
(d) Intravesical BCG

92. **5-aminolevulinic acid, when administered intravesically in conjunction with fluorescent cystoscopy uses which light?**
(a) Red (b) Blue
(c) Green (d) White

93. **Most important determinant of urethral tumor recurrence after radical cystectomy in TCC:**
(a) Carcinoma in situ
(b) Stage
(c) Prostatic stomal involvement
(d) Grade

94. **Following is absolute contraindication of partial cystectomy:**
(a) Urachal carcinoma
(b) Cancer in diverticula
(c) Carcinoma in situ
(d) Pheochromocytoma

95. **Cranial limit of extended pelvic lymph node dissection in bladder malignancy is:**
(a) Bifurcation of aorta
(b) Bifurcation of common iliac
(c) Origin of superior vesical artery
(d) Origin of superior mesenteric artery

96. **T2 N0 M0 TCC bladder after radical cystectomy. Diseases free survival:**
(a) <40% (b) 40-60%
(c) 60-80% (d) 80-90%

97. **Most common sarcoma of kidney:**
(a) Leiomyosarcoma
(b) Liposarcoma
(c) Rhabdomyosarcoma
(d) Osteosarcoma

98. **Classic cystoscopic surveillance for superficial low grade bladder carcinoma is all *except*:**
(a) At 3 months on initial resection
(b) Annually if no recurrence on initial resection
(c) No need for upper tract imaging
(d) Six monthly if recurrence occurs

99. **Which of the following is not a tumor suppressor gene?**
(a) TP-53 (b) Rb
(c) VHL (d) BRCA-1

100. **The organism most commonly cultured from an infected urachal cyst is:**
(a) Staphylococcus aureus
(b) Pseudomonas
(c) Klebsiella
(d) Candida albicans

101. **Which of the following associations in the bladder is not correct?**
(a) Nephrogenic adenoma – Adenocarcinoma
(b) Cystitis glandularis – Adenocarcinoma
(c) Cystitis follicularis – Lymphoma
(d) von Brunn's nests – Transitional cell carcinoma

102. What % of bladder wall is composed of collagen?

(a) 50% (b) 60%
(c) 30% (d) 20%

103. Latent pacemaker cells are present in:

(a) Upper ureter (b) Middle ureter
(c) Lower ureter (d) All of the above

104. Most common cause of gross hematuria in > 50 years male:

(a) RCC (b) Ca bladder
(c) Ca prostate (d) Hypercalciuria

105. In a postmenopausal women with T2 bladder carcinoma planned for surgery. Which of the following structure is not removed?

(a) Ovaries (b) Uterus
(c) Vagina (d) All of the above

106. Use of cyclophosphamide increases the bladder cancer manifold due to a metabolite called:

(a) Prolins (b) Hydrocarbons
(c) Free radicals (d) Acrolene

107. Congenital bladder diverticula are associated with the following conditions *except*:

(a) Menkes syndrome
(b) Williams syndrome
(c) Ehlers-Danlos syndrome
(d) Youssef's syndrome

108. Which of the following is not a risk factor for the development of squamous cell carcinoma of urinary bladder?

(a) Chronic indwelling vesical calculus
(b) Schistosoma hematobium
(c) Analgesic abuse
(d) Lynch syndrome

109. The preferred initial therapy for carcinoma-in-situ of urinary bladder is:

(a) BCG (b) Mitomycin
(c) Epirubicin (d) Gemcitabine

110. The boundaries for standard pelvic lymphadenectomy in carcinoma bladder are the following *except*:

(a) Aortic bifurcation
(b) Genitofemoral nerve
(c) Endopelvic fascia
(d) Urinary bladder

111. The Gold Standard treatment for muscle-invasive bladder tumor is:

(a) Radiation therapy
(b) Radical cystectomy
(c) Intravesical instillation with BCG
(d) Combination chemotherapy with radiation

112. Which of the following may predispose to Transitional cell carcinoma of the bladder?

(a) Smoking cigarettes
(b) Obesity
(c) Exposure to aluminum industry
(d) Chronic cystitis

113. Most common cause of gross hematuria in a 50-year-old patient is:

(a) Urolithiasis
(b) Renal pelvic tumor
(c) IgA nephropathy
(d) Bladder cancer

114. Most preferred intravesical chemotherapy to prevent recurrence after TURBT:

(a) BCG (b) Mitomycin
(c) Thiotepa (d) Adriamycin

115. Most definitive treatment of muscle invasive TCC:

(a) Radical cystectomy
(b) Chemotherapy
(c) Radiotherapy
(d) TURBT

116. Muscle invasive carcinoma bladder at presentation:

(a) 20% (b) 30%
(c) 40% (d) 5-10%

117. Urothelial carcinoma most common site:
(a) Upper (b) Middle
(c) Lower (d) Renal pelvic

118. Incidence of upper tract cancer in patient of bladder carcinoma:
(a) 60-70% (b) 20-30%
(c) 5-10% (d) 2-4%

119. Route of instillation of BCG:
(a) Intravenous
(b) Subcutaneous
(c) Intradermal
(d) Intravesical

120. Extraperitoneal rupture of bladder, investigation of choice:
(a) Cystogram with postvoid film
(b) RGU
(c) IVP
(d) USG

121. The most common lymph node involved in carcinoma bladder:
(a) Obturator
(b) Internal iliac
(c) External iliac
(d) Internal pudendal

122. Urachal carcinoma is:
(a) Adenocarcinoma
(b) Squamous cell carcinoma
(c) TCC
(d) Adenosquamous carcinoma

123. Most common type of malignancy in ectopia vesicae:
(a) Adenocarcinoma
(b) Squamous cell carcinoma
(c) TCC
(d) Sarcoma botryoid

124. First lymph node involved in carcinoma bladder:
(a) Obturator (b) External iliac
(c) Internal iliac (d) Para-aortic

125. Best treatment for superficial carcinoma bladder:
(a) TURBT
(b) Intravesical BCG
(c) Intravesical mitomycin
(d) Radical cystectomy

126. Carcinoma in situ bladder, all are true *except:*
(a) Poorly defined TCC confined to urothelium
(b) Urine cytology is positive in 80%
(c) Endoscopically visible
(d) The initial tumor-free response rate after BCG therapy is as high as 80%

127. All are contraindications of BCG *except:*
(a) Total incontinence
(b) UTI
(c) Immunosuppression
(d) Stress incontinence

128. Intravesical BCG therapy is indicated in all *except:*
(a) CIS
(b) Multifocal carcinoma
(c) Diffuse carcinoma
(d) Invasive carcinoma

129. Most common malignancy arising from bladder diverticula:
(a) Squamous cell carcinoma
(b) Transitional cell carcinoma
(c) Adenocarcinoma
(d) Verrucous carcinoma

130. Most common site for urothelial tumor is:
(a) Renal pelvis (b) Upper ureter
(c) Middle ureter (d) Lower ureter

131. All of these are used as intravesical agents *except:*
(a) Mitomycin C (b) Doxorubicin
(c) Gemcitabine (d) Cisplatin

132. The lateral limit of dissection in pelvic lymphadenectomy for carcinoma bladder is:
(a) External iliac vein
(b) External iliac artery

(c) Genitofemoral nerve
(d) Obturator nerve

133. Indications for partial cystectomy include all *except:*
(a) Solitary tumor in the region of the dome
(b) Urachal adenocarcinoma in the dome
(c) Primary pheochromocytoma
(d) Carcinoma in situ

134. Irrigation fluid in TURBT may be:
(a) DW (b) 1.5% glycine
(c) 0.9% NaCl (d) 10% mannitol
(e) 10% dextrose

135. Most common cause of gross hematuria in > 50 years male:
(a) RCC
(b) Carcinoma bladder
(c) Carcinoma prostate
(d) Hypercalciuria
(e) BPH

136. Bladder preservation criteria all *except*:
(a) HDN
(b) Muscle invasion
(c) Normal urinal analysis
(d) Normal KFT

137. Which of the following regarding the inguinal canal is correct?
(a) The external oblique muscle forms the roof and posterior wall of the canal
(b) The conjoint tendon reinforces the posterior wall at the superficial ring
(c) The cord structures enter medial to the inferior epigastric vessels
(d) The internal inguinal ring lies at the level of anterior superior iliac spine

138. Which of the following is a branch of the posterior division of the internal iliac artery?
(a) Internal pudendal artery
(b) Obturator artery
(c) Ascending lumbar artery
(d) Inferior vesicle artery

139. Which of the following deletion is most commonly associated with low grade papillary urothelial cancer?
(a) 2q deletion (b) 5q deletion
(c) 9q deletion (d) 10q deletion

140. Which of the following urinary marker has the highest sensitivity in the detection of urothelial cancer?
(a) BTA stat (b) BTA trak
(c) NMP 22 (d) CYFRA 21-1

141. Which of the following is true regarding the management of bladder tumor?
(a) ReTURBT is usually appropriate in the evaluation of T1 tumors as it will demonstrate worse prognostic findings in up to 25% of specimens
(b) All intraperitoneal and extraperitoneal perforations need emergency closure
(c) Random biopsies are indicated in low and high risk tumors, after resection
(d) 10–20% of CIS will develop muscle invasive tumours if untreated

142. Which of the following intravesical therapy is approved for BCG refractory bladder CIS?
(a) Mitomycin C (b) Thiotepa
(c) Valrubicin (d) Gemcitabine

143. Which of the following is correct regarding immediate intravesical instillation soon after bladder tumor resection?
(a) Either mitomycin or BCG are commonly administered
(b) 15–38% reduction in recurrence rates is documented
(c) Reduction in progression is the primary reason for instillation
(d) Doxorubicin should not be used for intravesical administration

144. Which of the following is correct regarding cystitis glandularis?
(a) It is a post-radiation change
(b) Transurethral resection is contraindicated

(c) Most common presentation is recurrent hematuria
(d) It may transform into adenocarcinoma

145. The following chemotherapeutic agent has been proven to cause bladder cancer:
(a) Cyclophosphamide
(b) Bleomycin
(c) Cisplatin
(d) Mitomycin

146. Which of the following is true regarding stapled bowel anastomosis?
(a) Tissues of 3–5 mm thickness are ideal for stapled anastomosis
(b) The TA stapler is for end to end circumferential anastomosis
(c) The TA stapler inverts the suture line
(d) Leak and fistula rates are similar for stapled and sutured anastomosis

147. With bowel interposition in the urinary tract, elevated renin and angiotensin is associated with which bowel segment?
(a) Stomach (b) Jejunum
(c) Ileum (d) Colon

148. As compared to open prostatectomy, TURP has:
(a) More blood loss
(b) More TUR syndrome
(c) More complete removal of prostate tissue
(d) Less retreatment rate

149. Intravesical treatment for carcinoma bladder:
(a) Gemcitabine
(b) Cyclophosphamide
(c) Cisplatin
(d) MMc
(e) Doxorubicin

150. T1G3 true are:
(a) Superficial low grade
(b) Muscle invasive low grade
(c) Superficial high grade
(d) CIS
(e) Muscle invasive high grade

151. Lymphatic drainage of bladder is via:
(a) EILN (b) Inguinal
(c) Para-aortic (d) IILN
(e) Obturator

152. About intravesical therapy true is:
(a) BCG should be started as early as possible to increase efficacy
(b) Induction BCG is the TOC for low grade
(c) Intravesical chemotherapy decrease recurrence in low grade tumors
(d) Traumatic catheterization is contraindication for BCG
(e) Intravesical chemotherapy is equivalent to BCG

ANSWERS

1.	C	32.	TFTTF	63.	FFTTT	94.	C	125.	A
2.	B	33.	TTTTT	64.	C	95.	A	126.	D
3.	D	34.	TTFTT	65.	E	96.	C	127.	D
4.	A	35.	TTTTT	66.	ABCD	97.	A	128.	D
5.	D	36.	TTTTF	67.	ABC	98.	D	129.	B
6.	B	37.	FTTTF	68.	C	99.	D	130.	A
7.	D	38.	TFTTT	69.	E	100.	A	131.	D
8.	D	39.	FFFTT	70.	ABCE	101.	D	132.	C
9.	A	40.	FFTTT	71.	BDE	102.	A	133.	D
10.	D	41.	TTFFT	72.	AD	103.	D	134.	B
11.	B	42.	FTFTT	73.	A	104.	B	135.	B
12.	B	43.	TFTTT	74.	A	105.	C	136.	A
13.	C	44.	FFTTT	75.	ABDE	106.	D	137.	B
14.	C	45.	TTTFT	76.	ABCDE	107.	D	138.	C
15.	D	46.	FTFFF	77.	AB	108.	D	139.	C
16.	B	47.	TTTTT	78.	ACDE	109.	A	140.	C
17.	FTTTF	48.	TTTTT	79.	ABDE	110.	A	141.	A
18.	TTFTF	49.	TTFTT	80.	ABDE	111.	B	142.	C
19.	TFTTF	50.	TTTTF	81.	ACE	112.	A	143.	B
20.	FFFFF	51.	TTTTF	82.	AC	113.	D	144.	D
21.	TTFTT	52.	TTFTT	83.	ABD	114.	A	145.	A
22.	FTFTT	53.	TTTTT	84.	C	115.	A	146.	D
23.	TFTFF	54.	FFTTT	85.	A	116.	A	147.	B
24.	FFFTT	55.	TTTTT	86.	A	117.	D	148.	B
25.	TTTTT	56.	TFTTT	87.	A	118.	D	149.	ADE
26.	FFTTF	57.	FTTTT	88.	A	119.	D	150.	C
27.	TFTFT	58.	TFTTF	89.	C	120.	A	151.	ADE
28.	TTFTF	59.	FFTTF	90.	C	121.	A	152.	BCD
29.	TTFTF	60.	FTTTT	91.	A	122.	A		
30.	FFFFF	61.	TFTTT	92.	B	123.	A		
31.	TTTTF	62.	TFTTT	93.	C	124.	A		

CHAPTER 14

Prostate

1. **Which of the following biomarkers is not characteristic of prostate stem cells?**
   (a) PSA (b) Trop 2
   (c) CD49 f (d) Keratins 5/14
2. **Benign prostatic hyperplasia originates in:**
   (a) Transition zone
   (b) Peripheral zone
   (c) Anterior zone
   (d) Transition zone and periurethral zone
3. **Which alpha-I subtype mediates prostate smooth muscle tension?**
   (a) α 1 (b) α 1A
   (c) α 1β (d) α 1C
4. **Which of the following is the likely mechanism for dizziness adrenergic blocker therapy?**
   (a) Vascular
   (b) Central nervous system
   (c) Carotid baroreceptors
   (d) Psychological factors
5. **The retrograde ejaculation is most commonly seen with:**
   (a) Terazosin (b) Tamsulosin
   (c) Alfuzosin (d) Prazosin
6. **Serum PSA elevations are specific for prostate:**
   (a) Cancer (b) Enlargement
   (c) Inflammation (d) None of the above
7. **The prostate gland has arterial supply through which of the following arteries?**
   (a) Pudendal (b) Superior vesical
   (c) Obturator (d) Inferior vesical
8. **The main parasympathetic efferent innervations to the pelvic plexus arises from:**
   (a) S_1 (b) S_2-S_4
   (c) T_{11}-L_2 (d) L_3-S_1
9. **The neurovascular bundle lies between which of the two periprostatic fascial planes?**
   (a) Prostate capsule and prostatic fascia
   (b) Prostate capsule and levator fascia
   (c) Prostatic fascia and levator fascia X
   (d) Denonvilliers fascia and endopelvic fascia
10. **The characteristic appearance of frozen tissue on ultrasound has:**
    (a) Mixed echogenicity
    (b) Hyperechogenicity
    (c) Anechogenicity
    (d) Hypoechogenicity
11. **All of the following are branches of posterior trunk of internal iliac artery *except:***
    (a) Superior vesical (b) Lateral sacral
    (c) Superior gluteal (d) Ascending lumbar
12. **Which of the following was not defined as clinical progression in the MTOPS study?**
    (a) Recurrent hematuria
    (b) Renal failure
    (c) Increase of 4 points in the AUA symptom score
    (d) Urinary incontinence
13. **Embryological origin of the transition zone:**
    (a) Mesoderm (b) Endoderm
    (c) Ectoderm (d) Mullerian duct
14. **Which vessels serve as macroscopic landmark to aid in the identification of the microscopic branches of the pelvic plexus?**

(a) Capsular arteries (b) Urethral arteries
(c) Pudendal artery (d) Cavernosal artery

15. Most common indication for TURP:
(a) Bothersome LUTS
(b) Recurrent hematuria
(c) Recurrent UTI
(d) Acute urinary retention

16. Carcinoma prostate commonly arises from:
(a) Central zone
(b) Peripheral zone
(c) Transitional zone
(d) Fibromuscular zone

17. Patients with prostatitis, especially acute suppurative prostatitis, true is:
(a) Should have residual urine measured by intermittent catheterization
(b) Should have bladder decompression by urethral catheter
(c) Should have repeated prostatic massage
(d) Should have no transurethral instrumentation if possible

18. Which one of the following is not the sex accessory tissues?
(a) Seminal vesicle
(b) Ampullary glands
(c) Bulbourethral glands
(d) Ejaculatory ducts

19. When compared with TURP, open prostatectomy offers all the advantages *except:*
(a) Lower retreatment rate
(b) More complete removal of the prostatic adenoma under direct vision
(c) Avoids the risk of dilutional hyponatremia
(d) Decreased potential for perioperative hemorrhage

20. Which statement regarding 5α-reductase enzyme is not correct?
(a) The type I enzyme is in the skin and in the adult scalp and is believed to be involved in hair formation
(b) The type I enzyme is the dominant isoform present in the prostate gland
(c) The type II enzyme appears in the basal cells of the epithelium and in the stromal cells
(d) The type II enzyme is absent in the secretory epithelial cells

21. Half life of serum PSA is:
(a) 2-3 seconds (b) 2-3 minutes
(c) 2-3 hours (d) 2-3 days

22. Men with obstructive LUTS and prostate 50 cc started on alpha blockers but no relief, after 3 months management will be:
(a) Redo TURP
(b) TRUS guided biospy
(c) CECT to rule out urothelial malignancy
(d) Continue medication for 3 more months

23. Most common site of rectal injury during RRP:
(a) Posteriorly while dissecting apex
(b) Posteriorly while dissecting seminal vesicles
(c) While dissecting posterior laterally
(d) During division of bladder neck

24. Enzalutamide false:
(a) Used in CRPC
(b) Not approved as FDA approved
(c) Inhibit breast cancer cell growth
(d) Formerly known as MDV 3100

25. False about Denosumab:
(a) Requires dose modifications in renal failure
(b) RANKL inhibitors
(c) Given for bone pain
(d) Does not have jaw bone necrosis

26. About silodosin all are true *except*:
(a) More cardiovascular side effects
(b) More selective for 1 α d
(c) Retrograde ejaculation present
(d) Dose titration not required in renal failure

27. Most common cause of storage LUTS:
(a) Carcinoma prostate

(b) CIS bladder
(c) Bladder diverticulum
(d) RCC

28. Patient with T2b carcinoma prostate with 20 PSA underwent radical prostatectomy, now has rising PSA of 2 what is next management?
(a) Should undergo RT
(b) Observation
(c) Adjuvant ADT
(d) Redo surgery

29. True about TURP using Bipolar cautery:
(a) Glycine can be used
(b) Cautery plate applied over the chest
(c) Cautery plate applied over the calves
(d) Cautery plate not required

Mention True and False respective to each statement (Q. No. 30 to 88)

30. Regarding free PSA:
(a) Half life 2-3 days
(b) Excretion mostly through kidney
(c) Subclinical prostatitis increases levels
(d) DRE significantly increases levels
(e) PSA liquify seminogelin I and II

31. Medical management of BPH:
(a) Tamsulosin is $\alpha\ 1_a$ selective
(b) Doxazosin T1/2 is 13 hours
(c) Terazocin Tl/2 is 12 hours
(d) Finasteride most common side effect is sexual dysfunction
(e) Most common dose used for finasteride is 10 mg

32. Pelvic innervations:
(a) Hypogastric nerve enters the sympathetic chain at T10-L2
(b) Presynaptic parasympathetic arises from inter-mediolateral column of sacral cord
(c) Pudendal nerve is a branch of sacral plexus
(d) Superior hypogastric plexus is formed by celiac plexus and 1st lumbar splanchnic
(e) Genital branch of genitofemoral nerve supplies posterior scrotum

33. Regarding TURP:
(a) 1.5% glycine isotonic and provide better vision than normal saline
(b) In bipolar TURP, normal saline can be used
(c) In laser TURP, normal saline can be used
(d) Distilled water can be used for small glands
(e) 100 ml of 3% NS provides 76 Meq of Na^+

34. α-blocker in BPH:
(a) Tamsulosin has same efficacy on α_{1b} and α_{1a}
(b) Doxazocin $T_{1/2}$ is more than that of terazosin
(c) In men with poorly controlled medically treated hypertension, terazosin, significantly lowered blood pressure
(d) Benefit of tamsulosin is that titration of dose is not required
(e) With terazosin peak flow is dose dependent

35. PVR:
(a) High value indicate poor surgical outcome
(b) Most common determinant of surgical outcome
(c) Significant high value indicate upper tract damage
(d) Has intraindividual variability
(e) Transabdominal USG is best method to predict PVR

36. Regarding carcinoma prostate with metastasis:
(a) LHRH agonist has better survival then bilateral orchidectomy
(b) LHRH achieves 100% castration levels
(c) Overall survival significantly favors the immediate ADT group compared with the delayed ADT in LN metastatic prostate cancer
(d) Androgen independent is same as hormone resistant carcinoma
(e) In D2, Taxanes + steroids improves overall survival

37. Regarding PSA:
(a) DRE increases PSA by 4 fold
(b) Free PSA metabolised in liver
(c) Free PSA increased in carcinoma prostate
(d) PSA is a serine protease that liquefies semenogelin I and II
(e) Chromosome of PSA is on long arm of 13

38. Patient with 40 gram prostate and pacemaker undergoing TURP:

(a) Ideal solution is normal saline
(b) Mode of pacemaker has to be changed
(c) Furosemide can worsen TUR syndrome by decreasing Na^+
(d) TUR syndrome can occur with $Na^+ < 125$ mEq/l
(e) 3% NaCl 100 ml solution will give 76 mEq of Na^+

39. Pelvic nerve supply:

(a) Parasympathetic preganglion arises from sacral inferomedial column
(b) Pudendal nerve arises from sacral plexus
(c) Iliohypogastric root value L1
(d) Sympathetic hypogastric plexus formed by celiac plexus and 1st lumbar splanchnic nerve
(e) Posterior femoral cutaneous nerve (S3) gives a perineal branch to supply the scrotum and perineum

40. Freyer's prostatectomy:

(a) Done transperitoneally
(b) At the apex, the prostatic urethra is transected using a pinch action of two fingertips
(c) Malament sutures are placed around bladder neck and is brought out through skin
(d) PSA done in all patients preoperatively
(e) Regional anesthesia may reduce intra-operative blood loss

41. Uroflowmetry:

(a) 150 ml of urine is must
(b) Qmax > 15 ml/sec is suggestive of obstruction
(c) PFR more specifically indentifies patients with BPH than does Q ave
(d) Normal urodynamic curve is bell shaped
(e) High AG suggest obstruction

42. AUA score 23, Qmax 13 ml/sec with LUTS and PSA is 8 mg/ml:

(a) Initial treatment includes antibiotics and repeat PSA after 4 weeks
(b) LUTS cannot be treated with medical management
(c) If first biopsy is negative for malignancy, next biopsy should be done
(d) Pressure flow study is must to document obstruction
(e) Cystoscopy is must before surgery

43. Regarding metastatic carcinoma prostate:

(a) Strontium 89 is used for localized metastasis with pain
(b) Impending paraparesis, steroids should not be used
(c) Zoledronic acid not recommended in patients with renal insufficiency
(d) Patient on LHRH analogue with rising PSA, LHRH analogue should be stopped
(e) Testosterone > 50 microgm/dl second line hormonal therapy should be started

44. Carcinoma prostate:

(a) Free PSA metabolised in kidney
(b) Free PSA is raised in carcinoma prostate
(c) PSA synthesis increased in carcinoma prostate
(d) Taxanes and steroid has survival advantage in HRPC
(e) LHRH agonist causes castrate level testosterone in 100%

45. TUR syndrome:

(a) Hyperammonemia is a cause
(b) Dilusional hyponatremia is a cause
(c) Water intoxication
(d) Syndrome can be reduced by administration of 3% saline
(e) Hyperkalemia is a cause

46. PSA:

(a) 33 KD serine protease
(b) Disease specific
(c) Increase PSA production in carcinoma prostate
(d) Liquifies semenogelin
(e) Free PSA increased in carcinoma prostate

47. TUR syndrome:
(a) Due to hyperkalemia
(b) Due to fluid absorption by bladder mucosa
(c) Height of glycine irrigant should be < 60 cm
(d) $Na^+ < 125$–correction of Na should be done
(e) Chances of syndrome increases if gland size is more than 45 gms and duration of surgery is more than 90 minutes

48. Zoledronic acid:
(a) Dose is 8 mg
(b) Causes nephrotoxicity
(c) Contraindicated in renal insufficiency
(d) Given as short I.V. infusion
(e) Given only in hormone resistant carcinoma prostate

49. Uroflowmetry:
(a) Qmax >15 rule out obstruction
(b) Voided volume > 150 is must
(c) PVR–100 ml is significant
(d) The peak flow rate more specifically identifies patients with BPH than does the average flow rate
(e) A Qmax of less than 15 ml/s does not differentiate between obstruction and bladder decompensation

50. BPH:
(a) Bladder stone is eight times higher in patients with BPH
(b) Prostatic infarction has been suggested as an underlying even causing AUR
(c) The risk for AUR increases with increasing serum PSA as well as prostate volume
(d) Bipolar TURP–NS can be used
(e) Strong correlations exists between measures of symptom severity, (I-PSS score), bother and disease-specific HRQOL

51. Regarding TUR syndrome:
(a) Due to hyperkalemia
(b) Seen usually with $Na^+ < 135$
(c) Fluid absorption from bladder mucosa
(d) Can be prevented by keeping fluid column < 60 cm
(e) Can be prevented by performing surgery < 90 min

52. PSA:
(a) 33 KDA
(b) Liquify seminogelins
(c) Free PSA T ½ 2-3 hours, metabolize by liver
(d) It is disease specific
(e) DRE increases PSA by 3 times

53. BPH:
(a) AUR is rare in natural history
(b) Good drainage by large bore catheter for AUR
(c) Patients with severe symptoms should not be offered medical treatment
(d) Foley's bulb to be inflated till capacity
(e) Indicates benign prostatic hypertrophy

54. BPH–Medical management:
(a) T½ of Doxazocin – 12 hours
(b) T½ of Terazosin – 2 hours
(c) Tamsulosin causes abnormal ejaculation
(d) Dutasteride 10 mg drug of choice
(e) Most common side effect of finasteride is sexual dysfunction

55. Endourological procedure:
(a) 1.5% glycine is fluid of choice for TURP
(b) TCC at ureteric orifice–coagulation current is used
(c) Increase in height of irrigation fluid increases absorption
(d) Bipolar TURP minimize risk of obturator reflex
(e) Distilled water can be used for small procedures

56. Regarding prostate:
(a) EGF is important for stromal growth
(b) TGF-β is responsible for epithelial growth in BPH
(c) Type II α reductase more in prostate stroma
(d) Type I α reductase is more than type II α reductase overall in prostate
(e) Dutasteride decreases DHT levels by 90%

57. Anatomy of prostate:
(a) Main blood supply from obturator artery
(b) TZ arises from ectoderm

(c) α_1 b is more common in prostatic stroma
(d) Endothelin in prostate causes vasoconstriction, HTN and stromal constriction
(e) Major production of neuroendocrine cell–TSH

58. Regarding PSA:
(a) Free PSA metabolize in liver
(b) Prostate cancer cells make less PSA than normal prostatic tissue
(c) DRE increases PSA by 4 times
(d) PSA chromosome is located on long arm of 19
(e) PSA liquify seminogelin I and II

59. Regarding TRUS:
(a) Bleeding PR is most common complication of TRUS biopsy
(b) In TRUS biopsy–Enema is prerequisite
(c) 18-gauge needle core biopsy device or biopsy gun
(d) Aspirin/NSAIDs should be stopped 7 to 10 days before prostate biopsy
(e) Antibiotic therapy should be continued for 2 to 3 days after biopsy

60. Carcinoma prostate and bone metastasis in 60 years male:
(a) LHRH agonist has survival advantage over orchidectomy
(b) For D2–Bicalutamide has survival advantage over orchidectomy
(c) Androgen independent and hormone refractory are same
(d) Taxanes and steroid has survival advantage in HRPC
(e) LHRH agonist causes castrate level testosterone in 100%

61. Regarding TURP:
(a) 3% hypertonic saline–contains 513 mEq/l of Na^+
(b) NS is best suited for TURP
(c) Na < 125 mg/l always causes TUR syndrome
(d) Pacemaker settings are not changed during TURP
(e) TUR syndrome is treated with diuretics

62. Prostate development:
(a) Most important determinant for inhibitor of epithelial growth is TGF β
(b) Estrogen causes squamous metaplasia
(c) 90% of epithelial cell loss occurs after orchidectomy
(d) Neuroendocrine tumors have undetectable PSA
(e) α1 is an adrenoceptor in smooth muscle

63. 50 years old male–presented with LUTS:
(a) PSA is mandatory
(b) TRUS is done to detect prostate malignancy
(c) Urine routine examination should be done
(d) Upper urinary tract imaging is not recommended in the routine evaluation of men with LUTS
(e) Pressure flow study should be done in all patients

64. PSA is specific for:
(a) Prostate disease
(b) Prostate cancer
(c) Prostate enlargement
(d) Prostatic cyst
(e) BPH

65. TUR syndrome:
(a) 300 ml/min of fluid is needed for a good vision field
(b) Common if resection time > 90 min
(c) Absorption is from bladder mucosa
(d) If height of irrigation fluid is < 60 cm incidence is decreased
(e) Is due to hyponatremia < 125 mmol/l

66. 60-year-old + urinary retention + coronary artery disease:
(a) Voiding trial before surgery should be given
(b) Increase PSA level can change the treatment
(c) Medical treatment should be attempted first
(d) If TWOC, fails, it's an indication for surgery
(e) If patient also has recurrent UTI, it's an indication for surgery

67. PSA:
(a) 33 KD serine protease
(b) DRE–Increases PSA by 7 times
(c) Disease specific marker for prostate
(d) Liquifies semen by acting on semenogelin
(e) Free PSA ½ life is 2-3 hours and is metabolised in liver

68. BPH:
(a) Patients castrated prior to puberty or who are affected by a variety of genetic diseases that impair androgen action or production do not develop BPH
(b) Type 1, 5 α reductase is important in BPH
(c) Type II, 5 α reductase mainly in stromal cells
(d) Intraprostatic testosterone concentration increased by 5α reductase inhibitor
(e) Prostate, maintains its ability to respond to androgens throughout life

69. Patient with BPH and hypertension with CAD:
(a) TURP is contraindicated because of CAD
(b) Predominant median lobe enlargement–dutasteride and α blocker is most effective
(c) In HPE report of prostate chips→ negative for carcinoma prostate – Rules out carcinoma of prostate if PSA is 4
(d) Spinal anesthesia is most appropriate for TURP
(e) A mild symptom denotes mild obstruction

70. TRUS:
(a) Probe of 7 MHZ
(b) Most hypoechoic lesion are carcinoma
(c) Precisely evaluate microscopic extra-capsular extension
(d) Clinically impalpable > 1 cm hypoechoic lesion are not detected in 50% of cases
(e) Used for planning of brachytherapy

71. BPH:
(a) Serum PSA can change the management
(b) Pressure flow study–most accurate for management
(c) Poor flow with increase PVR→ Indication of surgery
(d) Cystoscopy is used for diagnosis of BPH
(e) AUA–symptoms score related with severity of obstruction

72. PSA:
(a) If > 50–75% have LN present
(b) If >20 get bone scan
(c) Gene lies on chromosome-1
(d) 25% of patients with carcinoma prostate have PSA < 4 ng/ml
(e) BPH presents with PSA 15 ng/ml

73. Endothelin:
(a) 11 amino acid polypeptide
(b) Least potent vasoconstrictor
(c) Secreted by basal cells
(d) Also secreted by mesangial cells
(e) Act via G protein couple receptor

74. Regarding PSA:
(a) DRE test increases 4 times
(b) Molecular weight–33000 D
(c) Exclusively secreted by prostatic epithelial cells
(d) It is h KLK3
(e) Half life is 2-3 days

75. Anatomy of prostate:
(a) Weight–5 g
(b) Peripheral zone smallest
(c) Biopsy of prostatic urethra essential before planning orthotopic bladder reconstruction
(d) Orthotopic bladder reconstruction contraindicated if biopsy positive
(e) Asymptomatic patients with E. coli culture positive – prophylaxis needed

76. Carcinoma prostate:
(a) Biopsy of prostate not needed if PSA <4
(b) Transitional zone biopsy included in10 core biopsy
(c) Rectal enema prerequisite for prostatic biopsy
(d) Gleason's score grade 1-2 most common
(e) Gleason system is based on the glandular pattern of the tumor as identified at relatively low magnification

77. PSA:
(a) 33 KD serine protease
(b) Specific disease marker for prostate
(c) Liquify semen by acting on seminogelin
(d) Increases in DRE by 3 times
(e) Free PSA has T/½ of 2-3 months

78. Prostatic biopsy:
(a) In elderly with age 82 years should be done if PSA is 12
(b) If nodule is palpable no need to sextant biopsy
(c) TRUS does not increase serum PSA
(d) Most common complication is hematoma
(e) If hypoechoic lesion found on TRUS, chances of malignancy is 16-33%

79. Medical treatment of BPH:
(a) Finasteride is competitive inhibitor of Type I 5α reductase
(b) Finasteride causes 50% reduction in PSA
(c) Finasteride causes 20% reduction in prostate volume
(d) Better than α-blocker in BPH
(e) Most common side effect is sexual dysfunction

80. Medical treatment of BPH:
(a) T ½ doxazocin is 22 hours
(b) T ½ terazoin is 12 hours
(c) Dose of finasteride is10 mg/day
(d) Tamsulosin is α_{1a} subtype selective
(e) Finasteride is used for post TURP bleeding

81. Residual urine:
(a) PVR does not have significant intra individual variability
(b) High PVR is indication for surgery
(c) PVR can predict outcome of surgery
(d) PVR can be measured accurately by abdominal USG
(e) High PVR has effect on upper tracts

82. Uroflowmetry:
(a) Flow rate is inaccurate if voided volume is < 135–150 ml
(b) Average flow rate more specific than peak flow rate
(c) With advancing age Qmax decreases in females
(d) If Qmax <15, it does not differentiate between BPH and hypocontractile bladder
(e) In low flow rates results of surgery is not good

83. Regarding TURP:
(a) Approximately 300 ml/min of fluid was needed for a good vision field
(b) If after traction, bleeding does not stop prostate fossa packing is done
(c) If height of the fluid was changed from 60 to 70 cm, fluid absorption was greater than two-fold
(d) Glands weighing less than 30 g, incise the bladder neck with a Colling's knife at the 12 O'clock position
(e) Small bladder tumor resection can be done in NS

84. TURP:
(a) 15% glycine isotonic and provide better vision than NS
(b) In bipolar TUR, NS can be used
(c) In laser ablation, NS can be used
(d) If NS used in TUR it can prevent hypo-natremia
(e) IPSS can determine treatment modality

85. TRUS:
(a) 7.0 MHz probe
(b) 50% nonpalpable, >1 cm prostatic lesion cannot be detected by TRUS
(c) Most of the hypoechoic lesion on TRUS are carcinoma
(d) TRUS can detect microscopic extra-capsular extension
(e) TRUS can be used in planning for brachytherapy

86. Regarding prostate anatomy:
(a) Receive supply from pudendal artery
(b) NVB is present at 5 and 7 O' clock position at membranous urethra

(c) NVB is present between levator fascia and Denonviller's fascia
(d) The deep dorsal vein leaves the penis under Buck's fascia between the corpora cavernosa
(e) Capsular vessels provide the macroscopic landmark to aid in the identification of the microscopic branches of the pelvic plexus

87. Regarding TURP:
(a) 1.5% glycine isotonic and provide better vision than normal saline
(b) In bipolar TURP, normal saline can be used
(c) In laser TURP, normal saline can be used
(d) Distilled water can be used for small glands
(e) IPSS scoring can predict the need of HOLEP/ conventional TURP

88. Regarding TRUS:
(a) Probe frequency is 7 MHz
(b) Fifty percent non-palpable, < 1 cm tumor cannot be detected by TRUS
(c) Most of hypoechoeic lesion on TRUS is carcinoma
(d) TRUS can detect microscopic extracapsular extension
(e) TRUS can be used for the planning of brachytherapy

Which of the following statement is correct?

89. PSA:
(a) Member of kallikrein family
(b) Free PSA– $T_{1/2}$- 2-3 days
(c) Liquify semen
(d) Controversial in screening
(e) Cancer cells produce more PSA

90. Which are not the branch of anterior internal iliac artery?
(a) Superior gluteal artery
(b) Middle rectal artery
(c) Inferior vesical artery
(d) Gonadal
(e) Obturator

91. BPH treatment laser used:
(a) Ho-YaG (b) KTP
(c) Argon (d) CO_2
(e) Diode

92. TUR syndrome associated with:
(a) Tachycardia
(b) Bradycardia
(c) Hypertension
(d) Altered sensorium
(e) Hypotension

93. Hormone naïve prostatic carcinoma–anti-androgen used are:
(a) Bicalutamide (b) Flutamide
(c) Ketoconazole (d) Nilutamide
(e) Thalidomide

94. α1 receptors are mainly present in:
(a) Bladder neck
(b) Prostatic stroma and smooth muscle
(c) Bladder dome
(d) EUS
(e) Lower ureter

95. TRUS guided biopsy in carcinoma prostate – true is:
(a) Antibiotics not indicated before biopsy
(b) Sextant is not considered adequate
(c) Hematospermia is a complication
(d) Seminal vesical biopsy routine done
(e) Carcinoma can be diagnosed with certainty by hypoechoic lesions

96. Which of the following are anti-androgen?
(a) Spironolactone
(b) DES
(c) Ketoconazole
(d) Cyproterone acetate
(e) Clonidine

97. PSA not raised in:
(a) Adenocarcinoma prostate
(b) HRPC
(c) Undifferentiated prostate carcinoma
(d) Metastatic prostate carcinoma
(e) Neuroendocrine carcinoma of prostate

98. Carcinoma prostate extent can be evaluated by all *except*:
(a) DRE (b) PSA
(c) MRI (d) Bone scan
(e) Gleason's score

99. Carcinoma prostate true statement:
(a) Gleason's grade independent prognostic marker
(b) IVU done for diagnosis
(c) Seminal vesical involvement, stage is T4
(d) GnRH given for treatment of metastasis
(e) Hot flushes can be the side effect of GnRH agonist

100. Complication of radical prostatectomy all *except*:
(a) Priapism
(b) ED
(c) Urinary incontinence
(d) Bladder neck contracture
(e) Obturator nerve injury

101. Flare up phenomenon seen in:
(a) Goserelin
(b) Cetrorelix
(c) Triptorelin
(d) Cyproterone acetate
(e) Methotrexate

102. Batson's plexus associated with all *except*:
(a) Urinary bladder (b) Base of skull
(c) Prostate (d) Brain
(e) Lung

103. Carcinoma prostate histopathology:
(a) Gleason sum–6 to 10
(b) Gleason's grading–3 grades
(c) Perineural invasion in RP–worst prognosis
(d) Metastatic prostate – immunoperoxidase staining is helpful
(e) Transitional zone–most common

104. Regarding TRUS in carcinoma prostate as a screening tool:
(a) 50% non-palpable >1 cm tumor are not seen
(b) All hypoechoic lesions are not cancer
(c) Prostate cancer is mostly hyperechoic
(d) TRUS is not reproducible
(e) 7 MHz probe is used

105. Late complications in radical prostatectomy:
(a) Pulmonary embolism
(b) Infertility
(c) Erectile dysfunction
(d) Urinary incontinence
(e) Urinary retention (bladder neck contracture)

106. Carcinoma prostate involving rectal wall in palpation, further investigation required:
(a) Liver and spleen scan
(b) GI evaluation
(c) CT chest
(d) CT whole abdomen
(e) Gallium scan

107. PSA increased in:
(a) Large prostate adenocarcinoma
(b) Acute bacterial prostatitis
(c) Chronic abacterial prostatitis
(d) Granulomatous prostatitis
(e) BPH

108. Osteoblastic metastasis is seen in all *except*:
(a) Carcinoma prostate
(b) Medullary carcinoma thyroid
(c) RCC
(d) Breast cancer
(e) Neuroblastoma

109. Prostate is supplied by:
(a) Inferior vesical
(b) Middle rectal
(c) Bulbar
(d) Internal pudendal
(e) Superior vesical

110. Fluid not used in TURP:
(a) Glycine (b) Normal saline
(c) RL (d) Mannitol
(e) Glucose

111. Complication of prostatic biopsy:
(a) Hematoma (b) Bacterial sepsis
(c) Rectal bleeding (d) Perianal abscess
(e) Anal stenosis

112. In case of AUR, failure of attempt of gentle catheterization – next best option:
(a) Try catheterization with stiff catheter
(b) Suprapubic cystostomy
(c) DVIU
(d) Plan for prostatectomy
(e) End to end urethroplasty

113. In TURBT possible complications are:
(a) Perforation
(b) Clot retention
(c) Ureteric orifice fibrosis
(d) TUR syndrome
(e) Tumor dissemination

114. Late complication of radical prostatectomy in organ confined carcinoma prostate:
(a) Erectile dysfunction
(b) Infertility
(c) Incontinence
(d) Anastomotic stricture at vesicourethral anastomosis
(e) Thromboembolism

115. For screening of cancer prostate:
(a) DRE + PSA
(b) TRUS + PSA
(c) Sextant biopsy + PSA
(d) PSA + Endoluminal MRI
(e) DRE + Endoluminal USG

116. For carcinoma prostate screening–most effective:
(a) PSA + DRE
(b) PSA + MRI
(c) PSA + TRUS
(d) TRUS
(e) PSA

117. Limitation of TRUS:
(a) TRUS can add staging information over that gained with DRE
(b) Most of hypoechoic is not malignant
(c) More than 50% of <1 cm not detected
(d) Painful procedure requires regional anesthesia
(e) Corpora amylacea highlight plane between PZ and TZ

118. Osteoblastic secondary seen in all *except*:
(a) Prostate carcinoma
(b) Medullary thyroid carcinoma
(c) Carcinoma breast
(d) Renal cell carcinoma
(e) Rhabdomyosarcoma

119. TURP – HPE showing striated muscles chips. This can lead to:
(a) Urinary incontinence
(b) Impotency
(c) Extravasation
(d) No major bleeding
(e) No complication

120. Vascular supply of prostate:
(a) Superior vesical artery
(b) Inferior vesical artery
(c) Internal pudendal artery
(d) Middle rectal
(e) External iliac artery

121. PSA:
(a) Coagulate semen
(b) Specifically secreted by prostatic luminal epithelial cells
(c) Increased after DRE
(d) In seminal fluid concentration is 1-4 mg/ml
(e) PSA gene – hk3

122. PSA all *except*:
(a) Increase concentration in seminal plasma
(b) Glycoprotein
(c) Exclusively secreted by epithelial cells
(d) Increased by DRE
(e) Mainly bound to $\alpha 2$ microglobulin and macroglobulin

123. Abiraterone-drug used in castration-resistant prostate cancer, it inhibits:
(a) 21 α-hydroxylase
(b) 11 α-hydroxylase
(c) 17 α-hydroxylase
(d) 17 α-hydroxylase and C17, 20 lyases

124. **Blood supply to prostate all *except*:**
(a) Middle hemorrhoidal
(b) Inferior vesical
(c) Obturator
(d) Pudendal

125. **False about pelvic plexus:**
(a) Sagittal plane–lateral to rectum
(b) Starts at midpoint of seminal vesicles
(c) Pierced by minor vessels of prostate and rectum
(d) Both sides do not communicate with each other

126. **To preserve potency after radical cystectomy lateral and posterior pedicle tied:**
(a) At origin of bifurcation of CIA
(b) At origin from IIA
(c) Near bladder surface
(d) At crossing of ureter

127. **The zone affected most by chronic prostatitis is:**
(a) Anterior (b) Posterior
(c) Central (d) Transition

128. **Most abundant androgen in prostate:**
(a) DHEA
(b) Testosterone
(c) DHT
(d) Epiandrosterone

129. **Immediate precursor of Estrogen:**
(a) Progesterone (b) Testosterone
(c) DHEA (d) Estrone

130. **Epigenetic modification in carcinoma prostate:**
(a) GTPS1 methylation (b) AMACR
(c) UROC28 (d) Hepsin

131. **Seventy years old man wish to undergo open prostatectomy. Which is justified criterion?**
(a) Patient worry about cancer and wish to get his whole prostate removed
(b) More than 90 gms prostate
(c) He is on antiplatelets and do not want to stop
(d) Less erectile dysfunction

132. **Perineal pain with tender prostate PSA is 7.5:**
(a) Repeat PSA
(b) TURP
(c) Analgesic and antibiotics
(d) TRUS guided biopsy

133. **Hereditary prostate cancer in <55 years of age accounts for:**
(a) 0-20% (b) 20-40%
(c) 40-60% (d) 60-80%

134. **For preserving continence during TURP, sphincter preserved is:**
(a) Rhabdosphincter
(b) Lissosphincter
(c) Urethral smooth muscle
(d) Bladder neck

135. **Mortality due to prostate cancer is highest in:**
(a) Asia (b) UK
(c) USA (d) Sweden

136. **False about PSA:**
(a) > 100 ng/ml highly specific for prostate cancer
(b) Useful for screening in India
(c) PSA screening has equivocal result in prostate cancer specific mortality
(d) Increased after prostate biopsy

137. **5α reductase converts:**
(a) DHT → T (b) E → DHT
(c) E → T (d) T → DHT

138. **Not given in BPH:**
(a) Flutamide (b) Finasteride
(c) Alfuzosin (d) Terazosin

139. **Most of important determinant of uroflometry in BPH:**
(a) Peak flow rate
(b) Average flow rate
(c) Residual volume
(d) Voided volume

140. **In radical prostatectomy to prevent incontinence what is to be preserved:**
(a) Rhabdosphincter
(b) Transverse perineal muscles
(c) Perineal muscles
(d) Internal striated sphincter

141. **Perineal prostatectomy done by:**
(a) Freyer (b) Walsh
(c) Young (d) Millin

142. **Not a subtype of alpha receptor:**
(a) α 1a (b) α 1b
(c) α 1d (d) α 1g

143. **In men with post prostatectomy cuff of AUS is placed at:**
(a) Bulbous urethra
(b) Penile urethra
(c) Perineum
(d) Membranous urethra

144. **Which is a 5α reductase inhibitor?**
(a) Tamsulosin (b) Terazosin
(c) Dutasteride (d) Dicyclomine

145. **Dose of tamsulosin is:**
(a) 0.4 mg HS (b) 5 mg BD
(c) 10 mg OD (d) 12.5 mg OD

146. **Advantages of alfuzosin over tamsulosin:**
(a) Less retrograde ejaculation
(b) Less blue green vision
(c) Lesser cost
(d) Lesser schedule of dosing

147. **After transurethral resection of prostate, radical prostatectomy is done after:**
(a) 4 weeks (b) 8 weeks
(c) 12 weeks (d) 20 weeks

148. **Most common complication of prostatic biopsy:**
(a) Bleeding (b) AUR
(c) Infection (d) Septicemia

149. **Vaccine used in carcinoma prostate:**
(a) Gilivenge (b) Provenge
(c) Avenge (d) All of the above

150. **4 weeks after TURP, patient presented with stress urinary incontinence – treatment plan:**
(a) Deflux (b) AUS
(c) Male sling (d) Observation

151. **Half life of free PSA:**
(a) 2-3 days (b) 2-3 hours
(c) 7-10 days (d) 5-6 months

152. **Sixty-year-old male with radical prostatectomy, Gleason-9, margins negative, post-prostatectomy at 3 months–PSA-0, 6 months–PSA-1 ng/ml, 1 year –PSA-3 ng/ml, treatment:**
(a) Local radiotherapy (b) Chemotherapy
(c) Observation (d) Orchidectomy

153. **70-year-old male, history of CABG 4 years back, T1c tumor on prostatic biopsy, Gleason's score 3+3, > 10% tumor on one core, treatment plan:**
(a) Radical prostatectomy
(b) Robotic
(c) Observation
(d) Cyber knife

154. **Patient with carcinoma prostate, on LHRH analogue for 24 months with locally advanced carcinoma prostate initial metastatic work-up, negative. Now has rising PSA:**
(a) Check testosterone
(b) Add antiandrogen
(c) CECT pelvis
(d) Bone scan

155. **Patient with small cell carcinoma prostate – T3 stage. Treatment is:**
(a) Chemotherapy
(b) Local RT
(c) Androgen deprivation
(d) Radical prostatectomy

156. **Fifty-year-old smoker with hematuria normal DRE, cytology and CECT negative, what is to be done?**
(a) Finasteride (b) TURP
(c) Cystoscopy (d) Observation

157. **Chance of improvement of patients symptoms after a TURP is:**
(a) 98% (b) 88%
(c) 78% (d) 68%

158. **Most potent α blocker:**
(a) Alfuzosin (b) Tamsulosin
(c) Terazocin (d) Prazocin

159. **Tamsulosin mechanism of action is:**
(a) α_{1a} (b) α_{1b}
(c) α_{1d} (d) α_2

160. **In prostate cancer chemoprevention trial is done with:**
(a) Finasteride (b) Dutasteride
(c) Tamsulosin (d) Alfuzocin

161. **Finasteride for hematuria is used in:**
(a) BPH
(b) BPH and prostrate cancer
(c) Prostrate cancer alone
(d) None of the above

162. **Regarding PIN which of the following is true?**
(a) Low grade should not be reported in needle biopsies
(b) High grade is present in 7-10% of biopsies
(c) PSA levels, DRE, and TRUS findings do enhance the prediction of who is more likely to have carcinoma on repeat biopsy
(d) Patients diagnosed with high-grade PIN on extended initial core sampling, a repeat biopsy within the first year is necessary

163. **Mechanism of action of TUNA:**
(a) Radiofrequency (b) Ultrasonic
(c) Laser (d) Electrosurgical

164. **Temperature within the prostate in TUMT is:**
(a) < 40 °C (b) 44–70 °C
(c) 70–95 °C (d) > 100 °C

165. **Most important determinant of uroflowmetry in BPH:**
(a) Peak flow rate
(b) Average flow rate
(c) Residual volume
(d) Voided volume

166. **5α reductase converts:**
(a) Testosterone to dihydrotestosterone
(b) DHT to testosterone
(c) DHT to DHEA
(d) DHEA to DHT

167. **Present in maximum concentration in prostrate:**
(a) Dihydrotestosterone
(b) Testosterone
(c) DHEA
(d) Androstenedione

168. **Castration will cause:**
(a) 90% decrease in prostatic epithelial cells
(b) 90% decrease in prostatic stromal cells
(c) 40% decreases in prostatic epithelial cells
(d) 60% decrease in prostatic stromal cells

169. **Disadvantage of bilateral orchidectomy, which of the following is true?**
(a) More expensive than LHRH
(b) Onset of action delayed
(c) Can't produce intermittent androgen deprivation
(d) Less effective than LHRH analogues

170. **Why does BPH not cause urinary symptoms in dogs?**
(a) Urethra is eccentric
(b) Does not occur in transition zone
(c) Does not have a capsule
(d) Has a different histopathology

171. **Which of the following is not true?**
(a) 70% of cancer in peripheral zone
(b) Central zone surrounds ejaculatory duct
(c) Anterior fibromuscular zone has no glandular element
(d) Transitional zone is the largest gland

172. **All are suggestive of carcinoma prostate *except*:**
(a) Serum PSA density >0.15

(b) PSA velocity >0.75 ng/ml per year
(c) Free/total PSA >0.18
(d) PSA > 4 ng/ml

173. The zone forming the bulk of prostatic glandular tissue:
(a) Transitional (b) Central
(c) Peripheral (d) Anterior

174. The most common cause of mortality following TURP is:
(a) TUR syndrome
(b) Myocardial infarction
(c) Sepsis
(d) Hemorrhage

175. The drug that is used in the prostate cancer prevention trial study:
(a) Lycopene (b) Finasteride
(c) Flutamide (d) Pyridoxine

176. Which drug produces flare phenomenon during treatment of carcinoma prostate?
(a) Bicalutamide (b) Zoledronic acid
(c) Leuprolide (d) Dutasteride

177. The most commonly used isotope for permanent brachytherapy for carcinoma prostate is:
(a) I^{125} (b) I^{131}
(c) P^{12} (d) Tc99m

178. In prostate glandular volume contributes what % of total volume?
(a) 30% (b) 40%
(c) 60% (d) 70%

179. Prostate volume highly correlates with:
(a) PSA
(b) Urine flow rate
(c) Post void residual volume
(d) Histological grade

180. Gleason system for carcinoma prostate is based on the:
(a) Nuclear pattern of the cells
(b) Cell size
(c) Cell polarity
(d) Glandular pattern

181. Which of the following statements regarding the peripheral zone of prostate is false?
(a) Constitutes about 30% of the glandular tissue
(b) Covers the posterior and the lateral aspects of the gland
(c) 70% of prostate cancer arises in this zone
(d) This zone is most commonly affected by chronic prostatitis

182. International prostate symptom score questionnaire includes the following *except*:
(a) Frequency (b) Urgency
(c) Hesitancy (d) Straining

183. BPH arises in:
(a) Peripheral zone
(b) Transitional zone
(c) Anterior fibromuscular stroma
(d) Central zone

184. Usage of Finasteride:
(a) Is best for prostate >30 gm weight
(b) Is best used in conjunction with an alpha blocker
(c) Causes increased intraprostatic testosterone
(d) Causes impotence in 20% men

185. The neurovascular bundle of Walsh is most vulnerable during radical prostatectomy at:
(a) Prostatic base near bladder neck
(b) Prostatic apex at 3 and 9 O' clock position
(c) Prostatic apex at 5 and 7 O' clock position
(d) Membranous urethra

186. Prostate is composed of:
(a) 70% glandular and 30% fibromuscular stroma
(b) 30% glandular and 70% fibromuscular stroma
(c) 50% glandular and 50% fibromuscular stroma
(d) 60% glandular and 40% fibromuscular stroma

187. PSA – role is:
(a) Lyses semen (b) Nourishment
(c) Sperm motility (d) Provide volume

188. Most potent α-1 antagonist:
(a) Tamsulosin (b) Terazosin
(c) Prazosin (d) Doxazocin

189. 70% of prostate is composed of:
(a) Glandular
(b) Fibrous stroma
(c) Muscular stroma
(d) Fibromuscular stromal

190. T2b carcinoma prostate:
(a) Bilateral lobe involvement within capsule
(b) Same with extracapsular invasion
(c) Tumor involves more than half of one lobe
(d) PSA only increased

191. Highest PSA levels seen in:
(a) Metastatic carcinoma prostate
(b) Prostate adenoma >150 g
(c) Prostatic infection
(d) Semen of young male

192. Volume of prostate size that will decrease with androgen ablation with LHRH analogs is:
(a) 80% (b) 60%
(c) 70% (d) 30%

193. In prostatic abscess with retention, treatment is by:
(a) Perurethral catheterization
(b) Suprapubic catheterization
(c) Perineal urethrostomy
(d) PCN

194. Chronic prostatitis–long-term treatment of choice:
(a) Ciprofloxacin (b) Tetracycline
(c) Amikacin (d) Ampicillin

195. Median survival of extensive prostatic carcinoma with bone metastasis is:
(a) 11 months (b) 24 months
(c) 3 years (d) 4 years

196. Which of the following drug is not given in BPH routinely?
(a) Phenoxybenzamine (b) Tamsulosin
(c) Terazosin (d) Finasteride

197. Indication of upper tract study in BPH:
(a) Increased creatinine
(b) Residual urine >100 ml
(c) UTI
(d) History of previous urinary tract surgery

198. Prostate carcinoma most commonly arises from:
(a) Central (b) Peripheral
(c) Transitional (d) Periurethral zone

199. Which of the following is used for hormone-resistant metastatic carcinoma of prostate?
(a) Docetaxel (b) Cisplatin
(c) Bleomycin (d) 5-FU

200. Which of the following is not an appropriate option for chemical castration?
(a) Cyproterone acetate
(b) Finasteride
(c) LHRH agonist
(d) Bicalutamide

201. Most specific finding of nodal involvement by metastasis:
(a) Enhancement
(b) Central necrosis
(c) Size > 8-10 mm
(d) Multiple lymph nodes

202. Median survival of patients with extensive disease showing progression by PSA and bone scan both is:
(a) 40 months (b) 23 months
(c) 18 months (d) 11 months

203. The neurovascular bundle of Walsh consists of:
(a) Dorsal nerve of penis and deep dorsal artery of penis
(b) Cavernosal artery and cavernosal nerve

(c) Cavernosal nerve and prostatic capsular branch of inferior vesical artery
(d) Dorsal nerve of penis and cavernosal arrtery

204. Puboprostatic ligament is formed by:
(a) Parietal layer of pelvic fascia
(b) Visceral layer of pelvic fascia
(c) Prostatic capsule
(d) Superior fascia of pelvic diaphragm

205. The following fluid is not recommended for irrigation in TURP:
(a) Distil water (b) NS
(c) 5% dextrose (d) Glycine

206. Action of 5α reductase is:
(a) Conversion of testosterone to DHT
(b) Conversion of DHT to testosterone
(c) Conversion of testosterone to estrogen
(d) Conversion of estrogen to testosterone

207. Which of the following test is mandatory before starting 5α reductase therapy?
(a) Serum creatinine
(b) Serum PSA
(c) Acid phosphatase
(d) All of the above

208. Which one of the following is not the side effect of 5-ARI?
(a) Impotence
(b) Retrograde ejaculation
(c) Loss of libido
(d) Asthenia

209. After radical prostatectomy, the chance of recurrence is indicated by PSA levels above:
(a) 0.2 ng/ml (b) 0.3 ng/ml
(c) 0.4 ng/ml (d) 0.5 ng/ml

210. The principal blood supply to prostate is:
(a) Superior vesical artery
(b) Inferior vesical artery
(c) Internal pudendal artery
(d) External iliac artery

211. In TRUS which lesion has maximum chances of malignancy:
(a) Isoechoic
(b) Hypoechoic
(c) Hyperechoic
(d) All of the above has similar incidence

212. In prostate cancer pelvic CT is indicated in all *except:*
(a) In a patient with PSA > 20 ng/ml
(b) Young patient with age of onset < 40 years
(c) Advanced disease on DRE
(d) High grade carcinoma prostate (poor histology)

213. Bladder trabeculation on cystoscopy is seen in:
(a) Thimble bladder
(b) Bladder outlet obstruction
(c) Ureterocele
(d) Ectopic ureter

214. All of the following are absolute indication for TURP *except:*
(a) > 100 gm prostate
(b) Refractory retention
(c) Failure of medical treatment
(d) Recurrent UTI

215. Most common cause of TUR syndrome:
(a) Dilutional hyponatremia
(b) Glycine metabolized to NH_3
(c) Hemolysis
(d) Fluid overload

216. True about finasteride use in BPH:
(a) Selective inhibitor of type 2, 5α reductase
(b) Prostate volume decrease by 30% at 12 weeks
(c) Increase libido
(d) Increases PSA

217. True about cyproterone acetate, are all *except:*
(a) Decrease libido
(b) Gynecomastia

(c) Fluid retention
(d) It is steroidal antiandrogen

218. True about PSA, all *except:*
(a) It is a glycoprotein
(b) Affected by carcinoma prostate
(c) Exclusively secreted by epithelial cells of prostate
(d) Also called Hk2

219. True about BPH:
(a) It is pre-malignant
(b) 30% incidence in the 4th decade of life
(c) Best initial treatment is trial of GnRI-analogues
(d) Surgery is mainstay treatment option

220. Upper tract imaging is done in BPH in all *except:*
(a) UTI
(b) Previous surgery of upper tract
(c) Impaired renal function
(d) Severe LUTS

221. Richest source of prostaglandin is:
(a) Liver (b) Seminal vesicles
(c) Brain (d) Prostate

222. Which structure of urethra is unattached to any fixed structures?
(a) Penile (b) Bulbar
(c) Membranous (d) Prostatic urethra

223. 5-alpha reductase is not necessary for the development of:
(a) Acne (b) Hirsutism
(c) BPH (d) Seminal vesicles

224. Which of the following not an indication of BPH surgery?
(a) PVR > 150 ml
(b) Recurrent UTI
(c) Bladder stones
(d) Recurrent hematuria

225. During prostatectomy cavernosal nerves most likely to be damaged at:
(a) Base (b) Sides
(c) Apex (d) Bladder neck

226. How much % of early carcinoma prostate patients have PSA values < 4 ng/ml?
(a) 0 (b) 15
(c) 25 (d) 40

227. A patient presented with LUTS, on examination there is 120 g prostate and a 4 cm bladder calculus. Management of choice includes:
(a) Open supra pubic prostatectomy
(b) Open retropubic prostatectomy
(c) TURP
(d) Perineal prostatectomy

228. A patient taking finasteride since 12 months now the PSA value is 7, what could be the PSA levels before starting this drug?
(a) 3.5 (b) 14
(c) 21 (d) 49

229. Most common complication of TRUS biopsy:
(a) Infection
(b) Bleeding per rectum
(c) Rectourethral fistula
(d) Hematospermia

230. Richest source of prostaglandins in the body:
(a) Kidney (b) Skeletal muscle
(c) Liver (d) Seminal vesicles

231. What is the embryological origin of the transition zone?
(a) Mesoderm (b) Ectoderm
(c) Endoderm (d) Mullerian duct

232. Which drug has the association with flare phenomenon?
(a) Dutasteride (b) Bicalutamide
(c) Goserelin acetate (d) Abarelix

233. Which adrenoreceptor subtype mediates prostatic smooth muscle contraction?
(a) α_{1a} (b) α_{1b}
(c) α_2 (d) α_{2c}

234. Richest source of prostaglandins:
(a) Prostate (b) Seminal vesicle
(c) Adrenal (d) Epididymis
(e) Testis

235. Screening of prostate adenocarcinoma is done in:
(a) 60 years male with HTN and poorly controlled DM
(b) 60 years male with HTN with medication
(c) 55 years male with family history of carcinoma prostate
(d) 59 years male with family history of chronic severe COPD
(e) 69 years male with unstable angina

236. In prostate glandular volume contributes what % of total volume?
(a) 30% (b) 40%
(c) 60% (d) 70%
(e) 80%

237. If PSA >100, true is:
(a) Near 100% incidence of prostate malignancy with bone metastasis
(b) Can occur after DRE
(c) Can occur in acute prostatitis
(d) Can occur in chronic prostatitis
(e) In BPH >100 gm

238. Late complication of radical prostatectomy:
(a) Stricture
(b) Incontinence
(c) ED
(d) Bladder neck contracture
(e) Osteoporosis

239. Prostatic biopsy complication includes all *except*:
(a) Anal stenosis (b) Rectal bleeding
(c) Perianal abscess (d) Bacterial sepsis
(e) Hematuria

240. Regarding the anatomy of the prostate:
(a) The urethra is closest to the posterior surface of the prostate gland
(b) Approximately one third is composed of glandular elements
(c) 70% of the gland is made up of the peripheral zone
(d) The lobes of prostate have distinctly different histological difference

241. The ProVu device for BPH is a form of:
(a) Transurethral microwave therapy
(b) Transurethral needle ablation (radiofrequency)
(c) Urethral stent
(d) Laser prostatectomy

242. For prostate cancer prevention, which one of the following was used in the SELECT trial?
(a) Dutasteride (b) Statins
(c) Vitamin E (d) Lycopene

243. Which of the following is true about prostatic carcinoma?
(a) Mucinous adenocarcinoma is more aggressive than non mucinous cancer
(b) Primary urothelial carcinoma of prostate often presents early because of hematuria
(c) Pure primary squamous carcinoma has very good survival
(d) Average survival with small cell carcinoma is one year

244. Regarding imaging following the diagnosis of prostate cancer:
(a) Bone scans are recommended when PSA is greater than 10 ng/ml
(b) Radionuclide bone scan is more sensitive than bone survey skeletal radiography
(c) Prostascint is highly sensitive in detecting nodal metastasis
(d) MRI of pelvis is mandatory before radical prostatectomy

245. TUR syndrome can be seen in:
(a) Freyer's prostatectomy
(b) Unipolar TUR
(c) Bipolar TUR
(d) Laser enucleation of prostate
(e) Green light prostatectomy

246. Drugs cannot be used in CRPC:
(a) Docetaxel (b) Ketoconazole
(c) Abiraterone (d) Bicalutamide
(e) Enzalutamide

247. Following are obstructive symptoms:
(a) Frequency
(b) Dysuria
(c) Hesitancy
(d) Postvoid dribbling
(e) Urgency

248. Most efficient in obtaining anterior lobe prostatic biopsy:
(a) Transurethral biopsy
(b) Saturated biopsy
(c) 12 core biopsy
(d) 10 core biopsy
(e) Transperineal biopsy

249. Alpha 1 receptor mainly seen in:
(a) Striated spicture (b) Prostatic strama
(c) Dome of bladder (d) Lower ureter
(e) Bladder neck

250. Which of the following to be given in hormone naive carcinoma prostate?
(a) Bicalutamide (b) Flutamide
(c) Nilutamide (d) Thalidomide
(e) Ketoconazole

251. When not to use LHRH agonist:
(a) Ileal vein compression
(b) Iliac bone involvement
(c) Impending spinal cord compression
(d) Hypersensitivity
(e) Extensive liver metastasis

252. ALP increases in:
(a) Liver mets
(b) Bone mets
(c) Hyperthyroidism
(d) Hypoparathyroidism
(e) Obstructive jaundice
(f) All of the above

253. Old man with LUTS, recommended investigations:
(a) Urodynamics
(b) Uroflow + PVR
(c) Creatinine and RBS
(d) R/E
(e) DRE

254. About BPH anatomy true are:
(a) Increase curvature of prostatic urethra
(b) Anatomical narrowing of urethra
(c) Urethral lengthening
(d) If PFR <20, TURP should be done
(e) Peripheral zone sub mucosal glands

255. TUR syndrome all are seen *except*:
(a) Altered sensorium (b) Hypotension
(c) Hypertension (d) Bradycardia
(e) Tachycardia

256. A 60 years old man with LUTS diagnosed to have T3 carcinoma prostate, on biopsy small cell carcinoma, no metastasis, no comorbidity, next step of management:
(a) Radical prostatectomy
(b) Cystoprostatectomy
(c) Chemotherapy
(d) LHRH agonist
(e) EBRT

257. Most common site of metastasis from carcinoma prostate are:
(a) Lungs (b) Liver
(c) Bone (d) Adrenal
(e) Pleura

258. True regarding clinical state of rising PSA:
(a) RT is given in all
(b) Rising PSA after definitive local treatment in absence of any apparent metastasis
(c) Nomograms should be followed to determine local vs. systemic
(d) Treatment is standardized
(e) PSADT and Gleason's score is highly prognostic

259. Which of the following are not alpha blockers?
(a) Bicalutamide (b) Alfuzosin
(c) Dutasteride (d) Silodosin
(e) Propranolol

260. Which zone of prostate is affected by chronic prostatitis?
(a) Anterior-Fibromuscular
(b) Central
(c) Peripheral
(d) Transitional

ANSWERS

1.	A	26.	A	51.	FFFTT	76.	FFTFT	101.	AC
2.	D	27.	B	52.	TTFFF	77.	TFTFF	102.	E
3.	A	28.	C	53.	TTFFF	78.	FFFFF	103.	ABD
4.	A	29.	D	54.	FFTFT	79.	FTTFT	104.	ABE
5.	B	30.	FTTFT	55.	TFTTF	80.	TTFTT	105.	ACDE
6.	D	31.	TFTTF	56.	FFTFT	81.	FFFTF	106.	D
7.	D	32.	TTTFF	57.	FTFTF	82.	TFFTF	107.	ABCDE
8.	B	33.	FTTTF	58.	FTFTT	83.	TTTFF	108.	ADE
9.	B	34.	FTTTT	59.	FTTTT	84.	FTTFF	109.	AD
10.	B	35.	FFFTT	60.	FFFTF	85.	TTTFT	110.	BCE
11.	A	36.	FFTFF	61.	TFFFT	86.	TFFFT	111.	ABC
12.	A	37.	FFFTF	62.	TTTTT	87.	FTTTF	112.	B
13.	A	38.	FTFTF	63.	FFTTF	88.	TTFFT	113.	ABCDE
14.	A	39.	TTTFT	64.	FFFFF	89.	ACD	114.	ACDE
15.	A	40.	TTTTT	65.	TTFTT	90.	BCDE	115.	A
16.	B	41.	TFTTT	66.	TTTTT	91.	ADE	116.	A
17.	D	42.	TFTFT	67.	TFFTF	92.	BCD	117.	ABCDE
18.	D	43.	FFTTT	68.	TFTTT	93.	ABCD	118.	AC
19.	D	44.	TFFTF	69.	FTFTF	94.	AB	119.	AC
20.	B	45.	TTTTF	70.	TTFTF	95.	BC	120.	BC
21.	D	46.	TFFTF	71.	TFFFF	96.	ABCDE	121.	BCDE
22.	A	47.	FFTTT	72.	TTFTF	97.	E	122.	ABCDE
23.	A	48.	FTTTF	73.	FFTTT	98.	E	123.	D
24.	B	49.	TTFTT	74.	FTTTT	99.	ADE	124.	C
25.	A	50.	TTTTT	75.	FFTTF	100.	BCDE	125.	D

126.	C	154.	A	182.	C	210.	C	238.	E
127.	B	155.	A	183.	B	211.	B	239.	A
128.	C	156.	C	184.	C	212.	B	240.	C
129.	D	157.	B	185.	C	213.	B	241.	B
130.	A	158	B	186.	A	214.	A	242.	C
131.	B	159.	A	187.	A	215.	A	243.	D
132.	C	160.	A	188.	A	216.	A	244.	D
133.	C	161.	A	189.	D	217.	C	245.	BDE
134.	A	162.	D	190.	C	218.	D	246.	BDE
135.	D	163.	A	191.	A	219.	B	247.	C
136.	B	164.	B	192.	D	220.	D	248.	E
137.	D	165.	A	193.	B	221.	B	249.	BDE
138.	A	166.	A	194.	A	222.	C	250.	ABCE
139.	A	167.	A	195.	A	223.	D	251.	CD
140.	A	168.	A	196.	A	224.	A	252.	F
141.	C	169.	C	197.	D	225.	C	253.	BDE
142.	D	170.	C	198.	B	226.	C	254.	AC
143.	A	171.	D	199.	A	227.	B	255.	ABCD
144.	A	172.	C	200.	B	228.	B	256.	CE
145.	A	173.	C	201.	B	229.	B	257.	AC
146.	A	174.	D	202.	D	230.	D	258.	BCE
147.	C	175.	B	203.	C	231.	C	259.	ACE
148.	A	176.	C	204.	D	232.	C	260.	C
149.	B	177.	A	205.	B	233.	A		
150.	D	178.	D	206.	A	234.	B		
151.	B	179.	A	207.	B	235.	C		
152.	A	180.	D	208.	B	236.	D		
153.	C	181.	A	209.	C	237.	A		

CHAPTER 15

Pediatric Urology

1. **The indication for prophylactic gonadectomy is in:**
   (a) Klinefelter's syndrome
   (b) Kallman's syndrome
   (c) Down's syndrome
   (d) Testicular feminization syndrome

2. **Which of the following will not be a feature of testicular feminization syndrome?**
   (a) Testis are present
   (b) XY genotype
   (c) Primary amenorrhoea
   (d) Uterus present

3. **Polyuria can occur with all of the following *except:***
   (a) Hypokalemia
   (b) Hypocalcemia
   (c) Lithium toxicity
   (d) ADH deficiency

4. **Which of the following chromosomes are involved in autosomal dominant polycystic kidney disease?**
   (a) 6 and 11 (b) 4 and 16
   (c) 4 and 12 (d) 4 and 17

5. **Unilateral renal agenesis is associated with:**
   (a) Polycystic disease of pancreas
   (b) Hiatus hernia
   (c) Hypogonadism
   (d) Single umbilical artery

6. **Which of the following is the first manifestation of Alport's syndrome?**
   (a) Microscopic hematuria
   (b) Proteinuria
   (c) Oliguria
   (d) Sensorineural deafness

7. **Medullary cystic disease of the kidney is best diagnosed by:**
   (a) Urography (b) CT scan
   (c) Nuclear scan (d) Biopsy

8. **Which of the following is incorrect regarding the medullary sponge kidneys?**
   (a) Autosomal dominant
   (b) Nephrocalcinosis
   (c) Minimal proteinuria
   (d) More common in females

9. **The nephrogenesis is completed in the human foetus by:**
   (a) 34 to 36 weeks (b) 30 to 32 weeks
   (c) 24 to 28 weeks (d) 20 weeks

10. **Urethral meatus stenosis occurs in newborn:**
    (a) As a result of birth trauma
    (b) A sequelae to urinary tract infection
    (c) From undergarment irritation
    (d) After healing of the inflamed, denuded glans after circumcision

11. **Which of the following is a characteristic sign of mature renal scarring on DMSA renogram?**
    (a) Polar areas of diminished uptake
    (b) Diffuse renal enlargement
    (c) Wedge shaped areas of increased uptake
    (d) Focal circular areas of diminished uptake

12. **The most common cause for a 5-year-old girl with hydronephrotic pelvic kidney is:**
    (a) Vesicoureteric reflex
    (b) Malrotation
    (c) Ureterovesical junction obstruction
    (d) Ureteropelvic junction obstruction

13. Bilateral renal agenesis is associated with mutations of:
(a) GFR α 1 (b) GDNF
(c) RET (d) Pax 2

14. Normal rotation of the kidney towards midline to attain its orthotopic position involves 90 degrees of medial rotation. This happens between:
(a) 6th and 9th week
(b) 10th and 12th week
(c) 3rd and 5th week
(d) 16th and 20th week

15. Which of the following is true about congenital renal A-V fistulas? They are:
(a) Usually bilateral
(b) Cirsoid in configuration
(c) Symptomatic before the 3rd decade
(d) Usually located in lower pole

16. Which of the following features is associated with ASK-Upmark kidney (segmental hypoplasia)?
(a) Hypertension
(b) Renal artery intimal disease
(c) Found in boys
(d) All of the above

17. Renal sinus cysts are most likely derived from:
(a) Vascular elements
(b) Renal parenchyma
(c) Lymphatic system
(d) Nephrogenic rests

18. Blood volume in children can be most closely estimated as:
(a) 55 ml/kg (b) 25 to 50 ml/kg
(c) 70 to 80 ml/kg (d) 100 ml/kg

19. Hypothermia during laparoscopy in all infants is caused by:
(a) Evaporation
(b) Abdominal irrigation
(c) High frequency ventilation
(d) Room temperature insufflation

20. An ectopic ureter in a female may drain at any of the following sites *except:*
(a) Urethra (b) Fallopian tube
(c) Ovary (d) Vagina

21. All of the following may contribute to vesicoureteral reflux *except:*
(a) Lateral ureteral insertion
(b) Lax bladder neck
(c) Poorly developed trigone
(d) Short intramural tunnel

22. Which of the following is least likely to be caused by a ureterocele?
(a) Bladder outlet obstruction
(b) Upper pole obstruction
(c) Ipsilateral lower pole reflux
(d) Urinary incontinence

23. The estimated prevalence of vesicoureteral reflux in children with primary UTI is:
(a) 30% (b) 13%
(c) 5% (d) 10%

24. The live birth incidence of classic bladder exstrophy is:
(a) 1 in 100,000 (b) 1 in 60,000
(c) 1 in 50,000 (d) 1 in 70,000

25. Which of the following would be the most common finding while performing urodynamic studies on children with nocturnal enuresis?
(a) Low leak point pressure
(b) Marked reduction in bladder emptying efficiency
(c) Poor bladder compliance
(d) Reduced functional bladder capacity

26. Enuresis persists in about what percentage of children at age 5?
(a) 25% (b) 15%
(c) 45% (d) 5%

27. Sex reversal syndrome:
(a) 46 XX (b) 47 XYY
(c) 45 X0 (d) 47 XXY

28. Which gestational day does metanephros development begin?

(a) 20th day (b) 24th day
(c) 28th day (d) 36th day

29. In females remnants of mesonephric ducts includes all *except:*
(a) Epoophoron
(b) Paroophoron
(c) Hymen
(d) Gartner duct cysts

30. All of the following statements about SRY gene are true *except:*
(a) Its expression triggers the primitive sex cord cells to differentiate to sertoli cells
(b) Approximately 25% of the sex reversal conditions in humans are attributed to SRY mutations
(c) It is located on short arm of Y chromosome
(d) It causes regression of mesonephric ducts

31. GFR at birth is ..... % of normal adult value.
(a) 5-10% (b) 10-15%
(c) 15-20% (d) 20-25%

32. All of the following are seen in nephrotic syndrome *except:*
(a) Hyperalbuminemia
(b) Hyperlipidemia
(c) Heavy proteinuria
(d) Oedema

33. What percentage of patients of IgA nephropathy develop ESRD after 10 years of age?
(a) 30% (b) 20%
(c) 15% (d) 5%

34. Renal dysplasia associated with obstruction is characterized by:
(a) Renal atrophy
(b) Glomerular cysts
(c) Fibromuscular collars
(d) All of the above

35. Definition of severe antenatal hydronephrosis by anteroposterior diameter is:
(a) >5mm (b) >8mm
(c) >10mm (d) >15mm

36. Fetal ultrasound findings of posterior urethral valves include:
(a) Bilateral hydroureteronephrosis
(b) Thick walled bladder
(c) Dilated posterior urethra
(d) All of the above

37. Adrenal hemorrhage is estimated to occur in ..... % of healthy infants.
(a) 1-2% (b) 3-5%
(c) 5-7% (d) 10-15%

38. Cause of bilateral hydronephrosis in infants include:
(a) Posterior urethral valves
(b) Bilateral VUR
(c) Bilateral PUJ obstruction
(d) All of the above

39. The findings of multiple non-communicating cysts, minimal or absent renal parenchyma, absence of central cyst is diagnostic of:
(a) Unilateral hydronephrosis
(b) MCDK
(c) ADPKD
(d) ARPKD

40. The most common malignant abdominal tumour in infants is:
(a) Wilms' tumor
(b) Rhabdomyosarcoma
(c) Neuroblastoma
(d) Nephroblastoma

41. In case of testicular torsion, significant ischemic damage is known to occur after .....
(a) 0-2 hours (b) 2-4 hours
(c) 4-8 hours (d) 10-12 hours

42. Optimal timing of spinal ultrasonography during screening for occult spinal dysraphism is:
(a) Before 6 months of age
(b) 6 months –1 year of age
(c) Between 1 and 6 years of age
(d) After puberty

43. Urethral meatal stenosis in a newborn male is commonly due to:
(a) Birth trauma
(b) Undergarment irritation
(c) UTI
(d) After circumcision

44. Characteristics of bacteria more likely to infect kidneys include:
(a) MRHA characteristics
(b) Urease production
(c) P-blood group specific adhesions
(d) MRHA characteristics and P-blood group specific adhesions

45. Approximately..... of children with pyelonephritis acquire renal scarring.
(a) 7% (b) 10%
(c) 13% (d) 17%

46. Bilateral renal agenesis is associated with mutations of:
(a) GDNF (b) WNT
(c) Pax 2 (d) RET

47. Incidence of unilateral renal agenesis is:
(a) 1:500 (b) 1:5000
(c) 1:1100 (d) 1:11000

48. Congenital renal arteriovenous fistulas are:
(a) Usually bilateral
(b) Cirsoid in configuration
(c) More common in males
(d) Usually bilateral and more common in males

49. Bilateral megacalycosis is:
(a) More common in females
(b) Increased number of dilated calyses
(c) Associated with ureteral dilatation
(d) More common in females and associated with ureteral dilatation

50. Extra renal manifestations of ADPKD include all *except:*
(a) Hepatic cysts
(b) Cerebellar hemangiomata
(c) Colonic diverticula
(d) Mitral valve prolapsed

51. Two major genetic forms of ADPKD - PKD1, PKD2 are located on ..... chromosomes respectively.
(a) 16, 4 (b) 4, 16
(c) 6, 12 (d) 12, 6

52. Contralateral pelviureteric junction abnormality found in infants with MCDK (multicystic dysplastic kidney) in:
(a) 18-43% (b) 3-12%
(c) 0-2% (d) 40-80%

53. Bouquet of flowers appearance on IVP is seen in:
(a) Ask-upmark kidney
(b) Medullary sponge kidney
(c) Multicystic dysplastic kidney
(d) Horseshoe kidney

54. Blood volume in children can be estimated as:
(a) 55 ml/kg body weight
(b) 65-70 ml/kg body weight
(c) 70-80 ml/kg body weight
(d) 100 ml/kg body weight

55. Excisional tapering for more severely dilated mega ureters is named after:
(a) Kalicinski's (b) Bakker's
(c) Parrott's (d) Hendren's

56. All of the following are possible drainage sites for an ectopic ureter in females *except:*
(a) Ovary (b) Vagina
(c) Uterus (d) Fallopian tube

57. Most common form of ureteral triplication is:
(a) All 3 ureters joining to terminate in a single bladder orifice
(b) 3 ureters joining to form two ureteral orifices
(c) 3 ureters draining as 3 separate ureteral orifices
(d) None

58. Obstruction in a case of preureteral iliac artery occurs at a level of:
(a) L_2-L_3 (b) L_3-L_4
(c) L_4-L_5 (d) L_5-S_1

59. Estimated prevalence of vesicoureteral reflux in children with UTI:
(a) 1% (b) 3%
(c) 10% (d) 30%

60. Ratio of tunnel length to ureteral diameter found in normal children without reflux is:

(a) 5:1 (b) 4:1
(c) 3:1 (d) 2:1

61. Findings common in prune-belly syndrome include all *except:*
(a) Deficient abdominal wall musculature
(b) Palpable undescended testes
(c) Urinary tract dilatation
(d) Urachal pseudodiverticulum

62. Most commonly involved abdominal wall compartment in prune-belly syndrome:
(a) Medial (b) Inferior
(c) Lateral (d) Medial and lateral

63. Incidence of omphalocele associated with cloacal extrophy:
(a) 20% (b) 40%
(c) 60% (d) 95%

64. Fetal bladder can first be detected on ultrasound at ..... of gestational age.
(a) 10th week (b) 11th week
(c) 12th week (d) 13th week

65. Most common cause of mortality in patients with posterior urethral valves today is:
(a) Renal failure in newborn period
(b) Renal failure in mid childhood
(c) Pulmonary insufficiency in newborn
(d) Renal insufficiency in adolescence

66. Percentage of neonatal ascites caused by urinary conditions:
(a) 20% (b) 40%
(c) 60% (d) 80%

67. Valve bladder/Full valve bladder are terms coined by:
(a) Austin (b) Glassberg
(c) Mitchell (d) Ghanem

68. What percentage of uncircumcised boys will have persistent phimosis by 17 years of age?
(a) <1% (b) 5%
(c) 10% (d) 20%

69. Bladder dysfunction during emptying is seen in:
(a) Hinman's syndrome
(b) Ochoa's syndrome
(c) Both
(d) None

70. Koff's formula for calculating bladder capacity is:
(a) Age in years +2 × 30
(b) Age in years +3 × 30
(c) Age in years +4 × 30
(d) Age in years +6 × 30

71. Denys Drash syndrome includes all *except:*
(a) Male pseudo hermaphroditism
(b) Nephroblastoma
(c) Renal mesangial sclerosis
(d) Neuroblastoma

72. Risk of developing Wilms' tumor in a patient with Horseshoe kidney is:
(a) No risk (b) 3-fold
(c) 5-fold (d) 7-fold

73. Most aggressive and lethal childhood renal tumor is:
(a) Nephroblastoma
(b) Wilms' tumor
(c) Mesoblastic nephroma
(d) Rhabdoid tumor

74. Tuberous sclerosis complex is associated with chromosomal abnormality (TSC1, TSC2):
(a) 9, 16 (b) 16, 9
(c) 4, 16 (d) 16, 4

75. According to Divine-Horton's classification of congenital penile curvature, "congenital short urethra" refers to:
(a) Type 1 (b) Type 2
(c) Type 3 (d) Type 5

76. Diagnostic modality of choice in a 5 years old child with posterior urethral valve:
(a) USG pelvis (b) MR urography
(c) RGU (d) MCU

77. Most common cause of urinary ascities in children:
(a) Posterior urethral valve
(b) Trauma

(c) Renal calculus disease
(d) Idiopathic

78. What percentage of undescended testes are nonpalpable at presentation?
(a) 20% (b) 30%
(c) 50% (d) 80%

79. What is the most common cause of micropenis?
(a) Hypergonadotropic hypogonadism
(b) Hypogonadotropic hypogonadism
(c) Idiopathic
(d) Androgen insensitivity syndrome

80. AML associated with:
(a) Neurofibromatosis
(b) Tuberous sclerosis
(c) Hereditary nonpolyposis colon cancer
(d) Birt Hogg Dube syndrome

81. To maximize fertility potential, orchidopexy for cryptorchidism should be done before:
(a) Age of 20 years (b) Age of 12 years
(c) Before marriage (d) Age of 2 years

82. In Alports syndrome..........all are true *except.*
(a) Usually autosomal recessive
(b) Bilateral anterior lenticonus is the usual eye manifestation
(c) Sensory neural deafness usually to high tone first
(d) The pathological hallmark is progressive degeneration of the glomerular basement membrane

83. Androgen receptor gene is located on:
(a) Short arm of the Y chromosome
(b) Long arm of the Y chromosome
(c) Short arm of the X chromosome
(d) Long arm of the X chromosome

84. All are methods of urethral plication *except:*
(a) Henderson (b) Starrz
(c) Kallinski (d) Kroops

85. True about ADPKD are all *except*:
(a) Higher chances of malignancy
(b) Berry aneurysm is seen in 10-40%
(c) Present at 30-50 years of age
(d) Chromosome 16 and 4

86. AML with tuberous sclerosis:
(a) AD 16 and 9 (b) AD 16 and 4
(c) AR 16 and 9 (d) AR 16 and 4

87. All are true about CAH *except:*
(a) 46XY DSD
(b) 95% deficiency in 21 hydroxylase
(c) 11 α hydroxylase deficiency does not cause hypertension
(d) Female pseudohermaphrodite

88. All are true regarding persistent mullerian duct syndrome *except:*
(a) Intra-abdominal testes
(b) Ovary at normal position
(c) Ambiguous genitalia
(d) Uterus and fallopian tube may be present

89. False about Unilateral Renal Agenesis:
(a) More common in females
(b) Incidence <1100
(c) Mullerian abnormality present
(d) Vas may be absent on the same side

90. Percentage of children bedwetting at age of 15:
(a) 1 (b) 5
(c) 10 (d) 15

Mention True and False respective to each statement (Q. No. 91 to 158)

91. Klinefelter's syndrome:
(a) Extra X is hallmark
(b) Mental retardation in some
(c) Usually due to meiotic nondisjunction
(d) Triad is low gonadotropins, gynecomastia and small testis
(e) LH can be normal

92. Prune-belly syndrome:
(a) Bilateral cryptorchidism is rule
(b) VUR in 10%
(c) Bladder is massively enlarged
(d) Renal dysplasia
(e) Fertility with assisted reproductive techniques may be feasible

93. Regarding renal development:
(a) Kidney ascends between 6-9 weeks
(b) Nephrogenesis occurs before 34 weeks of gestation

(c) Ureteric bud arises from distal portion of nephric duct
(d) Ureteric bud comes in contact with condensing blastema of metanephric mesenchyme at 28th day
(e) Definitive kidney arise from metanephros

94. On prenatal USG:
(a) Fetal urine form most of amniotic fluid at 20 weeks
(b) Pulmonary hypoplasia if oligohydramnios occurs after 30 weeks
(c) Oligohydramnios due to urinary tract obstruction is evident after 20 weeks of gestation
(d) Pulmonary hypoplasia in renal agenesis is due to oligohydramnios
(e) Key hole sign–ureteric calculi

95. Neuroblastoma:
(a) Local excision–Stage I
(b) Local excision–Stage II
(c) Local excision–Stage III
(d) Local excision + Chemotherapy–Stage IV
(e) Local excision is sufficient in Stage IVS

96. Creatinine clearance in children:
(a) Schwarz formula includes weight of child
(b) MDRD creatinine clearance formula includes age and length
(c) Creatinine clearance overestimates GFR
(d) Marked variation in production rates between individuals
(e) Creatinine clearance depends on muscle mass and age

97. Voiding dysfunction in children:
(a) Male > Female
(b) Associated with diurnal and nocturnal incontinence
(c) Associated with constipation
(d) Pelvic floor exercise has no role
(e) Associated with UTI

98. MCDK:
(a) Bilateral cases reach puberty
(b) Malignant transformation is common
(c) Increased uptake of DMSA
(d) If diagnosed then nephrectomy
(e) 40% of MCDKs will spontaneously involute

99. Ascent of kidney:
(a) Occur at 7-10 weeks
(b) Differential growth of the lumbar and sacral regions of the embryo plays a major role
(c) Vessels stretch along with ascent
(d) In HSK during ascent, the fused lower pole becomes trapped under the SMA
(e) Adrenal gland also ascend alongside kidney

100. Regarding infant:
(a) All infant voids within 12 hours
(b) Oliguria–Less than 2 ml/kg/hour
(c) Polyuria – > 1000 ml/1.73 m^2
(d) Fetus produces hypotonic urine
(e) GFR at birth ½ of adult

101. Creatinine clearance in child:
(a) Over estimates GFR
(b) Protein content increases the value
(c) Muscle mass changes the value
(d) Schwartz formula uses weight of child
(e) Nephrogenesis is complete by 34 weeks of gestational age in the fetus

102. Anion gap:
(a) The anion gap is defined as the difference between the levels of routinely measured cations and anions in blood
(b) Unmeasured anions include calcium, magnesium and gamma globulins
(c) Ureterosigmoidostomy has normal anion gap
(d) Lactic acidosis increases anion gap
(e) The normal range is 9 to 14 mEq/l

103. Renal ectopic:
(a) Most common on left side
(b) Pelvic is the most common type
(c) > 50% is hydronephrotic
(d) More incidence of disease
(e) Least chances of VUR

104. Ectopic ureter:
(a) Most common site is in posterior urethra
(b) Genital abnormalities not seen
(c) If the ureteric bud arises more proximally on the mesonephric duct than normally, it results in a ureteral orifice more medial and caudal than is usual
(d) In males, most ectopic ureters drain single systems
(e) The segment of mesonephric duct proximal to the ureteric bud is the common excretory duct

105. VUR:
(a) Lich Greigor is intravesical approach
(b) Cohen is extravesical approach
(c) Glenn-Anderson technique is infrahiatal approach
(d) The length: Diameter ratio of the submucosal tunnel should be 3:1
(e) Cohen's technique is particularly well suited for small bladders or thick-walled bladders

106. Klinefelter's syndrome:
(a) Extra X is hallmark
(b) Mental retardation may be present in some cases
(c) Triad–Gynecomastia, reduced urinary gonadotropin and small testis
(d) Represents the most common major abnormality of sexual differentiation
(e) LH levels are mildly elevated

107. Regarding absent testis:
(a) Blind ending spermatic vessels
(b) Blind ending vas
(c) Unilateral renal agenesis
(d) XY/XO
(e) Contralateral testicular hypertophy is reliable sign

108. Pediatric urology:
(a) Keyhole is a sign of ureterocele
(b) Lower pole HDN is associated with ureterocele
(c) Cobra head appearance is seen with PUV
(d) Malignancy is common sequelae of MCDK
(e) Increase DMSA uptake in MCDK

109. Pediatric urology:
(a) Neonatal GFR is dependent on gestational age and doubles in the first 2 weeks of life
(b) AF is fetal urine at 20 weeks
(c) Nephrogenesis is complete by 34 weeks of gestational age in the fetus
(d) Urine production in human kidney begins at 10-12 weeks
(e) The fetus produces hypotonic urine with high sodium content and in large volumes

110. Infertility/Testicular failure:
(a) Deficiency of steroid 21-hydroxylase is responsible for 95% of cases of CAH
(b) MRKH syndrome is most common cause of primary amenorrhea
(c) Presence of an extra Y chromosome is the genetic hallmark for Klinefelter's syndrome
(d) Klinefelter's syndrome is the most common major abnormality of sexual differentiation
(e) Most common cause of ambiguous genitalia–CAH

111. In impalpable left testis in 11-year-old child, testicular absence can be confirmed by:
(a) Blind ending vas
(b) Blind ending vessels
(c) Absent left kidney
(d) XY/XO–Karyotype
(e) Contralateral testicular hypertrophy is reliable sign

112. Predisposing factor to VUR:
(a) Laterally placed ureteric orifice
(b) Short intravesical length
(c) High compliant flaccid bladder
(d) Hyperreflexia bladder
(e) DESD

113. A 4 years old female with right hydronephrosis, fever and recurrent UTI:

(a) Differential diagnosis is – PUJO, VUR, megaureter
(b) Antenatal VUR always require surgical correction
(c) Grade II VUR require surgical correction
(d) MCU is not required in HDN
(e) DMSA scan is used to detect scarring

114. MCDK:
(a) Mean age at the time of antenatal diagnosis is about 28 weeks
(b) Mostly regress by age and even disappear
(c) Not reniform in shape
(d) Central large cyst
(e) Without visible communication between cyst

115. Embryology of kidney:
(a) In mammals three sets of kidney develops
(b) Usually arises from intermediate mesoderm
(c) Glomerulus arises from metanephric mesenchyme
(d) Seminal vesicle originate from distal mesonephric duct at 12 weeks
(e) Mesonephros forms definitive kidney

116. Regarding paramesonephric duct:
(a) Mullerian duct forms female internal genitalia
(b) Mullerian duct gives rise to appendix testis
(c) MIS is produced by leydig cells
(d) MIS production is regulated by 'SRY' gene
(e) Mullerian duct give rise to vas deferens

117. Regarding genitourinary embryology:
(a) Wolffian duct give rise to epoophoron in females
(b) Mesonephric duct forms vas deferens
(c) Prostatic utricle arise from mesonephric duct
(d) In 20% male ectopic ureter opening is below membranous urethra
(e) The fault in URA lies with ureteric bud

118. Sacral agenesis:
(a) Last two vertebra are completely absent
(b) Low gluteal cleft with flat buttocks
(c) Loss of perianal sensation
(d) Equal distribution of both UMN and LMN
(e) Babies of IDDM mother have 1% chance for this condition

119. Prune-belly syndrome:
(a) Hypoplasia of abdominal muscles
(b) Hypercontractile bladder
(c) Unilateral dilation of ureter
(d) Dilated posterior urethra
(e) Bilateral cryptorchidism

120. Ectopic ureter:
(a) Of all ectopic orifices, 80% are associated with a duplicated collecting system
(b) In the male, the posterior urethra is the most common site of termination of an ectopic ureter
(c) Drainage into the genital tract involves the seminal vesicle three times more often than the ejaculatory duct and vas deferens combined
(d) In the female, the urethra and vestibule are the most common sites
(e) If the ureteric bud arises more proximally on the mesonephric duct than normally, it results in a ureteral orifice more medial and caudal than is usual

121. Regarding hypertension in children:
(a) 3-10% of children referred for the evaluation of severe hypertension are subsequently found to have clinically significant renovascular lesions
(b) Renovascular hypertension is the second most common cause of correctable hypertension in children
(c) Focal scarring always produce HTN
(d) In India Takayasu disease is the most important cause of renovascular hypertension
(e) Bilateral renal artery disease is more common than unilateral

122. Voiding dysfunction in children:
(a) More in boys

(b) Diarrhea always associated
(c) Pelvic floor exercise is not usually effective
(d) Nocturnal and diurnal incontinence is common
(e) UTI is always present

123. Funguria in children:
(a) Candida is most common
(b) Usually stone associated
(c) Change of catheter will not help
(d) Parenteral nutrition leads to funguria
(e) Asymptomatic funguria do not require treatment

124. VUR:
(a) Reflux may be present in upto 70% of infants with UTI
(b) Stage IV – Spontaneous resolution is 10%
(c) Dilated pelvis usually predicts PUJO
(d) Antenatally more common in boys
(e) USG can diagnose VUR

125. Wilms' tumor:
(a) IVC involvement in 5%–10%
(b) 60% of all childhood tumor
(c) Speckled calcification
(d) Arises from distal tubules
(e) Stage 1 with anaplasia–surgery only sufficient

126. Neuroblastoma:
(a) Stage I – Surgery only sufficient
(b) Stage II – Surgery only sufficient
(c) Stage III – Surgery only sufficient
(d) State IV – Surgery + Adjuvant chemotherapy
(e) Stage IVS – Local excision sufficient

127. Megaureter:
(a) Routine surgical correction in newborns and infants with grade IV or V reflux is appropriate
(b) Increase in collagen
(c) IVP is better scan for detection of function
(d) To differentiate from VUR, VCUG is done
(e) Plication of ureters greater than 1.75 cm in diameter has been associated with more complications

128. VUR spontaneous resolution occurs in:
(a) Grade 1 – 90%
(b) Grade 2 – 90%
(c) Grade 3 – 80%
(d) Grade 4 – 70%
(e) Grade 5 – 40%

129. Regarding retractile testis:
(a) Follow up is not required
(b) Should not be treated at 1 year of age
(c) 90% are cured by puberty
(d) Scrotal support is usually helpful
(e) Encountered between 3-5 years of age

130. MCDK:
(a) Malignancy is always sequelae
(b) DMSA shows increase uptake
(c) Nephrectomy is required if HTN present
(d) Bilateral MCDK–Patient can live upto puberty
(e) Unilateral MCDK associated with pulmonary hypoplasia

131. Regarding renal embryogenesis:
(a) Pronephros degenerate by 5th week
(b) Mesonephros disappear at 9th week
(c) Ureteric bud appears at 4th week
(d) Kidney forms at sacral region
(e) Ureteric bud comes in contact with condensing blastema of metanephric mesenchyme at 28th day

132. 4 years old girl and right HDN:
(a) PUJO, VUR, Megaureter are the differential diagnosis
(b) Grade II reflux is treated by surgery
(c) If prenatal USG shows HDN – surgical intervention is done in all cases
(d) She can be observed if on DTPA function is not deteriorating
(e) Most common anomaly will be PUJ obstruction

133. Ureteric development:
(a) Ureteric bud develops from mesonephric duct at 4th week of development
(b) The first signs of ureteral muscularization and development of elastic fibers are seen at 12 weeks of gestation
(c) If the ureteric bud arises more proximally on the mesonephric duct than normally, it results in a ureteral orifice more medial and caudal than is usual
(d) 20% of male ectopic ureter is distal to membranous urethra
(e) Collecting ducts, calyces, pelvis and ureter are derived from ureteric bud

134. Horseshoe kidney:
(a) Most common fusion anomaly
(b) Incidence is 1: 1000
(c) Occur usually due to fusion of lower and mid pole
(d) Isthmus is usually at the level of L_{3-4}
(e) Ureter is placed posteriorly

135. Megaureter:
(a) Secondary to UTI
(b) Non-obstructing non refluxing megaureter is due to prune belly syndrome
(c) Plication of ureters >1.75 cm in diameter has been associated with more complication
(d) Normal ureteral diameter is rarely greater than 5 mm
(e) True obstruction is present

136. Regarding ectopic ureter:
(a) Can open in ejaculatory duct and seminal vesicle
(b) Males can be incontinent
(c) Upper pole segments is always normal
(d) Of all ectopic orifices, 80% are associated with a duplicated collecting system
(e) In females most common site is urethra

137. 3 years old child undergoing open pyeloplasty:
(a) Out of drain, nephrostomy and stent drain last to be removed
(b) Nephrostomy tube is preferred to internal stent because it avoids further anesthesia for stent removal
(c) In case of failed pyeloplasty with large pelvis, endopyelotomy is the best option
(d) Lumbotomy incision can be used
(e) PUJO with short intrarenal pelvis and antegrade drainage endopyelotomy is treatment of choice

138. Prune-belly syndrome:
(a) Hypoplastic abdominal wall
(b) Bilateral cryptorchidism
(c) Unilateral dilated ureter
(d) Hyperreflexic bladder
(e) Dilated posterior urethra

139. Klinefelter syndrome:
(a) Extra X hallmark
(b) Nondisjunction of the meiotic chromosomes of the gametes of either parent
(c) Classic triad of gynecomastia, low gonadotropin and small testis
(d) Some are mentally retarded
(e) 50 times increase risk of breast cancer

140. In duplex kidney:
(a) If two separate ureteric buds originate from the mesonephric duct, two complete and separate interactions will develop between the ureter and the metanephric blastema
(b) Upper moiety–reflux more common
(c) Lower moiety–ureterocele more common
(d) More prone to tumor
(e) If the ureteric bud arises more proximally on the mesonephric duct it results in a ureteral orifice more medial and caudal than is usual

141. In ectopic kidney:
(a) Often symptomatic
(b) Malrotation common
(c) More prone to malignancy
(d) Mostly presents in childhood
(e) Most common location is in the pelvis

142. Fetal kidney:
(a) Lobulated surface
(b) Every infant voided within the first 1 hour of life regardless of gestational age
(c) Urine production start at 10th week
(d) The fetus produces hypotonic urine with high sodium content and in large volumes
(e) Doubles in the first 2 weeks of life

143. Infantile recessive polycystic disease:
(a) Hypoplastic
(b) Aplastic
(c) Dysplastic
(d) Hydronephrotic
(e) *PKHD1*, located on chromosome 6, is responsible for the disease

144. Regarding prune-belly syndrome:
(a) Dysplastic flabby abdominal musculature
(b) Dilated posterior urethra
(c) Bilateral cryptorchidism
(d) Bladder outlet obstruction
(e) Renal splasia in 50% of cases

145. Megaureter:
(a) Bilateral in 10-15% cases
(b) More common on left side
(c) Most common finding is an aperistaltic juxta vesical (adynamic) ureteral segment
(d) Many cases of antenatally diagnosed MGU will resolve spontaneously
(e) Associated with lithogenesis

146. Prune-belly syndrome:
(a) Bilateral cryptorchidism is a rule
(b) Megalourethra is common
(c) Most patients void spontaneously with normal voiding pressures, normal flow rates and low PVR
(d) Reflux positive in <10%
(e) Retrograde ejaculation due to incompetent bladder neck

147. Distal RTA:
(a) Hypokalemic, hypochloremic metabolic acidosis
(b) Hypokalemic periodic paralysis can be presenting feature
(c) In adult stone present in 10-15%
(d) Hypercalcemia is most important cause of stone formation
(e) Calcium phosphate stone is present

148. Ectopic ureter:
(a) Lower pole orifice is cranial and lateral
(b) Upper pole moiety is always normal
(c) Reflux is usually in lower pole ureter
(d) It can open in seminal vesicle and vas deferens
(e) In males may lead to incontinence

149. VUR:
(a) Golf hole ureteric orifice
(b) Laterally placed ureteric orifice more prone to VUR
(c) Small intravesical ureter
(d) Bladder overactivity may lead to VUR
(e) The most common anatomic obstruction of the bladder leading to VUR in pediatric population is PUV

150. Cryptorchidism:
(a) In recent series 3 to 14% chances of testicular tumor
(b) 5-10% chances of tumor in opposite testis
(c) Birth weight alone is the principal determinant of cryptorchidism at birth
(d) Risk for an undescended testis in a newborn male if a family member is already affected is 3.6-fold
(e) Isolated cryptorchidism affects 3% of full-term male newborns

151. Features suggestive of absent testis:
(a) Blind ending spermatic vessels
(b) Blind ending vas
(c) Empty scrotum
(d) Ipsilateral renal agenesis
(e) Right sided testicular hypertrophy is reliable sign

152. Embryogenesis of kidney:
(a) Ureteric bud arises from distal portion of nephric duct

(b) Bud fuses with metanephric blastema at 6 weeks
(c) Ascends by 6–8 weeks
(d) Nephrogenesis complete by 36 weeks
(e) During ascent, arteries elongate to follow the ascending kidney

153. Regarding embryology:
(a) At the 3rd week of gestation, the cloacal membrane remains a bilaminar structure composed of endoderm and ectoderm
(b) Uroretal septum divides at 8-10th week
(c) Gubernaculum appear in 7th week
(d) Urachus arises forms median umbilical ligament
(e) Definitive kidney is metanephros

154. Regarding UDT:
(a) 90% associated with epididymal anomalies
(b) 40 times increase risk of carcinoma testis
(c) Associated with contralateral CIS 5–10%
(d) 3% in normal full term infant
(e) Testicular descent occurs by 2nd trimester

155. A 2 years child with high grade fever and abdominal lump:
(a) MCU should be the first investigation
(b) If bilateral VUR (+) and PUV→ Do vesicostomy
(c) If bilateral HDN → do bilateral PCN
(d) Fulguration of valve done at 5 and 7° O' clock
(e) Neuroblastoma should be kept as differential diagnosis

156. Regarding embryogenesis of kidney:
(a) Ureteric bud arises from distal portion of nephric duct
(b) Fuses with metanephric blastema at 6 weeks
(c) Ascends by 6-9 weeks
(d) Nephrogenesis is completed before birth
(e) Intrarenal cyst is detachment of nephron moiety

157. Regarding embryology:
(a) UGS arises from anterior part of cloaca
(b) Female distal vagina arises from posterior part of urogenital sinus
(c) Urorectal septum divides at 8th to 10th week
(d) Gubernaculum appears at 7th week
(e) Umbilical artery lies in medial umbilical ligament

158. Regarding undescended testis (UDT):
(a) 90% associated with hernia
(b) 40 times increase risk for malignancy
(c) Definitive treatment of an undescended testis should take place between 6 and 12 months of age
(d) 3% in normal full term at birth
(e) In most cases testicular descent is complete between the 30th and 32nd week

Which of the following statement is correct?

159. A child after awakening complaints of severe scrotal pain. History of similar episodes in past. On lifting testis pain increases. Next step:
(a) IV fluids with antibiotics–Observe
(b) USG for diagnosis
(c) Immediate exploration
(d) Evaluate for vascularity
(e) Contralateral testis should be explored

160. Renal ectopia:
(a) Left > right
(b) The renal pelvis is usually anterior to the parenchyma because the kidney has incompletely rotated
(c) Left-to-right ectopia is seen three times more frequently than right-to-left ectopia
(d) The length of the ureter is according to the position of the kidney
(e) Ectopic kidney is usually smaller, and it may not conform to the usual reniform shape

161. Differentiation between testicular torsion and epididymo-orchitis is by:
(a) Age at presentation
(b) Tenderness on clinical examination
(c) Radionuclide scan

(d) Doppler scan
(e) Epididymal swelling

162. True hermaphrodite, all *except*:
(a) The ovarian portion of the ovotestis is frequently normal, whereas the testicular portion is typically dysgenetic
(b) Most common karyotype 46XX
(c) Most common karyotype 46XY
(d) Both ovary/testis present
(e) Perineoscrotal hypospadiasis present

163. ARPKD all are true *except*:
(a) Most die within first few days
(b) All have congenital hepatic fibrosis
(c) Homogeneous echogenic kidney
(d) Sibling of either sex has 1/2 chance of getting affected
(e) Associated with potter's syndrome

164. PUV all are true *except*:
(a) Most common cause of BOO in infants
(b) Incidence–One in one lakh
(c) Type 1 is most common
(d) Voiding cystourethrography most important study in diagnosis
(e) Type 1 has central diaphragm distal to veru

165. Palpable kidney in childhood–unlikely cause:
(a) Neuroblastoma (b) VUR
(c) Wilms' tumor (d) PUJO
(e) MCDK

166. 40-year-old lady, 3 children, presents with incontinence since 8 years (birth of last child) with normal voiding (4-5) times per day:
(a) VVF involving trigone and bladder neck
(b) Supratrigonal VVF
(c) Ureterovaginal fistula
(d) Stress incontinence
(e) Ectopic ureter

167. 12-year-old boy with right non-viable testis and left non-palpable testis:
(a) Right orchidectomy with localization and management of left testis on a later date
(b) Right orchidectomy with immediate left orchidopexy
(c) Only left orchidopexy
(d) Right testicular prosthesis
(e) Hormonal stimulation

168. Unilateral renal agenesis associated with:
(a) Bladder hemitrigone
(b) Adrenal absent
(c) Ureter absent in >50%
(d) Uterine anomalies
(e) Undescended testis

169. Which of the following is true for MCDK?
(a) Bilateral loin mass in newborn – most common presentation
(b) Kidney has the appearance of "a bunch of grapes"
(c) Bilateral is incompatible with life
(d) Blood supply is variable
(e) May be small or large

170. Regarding Weigert Meyer rule, which statement is/are correct?
(a) Lower pole orifice is lateral at bladder
(b) Lower pole orifice is cranial at bladder
(c) Lower pole orifice is caudal at bladder
(d) Upper pole orifice is caudal at bladder
(e) Upper pole orifice is medial at bladder

171. Unilateral renal agenesis:
(a) Ureter absent in >50%
(b) Adrenal absent
(c) Associated uterine anomaly
(d) Ipsilateral UDT
(e) Contralateral ectopic or malrotated kidney

172. GFR in children reach adult value by:
(a) 9 months (b) 6 months
(c) 1 year (c) 2 years
(e) 4 years

173. 2-year-old child with recurrent UTI, next investigation is:
(a) DMSA (b) DTPA
(c) MCU (d) MAG
(e) Gallium scan

174. 4-year-old boy with unilateral scrotal pain all *except*:
(a) Testicular tumor suspected

(b) Doppler useful
(c) Early exploration if testicular torsion suspected
(d) Irreversible ischemic injury to the testicular parenchyma may begin as soon as 1 hour after occlusion of the cord
(e) "Blue dot sign" is seen in torsion of testicular appendages

175. MCDK true is:
(a) One of the most common cause of abdominal mass in infants
(b) Kidneys can be large or small in size
(c) Bilateral incompatible with life
(d) DMSA uptake is present
(e) Most common cystic disease

176. Renal agenesis all *except*:
(a) UDT commonly seen
(b) Hemitrigone is present in some cases
(c) Adrenal usually seen normally
(d) Ureter absent in half the cases
(e) Genitourinary abnormalities more common in female

177. Adult polycystic kidney disease:
(a) 100% prevalence
(b) Between 30-50 years
(c) Gene defect is on chromosome 3
(d) 2 genes
(e) All children of affected parents suffer from this disease

178. Remnant of paramesonephric duct:
(a) Appendix of testes
(b) Bulbourethral gland
(c) Prostatic utricle
(d) Gartner's duct cyst
(e) Appendix of epididymis

179. Klinefelter syndrome:
(a) Extra X chromosome
(b) Increased gonadotropin
(c) Small firm testes
(d) No therapy to improve spermatogenesis
(e) Gynecomastia

180. Congenital adrenal hyperplasia:
(a) Increased cortisol
(b) Early fusion of epiphysis
(c) Increased adrenal size
(d) Increased testosterone
(e) Virilization in male and female

181. An 84-year-old female with large lower abdominal mass, USG suggestive of mass between rectum and bladder – diagnosis is:
(a) Sacrococcygeal teratoma
(b) Fluid filled vagina
(c) Hematocolpos
(d) Ovarian tumor
(e) Prolapse ureterocele

182. Posterior urethral valve:
(a) At veru–type 1
(b) Near bladder neck–type 2
(c) Above veru–type 1
(d) Below veru–type 3
(e) Most common variant–type 1

183. Prenatal USG, PUV features:
(a) Thickened bladder wall
(b) Dilated bladder neck and posterior urethra
(c) Oligohydramnios
(d) Bilateral hydroureteronephrosis
(e) Normal kidney

184. Ureterocele:
(a) Present as prolapsing mucosa in female
(b) Can have stone in it
(c) Endoscopic treatment never successful
(d) May cause contralateral reflux
(e) Most ureteroceles arise from the upper poles of duplicated systems

185. Ectopic ureter in female may present as:
(a) Continuous incontinence with otherwise normal voiding
(b) May open in proximal urethra/distal urethra/vestibule/vagina
(c) Reflux and infection is common
(d) For functional integrity of upper pole in duplex system – DTPA better than DMSA

(e) If the ectopic ureter terminates proximal to the urinary sphincter, endoscopic dilation of the insertion site can relieve obstruction

186. One day old female lower abdominal lump on USG:
(a) Sacrococcygeal teratoma
(b) Neuroblastoma
(c) Ovarian mass
(d) Hydrometrocolpos
(e) Fluid filled vagina

187. PUV on prenatal USG – diagnostic feature:
(a) Thickened urinary bladder
(b) Bilateral HDUN
(c) Dilated posterior urethra
(d) Thin renal cortex
(e) Polyhydramnios

188. In USG postnatal dilated PCS and dilated ureter – most important diagnosis is:
(a) VUR
(b) PUV
(c) Prune-belly syndrome
(d) VUJ obstruction
(e) PUJ obstruction

189. Horseshoe shaped kidney associated with:
(a) Turner's syndrome
(b) Down syndrome
(c) Tuberous sclerosis
(d) VHL

190. Metanephros develops on:
(a) 14 days (b) 28 days
(c) 14 weeks (d) 28 weeks

191. Male with CAH with precocious puberty, most common enzyme deficiency:
(a) 21 hydroxylase
(b) 17 hydroxylase
(c) 3β-Hydroxysteroid dehydrogenase deficiency
(d) StAR deficiency

192. Klinefelter syndrome:
(a) Extra X chromosome from mother
(b) Extra X chromosome from father
(c) Extra mitosis of X chromosome in mother
(d) Extra mitosis of X chromosome in father

193. Renal cystic disease developing before formation of nephron:
(a) ARPKD
(b) Multicystic kidney diseases
(c) ADPKD
(d) Juvenile nephropathy

194. 12-year-old boy with scrotal pain, palpation not possible due to pain, upper scrotum shows blue color dot over upper testis next step is:
(a) Immediate exploration
(b) Orchidectomy
(c) De rotation
(d) Observation

195. ADPKD female with acute pain and fever. Treatment is given for E. coli but continues to have fever. Urine culture is negative. Diagnosis is:
(a) Ruptured cyst
(b) Passage of stones
(c) Renal abscess
(d) Infected hydronephrosis

196. Not used in VUR:
(a) Teflon
(b) Deflux
(c) Durasphere
(d) Cross linked bovine collagen

197. Bladder is:
(a) Epidermal in origin
(b) The bladder body is endodermal in origin while trigone is mesodermal in origin
(c) The bladder body is mesodermal in origin while trigone is endodermal in origin
(d) The bladder body is epidermal in origin while trigone is mesodermal in origin

198. Not true about Rokitansky–Kuster Hauser syndrome:
(a) Most common presentation is primary amenorrhea
(b) Atypical forms of MRKH syndrome have been described in up to 10% of cases

(c) Urinary tract anomalies occur more commonly in patients with the atypical form
(d) Upper urinary tract anomalies occur in approximately two third of patients

199. DAZ gene is located on which chromosome?
(a) 21 (b) 22
(c) X (d) Y

200. Most common clinical presentation in CAH:
(a) Male pseudohermaphroditism
(b) Female pseudohermaphroditism
(c) Virilization
(d) Salt wasting

201. Most common type of PUV:
(a) Type III (b) Type II
(c) Type I (d) Type IV

202. Potter facies in BRA occurs due to:
(a) Oligohydramnios
(b) Multiple organ system defects
(c) Polyhydramnios
(d) Pulmonary dysplasia

203. Distal hypospadias is repaired with:
(a) MAGPI
(b) OIF
(c) TPIF
(d) Double onlay preputial flap

204. TIP repair is described by:
(a) Snodgrass
(b) Heineke-Mikulicz
(c) Barcat
(d) Mathieu

205. Artificial erection was described by:
(a) Duckett
(b) Gittes and McLaughlin
(c) Mathieu
(d) Heineke-Mikulicz

206. Investigation to detect PUV:
(a) MCU (b) RGU
(c) RGP (d) Cystogram

207. Gold standard in diagnosis of undescended testis:
(a) Laparoscopy (b) CT
(c) MRI (d) USG

208. Most common cause of testicular torsion:
(a) Spontaneous
(b) Sports activity
(c) Trauma
(d) Cremasteric spasm

209. Most common testicular tumor below age of 1 year:
(a) Yolk sac tumor (b) Teratoma
(c) Seminoma (d) Leydig cell tumor

210. Regarding Ask-Upmark all are correct *except*:
(a) Segmental hypoplasia
(b) Most patients are 10 years of age or older at diagnosis
(c) The Ask-Upmark kidney is smaller than normal
(d) In patients with unilateral disease, partial nephrectomy may control the hypertension

211. Multilocated cystic nephroma all are true *except*:
(a) Occurs in young females and older male
(b) The only way to determine the diagnosis is by surgical excision
(c) The bleeding is secondary to herniation of the cyst through the transitional epithelium into the renal pelvis
(d) In children, an asymptomatic flank mass is the most common finding

212. History of surgery for left undescended testis (orchidopexy) at 8 years age. Now underwent right hernioplasty. Post hernioplasty – infertility. Vasography shows vas obstruction in right groin. Couple does not want IVF, best option:
(a) Vasovasostomy
(b) IUI
(c) Donor insemination
(d) Only treatment is IVF

213. Child with abdominal mass (2-year-old) one side limb longer than other, most probable diagnosis:
(a) Wilms' tumor
(b) Neuroblastoma
(c) Embryonal rhabdomyosarcoma
(d) RCC

214. Investigation of choice for medullary sponge kidney:
(a) IVP (b) CT
(c) MRI (d) USG

215. Worst prognostic marker for nephroblastoma:
(a) Stage III clear cell sarcoma
(b) Stage III Wilms' tumor
(c) Stage IV favorable histology
(d) Bilateral stage IV favorable histology

216. Worst prognosis for:
(a) Congenital mesonephric blastoma
(b) Clear cell sarcoma
(c) Rhabdoid tumor
(d) Anaplastic Wilms' tumor

217. Which is not true regarding anaplastic variant in Wilms' tumor?
(a) Tumor with anaplastic features are rare in patients <2 years of age
(b) When anaplasia is completely removed, prognosis is still poor
(c) Anaplasia is marker for chemoresistant
(d) Anaplasia is further divided into focal and diffuse patterns

218. Mullerian derivative all *except*:
(a) Uterus
(b) Cervix
(c) Upper two-third of vagina
(d) Lower third of vagina

219. Which is false regarding horseshoe kidney?
(a) 0.25% incidence
(b) Most common of all renal fusion anomalies
(c) Isthmus is located adjacent to the L1 or L2 vertebra
(d) Associated rate of renal calculi is 20%

220. Braca's II procedure is used for:
(a) Proximal hypospadias
(b) Distal penile hypospadias
(c) Clitoral reduction
(d) Peyronies disease

221. Investigation of choice for thrombus in IVC in Wilms' tumor:
(a) MRI (b) CT
(c) USG (d) TEE

222. Testicular descent caused by:
(a) TSH (b) FSH
(c) DHT (d) DHEAS

223. Reduction or spontaneous resolution is seen in which tumor?
(a) Nephroblastoma
(b) Neuroblastoma
(c) Bladder carcinoma
(d) Prostate carcinoma

224. Most common extracranial tumor in a neonate:
(a) Neuroblastoma
(b) Nephroblastoma
(c) RCC
(d) Rhabdomyosarcoma

225. Origin of Wilms' tumor is from:
(a) Epithelial (b) Blastemal
(c) Stromal (d) All of the above

226. Which is the most common abnormality associated with complete ureteral duplication?
(a) Ureteropelvic junction obstruction
(b) Ureterocoele
(c) Vesicoureteric reflux
(d) Obstructive megaureter

227. Hematogenous metastasis in Wlims' tumor stage is:
(a) V (b) II
(c) III (d) IV

228. Incidence of undescended testis at birth:
(a) 1% (b) 5%
(c) 3% (d) 7%

229. Glial cell derived neutrophilic factor is required in development of:

(a) Ureteric bud (b) Prostate
(c) Testis (d) Urinary bladder

230. In female which gland is homologous to prostate?
(a) Skene's (b) Camper
(c) Prostatic utricle (d) Mucous gland

231. Congenital absence of vas deferens is best diagnosed by:
(a) TRUS
(b) Palpation
(c) Scrotal USG
(d) Surgical exploration

232. Most common malignant tumor of infancy:
(a) Neuroblastoma
(b) Nephroblastoma
(c) RCC
(d) Embryonal rhabdomyosarcoma

233. Tumor most commonly present in horseshoe kidney is:
(a) Wilms' tumor
(b) RCC
(c) Pelvic epithelial tumor
(d) Neuroblastoma

234. The following statements about appendix testis are correct *except*:
(a) Torsion produces the blue dot sign
(b) Is a mullerian duct remnant
(c) Is a Wolffian duct remnant
(d) Torsion can mimic torsion testes

235. A 42-year-old lady with CRF is on hemodialysis for 4 years. Ultrasound showed both kidneys of 7 cm and containing multiple cysts. She is suffering from:
(a) Adult polycystic kidney disease
(b) Renal artery stenosis
(c) Medullary sponge kidney
(d) Acquired renal cystic disease

236. The following statements about acquired renal cystic disease are correct *except*:
(a) Seen in ESRD patients on dialysis
(b) Predisposition to renal cell carcinoma
(c) Bilaterally large kidneys with multiple cysts
(d) Presents with pain and hematuria

237. The pathological finding with the worst prognosis in Wilms' tumor is:
(a) Smooth muscle cells
(b) Anaplasia
(c) Striated muscle fibers
(d) Cellular calcification

238. The most common renal tumor in the first six months of life is:
(a) Congenital mesoblastic nephroma
(b) Nephroblastoma
(c) Extra adrenal neuroblastoma
(d) Rhabdomyosarcoma

239. Pseudovaginal perineoscrotal hypospadias is a feature of:
(a) Complete androgen deficiency
(b) Partial androgen deficiency
(c) Persistent mullerian duct syndrome
(d) 5α-Reductase deficiency

240. A child with ambiguous genitalia is found to have a streak gonad on one side and contralateral intraabdominal testis on the opposite side. The child has:
(a) True hermaphroditism
(b) Mixed gonadal dysgenesis
(c) Male pseudohermaphroditism
(d) Female pseudohermaphroditism

241. Which of the following is false when Tc 99 scan is used to differentiate hydronephrosis (HDN) from multicystic kidneys (MCDK)?
(a) Multicystic kidneys rarely reveal concentration of this isotope
(b) Kidneys with UPJ obstruction generally exhibit good concentration of the isotope
(c) In UPJ uptake of the isotope will be seen peripherally in the cortex
(d) In MCDK more peripheral enhancement than medial

242. Other name for "sertoli cell only syndrome":
(a) Hypospermatogenesis

(b) Maturation arrest
(c) Germinal cell aplasia
(d) End stage testis

243. Incidence of unilateral renal agenesis:
(a) 1/1100 (b) 1/2200
(c) 1/1600 (d) 1/45

244. Reflux of urine into non-dilated ureter, pelvis corresponds to VUR:
(a) Grade 2 (b) Grade 3
(c) Grade 4 (d) Grade 5

245. False about Klinefelter's syndrome:
(a) Eunuchoidism
(b) Gynecomastia
(c) Azoospermia
(d) Decreased gonadotropin levels

246. Transverse plication of redundant ureter is:
(a) Kalisinki plication
(b) Starr plication
(c) Polatino – lead better method
(d) Hendren plication

247. Medullary sponge kidney true is:
(a) Common in male stone farmers than female
(b) Is a rare cause of hypercalciuria
(c) Is a rare cause of hypertension
(d) Is inheritable

248. Persistence of hydronephrosis in immediate post operative period after surgical correction of VUR is commonly due to:
(a) UPJO
(b) UVJO
(c) Non-obstructive hydronephrosis
(d) Infravesical obstruction

249. Most common crossed renal ectopia:
(a) Crossed renal ectopia without fusion
(b) Crossed renal ectopia with superior fusion
(c) Crossed renal ectopia with inferior fusion
(d) Solitary crossed renal ectopia

250. True about thoracic kidney:
(a) Most commonly associated with diaphragmatic hernia
(b) Renal arteries commonly derived from thoracic aorta
(c) Renal rotation is usually complete
(d) Frequently associated with ascent of other intra abdominal structures

251. False after ureteroneocystostomy for correction of VUR:
(a) Early reflux is common
(b) Contralateral reflux is more common than ipsilateral
(c) Early reflux spontaneously resolves by 1 year
(d) Prophylactic bilateral reimplantation for unilateral reflux, to avoid contralateral reflux, is not warranted

252. All of the following abnormalities are predisposing causes for torsion of the testis *except*:
(a) Inversion of testis
(b) Low investment of tunica vaginalis
(c) High investment of tunica vaginalis
(d) Separation of the epididymis

253. By how many weeks of gestation does the fetal testis secretes testosterone?
(a) 9 weeks (b) 10 weeks
(c) 11 weeks (d) 12 weeks

254. Regarding Klinefelter's syndrome the following statements are true *except*:
(a) It occurs as a result of nondisjunction during meiosis
(b) Serum gonadotropins levels are low
(c) Most of these patients are azoospermic
(d) They have increased risk of development of breast carcinoma

255. The mesonephros degenerates by:
(a) 7 to 8 weeks of gestation
(b) 9 to 10 weeks of gestation
(c) 11 to 12 weeks of gestation
(d) 13 to 16 weeks of gestation

256. Every infant voids within the first:
(a) 6 hours of life (b) 12 hours of life
(c) 18 hours of life (d) 24 hours of life

257. **Features of Potter's syndrome include the following *except*:**
(a) Oligohydramnios
(b) Limb contractures
(c) Compressed facies
(d) Absent ears

258. **The most common renal fusion anomaly is:**
(a) Horseshoe kidney
(b) Unilateral fused kidneys
(c) Crossed renal ectopia
(d) Sigmoid kidney

259. **The autosomal dominant polycystic kidney disease, cysts are derived from:**
(a) Proximal tubule (b) Distal tubule
(c) Collecting duct (d) Entire nephron

260. **In autosomal recessive polycystic kidney disease, the abnormal gene is located on:**
(a) Chromosome 4 (b) Chromosome 6
(c) Chromosome 16 (d) Chromosome 19

261. **The percentage of nephrons developing cysts in autosomal dominant polycystic kidney disease is:**
(a) 1% (b) 3%
(c) 6% (d) 9%

262. **The most common presentation of medullary sponge kidney is:**
(a) Urinary tract infection
(b) Gross hematuria
(c) Renal colic
(d) Hypertension

263. **The most common site of termination of an ectopic ureter in the male is:**
(a) Posterior urethra (b) Seminal vesicle
(c) Ejaculatory duct (d) Vas deferens

264. **Moderate ureteral tortuosity and dilatation of the pelvis and calyces indicate:**
(a) Grade I vesicoureteral reflux
(b) Grade II vesicoureteral reflux
(c) Grade III vesicoureteral reflux
(d) Grade IV vesicoureteral reflux

265. **The incidence of vesicoureteric reflux associated with ureteropelvic junction obstruction ranges from:**
(a) 9% to 18% (b) 18% to 27%
(c) 27% to 36% (d) 36% to 45%

266. **All the following are involved in the descent of testis *except:***
(a) Genitofemoral nerve
(b) INSL3
(c) Androgens
(d) Ilioinguinal nerve

267. **In hypospadias:**
(a) Urethral opening is on dorsal side of penis
(b) Hypospadiac newborn should not be circumcised
(c) Penis is larger due to chordee
(d) Majority are penoscrotal or perineal

268. **Second most common site of ectopic ureter in male:**
(a) Seminal vesicle (b) Prostatic urethra
(c) Ejaculatory duct (d) Vas deferens

269. **Deafness + GN seen in:**
(a) Alport's syndrome
(b) Fabry's disease
(c) Takayasu syndrome
(d) Kawasaki syndrome

270. **Urine production in intrauterine starts at:**
(a) 10 – 12 weeks (b) 20 – 30 weeks
(c) 15 – 18 weeks (d) After delivery

271. **Vas deferens is derived from:**
(a) Mullerian duct
(b) Tail of lockwood
(c) Paramesonephric duct
(d) Wolffian duct

272. **In Turner syndrome chromosomal anomaly is:**
(a) 45X (b) 46X
(c) 46XY (d) 46XX

273. **Most common perineal protuberant mass in newborn female:**
(a) Periurethral cyst
(b) Prolapsed ureterocele
(c) Imperforated hymen
(d) Prolapsed urethra

274. Kidney develops from:
(a) Axial mesoderm
(b) Lateral plate mesoderm
(c) Intermediate mesoderm
(d) Neural tube

275. Torsion of testis most commonly involved:
(a) Hydatid of morgagni
(b) Appendix of epididymis
(c) Upper paradidymis
(d) Lower paradidymis

276. Most common fusion anomaly:
(a) Horseshoe kidney
(b) Sigmoid kidney
(c) Disk kidney
(d) Inferior ectopic kidney

277. Oliguria in full term baby is less than:
(a) 1 ml/hr (b) 2 ml/hr
(c) 3 ml/hr (d) 4 ml/hr

278. Most common site of metastasis from Wilms' tumor:
(a) Lung (b) Liver
(c) Bone (d) Brain

279. Nephrogenesis is complete from:
(a) 30 weeks of gestation
(b) 34 weeks of gestation
(c) At birth
(d) 6 weeks after birth

280. Circumcision is avoided in:
(a) Coronal hypospadias
(b) Phimosis
(c) Recurrent balanitis
(d) Meatal stenosis

281. Which of the following is not a benign tumor of kidney?
(a) Nephroblastoma
(b) Angiomyolipoma
(c) Angioma
(d) Adenoma

282. A 20 days old neonate with right hydronephrosis with dilated calyces (20 mm) management is:
(a) VCUG
(b) Observation for 6 months
(c) Radioisotope scan
(d) Cystourethroscopy

283. Most common cause of hydronephrosis in newborns:
(a) PUJ obstruction (b) PUV
(c) Oligohydramnios (d) Megaureter

284. Non-obstructed enlarged calyx is known as:
(a) Hydrocalycosis
(b) Megacalycosis
(c) Hydronephrosis
(d) Calyceal diverticulum

285. All of the following are true about retractile testis *except:*
(a) Most common age of occurrence is 5-7 years
(b) Usually found in the inguinal region
(c) Should be corrected before 2 years of age
(d) It is due to hyperactive cremasteric reflex

286. In undescended testis, best hormonal option available is:
(a) Intramuscular hCG
(b) Intranasal GnRH analogues
(c) Intravenous hCG
(d) Intramuscular placebo

287. The most common tumor developing in a cryptorchid testis is:
(a) Embryonal cell tumor
(b) Teratoma
(c) Seminoma
(d) Yolk sac tumor

288. Klinefelter's syndrome:
(a) 46XX (b) 47XXY
(c) 47XYY (d) 47XXX

289. Feedback inhibition of FSH is by:
(a) Testosterone (b) Inhibin
(c) Estrogen (d) ABP

290. Complete separation of cloaca and rectum by urorectal septum occurs by:
(a) 2-4 weeks (b) 4-6 weeks
(c) 6-8 weeks (d) 8-10 weeks

291. Kidney develops from:
(a) Metanephros (b) Mesonephros
(c) Ureteric bud (d) Pronephros

292. Ureteric bud bifurcates four times, yielding approximately 16 branches by:
(a) 6th week (b) 8th week
(c) 4th week (d) 10th week

293. Ambiguous genitalia 46 XX with symmetrical gonads:
(a) Undervirilized male
(b) Overvirilized female
(c) Mixed gonadal dysgenesis
(d) Ovotesticular disorder of sex differentiation

294. Cremasteric reflex most pronounced at:
(a) Birth
(b) 5th-6th years
(c) Puberty
(d) After 20 years of age

295. ADPKD with stone disease, risk of malignancy is:
(a) Increased risk (b) Same risk
(c) Decrease risk (d) No risk

296. In modern stage repair of bladder exstrophy, epispadias repair is done at:
(a) Birth (b) 0-6 months
(c) 6-12 months (d) 5 years

297. Anaplasia in Wilms' tumor is seen at age:
(a) Less than 1 year
(b) Less than 2 years
(c) More than 5 years
(d) More than 2 years

298. Investigation of choice for intracaval and atrial thrombus in Wilms' tumor:
(a) CT scan (b) MRI
(c) USG (d) PET scan

299. Poor outcome in Wilms' tumor is suggested by:
(a) Stage III
(b) Stage III with clear cell sarcoma
(c) Stage IV with favourable histology
(d) Bilateral Wilms' tumor with favourable histology

300. Neuroblastoma with high risk prognosis:
(a) Stage IV with N-myc amplification
(b) State IV without N-myc amplification
(c) Cystic lesions
(d) Cervical neuroblastoma

301. Most aggressive and lethal childhood renal neoplasm:
(a) Rhabdoid tumor
(b) Clear cell tumor
(c) Anaplastic Wilms' tumor
(d) Rhabdomyosarcoma

302. Bracka's procedure done for:
(a) Proximal hypospadias
(b) Distal hypospadias
(c) Clitoral reconstruction
(d) Congenital curvature of penis

303. Rupture of the cloacal membrane after complete separation of the genitourinary and GI tracts results in:
(a) Bladder exstrophy
(b) Anorectal malformations
(c) Cloaca
(d) Epispadias

304. Nephroblastoma is derived from:
(a) Metanephros (b) Mesonephros
(c) Pronephric tissue (d) Neuroectoderm

305. Lowest grade of VUR when reflux is upto PUJ:
(a) I (b) II
(c) III (d) V

306. Most common solid tumor of neonates:
(a) Neuroblastoma
(b) Rhabdomyosarcoma
(c) Sacrococcygeal teratoma
(d) Wilms' tumor

307. Hormone causing testicular descent:
(a) FSH (b) LH
(c) DHT (d) DHEA-S

308. Size after which a dilated duct is called a cyst in the kidney:
(a) 50 microns (b) 100 microns
(c) 150 microns (d) 200 microns

309. True about horseshoe kidney are all *except:*
(a) Incidence of 0.25%
(b) Located at L3-L4 just above origin of IMA
(c) Generally isthmus is flimsy midline band
(d) About 1/3rd patients have PUJ obstruction

310. Calyceal diverticulum all are true *except:*
(a) Congenital
(b) Wide necked communicating with pelvicalyceal system
(c) Lined by non-secretory urothelium
(d) Present in 0.2-0.8%
(e) Stone incidence 9.5-50%

311. Horseshoe kidney all are true *except:*
(a) Most common congenital renal anomaly
(b) Early gestational fusion of mesonephros
(c) Associated UPJ obstruction causes infection and stone
(d) PNL can be used for large pelvic stone
(e) ESWL can be used for calyceal stone

312. Bilateral renal agenesis all are true *except:*
(a) Incidence is 1:4800
(b) 40% stillborn
(c) Male preponderance
(d) Increased incidence with increased maternal age
(e) Hyperkalemia is most common cause of death

313. Thoracic kidney all are true *except:*
(a) Most common in anterior mediastinum
(b) <5% ectopic kidney
(c) Long ureter
(d) Asymptomatic mostly
(e) Increased hemidiaphragm

314. Bifid renal pelvis all are true *except:*
(a) 10% incidence
(b) Normal variant
(c) Increased incidence of pelvic disease
(d) May be seen on IVU
(e) Yo-Yo effect on renal scan

315. Ask-Upmark kidney all are true *except:*
(a) Developmental anomaly
(b) Focal renal dysplasia
(c) Severe hypertension
(d) Proteinuria
(e) Severe hematuria

316. MCDK, all are true *except:*
(a) Kidneys are reniform shape with no calyceal drainage
(b) Kidney has the appearance of "a bunch of grapes", with little stroma between the cysts
(c) Haphazard distribution of cysts of various sizes
(d) No large central or medial cyst and without visible communications between the cysts
(e) Renal uptake is seldom seen in MCDK

317. CT findings of benign simple cyst are all *except:*
(a) Smooth outline and thin walled
(b) Round oval shape
(c) -10 to +20 HU
(d) Heterogeneous
(e) No contrast enhancement

318. Prune-belly syndrome all are true *except:*
(a) Absent abdominal musculature
(b) Bilateral intra-abdominal testes
(c) Bilateral HDUN
(d) Dilated prostatic urethra
(e) Trabeculated and thickened bladder wall

319. Congenital megacystis megaureter syndrome all are true *except:*
(a) Thin walled bladder
(b) Bilateral VUR
(c) Hypocontractile detrusor
(d) Wide and poorly developed trigone
(e) Lateral insertion of ureter

320. Acquired renal cystic disease all are true *except:*
(a) Seen in CRF patients on dialysis

(b) Associated only with benign tumors
(c) Seen in CRF patients on medical management
(d) Pain and hematuria most common presentation
(e) Increase incidence of RCC in these patients

321. Renal sinus cysts all are true *except:*
(a) Usually unilateral
(b) Usually multiple
(c) Associated with inflammation
(d) No parenchymal involvement
(e) Lymphatic origin (most common)

322. Walker criteria for VUR all *except:*
(a) Most cases resolve spontaneously
(b) High grade don't resolve spontaneously
(c) Sterile reflex is benign
(d) Extended prophylactic antibiotics not justified
(e) Very high success rate with surgery

323. Ureterocele all are true *except:*
(a) Female more commonly associated with duplicated system
(b) F: M = 2:1
(c) 80% involves upper moiety of duplicated system
(d) Simple ureterocele usually presents in adults
(e) 10% is bilateral

324. Anterior urethral valve all are true *except:*
(a) Less common than PUV
(b) In true sense it is a urethral diverticulum
(c) No defect in corpora spongiosum
(d) Diagnosed by MCU/urethroscopy
(e) Ballooning and diverticulum seen during voiding

325. PUV all are true *except:*
(a) Antenatal diagnosis possible
(b) USG-KUB most important study for the diagnosis of PUV
(c) Type 1 is most common type
(d) Pulmonary hypoplasia is most severe associated anomaly
(e) Varying degree of renal insufficiency

326. Nonautologous injectable material for VUR are all *except:*
(a) PTFE
(b) Deflux
(c) Polydimethylsiloxane
(d) Cross-linked bovine collagen
(e) Chondrocytes

327. Mitotic activity of gonocyte is detectable at:
(a) 36 weeks (b) 1-3 years
(c) 5-7 years (d) 7-9 years
(e) 15 years

328. Ascent of horseshoe kidney obstructed by:
(a) IMA (b) SMA
(c) Renal artery (d) Celiac plexus
(e) Gonadal artery

329. Principles of ureteric reimplantation includes all *except:*
(a) Detrusor hiatus opening is of no significance
(b) Submucosal tunnel length 5:1
(c) Bladder handled gently to reduced spasm and hematuria
(d) Distal ureteric blood supply to be preserved
(e) It is easy to form submucosal tunnel with good muscle backing in stomach

330. Largest glandular zone in prostate:
(a) Peripheral (b) Central
(c) Transition (d) Periurethral

331. Most common of the enzyme defects responsible for CAH is:
(a) Deficiency of 3-hydroxylase
(b) Deficiency of 11-hydroxylase
(c) Deficiency of 17-hydroxylase
(d) Deficiency of 21-hydroxylase

332. First sign of puberty growth in males:
(a) Appearance of pubic hair
(b) Breast enlargement

(c) Lengthening of penis
(d) Enlargement of testis

333. Hormone necessary for the development of Wolffian duct:
(a) DHT (b) Testosterone
(c) LH (d) GnRH

334. Which of the following is not a Wolffian duct derivative?
(a) Vas deferens (b) Epoophoron
(c) Prostatic utricle (d) Gartner's duct

335. False regarding ARPKD:
(a) Due to mutation in chromosome 6
(b) Autosomal recessive mode of inheritance
(c) Presence of hepatic fibrosis
(d) Multiple cysts visualized on USG

336. Horseshoe kidney most commonly associated with:
(a) Trisomy 18
(b) Turner's syndrome
(c) MRHK syndrome
(d) Tuberous sclerosis

337. "Bouquet of flowers" appearance on IVP is seen in:
(a) Medullary cystic disease
(b) Multicystic dysplastic kidney
(c) Medullary sponge kidney
(d) Multilocular cyst

338. False about PUV:
(a) Type 1 is most common type
(b) Type 2 most commonly causes obstruction
(c) Type 3 is due to incomplete dissolution of urogenital membrane
(d) There is no muscle within the valve

339. All are components of PBS *except:*
(a) Defective abdominal muscle
(b) Bilateral hydrouretero nephrosis
(c) Dilatation of bladder
(d) Presence of valves in posterior urethra

340. Which of the following physical examination finding is important in patients with ambiguous genitalia?
(a) Presence of hypospadias
(b) Length of penis
(c) Palpability of gonad
(d) Sacral dimple

341. Following should be suspected when there is transverse testicular ectopia:
(a) Complete androgen insensitivity syndrome
(b) Peno scrotal disproportion
(c) Persistent mullerian ducts syndrome
(d) 21 hydroxylase deficiency

342. The most common cause of mortality in a child with posterior urethral valve:
(a) Renal failure
(b) Sepsis
(c) Pulmonary hypoplasia
(d) Cardiac failure

343. Bilateral renal agenesis, all are true *except:*
(a) Incidence is more in males than females
(b) Complete ureteral atresia seen in 50% patients
(c) Absent or hypoplastic bladder
(d) Absent adrenal glands

344. Klinefelter's syndrome is associated with which of the following karyotype?
(a) 46XY (b) 47XYY
(c) 47XXY (d) 45X

345. In a horseshoe kidney further ascent of the kidneys is prevented by the:
(a) Superior mesenteric artery
(b) Inferior mesenteric artery
(c) Superior mesenteric vein
(d) Inferior mesenteric vein

346. The remnants of mullerian duct in males is:
(a) Appendix testis
(b) Prostatic utricle
(c) Appendix testis and prostatic utricle
(d) Appendix of the epididymis

347. Wilms' tumor has been linked to which of the following hereditary tumor syndromes?
(a) WAGR syndrome
(b) Denys-Drash syndrome
(c) Beckwith-Wiedemann syndrome
(d) All of the above

348. Pseudovaginal perineoscrotal hypospadias is seen in:
(a) Syndrome of partial androgen resistance
(b) Syndrome of complete androgen insensitivity
(c) Pure gonadal dysgenesis
(d) Partial gonadal dysgenesis

349. A child with ambiguous genitalia is found to have a streak gonad on one side and a testis on the opposite side. The child has:
(a) True hermaphroditism
(b) Mixed gonadal dysgenesis
(c) Male of pseudohermaphroditism
(d) Female pseudohermaphroditism

350. Repair of mid penile hypospadias can be achieved by all the following procedures *except:*
(a) Asopa (b) Snodgrass
(c) Mathieu (d) MAGPI

351. Structure which does not arise from paramesonephric duct:
(a) Appendix testis
(b) Appendix epididymis
(c) Prostatic utricle
(d) Upper vagina
(e) Fallopian tube

352. Chordee in hypospadias true is:
(a) Dorsal hood
(b) Ventral curvature
(c) Always associated with hypospadias even with glandular
(d) Treatment of choice–Incision and release
(e) Fibrosis limited to external meatal tip

353. Reflux of urine into non dilated ureter, pelvis corresponds to VUR:
(a) Grade 1 (b) Grade 2
(c) Grade 3 (d) Grade 4
(e) Grade 5

354. Not an autosomal dominant renal cystic condition:
(a) VHL
(b) Tuberous sclerosis
(c) Medullary sponge kidney
(d) MCDK
(e) Medullary cystic disease

355. Valve bladder term was coined by:
(a) Hugh Hampton Young
(b) Mitchell
(c) Marshall
(d) Youssif

356. Percent of nephrons involved in ADPKD:
(a) 1% (b) <15% (c) 15% (d) >15%

357. Pyelogenic cyst is also termed as:
(a) Ureteral duplication
(b) Parapelvic cyst
(c) Renal sinus cyst
(d) Calyceal diverticulum

358. Most common major abnormality of sexual differentiation:
(a) XXY
(b) XO
(c) Deletion of Chromosome Y
(d) XYY

359. Persistent mullerian duct syndrome all are true *except*:
(a) Transverse testicular ectopia
(b) Patients are phenotypic males
(c) MIC gene defect
(d) 46, XY karyotype and normal male external genitalia

360. Seminal vesicle development is from:
(a) Mesonephric duct
(b) Fallopian duct
(c) Wolffian duct
(d) Urogenital sinus

361. Nephroblastomatosis means:
(a) Multiple nephrogenic rest
(b) Disseminated malignancy
(c) Neuroblastoma
(d) Multicystic kidney disease

362. Blue dot sign is seen in:
(a) Torsion of testis
(b) Torsion of epididymis

(c) Orchitis
(d) Epididymitis

363. When does the kidney ascend to lumbar site during embryogenesis?
(a) 6–9 weeks (b) 9–12 weeks
(c) 12–14 weeks (d) 14–16 weeks

364. Which of the following is a suppressive factor in early kidney development?
(a) Glial cell line-derived neurotrophic factor
(b) Eya1
(c) Pax2
(d) FoxC

365. Which of the following is correct about neonatal renal function?
(a) GFR at birth is about 60% of normal adult values
(b) Urine concentrating ability is increased in the neonate which subsequently decreases
(c) Renal acidification is normal right from birth
(d) The fractional excretion of sodium (FE_{Na}) is higher than normal at birth

366. In horseshoe kidneys:
(a) Two third are fused at lower pole and one third at the upper pole
(b) Incidence is about one in 400
(c) Incidence of PUJ obstruction is similar to normal kidneys
(d) The calyces point anteriorly because of the fusion

367. In autosomal dominant polycystic kidney disease, which is true?
(a) Incidence of RCC is higher than in general population
(b) Hepatic cysts occur in all patients with ADPKD
(c) Half of the affected individuals have PKD gene 1 mutation
(d) USG criteria for diagnosis include at least two unilateral or bilateral cysts in individuals younger than 30 years

368. In pediatric pyeloplasties:
(a) One fifth of children with VATER anomaly have PUJ obstruction
(b) Success rate of antegrade endopyelotomy are comparable to open techniques
(c) Transmesocolic approach in laparoscopy is preferred for right side
(d) Non-dismembered techniques are preferred over dismembered techniques

369. Which of the following results in a pseudoureterocele?
(a) High grade VUR
(b) Primary obstructive megaureter
(c) Ectopic ureter
(d) Syringocele

370. A 4 years old boy is brought with right supra-scrotal testis. There is history of inguinal hernia surgery at the age of 2 years. This boy now has:
(a) Testicular retraction
(b) Secondary cryptorchidism
(c) Recurrent cryptorchidism
(d) Acquired cryptorchidism

371. Which of the following is an extravesical procedure for ureteric reimplantation?
(a) Cohen's technique
(b) Glenn-Anderson technique
(c) Lich Gregoir technique
(d) Leadbetter-Politano technique

372. IPGAM closure is described for:
(a) Hypospadias repair
(b) Epispadias repair
(c) Cloacal exstrophy
(d) Urethrocutaneous fistula

373. Which of the following does not cause bilateral hydroureteronephrosis?
(a) Prune-belly syndrome
(b) Posterior urethral valve
(c) Bilateral PUJ obstruction
(d) Vesicoureteral reflux

374. The following procedure is not indicated in proximal hypospadias:

(a) Snodgrass procedure
(b) Koyanagi procedure
(c) Ulaanbaatar procedure
(d) MAGPI procedure

375. True about embryologic origin:

(a) Seminal vesicle and vas deferens–Mesonephric duct
(b) Lower 1/3rd vagina–Urogenital sinus
(c) Upper 2/3rd vagina–Mullerian duct
(d) Gartner duct cyst in female—Mullerian duct
(e) Appendix of testis–Wolffian duct

376. True about testicular tumors in children:

(a) Yolk sac tumor primarily produces hCG
(b) Partial orchiectomy can be done for testicular teratoma
(c) Present most commonly in infancy
(d) Associated most commonly with cryptorchidism
(e) Present most commonly in retroperitoneum

377. Treatment option for VUR are:

(a) Transtriagonal ureteric reimplantation
(b) Boari flap
(c) Submucosal injection therapy
(d) Observation
(e) Extravesical Lich and Gregoir repair

378. Following about epispadias are true:

(a) Renal agenesis always present
(b) Incontinence always almost present
(c) Chordee always dorsal
(d) Children should be evaluated for VUR
(e) Adequate penile length is generally achievable

379. Regarding hypospadias:

(a) Surgery to be done before 2 years
(b) Proximal hypospadias–surgery for cosmosis only
(c) Full circumcision to compensate ventral chordee
(d) Perineal hypospadias most common
(e) Chordee decreases on erection

380. Newborn with fever with massive dilated bladder, no distal obstruction, no neurogenic components, true is:

(a) PUV resection
(b) Urethral dilatation
(c) Permanent vesicostomy
(d) Upper tract diversion
(e) Bilateral ureteric reimplantation

381. UDS in pediatric patients:

(a) Helps in management of neurogenic bladder
(b) Always done in supine position
(c) Urine culture should be sterile
(d) Easy to perform in children
(e) Does not help in diagnosis

382. Gonadal dysgenesis seen in A/E:

(a) CAH
(b) Mixed gonadal dysgenesis
(c) Swyer syndrome
(d) True hermaphroditism
(e) Turner's syndrome

383. True about true hermaphroditism:

(a) Perineoscrotal hypospadias seen
(b) Both testis and ovary present
(c) Uterus present
(d) 46+XX most common
(e) 46+XY most common

384. All are true for ureterocele all *except*:

(a) Ureterocele disproportion is seen associated with duplex system
(b) Only minority get diagnosed on antenatal USG
(c) Proposed mechanism is failure of disappearance of chwalla membrane
(d) Cecoureterocele means ureteric opening and ureterocele extending in urethra
(e) It is a form of ectopic ureter with cystic dilatation of distal ureter

385. Epispadias/exstrophy true is:
(a) Anorectal malformation
(b) HSK
(c) Open urethral plate
(d) Hypoplasia of tail gut
(e) Public diasthesis

386. True about ectopic ureter all *except*:
(a) Never open in triagone
(b) In female open anywhere, even urethra
(c) Associated with lower moiety in duplex
(d) In males opening above perineal floor
(e) Present with incontinence and normal voiding

387. Wolffian duct derivatives true are:
(a) Round ligament of uterus
(b) SFTH
(c) VD
(d) Uterine tube
(e) Urethra

388. ARPKD true is:
(a) Associated with trisomy 13
(b) Cyst due to enlarged Bowmen's
(c) Due to fibrocystine mutation
(d) Large distorted kidney
(e) Can be diagnosed on USG

389. Mechanism of VUR prevention are all *except*:
(a) No true space between bladder and ureter
(b) Mobile intramural ureter
(c) Effective ureteric peristalsis
(d) Fix ureteric orifice
(e) Neural mechanism

390. Regarding undescended testis:
(a) Bilateral undescended testis-lap to be done
(b) <1/3rd palpable
(c) To be repaired before 24 hours of life preferably
(d) Orchidectomy to be considered in unilateral UDT post puberty
(e) Unpalpable testis may be vanishing or absent

391. Which of the following is true about prune-belly syndrome?
(a) Anterior urethra dilated
(b) Ureter are usually normal though renal dysplasia present
(c) 95% occurs in male
(d) Triad of intra-abdominal testis, abdominal wall defect and renal anomalies
(e) Seminal vesical normal

392. Anterior urethral valve false are:
(a) More than 5% of patients progress to ESRD
(b) Prognosis of anterior urethral valve is better than posterior urethral valve
(c) Endoscopic incision is done
(d) Diagnosis depends on urethral mass irrespective of cystoscopic findings
(e) Antenatal HDN on USG seen in PUV not as common as AUV

393. True about PUV:
(a) Immediate PU catheterization is preferred initial treatment
(b) Valve ablation is the surgical therapy
(c) Hydronephrosis and VUR managed by PCN
(d) Renal and bladder function are variable throughout life and aggressive lifelong monitoring required
(e) Cutaneous vesicostomy done in all cases

394. Investigations for VUR:
(a) CT
(b) MRI
(c) DTPA
(d) VCUG
(e) USG

395. False about exstrophy:
(a) Internal rotation of the anterior segment
(b) External rotation of the anterior segment
(c) 30% lengthening is seen in anterior segment

(d) Pubic diastasis
(e) External rotation of posterior segment

396. About hypospadias:

(a) TIP repair (Glansplasty) is independent of urethral plate tubularization
(b) Preop hormonal stimulation is given to increase penile size and vascularity
(c) Prepuce is deficient dorsally
(d) Ventral chordee not commonly corrected by degloving and dartos dissection
(e) Hypospadias with bilateral cryptorchidism is s/o DSD

397. About ectopic kidney true is:

(a) First branches from median sacral artery
(b) Pelvic kidney most common
(c) Bilateral pelvic kidney in 60%
(d) Adrenal is present and in orthotopic position
(e) Thoracic kidney is due to delayed regression of mesonephros

398. A 13 years old girl with sexual infantilism and normal height on evaluation was found to have 46XX karyotype, bilateral streak gonad, normal female external genitalia and normal mullerian structures with absent Wolffian structures. This girl has:

(a) Turner's syndrome
(b) Noonan's syndrome
(c) 46XX pure gonadal dysgenesis
(d) Partial gonadal dysgenesis

399. The most critical finding on clinical examination in a neonate with ambiguous genitalia is:

(a) Size of phallus
(b) Position of external meatus
(c) Palpable gonads
(d) Presence of uterus on rectal examination

400. In prune-belly syndrome, the testes are usually found:

(a) At external ring
(b) Ectopic
(c) Over the iliac vessels
(d) In the inguinal canal

ANSWERS

1.	D	26.	B	51.	A	76.	D	101.	TTTFT
2.	D	27.	A	52.	B	77.	B	102.	TFTTT
3.	A	28.	C	53.	B	78.	A	103.	TTTFF
4.	B	29.	C	54.	C	79.	B	104.	TFTTF
5.	D	30.	D	55.	B	80.	B	105.	FFTFT
6.	A	31.	B	56.	A	81.	D	106.	TTFTT
7.	B	32.	A	57.	A	82.	A	107.	TFTTF
8.	C	33.	C	58.	D	83.	D	108.	FFFFF
9.	A	34.	C	59.	D	84.	D	109.	TFTTT
10.	D	35.	C	60.	A	85.	A	110.	TFTTT
11.	A	36.	D	61.	B	86.	A	111.	TFTTF
12.	D	37.	A	62.	D	87.	C	112.	TTTTT
13.	C	38.	D	63.	D	88.	C	113.	TFFFT
14.	A	39.	B	64.	A	89.	A	114.	TFTFT
15.	B	40.	C	65.	C	90.	A	115.	TTTTF
16.	A	41.	C	66.	B	91.	TTTTT	116.	TTFTF
17.	C	42.	A	67.	C	92.	TFTTT	117.	TTFFT
18.	C	43.	D	68.	A	93.	TTTTT	118.	TTFTT
19.	A	44.	D	69.	C	94.	TFTFF	119.	TFFTT
20.	C	45.	D	70.	A	95.	TTFTT	120.	TTTTT
21.	B	46.	D	71.	D	96.	FFTTT	121.	TTFTT
22.	D	47.	C	72.	D	97.	TTTFT	122.	FFTTF
23.	A	48.	B	73.	D	98.	FFFFT	123.	TFFTT
24.	C	49.	B	74.	A	99.	TTFFF	124.	TTTTF
25.	A	50.	B	75.	D	100.	FFFTF	125.	FFFFF

126.	TTFTT	155.	FTFFT	184.	ABDE	213.	A	242.	C
127.	FTFTT	156.	TFTTT	185.	ABCE	214.	A	243.	A
128.	TFFFF	157.	TTTFT	186.	ABCDE	215.	A	244.	A
129.	FTTFT	158.	TTTTT	187.	ABCD	216.	C	245.	D
130.	FFFFT	159.	BCDE	188.	ABCD	217.	B	246.	B
131.	TFTTT	160.	ABCDE	189.	A	218.	D	247.	C
132.	TFFTT	161.	ACD	190.	B	219.	C	248.	C
133.	TTTFT	162.	CE	191.	A	220.	A	249.	C
134.	TFTTF	163.	ABCE	192.	B	221.	A	250.	C
135.	TTTTF	164.	BE	193.	B	222.	C	251.	B
136.	TFFTT	165.	ACD	194.	D	223.	B	252.	D
137.	TTFTF	166.	C	195.	A	224.	A	253.	A
138.	TTFTT	167.	B	196.	C	225.	D	254.	B
139.	TTFTT	168.	ACD	197.	B	226.	C	255.	C
140.	TFFFT	169.	ABCDE	198.	D	227.	D	256.	D
141.	FTFFT	170.	ABDE	199.	D	228.	C	257.	D
142.	TFTTT	171.	AC	200.	B	229.	A	258.	A
143.	FFTFT	172.	D	201.	C	230.	A	259.	B
144.	TTTFT	173.	C	202.	A	231.	B	260.	B
145.	FTTTF	174.	D	203.	A	232.	A	261.	A
146.	TTTTT	175.	ABCE	204.	A	233.	B	262.	C
147.	FTFFT	176.	A	205.	B	234.	C	263.	A
148.	TFTTF	177.	ABD	206.	A	235.	D	264.	D
149.	TTTTT	178.	AC	207.	A	236.	C	265.	A
150.	TTTTT	179.	ABCDE	208.	A	237.	B	266.	D
151.	TFTTF	180.	BDE	209.	A	238.	A	267.	B
152.	TFTTF	181.	BCDE	210.	A	239.	B	268.	A
153.	TTFTT	182.	BDE	211.	A	240.	B	269.	A
154.	TTTTF	183.	ABCD	212.	A	241.	D	270.	A

271. D	293. B	315. E	337. C	359. C	381. ABC
272. A	294. C	316. A	338. B	360. A	382. D
273. A	295. D	317. D	339. D	361. A	383. BCD
274. C	296. C	318. E	340. C	362. B	384. BD
275. B	297. D	319. C	341. C	363. A	385. ACE
276. A	298. B	320. B	342. C	364. A	386. C
277. A	299. B	321. A	343. D	365. A	387. C
278. A	300. A	322. D	344. C	366. B	388. CE
279. B	301. A	323. B	345. B	367. D	389. AD
280. A	302. A	324. C	346. C	368. A	390. ADE
281. A	303. A	325. B	347. D	369. B	391. CD
282. B	304. A	326. E	348. A	370. B	392. ADE
283. A	305. B	327. D	349. B	371. C	393. ABD
284. B	306. A	328. A	350. D	372. A	394. DE
285. C	307. C	329. A	351. B	373. C	395. AC
286. B	308. D	330. B	352. B	374. D	396. ABDE
287. C	309. C	331. D	353. B	375. ABC	397. BDE
288. B	310. B	332. D	354. D	376. BC	398. C
289. A	311. B	333. B	355. B	377. ACDE	399. C
290. B	312. E	334. C	356. A	378. CDE	400. C
291. A	313. A	335. D	357. D	379. A	
292. A	314. C	336. B	358. A	380. AD	

General Surgery

1. **The following is true of Ewing's sarcoma *except:***
   (a) It presents with fever and malaise
   (b) 'Onion ring' type of periosteal elevation
   (c) It occurs in metaphysis
   (d) It occurs in flat bone
2. **Jefferson fracture is fracture of:**
   (a) Pedicle of C2 vertebra
   (b) Pedicle of C1 vertebra
   (c) Ring of C1 vertebra
   (d) Ring of C2 vertebra
3. **All are true in Hangman's fracture *except:***
   (a) It is caused by hyperextension of spine
   (b) It is fracture of pedicle of C2 vertebra
   (c) It constitutes 10% of cervical injuries
   (d) It is a fracture of pedicle of C1 vertebra
4. **Features in primary hyperparathyroidism are seen with following *except:***
   (a) Pathological fracture
   (b) Nephrocalcinosis
   (c) Dementia
   (d) Diarrhea
5. **In Cushing's syndrome ACTH-dependent cortisol excess is caused by:**
   (a) Microadenoma from anterior pituitary
   (b) Ectopic ACTH production from small lung cancers
   (c) From foregut carcinoid tumors
   (d) Adrenocortical adenomas
6. **Mycotic aneurysm is caused by:**
   (a) Actinomycosis
   (b) Nocardia madurae
   (c) By bacteria
   (d) They are most common in occurrence
7. **In carcinoid syndrome all are true *except:***
   (a) Reddish blue cyanosis
   (b) Asthmatic attacks
   (c) Flushing attacks
   (d) Mitral stenosis
8. **In Carney's triad all is true *except:***
   (a) Usually familial occurring in young men
   (b) Functioning paraganglioma
   (c) Gastric leiomyosarcoma
   (d) Pulmonary chondroma
9. **In multiple endocrine neoplasia 2-B all of following is found *except:***
   (a) Medullary cancer thyroid
   (b) Pheochromocytoma
   (c) Hyperparathyroidism
   (d) Cutaneous lichen amyloidosis
10. **Thymic carcinoma presents with the following features *except:***
    (a) Capsular invasion
    (b) Metastasis
    (c) Resembles squamous cell carcinoma
    (d) Associated with myasthenia
11. **All of following is true in carcinoma of esophagus *except:***
    (a) Squamous carcinoma occurs in lower third
    (b) Adenocarcinoma occurs in lower 3rd
    (c) Squamous carcinoma occurs in upper 2/3rd
    (d) Dysphagia is a late feature
12. **Which of the following is true of gastric polyps?**
    (a) Most common is metaplastic polyp
    (b) Inflammatory polyps are rare
    (c) Polyps have great malignant potential
    (d) Gastric carcinoids are found in large polyps
13. **All are true in gastric lymphoma *except:***
    (a) They occur in 6th decade
    (b) They are B cell derived

(c) Diagnosis can be made on endoscopic features
(d) Diagnosis can be made on endoscopic biopsy

14. In primary Sjögren's syndrome all are false *except:*
(a) Male to female ratio is 1: 10
(b) It occurs in middle age
(c) Underlying connective tissue disorders
(d) Severe xerostomia

15. The following is true of malignant melanoma *except:*
(a) Lentigo maligna is least malignant
(b) Acral lentiginous melanoma carries a very good prognosis
(c) Nodular melanoma occurs in younger people
(d) Amelanotic melanoma presents with regional nodes

16. In abdominal aneurysm the following is true:
(a) Anterior rupture of aortic aneurysm occurs in 20%
(b) Anterior rupture of aortic aneurysm occurs in 80%
(c) Posterior rupture in retroperitoneum occurs in 70%
(d) Posterior rupture occurs in retroperitoneum in 20%

17. In lymphedema precox all are true *except:*
(a) Onset is 1 to 35 years
(b) More common in males than females
(c) More likely to be bilateral
(d) Peak incidence is before menarche

18. In thyroglossal cyst all are true *except:*
(a) Frequently occurs beneath hyoid
(b) Occurs above hyoid
(c) Occurs in midline
(d) In thyroid cartilage region gets pushed to right

19. In Hirschsprung's disease all are true *except:*
(a) More common in females than males
(b) Absence of ganglion cells in neural plexus in intestinal wall
(c) Lower 2/3rd of patient's lower rectum/sigmoid colon is involved
(d) Severe symptoms are related to number of acetyl cholinesterase positive fibres

20. The following is true of dentate line *except:*
(a) It separates cuboidal epithelium above and squamous epithelium below
(b) Autonomic fibres above and spinal nerves below
(c) Portal system above and systemic venous system below
(d) Systemic venous system above and portal system below

21. In esophageal diverticula which of these is true?
(a) Pulsion diverticula are very rare
(b) Traction diverticula are very common
(c) Traction diverticula may not be due to pathology of adjacent nodes
(d) Pulsion diverticula are the most common

22. In Plummer-Vinson syndrome all are true *except:*
(a) It is associated with iron deficiency anemia
(b) Sideropenic dysphagia
(c) Brown Kelly Paterson syndrome
(d) Dysphagia occurs in distal esophagus

23. In toxic nodule what is not true?
(a) It is autonomous nodule
(b) High level of TSH is suppressed by high level of thyroxine
(c) Normal thyroid tissue surrounding the nodule is inactive
(d) Hypertrophy and hyperplasia is due to TSH-RAb

24. The following is not true in ulcerative colitis:
(a) It is a mucosal immunological reaction
(b) A weakened mucous barrier
(c) Defective mucosal metabolism of butyrates
(d) Smoking worsens disease

25. In familial adenomatous polyposis all are true *except:*
(a) Inherited and mendelian dominant
(b) Males and females equally affected
(c) Can occur sporadically
(d) Seldom associated with desmoids tumors

26. In hypernephroma all are true *except:*
(a) It is twice more common in men as in women

(b) Hematuria is usual presenting complaint
(c) Polycythemia can occur
(d) They occur frequently in lower pole

27. The following is not true in bladder rupture:
(a) Intraperitoneal rupture occurs in 20%
(b) Extraperitoneal rupture in 80%
(c) Intraperitoneal rupture occurs in distended bladder
(d) Intraperitoneal rupture occurs due to fracture pelvis

28. All are true about balanoposthitis:
(a) It can be associated with penile cancer
(b) It is inflammation of prepuce
(c) It may be associated with diabetes
(d) Monilial infection may be associated

29. The following is true in respiratory alkalosis:
(a) It occurs in hyperventilation
(b) In hyperpyrexia
(c) Occurs in high altitudes
(d) Rectified by oxygen insufflations

30. Which of the following is false?
(a) Hemophilia-A caused by deficiency of factor IX
(b) Hemophilia-B caused by deficiency of factor IX
(c) Hemophilia-B is called as Christmas disease
(d) Hemophilia manifests only in men

31. In dysphagia lusoria which of the following is true?
(a) Aberrant right subclavian artery
(b) Compression of aortic arch
(c) It can present in old age
(d) Compression by normal subclavian artery

32. In Zollinger-Ellison syndrome all are true *except:*
(a) Very high basal acid output with no response to pentagastrin
(b) Can be inherited as MEN type II
(c) Can be inherited as MEN type I
(d) Gastrin producing endocrine tissue is found in duodenum

33. All are true about volvulus of stomach *except:*
(a) Rotation occurs organoaxial
(b) Rotation occurs in mesenterico-caval
(c) It is associated with paraesophageal hernia
(d) Mesenterico-caval is the most common volvulus

34. In Budd-Chiari syndrome all are true *except:*
(a) Protein C or S deficiency may be found
(b) CT scan will show enlarged caudate lobe
(c) Hypertrophy of segment 3
(d) Patient goes for fulminant liver failure in acute thrombosis

35. The following is true in focal nodular hyperplasia:
(a) It contains hepatocytes only
(b) It contains Kupffer cells only
(c) Contains both Kupffer cells and hepatocytes
(d) Sulphur colloid scan is taken up by hepatocytes

36. In hereditary spherocytosis which is true?
(a) Defect transmitted as Mendelian recessive
(b) Females are more affected
(c) Cholesterol stones are formed
(d) Acholuric jaundice will be present

37. The length of common bile duct is:
(a) 6.5 cms (b) 9 cms
(c) 5.5 cms (d) 7.5 cms

38. In neuroma what is false?
(a) Ganglioneuroma is found in retroperitoneal space
(b) Neuroblastoma disseminates by blood stream
(c) In myelenic neuroma ganglion cells are absent
(d) In myelenic neuroma ganglion cells are present

39. Which is false in the following?
(a) Exudation cysts occur in thyroid
(b) Cystic hygroma is a distention cyst
(c) Distention cysts occur in ovary
(d) Bursa example of distention cysts

40. The following is true about grafts:
(a) Partial thickness graft contains epidermis only
(b) Full thickness contains all of epidermis and part of dermis

(c) Composite graft contains epidermis and entire dermis
(d) Graft can survive on periosteum and paratenon

41. In hidradenitis suppurativa what is not true?
(a) Suppuration caused by hyperplasia of the gland
(b) More common in women
(c) Staph aureus is the most common organism
(d) Bacteroides is the causative organism

42. About Bowen's disease what is true?
(a) Erythroplasia of queyrat is Bowen's disease of glans penis
(b) Bowen's disease occurs in young patients
(c) It is unrelated to solar radiation
(d) Not associated with arsenic ingestion

43. In Barrett's esophagus what is not true?
(a) Junction between gastric and esophageal mucosa moves proximally
(b) Endoscopy is difficult to distinguish hiatus hernia and Barrett's
(c) Peptic stricture occurs at squamocolumnar junction
(d) Barrett's ulcer occurs at squamocolumnar junction

44. In testicular tumor what is true?
(a) Teratoma differentiated is common
(b) Teratoma differentiated is uncommon
(c) Teratocarcinoma is uncommon
(d) Teratoma trophoblastic is least malignant

45. In sigmoid volvulus what is true?
(a) Acute form of sigmoid volvulus occurs in younger patients
(b) Vomiting is early feature
(c) Abdominal distension is late feature
(d) Very common in Europe and USA

46. In congenital atresia what is not true?
(a) Duodenum occurrence 15%
(b) Duodenum occurrence 35%
(c) Jejunum 15%
(d) Ileum 25%

47. In cavitron ultrasonic surgical aspirator, all are true *except:*
(a) Functions as acoustic vibrator and suction device at same time
(b) Used to dissect tissue with high fibre content
(c) Results in less blood loss
(d) Results in less collateral tissue injury

48. All about flail chest is true *except:*
(a) Two or more fracture of 3 or more consecutive ribs
(b) Paradoxical movement of chest wall inward on inspiration and outward on expiration
(c) Paradoxical movement of chest wall outward on inspiration and inward on expiration
(d) Flail chest results in respiratory failure

49. In motor disorder of esophagus all are true *except:*
(a) Motility disorder due to achalasia
(b) Collagen and neuromuscular disease
(c) Nutcracker esophagus
(d) Hypertensive LES

50. In MEN all are true *except:*
(a) In MEN 2B all patients have MTC
(b) All MEN 2B patients have mucosal neuromas
(c) MTC in MEN 2B presents at young age
(d) MEN 2B patients develop hyperparathyroidism

51. In esophageal motility all are true *except:*
(a) Primary peristaltic contraction moves at the rate of 2-4 cm/sec
(b) Secondary contractions occur to clear esophagus
(c) Tertiary contractions are monophasic
(d) Tertiary contractions are progressive/ monophasic and multiphasic

52. The following is true of alveolar hydatid *except:*
(a) Occurs in people of Alaska
(b) Caused by echinococcus multilocularis
(c) Mimic malignant growth
(d) Caused by echinococcus granulosus

53. The following is true of cysticercosis:
(a) It is caused by taenia solium
(b) It is caused by echinococcus granulosus
(c) It is caused by spirometra
(d) It never affects the CNS

54. All are true about sialolithiasis of parotid gland:
(a) Only 20% occur in parotid
(b) 80% occur in submandibular gland
(c) The stones are radiolucent
(d) The stones are radiopaque

55. The following is true of sialadenosis *except:*
(a) Seen in diabetes mellitus
(b) Bulemia
(c) Idiopathic
(d) It is inflammatory

56. The following in oropharynx is true *except:*
(a) Hodgkin's disease is common
(b) Most of them are B cell type
(c) They may not have the disease in rest of the body
(d) Hodgkin's disease is rare

57. All are true about chemodectoma:
(a) Occurs in people living in high altitudes
(b) 10% family history
(c) Associated with pheochromocytoma
(d) Associated with medullary carcinoma thyroid

58. The following is false in Mallory-Weiss tear:
(a) Occurs in gastroesophageal junction
(b) Tear occurs in lower esophagus
(c) It is a longitudinal tear
(d) It is caused by strenuous vomiting

59. The following is true about annular pancreas:
(a) May be associated with Down syndrome
(b) Vomiting is bile stained
(c) Treatment is duodenojejunostomy
(d) Resection of annular pancreas

60. The following is true about rectal prolapse:
(a) Complete rectal prolapsed is less common than partial prolapse
(b) It starts at the posterior wall of rectum
(c) It is very common in children
(d) Men are more affected than women

61. Which of these is true in thrombosed external hemorrhoids?
(a) Called as sentinel pile mass
(b) Called as perianal hematoma
(c) It never presents as emergency
(d) There is no role for conservative management

62. In Laugier's femoral hernia the following is true:
(a) It is associated with hip dislocation
(b) Occurs beneath fascia covering pectineus muscle
(c) It occurs due to gap in lacunar ligament
(d) The obstruction is due to the lacunar ligament itself

63. The following is true of lumbar hernia:
(a) It occurs in superior lumbar triangle
(b) It occurs in inferior lumbar triangle
(c) Primary lumbar hernia is most common
(d) Secondary lumbar hernia is rare

64. The following is true about obturator hernia:
(a) More common in women
(b) It causes swelling in Scarpa's triangle
(c) It passes through the greater sciatic foramina
(d) A Richter's hernia is very rare in this hernia

65. Cholesterosis is also called as:
(a) Porcelain gallbladder
(b) Strawberry gallbladder
(c) Adenomyomatosis of gallbladder
(d) Typhoid Mary's gallbladder

66. The following is true of retrosternal thyroid *except:*
(a) They arise from ectopic thyroid tissue
(b) The negative intrathoracic pressure draws the nodules in the mediastinum
(c) They can present with dyspnoea
(d) Can result in SVC obstruction

67. In hyperparathyroidism the indications for surgery the following is true *except:*
(a) Urinary tract calculi
(b) Markedly reduced bone density
(c) Serum calcium > 2.85 mmol
(d) Old age and mild hyperparathyroidism

68. The following is true of dry gangrene:
(a) Occurs due to slowing of bloodstream to the part
(b) Occurs due to sudden occlusion
(c) Crepitus may be felt
(d) Limb becomes discolored

69. The following is true about gallstones:
(a) Brown stones are rare in gallbladder
(b) Cholesterol stones are rare

(c) Black pigment stones are very common
(d) Brown stones are common

70. The following is true about insulinoma *except:*
(a) Incoordination of movement
(b) Hyperglycemia
(c) Sweating
(d) Slurred speech

71. Meconium peritonitis occurs in all are true *except:*
(a) Early intrauterine life
(b) Can present shortly after birth
(c) Meconium is sterile for 3 hours after birth
(d) It is suspected when baby has vomiting with tense abdomen

72. The following is true about periodic peritonitis:
(a) It is associated with familial mediterranean fever
(b) It is very common among Chinese
(c) It occurs due to colchicines
(d) It is associated with leucopenia

73. Enzyme activated in apoptosis is:
(a) Amylase
(b) Lactate dehydrogenase
(c) Caspase
(d) Carbonic anhydrase

74. Neovascularization in wound healing is maximal by:
(a) 8-9 days (b) 1-2 days
(c) 5-7 days (d) 3-4 days

75. The following are true about postmortem clots *except:*
(a) Show the upper yellow 'chicken fat' layer
(b) Not attached to vessel wall
(c) Show lines of Zahn
(d) Show dark red dependent portion

76. Inherited defect in glycoprotein fibrillin I is seen in:
(a) Marfan's syndrome
(b) Ehlers-Danlos syndrome
(c) Familial hypercholesterolemia
(d) Osteogenesis imperfecta

77. Examples of type III hypersensitivity reactions include the following *except:*
(a) Autoimmune hemolytic anemia
(b) Systemic lupus erythematosus
(c) Serum sickness
(d) Polyarteritis nodosa

78. Point mutation in KIT proto-oncogene is seen in the following *except:*
(a) Gastrointestinal stromal tumor
(b) Hepatocellular carcinoma
(c) Seminoma
(d) Leukemia

79. Mucormycosis shows:
(a) Septate hyphae
(b) Irregularly wide hyphae
(c) Acute angle branching of hyphae
(d) Fruiting bodies

80. Punctate basophilic stippling of RBC is seen in poisoning due to:
(a) Mercury (b) Arsenic
(c) Cadmium (d) Lead

81. Acrodermatitis enteropathica is seen in deficiency of:
(a) Copper (b) Selenium
(c) Fluoride (d) Zinc

82. Which of the following is most likely to occur within 5 minutes of the accidental insertion of an endotracheal tube into the right main bronchus of a ventilated patient?
(a) Hypotension
(b) Severe bradycardia
(c) An increase in the requirement for the volatile agent
(d) An increased inflation pressure

83. For heat moisture exchanger for humidification, which is not true?
(a) Exchange of heat and moisture between gases and surface over which it flow
(b) May be a cause of rebreathing
(c) HME should be placed in the breathing system as far as possible from the patient
(d) A cause of auto PEEP

84. A pressure-volume curve can be used for measuring:
(a) The work of breathing
(b) Functional residual capacity
(c) Anatomical dead space
(d) Respiratory quotient

85. Treatment of hypoxemia during one lung anesthesia include all *except:*
(a) Resume two lung ventilation
(b) Do not apply PEEP
(c) Increase FiO_2
(d) Recruitment can be done

86. Criteria for brain death include all *except:*
(a) Apnea test present
(b) Spinal reflexes absolutely absent
(c) Contrast angiography shows nonfilling of the intracranial arteries at the entry to the skull
(d) Absent gag reflex

87. With regard to endotracheal tube standard specify:
(a) Area of Murphy's eye must be less than 50% of cross-sectional area of tube lumen
(b) Tube with hole in the wall at distal end is called Magill's eye
(c) A radius of curvature from 12 to 16 cm
(d) The angle of bevel is obtuse angle between the bevel and the longitudinal axis of the tracheal tube

88. What is true with Mapleson "F" circuit?
(a) It has no bag with mechanism for venting the gas from exhalation limb
(b) Functionally it is like Magill system
(c) Respiration is only spontaneous
(d) Also called Jackson Re-modification of the T piece system

89. Complication of neurosurgery in sitting posture include *except:*
(a) Venous air embolism
(b) Cardiac instability
(c) Cervical cord ischemia
(d) Increased surgical bleeding

90. Stimulation of alpha adrenergic receptors will cause all, *except:*
(a) Vasoconstriction of the coronary arteries
(b) Increased tone in the bladder neck muscle
(c) Increased platelet aggregation
(d) Bronchodilation

91. 60 years with painless jaundice and palpable gallbladder all *except:*
(a) Carcinoma gallbladder
(b) Periampullary carcinoma
(c) Carcinoma head of pancreas
(d) Hilar cholangiocarcinoma
(e) GB stricture with CBD stricture

92. True about post transplant immunosuppression:
(a) CMV infection reactivation is a concern
(b) Adrenal steroids used for induction
(c) Cardiovascular related mortality common
(d) Not required for cardiac transplant
(e) Increased risk of viral related malignancies

93. Esophagus anatomy:
(a) Enters diaphragm at T12
(b) Upper 1/3rd supplied by inferior thyroid artery
(c) Lower 1/3rd lymphatic drainage to celiac node
(d) Foreign body impaction in adults at 15 cm, 25 cm, 40 cm from incisor
(e) Infrahiatal esophagus lined by peptic and oxyntic cells

94. Increased CVP is seen in:
(a) Septic shock
(b) Neurogenic shock
(c) Hypovolemic shock
(d) Cardiogenic shock
(e) Constrictive pericarditis

95. Features of endotoxic shock:
(a) Increased CVP
(b) Peripheral vasodilatation
(c) Increased cardiac output in initial phase
(d) Metabolic acidosis
(e) Increased fluid requirement

96. Criteria for SIRS:
(a) Temp > 38, or < 35
(b) HR > 100/min
(c) SBP < 90 mm Hg
(d) Oliguria < 400 ml/Hr
(e) WBC > 12000 or < 4000

97. About SSI:
(a) Prevalence of SSI in clean contaminated wound is 1-5% acceptable
(b) More common cause is Staph aureus

(c) Patient preparation and surgeon preparation have role in reducing SSI
(d) Level I evidence suggest chlorhexidine is better than povidone iodine solution
(e) Operative room design has no role in reducing SSI

98. Correct match:
(a) Skin infection – E coli
(b) Vaginal inf – Stap aureus
(c) Biliary – Streptococcus
(d) Colorectal – Bacteroides
(e) UTI–E fecalis

99. About wound infection:
(a) Thyroidectomy is a clean contaminated surgery
(b) Contaminated wound should be closed by primary delayed closure
(c) Prosthetic device infection most common by pseudomonas
(d) Acinobacter infection is commonly associated by hospital acquired pneumonia
(e) For MRSA treatment of choice is voriconazole

100. About secondary hemorrhage:
(a) Occurs after 7 to 10 days
(b) Occurs due slippage of ligature
(c) Occurs due to infection
(d) Herald by warning hemorrhage
(e) Sudden rise in post op BP is the cause

101. Tumor marker correct match:
(a) HCC-Beta HCG
(b) Follicular Carcinoma thyroid-calcitonin
(c) Ovary-Carcinoma 125
(d) Pancreas-Carcinoma 19.9
(e) Colon-CEA

102. About electrocautery:
(a) Heat generated is directly proportional to area of contact
(b) Intermittent current is used in cutting mode
(c) Lateral heat loss is more on monopolar cutting mode
(d) Coagulation is more in bipolar mode
(e) Ultrasonic dissection is similar to bipolar

103. Bone metastasis:
(a) Oral cavity carcinoma
(b) Carcinoma thyroid
(c) Carcinoma stomach
(d) Carcinoma breast
(e) Carcinoma prostate

104. Pressure sore:
(a) Ischium is common site
(b) Blanching and erythema is early sign
(c) Common in paraplegic patients
(d) Vacuum assisted closure is contraindicated
(e) Prevention is best treatment

105. Premalignant condition:
(a) Leukoplakia
(b) Barrett's esophagus
(c) Phimosis
(d) Villous adenoma of colon
(e) Chronic cervicitis

106. Elemental nutrition given in:
(a) Short bowel syndrome
(b) Sepsis
(c) Severe malnutrition
(d) Pancreatic insufficiency
(e) Renal failure

107. TPN:
(a) Minimal calorie provided by carbohydrate is 1000 Kcal
(b) Peripheral solution is hyperosmolar
(c) Non-protein calorie should contribute 70 to 80% of total calorie
(d) TPN contains dextrose, AA, lipids
(e) Femoral vein is most common site for access in TPN

108. An unconscious patient brought to emergency:
(a) GCS does not assess for papillary size and limb asymmetry
(b) Dolls eye movement is done to assess extra ocular movement
(c) DOC for persistent status epilepticus is phenytoin
(d) 50% dextrose is detrimental
(e) Hypernatremia > 155 mEq, mannitol contraindicated

109. Packed RBC transfused in:
(a) Hemodynamically stable patient with hemocrit 30%
(b) Stable patient with Hb <8 gm
(c) It improves wound healing
(d) CAD patient with Hb <12 gm
(e) If preop autologus blood is always preferred for transfusion

110. Long storage of blood:
(a) Decreased oxygen binding capacity
(b) Decreased 2, 3 DPG and ATP
(c) Decrease in potassium, ammonia and phosphates
(d) Vasoactive substance are released
(e) Hemolysis occurs

111. Perioperative management in diabetic patient:
(a) Metformin should be stopped in pre-op patient
(b) Patient using insulin pump should be weaned from it
(c) Patient should be put on long acting insulin
(d) Cardiogenic risk assessment should be done
(e) Pre-op glycemic control affects wound healing

112. Regarding dressing:
(a) Wound healing is better in occlusive than in absorptive dressing
(b) Goat skin is most commonly used in Xenograft
(c) Antibacterial ointment prevents wound infection
(d) Protease in wound decreases efficiency of locally applied growth factors
(e) Negative pressure enhances epithelisation

113. About chromosomal inheritance:
(a) Human cell contains 22 chromosomes and 1 sex chromosome
(b) Most common trisomy is present on chromosome 21
(c) FISH is most sensitive and reliable for trisomy 21
(d) Autosomal disease transmitted in subsequent progeny is 1 in 4
(e) X linked disease father to son transmission

114. Statistical test:
Apgar score in comparison in 80 twice –
(a) T paired test
(b) Chi-square test
(c) Log rank test
(d) Ceftriaxone acts on both gram positive and negative infections

115. About pain:
(a) Patients control analgesia should be used
(b) Propofol is most commonly used in analgesia
(c) First epidural dose is better than multiple dose
(d) Analgesia has no effect on catecholamine levels
(e) Pain control has favourable influence on metabolic changes (post-surgical trauma)

116. GI anastomosis:
(a) Single layer interrupted least chance of necrosis of edge
(b) Colon single layer and double layer closure have almost same chance of anastomotic leak
(c) Absorbable suture used for biliary anastomosis
(d) Single layer interrupted in esophagus is preferred
(e) Leak rate higher in anastomosis of stomach

117. Vein of Galen malformation is not associated with:
(a) Seizures
(b) Hydrocephalus
(c) Developmental delay
(d) Low output cardiac failure

118. Esophageal atresia and TOF are often associated with:
(a) ARM
(b) Renal dysplasia
(c) GI malformation
(d) Duodenal atresia

119. Papillary calcification is found in all *except:*
(a) Medullary sponge kidney
(b) Analgesic nephropathy
(c) SLE
(d) Hodgkin's lymphoma

120. Echinocandins are not effective against:
(a) Cryptococcus
(b) Candida albicans
(c) Candida glabrata
(d) Aspergillus

121. Hemobilia is not associated with:
(a) Sepsis
(b) Abdominal colic
(c) Upper GI hemorrhage
(d) Jaundice

122. Empty sella syndrome gland affected is:
(a) Thalamus (b) Pituitary
(c) Pons (d) Midbrain

123. About diverticulosis, all *except*:
(a) Bleeding stops spontaneously
(b) 25% present with obstruction, perforation and bleeding
(c) Asymptomatic doesn't require treatment
(d) Contrast CT is investigation of choice in acute episode of diverticulitis

124. Arc of Riolan is:
(a) Middle colic to left colic
(b) Right colic to left colic
(c) Celiac to SMA
(d) SMA to IMA

125. During I and D of ischiorectal abscess which nerve can get damaged?
(a) Superior rectal nerve
(b) Superior gluteal nerve
(c) Inferior rectal nerve
(d) Pelvic plexus

126. Most common ARM in females:
(a) Ano-vestibular fistula
(b) Recto-vaginal fistula
(c) Cloaca
(d) Recto-vestibular fistula

127. Most common R-L shunt is:
(a) Endocardial cushion defect
(b) TOF
(c) Tricuspid atresia
(d) Ebstein's anomaly

128. In recurrent laryngeal nerve palsy which muscle is not affected?
(a) Cricothyroid
(b) Thyroarytenoid
(c) Posterior cricoarytenoid
(d) Lateral cricoarytenoid

129. Most common bariatic surgery done:
(a) Biliopancreatic division
(b) Vertical band gastroplasty
(c) Adjustable gastric banding
(d) Roux-en-Y gastric bypass

130. Which one of the following complication is found more in Roux-en-Y as compared to biliopancreatic division with duodenal switch?
(a) Weight loss
(b) Vitamin deficiency
(c) Dumping syndrome
(d) GERD

131. Popcorn calcification on endoscopic USG:
(a) Insulinoma
(b) GIST
(c) GI carcinoid
(d) Ectopic pancreatic tissue

132. Most common site of carcinoid is:
(a) Appendix (b) Small intestine
(c) Colon (d) Stomach

133. In esophageal perforation false is:
(a) Gastrografin study is preferred contrast
(b) Mostly iatrogenic
(c) Mackler's triad is present in most patients
(d) Endoscopy has no role in the diagnosis of spontaneous esophageal perforation

134. Sushruta in nasal reconstruction used which flap?
(a) Forehead flap
(b) Cheek
(c) Forearm tube flap
(d) Radiolateral flap

135. Pneumothorax best visualised in:
(a) Inspiration (b) Expiration
(c) Decubitus (d) Prone

136. **CIC tube:**
(a) Sterile catheter used every time
(b) Sterile glove used every time
(c) Prophylactic antibiotic not always required
(d) Medical supervision always required

137. **Left gastric vein drains into:**
(a) Portal vein
(b) IVC
(c) Splenic vein
(d) Short gastric vein

138. **Esophageal web–false is:**
(a) Vit B_{12} deficiency is a common cause
(b) More common in females
(c) Associated with celiac disease
(d) Mainly observed in Plummer Vinson syndrome

139. **SIRS is defined by all *except*:**
(a) Temperature >38° C
(b) Heart rate >120/min
(c) Respiratory rate >20/min
(d) White cell counts > 12,000 cells/mm^3

140. **Folds of cystic duct are:**
(a) Spiral (b) Angular
(c) Parallel (d) Circumferential

141. **MALT lymphoma which is not true?**
(a) Associated with H pylori
(b) Surgery is main treatment
(c) Cancer originating from B cell
(d) Diagnosis is by biopsy of suspicious lesion

142. **Septic shock which is false?**
(a) Cold skin (b) Leukocytosis
(c) Tachycardia (d) Restlessness

143. **Carcinoid type I and II:**
(a) Type II is usually malignant
(b) Type I is most common
(c) Type I associated with pernicious anemia
(d) Type II associated with MEN syndrome

144. **80 years old male with duodenal perforation with localised tenderness what is done?**
(a) IV fluid with antibiotic only
(b) Gastrografin X-ray with NGT
(c) Surgery required in most cases
(d) H pylori treatment given

145. **Most common benign tumor of liver is:**
(a) Hemangioma
(b) Adenoma
(c) Focal nodular hyperplasia
(d) Hamartoma

146. **Which is not a predisposing factor for cholangiocarcinoma?**
(a) Recurrent hepatitis E infection
(b) Primary sclerosing cholangitis
(c) Thorotrast
(d) Liver flukes

147. **Chylothorax, which is false?**
(a) Fluid cholesterol >50 mg/dl
(b) Fluid triglyceride < 50 mg/dl
(c) Fluid protein >3 g/dl
(d) Predominantly chylomicrons

148. **Tubercular peritonitis, false is:**
(a) Fluid has high LDH
(b) SAAG ratio low
(c) Cholesterol raised
(d) High protein content

149. **In acute pancreatitis true is:**
(a) Microlithiasis is most common cause
(b) Acute fluid collection resolves spontaneously
(c) Pseudoaneurysm is most common cause of bleeding
(d) Requires CT evaluation to differentiate mild acute pancreatitis from severe necrotic pancreatitis

150. **Which of the following is least malignant?**
(a) FAP
(b) Gardner syndrome
(c) Turcot syndrome
(d) Hemangioma

151. **Which of the following is not a premalignant condition?**
(a) Medullary sponge kidney
(b) FAP
(c) VHL
(d) Neurofibroma

152. Sensitivity is:
(a) True negative (b) False negative
(c) True positive (d) False positive

153. Rule of nine is given by:
(a) Wallace
(b) Lynd and Broader
(c) Goodman
(d) Arthur Smith

154. ↑ T_3, T_4, ↓ TSH and decreased radionuclide iodine uptake is seen in:
(a) Hashimoto thyroiditis
(b) Graves' disease
(c) Toxic nodular goitre
(d) Subacute thyroiditis

155. Self retaining catheter:
(a) Nelaton (b) Robinson
(c) Pezzer (d) Coude

156. All are true regarding Hirschsprung's disease *except*:
(a) Hypertrophied ganglionic cells
(b) Rectal biopsy is the gold standard for diagnosis
(c) Delayed passage of meconium in history
(d) Lack of ganglion cells is in Auerbach's plexus

157. Investigation for lymphogranuloma venereum:
(a) Heaf test (b) Fries test
(c) Casoni's test (d) Mantoux test

158. Exstrophy bladder:
(a) External rotation of the posterior aspect of the pelvis by 12 degrees on each side
(b) Retroversion of the acetabulum
(c) Mean 18 degrees of external rotation of the anterior pelvis
(d) Mean 30% lengthening of the pubic rami

159. PSA > 20 may be found in:
(a) Organ confined adenocarcinoma
(b) Acute bacterial prostatitis
(c) Chronic bacterial prostatitis
(d) All of the above

160. True regarding scalp injury:
(a) Hematoma should be drained to avoid abscess
(b) Blood supply is between galea and periosteum
(c) Approximation should be done when possible
(d) Should be drained in case of extensive laceration

161. Maximum length of trachea can be resected is:
(a) 10% (b) 30%
(c) 50% (d) 60%

162. Bochdalek hernia:
(a) Also known as a posterolateral diaphragmatic hernia
(b) Majority on right side
(c) Most of newborns born with a Bochdalek hernia are immediately high risk
(d) Make up about 90% of all diaphragmatic hernia cases

163. Which of the following is absent in cubital fossa?
(a) Radial nerve
(b) Median nerve
(c) Ulnar nerve
(d) Tendon of biceps brachii

164. Loss of which function is associated with damage of popliteal nerve in fracture head of fibula?
(a) Inversion of foot
(b) Flexion of foot
(c) Extension of toes
(d) Loss of sensory supply of lateral aspect of thigh

165. After burns, RL is preferred over normal saline due to:
(a) Metabolic acidosis is corrected by RL
(b) RL has better tonicity than NS
(c) RL provides caloric nutrition
(d) High volume administration of normal saline produces hyperchloremic acidosis

166. Which of the following is correct?
(a) After 5 days if suturing is done it heals by secondary intention
(b) Keloid scar is more common in Caucasian

(c) Scarring is a natural part of the healing process
(d) Hypertrophic scar usually occur within 4 to 8 weeks following wound infection

167. False regarding vertical mattress suturing is:
(a) Provides closure for both deep and superficial layers
(b) Allows perfect eversion and vertical opposition of the superficial skin edges
(c) Low propensity to dig into skin
(d) Cause prominent stitch mark scars

168. False regarding tumor lysis syndrome:
(a) Hyperuricemia
(b) Hypercalcemia
(c) Hyperkalemia
(d) Hyperphosphatemia

169. Weight loss with fever is seen in all *except:*
(a) TB
(b) Thyrotoxicosis
(c) Renal cell carcinoma
(d) Pheochromocytoma

170. Which tumor is found exclusively in parotid?
(a) Mucoepidermoid carcinoma
(b) Warthin tumor
(c) Adenoid cystic tumor
(d) Pleomorphic adenoma

171. Left to right side shunt is seen in all *except:*
(a) ASD
(b) VSD
(c) PDA
(d) Coarctation of aorta

172. Bileaflet prosthetic heart valves is:
(a) TTK chitra
(b) Carpentier Edward
(c) Starr Edward
(d) ATS

173. In hydrocephalus, obstruction at which site causes dilatation of one ventricle only?
(a) Foramen of Monro
(b) Foramen of Magendie
(c) Foramen of Luschka
(d) Subarachnoid space

174. Grade II dysphagia:
(a) Unable to swallow solid
(b) Can swallow solid with help of liquids
(c) Unable to swallow liquid
(d) Can swallow liquid with valsalva maneuver

175. Transthoracic procedure for sliding hiatus hernia is:
(a) Heller's (b) Belsy
(c) Fontan (d) Ramstedt

176. Bacillary angiomatosis, true is:
(a) Bartonella
(b) Gardnerella
(c) Mycobacteria
(d) Not related to any of the above

177. Inner layer of hydatid is:
(a) Ectocyst (b) Pericyst
(c) Laminated layer (d) Germinal layer

178. Sternal angle is supplied by:
(a) T2 (b) T3
(c) T4 (d) T1

179. Radiolucent calculi:
(a) Uric acid (b) Cystine
(c) Phosphate stone (d) Oxalate

180. How many layers of lumbosacral fascia is present?
(a) 1 (b) 2
(c) 3 (d) 4

181. Condition causing dysphagia, regurgitation and halitosis:
(a) Zenker's diverticulum
(b) Achalasia
(c) GERD
(d) Globus hystericus

182. True regarding ulcerative colitis in pregnancy:
(a) Increase in extracolonic manifestation
(b) Abortion
(c) Congenital anomaly
(d) Flare of ulcerative colitis

183. Not seen in neurofibromatosis 1:
(a) Spina aperta
(b) Lisch nodule
(c) Optic glioma
(d) Sphenoid dysplasia

184. APC gene is located on:
(a) Short arm of chromosome 3
(b) Short arm of chromosome 5
(c) Long arm of chromosome 3
(d) Long arm of chromosome 5

185. Aztreonam false is:
(a) Effective against all gram negative
(b) Can be used in patients allergic to penicillin
(c) Not effective against gram positive
(d) Not effective against anaerobe

186. Colistin is not effective in:
(a) Acinetobacter (b) Klebsiella
(c) Pseudomonas (d) E coli

187. Blood supply to breast:
(a) Internal mammary artery
(b) Lateral thoracic artery
(c) Posterior intercostal artery
(d) Musculophrenic artery

188. Meckel's diverticulum all are true *except*:
(a) Arise from mesenteric border
(b) Individual blood supply
(c) Consists of three layers
(d) Heterotrophic mucosa

189. Sternocleidomastoid all are true *except*:
(a) Origin from clavicle and sternum
(b) Nerve supply from cranial part of spinal accessory
(c) Contraction causes bending of face to opposite side
(d) It is thick and narrow at its central part, but broader and thinner at either end

190. Most common intradural extramedullary tumor:
(a) Metastasis (b) Schwannoma
(c) Lipoma (d) Glioma

191. Sclerosing agent in cystic hygroma:
(a) Bleomycin
(b) Sodium tetradecyl sulphate
(c) Pure ethanol
(d) Ethanolamine

192. False regarding pressure sore:
(a) Ischemia has role in its pathology
(b) Stage I: Partial thickness loss of dermis presenting as a shallow open ulcer with a red pink wound bed, without slough
(c) Risk of developing bedsores can be determined by using the Braden scale for predicting pressure ulcer risk
(d) Necrotic tissue should be removed in most pressure ulcers

193. Role of CEA in carcinoma colon:
(a) Prognostic value
(b) Depends on stage
(c) Present in normal adult liver
(d) Increased with metastasis of liver

194. Total mesorectal excision, all *except*:
(a) Autonomic nerve preservation
(b) Increased anastomotic leak
(c) Sphincter preservation not possible
(d) Results in a lower recurrence rate than traditional approaches and a lower rate of permanent colostomy

195. Bloomer's shelf:
(a) Peritoneal metastasis on DRE
(b) Ovarian tumor in pelvis
(c) Supraclavicular lymph node
(d) Pouch of Douglas is area of metastatic disease

196. Virchow's triad all *except*:
(a) Hypercoagulability
(b) A-V fistula
(c) Endothelial injury
(d) Stasis

197. True about endoscopic ultrasound:
(a) Infection can occur during aspiration of fluid from cysts and antibiotics may be given before the procedure
(b) Good investigation for studying 'submucosal lesions' which may be hidden in the intestinal wall covered by normal appearing lining of the intestinal tract
(c) When FNA is performed complications occur more often (5.0%)

(d) Highly sensitive for detection of pancreatic cancer (90-95% sensitivity)

198. Continence grading given by:
(a) Truman (b) Mills
(c) Wexner (d) Billroth

199. Most common gastric malignancy is:
(a) Lymphoma
(b) Squamous cell carcinoma
(c) Adenocarcinoma
(d) Carcinoid

200. Predisposing factor for carcinoma stomach are all *except*:
(a) Menetrier disease
(b) Pernicious anemia
(c) Blood group B
(d) Smoking

201. Charcot's triad all *except*:
(a) Mental obtundation
(b) Fever
(c) Pain
(d) Indicator of acute cholangitis

202. Management of mucocele:
(a) Cholecystectomy
(b) Cholecystectomy with CBD drainage
(c) Percutaneous aspiration
(d) Oral dissolution therapy in obstructed gallbladders

203. Regarding heparin which statement is not true?
(a) One unit of heparin is an amount approximately equivalent to 0.002 mg of pure heparin
(b) The conformational change in AT on heparin-binding mediates its inhibition of factor Xa
(c) Protamine sulfate (1 mg per 100 units of heparin) acts as antidote
(d) Heparin is a naturally occurring anti-coagulant produced by eosinophils and mast cells

204. Primary sclerosing cholangitis, all are true *except*:
(a) Steroid responsive
(b) Male predominance
(c) Insidious onset
(d) Ursodeoxycholic acid increases survival

205. Splenic vein drains into:
(a) Right gastric
(b) Left gastric
(c) Right gastroepiploic
(d) Left gastroepiploic

206. Which vein does not drain into IVC?
(a) Left renal vein
(b) SMV
(c) IMV
(d) Left adrenal vein

207. False regarding sliding hernia:
(a) Internal organ makes wall of the hernial sac
(b) Most common organ involved is colon
(c) Usually associated with indirect inguinal hernia
(d) May occur in femoral hernia

208. Nosocomial infection, true is:
(a) Occurs at least 48 hours after admission
(b) Contact transmission is the most important and frequent mode of transmission
(c) Handwashing is single most important measure to reduce the risk of transmitting skin microorganisms
(d) UTI and pneumonia are most common

209. Corkscrew esophagus seen in:
(a) Diffuse esophageal spasm
(b) Achalasia
(c) Chagas disease
(d) Pseudoachalasia

210. Fat embolization occurs in all *except*:
(a) Orthopedic trauma
(b) Liposuction surgery
(c) Liver trauma
(d) Renal trauma

211. Most common presentation of fat embolism:
(a) Respiratory (b) Cardiovascular
(c) Hepatic (d) Renal

212. About ursodeoxycholic acid all are true *except*:
(a) Reduces biliary cholesterol
(b) Increases bile acid pool

(c) Causes liver damage
(d) Immunomodulatory role

213. Necrotizing fasciitis caused by all *except*:
(a) Clostridium (b) E. coli
(c) Staphylococcus (d) Bacteroides

214. For adequate pneumoperitoneum:
(a) Gas flow 1 l/min (b) Gas flow 2 l/min
(c) Gas flow 3 l/min (d) Gas flow 4 l/min

215. Most sensitive pancreatic function test:
(a) Serum trypsin
(b) Fecal elastase
(c) Endoluminal ultrasound (EUS)
(d) Secretin test

216. IVC filter indication all *except*:
(a) Iliofemoral thrombosis
(b) IVC obstruction
(c) Recurrent PE
(d) Not treated by anticoagulation

217. Acute acalculous cholecystitis can occur with, all *except*:
(a) Nephrectomy
(b) Bone marrow transplant recipient
(c) TPN
(d) Burns

218. Testicular artery arises from aorta:
(a) Above renal hilum
(b) Below origin of SMA
(c) Below origin of IMA
(d) Below origin of celiac plexus

219. False about hemorrhoids:
(a) Does not cause pruritus
(b) Can be felt on DRE
(c) Most common office procedure is band ligation
(d) Stapler hemorrhoidectomy reduces pain

220. Minimum length required to avoid permanent TPN:
(a) 60 to 90 cm of small intestine along with a portion of the colon
(b) 150 cm of combined jejunum and ileum if no colon is left
(c) Both of the above are true
(d) Both of the above are false

221. Anal continence factor, all are important *except*:
(a) Anorectal angle
(b) Rectal compliance
(c) Pressure at anal sphincter
(d) Consistency of stool and volume

222. Treatment of medullary carcinoma thyroid:
(a) Subtotal thyroidectomy
(b) Total thyroidectomy
(c) Partial thyroidectomy
(d) Radioiodine

223. Gallstone ileus, most common site:
(a) Ileum (b) Jejunum
(c) Colon (d) Duodenum

224. Bleeding through breast nipple most common cause is:
(a) Carcinoma breast (b) Duct papilloma
(c) Ductal ectasia (d) Adenoma

225. Carcinoma colon not true is:
(a) (Astler collen) B1: Tumor grows through muscularis mucosae but not through muscularis propria
(b) (Astler collen) C2: Stage B2 with regional lymph node metastasis
(c) (AJCC) N1: Metastasis to 1 to 5 regional lymph nodes
(d) (AJCC) T3: Tumor invades subserosa or beyond

226. Common cause of obscure lower GI bleed:
(a) Angiodysplasias of small intestine
(b) Celiac sprue
(c) Hemorrhoids
(d) GI polyps

227. Both diagnostic and therapeutic:
(a) Enteroclysis
(b) CT
(c) Capsule endoscopy
(d) Angiography

228. Most common complication following thyroidectomy:
(a) Hypercalcemia
(b) Hypocalcemia
(c) Respiratory difficulty
(d) Hoarseness of voice

229. Risk factor for SCC esophagus, all *except*:
(a) Barrett's esophagus
(b) Tylosis
(c) Tobacco
(d) Alcohol

230. Most common symptom of carcinoma esophagus:
(a) Weight loss
(b) Dysphagia
(c) Regurgitation
(d) Recurrent pneumonia

231. Classification of cholecystectomy wound is:
(a) Clean
(b) Clean contaminated
(c) Contaminated
(d) Dirty

232. Cholangiocarcinoma:
(a) Extrahepatic 20-25%
(b) Epithelial origin from bile duct
(c) Surgery can cure
(d) A Klatskin tumor occurs at the confluence of the right and left hepatic duct

233. Acute liver failure, all *except*:
(a) INR>1.5
(b) Pre-existing chronic liver disease
(c) Pre-existing normal liver before illness
(d) Encephalopathy

234. Not a child pugh criteria:
(a) Serum creatinine (b) Bilirubin
(c) Albumin (d) PT

235. PT is deranged in all *except*:
(a) Heparin administration
(b) Warfarin administration
(c) Aspirin administration
(d) Liver failure

236. NG tube, true all *except*:
(a) Increased pulmonary compliance
(b) Increased GE reflux
(c) Increased sinusitis
(d) Early recovery from paralytic ileus

237. The timing of stitches removal does not depend on:
(a) Stitches material
(b) Patient's chronic illnesses
(c) Patient's medications
(d) Wound location

238. Small bowel lymphoma, all are true *except*:
(a) Most common–B cell type
(b) Ileum most common site
(c) GI is most common extranodal site
(d) T cell type better prognosis than B cell type

239. Varices arise once portal pressure rises:
(a) 8 mm Hg (b) 10 mm Hg
(c) 12 mm Hg (d) 14 mm Hg

240. Colonic anastomosis best done by:
(a) Single layer extramucosal vicryl
(b) Two-layer chromic and silk
(c) Single layer monocryl
(d) Double layer silk

241. Cecal volvulus false:
(a) 20-40% of large gut volvulus
(b) Endoscopic treatment is curative in 25%
(c) Cecopexy is better than cecostomy
(d) Surgical resection is best treatment option

242. Which of the following is not the branch of thyrocervical trunk?
(a) Inferior thyroid artery
(b) Suprascapular artery
(c) Superior cervical artery
(d) Inferior cervical artery

243. Uterine artery is branch of:
(a) Internal iliac artery
(b) External iliac artery
(c) Common iliac artery
(d) Pudendal artery

244. Heparin all *except*:
(a) Molecular weight 10000 dalton
(b) Protamine is antagonist
(c) Bind to antithrombin-3
(d) CTVS surgery dose is 300 U/kg

245. Potassium sparing diuretics, all *except*:
(a) Furosemide (b) Spironolactone
(c) Triamterene (d) Amiloride

246. In surgical stress, which hormone decreases?
(a) Insulin (b) ACTH
(c) Growth hormone (d) AVP

247. Virchow's triad all *except*:
(a) A-V connection
(b) Alterations in normal blood flow
(c) Injuries to the vascular endothelium
(d) Alterations in the constitution of blood (hypercoagulability)

248. Gas in subcutaneous tissue is most commonly due to:
(a) Clostridium species (b) Klebsiella
(c) Pseudomonas (d) Proteus

249. Hemobilia, all *except*:
(a) Fever (b) Jaundice
(c) GI bleed (d) Colic

250. Pre-auricular lymph node does not drain:
(a) Parotid gland (b) Upper face
(c) Temporal region (d) Anterior pinna

251. Ranula all *except*:
(a) Due to obstruction of minor or sublingual gland
(b) Lined by epithelium limited to sublingual space
(c) Actually a pseudocyst
(d) Doesn't increase in size on chewing and swallowing

252. A mass showing alternating layers of soft tissue and fat:
(a) Intussusception (b) Cystic fibrosis
(c) Mesenteric cyst (d) Volvulus

253. Most common surgical presentation of bezoars:
(a) Obstruction
(b) Hemorrhage
(c) Asymptomatic mass
(d) Peritonitis

254. Scrotal metastasis most common from:
(a) Prostate (b) Lung
(c) Colon (d) Kidney

255. With intraarterial injection, all can be complications *except*:
(a) Complete pulse is not palpable
(b) Mottling
(c) Muscle necrosis with compartment syndrome
(d) Edema with muscle tenderness

256. Ulcer in DM, not primary site is:
(a) Head of metatarsal (b) Heal
(c) Tip of toe (d) Web space

257. Serous cystadenoma of pancreas all *except*:
(a) Almost always malignant
(b) The most common symptoms are very non-specific and include abdominal pain and vomiting
(c) Relatively large and well defined
(d) Usually found in the tail of the pancreas

258. Buerger's disease, all *except*:
(a) Complete cessation of smoking is the only true modality of treatment
(b) Unilateral involvement rare
(c) Segmental involvement of small to medium size artery and vein
(d) Superficial thrombophlebitis

259. Primary lymphedema true is:
(a) Skin ulcers are very common
(b) Treatment with diuretics is of little importance
(c) Lymph vesicles and fistula require operative treatment
(d) Milroy syndrome is an old term to describe hereditary congenital lymphedema

260. Following condition is appropriate for day care surgery:
(a) Recurrent inguinoscrotal hernia
(b) Inguinal hernia with BMI >35
(c) Strangulated hernia repair in 26-year-old male
(d) Hernia repair in man with well controlled angina

261. Papillary carcinoma true is:
(a) Secretes calcitonin
(b) Common in iodine deficient area
(c) Multifocal in upto 75%
(d) Presents with distant metastasis

262. True regarding intussusception in children:
(a) Can be treated with air enema only when there is no peritonitis
(b) Most common cause of small bowel obstruction in children <18 months of age

(c) Usually presents with brick red color stools
(d) Lead point is found in 80% of cases

263. True in gallstone disease is:
(a) Acute cholecystitis presents with perforation of gallbadder (GB)
(b) Acute cholecystitis presents with mucosal ulceration of GB
(c) >80% of cases are symptomatic in cholelithiasis
(d) Mucocele of GB contains infected bile

264. Child Pugh classification does not include:
(a) S. bilirubin
(b) S. albumin
(c) S. calcium
(d) Prothrombin time

265. Not an indication for surgery in ulcerative colitis:
(a) Presence of dysplasia on colonic biopsy
(b) Pancolitis
(c) Toxic megacolon
(d) Failure of acute colitis to respond on medical therapy

266. True for surgical treatment of rectal cancer:
(a) Irrigation of divided bowel ends with cytotoxic solution may reduce local recurrence
(b) Intramural spread is >4 cm
(c) Minimum of 5 cm distal resection margin is required
(d) Mesorectum is devoid of lymph nodes

267. Most common site of diverticula:
(a) Sigmoid
(b) Transverse colon
(c) Ascending colon
(d) Descending colon

268. Which of the following is true for colon cancer?
(a) Colon carcinoma inherited in 30% of cases
(b) Synchronous lesions seen in 1% of cases
(c) Metachronous lesions seen in upto 12% of cases
(d) Inevitable in untreated cases of FAP

269. During open cholecystectomy, Kocher's incision divides:
(a) Obturator fascia
(b) Anterior rectus sheath
(c) Rectus abdominis muscle
(d) T10 nerve

270. True for carcinoma gallbladder:
(a) Most commonly presents with obstructive jaundice
(b) 90% associated with gallstones
(c) 5 years survival 35%
(d) 30% has squamous cells

271. Regarding pseudocyst true is:
(a) Cyst wall lined by squamous cell lining
(b) Endoscopic treatment may be curative
(c) Always found in lesser sac
(d) Always occurs due to alcoholic pancreatitis

272. Regarding carcinoid appendix all are true *except*:
(a) 50% of GI carcinoid
(b) Most common at tip
(c) Carcinoid syndrome is rare
(d) Right hemicolectomy treatment of choice

273. Etiological factors for carcinoma stomach all *except*:
(a) Previous gastric surgery
(b) Atrophic gastritis
(c) Blood group B
(d) FAP

274. Most common site of duplication of intestine:
(a) Ileum (b) Duodenum
(c) Jejunum (d) Colon

275. In acoustic neuroma, nerve involved is:
(a) 5th (b) 6th
(c) 7th (d) 10th

276. Most common cause of death in Whipple's:
(a) Pancreatic anastomotic leak
(b) Gastric anastomotic leak
(c) CBD anastomotic leak
(d) Respiratory failure

277. Carcinoma esophagus:
(a) Adenocarcinoma most common in middle 1/3rd

(b) Barrett's esophagus can give rise to squamous cell carcinoma
(c) 5 years survival–25%
(d) EUS can accurately stage the disease

278. Gardner's syndrome includes all *except*:
(a) Brain tumor (b) Desmoid
(c) Bone tumors (d) Renal tumors

279. Mean total colon transit time is:
(a) 20 hours (b) 40 hours
(c) 60 hours (d) 80 hours

280. Percentage of carcinoma rectum presenting with obstruction:
(a) 5-10% (b) 25-30%
(c) 18-20% (d) >35%

281. Maximum gas produced by fermentation of:
(a) H_2 (b) H_2S
(c) Methane (d) CO_2

282. Not true regarding H. pylori is:
(a) 80 percent of individuals infected with the bacterium are asymptomatic
(b) It is anaerobic and does not require oxygen
(c) Most reliable method for detecting H. pylori infection is a biopsy check during endoscopy
(d) The standard first-line therapy is a one week "triple therapy"

283. Zygoma fracture includes:
(a) Also called as tripod or malar fracture
(b) Ecchymosis over zygoma
(c) Difficulty in opening mouth
(d) Diplopia

284. Achalasia cardia is:
(a) < 40 mm pressure at LES with aperistalsis
(b) Aperistalsis in body with delayed relaxation of LES
(c) Hyperperistalsis with LES >100 mm Hg
(d) Simultaneous peristalsis of upper and lower segment

285. Lipoma in GIT all are true *except*:
(a) Subserosal
(b) Submucosal
(c) Most common in cecum
(d) Squeeze sign in radiology

286. In case of trauma which hormone increases?
(a) Insulin (b) Thyroxine
(c) ACTH (d) FSH

287. Affected in cortical lesions:
(a) Pain
(b) Temperature
(c) Temperature and pain
(d) Proprioception and fine touch

288. Substrate level phosphorylation with production of ATP and GTP occurs from:
(a) Fumarate
(b) Aconitase
(c) Succinyl thiokinase
(d) LDH

289. Volvulus of sigmoid:
(a) Clockwise
(b) CECT diagnostic
(c) Rigid sigmoidoscopy is treatment
(d) Sigmoidectomy is usually not required

290. Incision during tracheostomy centered at:
(a) 1st or 2nd tracheal ring
(b) 2nd or 3rd tracheal ring
(c) 3rd or 4th tracheal ring
(d) 4th or 5th tracheal ring

291. Most common complication of pseudocyst:
(a) Infection (b) Rupture
(c) Hemorrhage (d) Compression

292. Treatment of choice for carcinoma esophagus:
(a) Esophagectomy
(b) External radiotherapy
(c) Internal radiotherapy
(d) Chemotherapy

293. Esophageal carcinoma is adequately assessed by:
(a) Barium swallow
(b) Endoscopy
(c) USG
(d) Barium swallow + endoscopy

294. Metabolic equivalent testing by:
(a) Echocardiography
(b) Angiography
(c) Stress exercise
(d) MRI

295. Physiological constrictors from incisor lies at all *except*:
(a) 10 cm (b) 40 cm
(c) 15 cm (d) 20 cm

296. Regarding flail chest, which statement is not true?
(a) Two adjacent ribs fracture at one site
(b) >4 ribs fracture at two sites
(c) The flail segment moves in the opposite direction to the rest of the chest wall
(d) Half of patients with flail chest die

297. Best prognosis in carcinoma gallbladder:
(a) Papillary (b) Adenoma
(c) Squamous (d) Melanoma

298. Most common site of diverticula:
(a) Sigmoid
(b) Transverse colon
(c) Ascending colon
(d) Descending colon

299. Forearm amputation, distance from olecranon is:
(a) 5-10 cm (b) 10-15 cm
(c) 15-20 cm (d) 20-25 cm

300. Crohn's disease least common complication:
(a) Acute free perforation
(b) SAIO
(c) Perforation with internal fistula
(d) Perforation with external fistula

301. Somatostatin:
(a) Inhibits exocrine secretion of pancreas
(b) Increases gastric motility
(c) Inhibits glucagon release
(d) Inhibits insulin release

302. Diarrhea is seen in all *except*:
(a) Medullary thyroid carcinoma
(b) Hyperparathyroidism
(c) Addison's disease
(d) Papillary thyroid carcinoma

303. Interleukin-12 is produced by:
(a) Anti-inflammatory cytokines
(b) T cell
(c) Proinflammatory cytokines
(d) Involves in apoptotic cell death

304. Acute intestinal obstruction–early features:
(a) Persistent abdominal pain
(b) Hypotension
(c) Metabolic acidosis
(d) Vomiting

305. Most common site of bowel malignancy:
(a) Ileum (b) Duodenum
(c) Jejunum (d) Large bowel

306. Boundary of ischiorectal fossa, which is not true?
(a) Anterior–Colles' fascia
(b) Lateral–obturator internus
(c) Medial–levator ani
(d) Inferior–rectus

307. In HUS syndrome true are all *except*:
(a) Micro-angiopathic hemolytic anemia
(b) Thrombocytopenia
(c) ARF
(d) Large vessels disease

308. Hypokalemia is associated with all *except*:
(a) Lethargy
(b) Weakness
(c) Clinical effects masked by extra fluid deficiency
(d) Hypokalemia is simultaneously corrected with volume replacement

309. Most common mixed metabolic acid-base disorder is:
(a) Metabolic acidosis and alkalosis
(b) Respiratory acidosis and alkalosis
(c) Metabolic acidosis and respiratory alkalosis
(d) Respiratory acidosis and metabolic alkalosis

310. In Barrett's esophagus epithelium seen is:
(a) Specialized interstitial epithelium
(b) Gastric epithelium
(c) Junctional epithelium
(d) Columnar epithelium

311. All are true of leiomyosarcoma of stomach *except*:
(a) Bleeding is present
(b) Most common sarcoma of stomach

(c) Metastasis to lung
(d) Proximal site is most common

312. **Most common tumor metastasis to small bowel is:**
(a) Uterus and cervix malignancies
(b) Melanoma
(c) Bladder carcinoma
(d) Bronchial carcinoma

313. **Most common ACTH producing tumor is:**
(a) Bronchial carcinoma
(b) Breast carcinoma
(c) Colon carcinoma
(d) Hepatocellular carcinoma

314. **Risk factor for skin cancer are all *except*:**
(a) Cigarette smoking
(b) Herpes infection
(c) Cyclophosphamide
(d) Nickle

315. **Predisposing cause for carcinoma of lung are all *except*:**
(a) Benzene
(b) Aromatic amines
(c) Cyclophosphamide
(d) Nickle

316. **Mammography radiation dose is:**
(a) <0.01 mSv (b) 0.01-0.1 mSv
(c) 0.1-1.0 mSv (d) 1-10 mSv

317. **Features on mammography suggestive of malignancy are all *except*:**
(a) Blotchy calcification
(b) Multiple small calcification
(c) Spiculate calcification
(d) Parenchymal asymmetry

318. **Prognosis of carcinoma breast depends on all *except*:**
(a) Age
(b) Size
(c) Histological grade
(d) Axillary LN status

319. **Dentigerous cyst arises from:**
(a) An unerupted tooth
(b) Apex of an infected tooth
(c) Nasopalatine cysts
(d) Solitary bone cysts

320. **Cowden syndrome is associated with:**
(a) GIT hamartoma with carcinoma cervix
(b) GIT hamartoma with carcinoma breast
(c) GIT hamartoma with carcinoma tonsil
(d) GIT hamartoma with carcinoma spinal cord

321. **In dermoid tumor true are all *except*:**
(a) Encapsulated
(b) Association with familial polyposis
(c) Association with trauma
(d) Association with old scar

322. **Plasma constitute what percent in a normal human being?**
(a) 5% (b) 20%
(c) 40% (d) 55%

323. **In child burn, resuscitation fluid is given according to the formula:**
(a) 3 ml/% burn/body weight
(b) 6 ml/% burn/body weight
(c) 8 ml/% burn/body weight
(d) 10 ml/% burn/body weight

324. **Most common cause of acquired tracheo-esophageal fistula is:**
(a) Trauma
(b) Malignancy
(c) Prolonged intubation
(d) Steroid

325. **Parabronchial diverticula, all are true *except*:**
(a) Site is mid esophageal
(b) False diverticula
(c) Motility defects
(d) Diagnosis by barium swallow

326. **Microsatellite instability is seen in:**
(a) HNPCC
(b) FAP
(c) Sporadic Ca colon
(d) Juvenile polyposis

327. **Esophagus passes through:**
(a) Central tendon (b) Right crus
(c) Left crus (d) Aortic hiatus

328. **Regarding Bochdalek hernia, which statement is not true?**
(a) Congenital
(b) 90% of all diaphragmatic hernia

(c) Chest X-ray can be done to examine abnormalities of lung, diaphragm and intestine
(d) More commonly on the posterior right side

329. Pre-malignant condition of esophagus are all *except*:
(a) Nut cracker esophagus
(b) Tylosis
(c) Caustic ingestion
(d) Achalasia

330. Most common anal margin carcinoma:
(a) Squamous cell carcinoma
(b) Basal cell carcinoma
(c) Adenocarcinoma
(d) Melanoma

331. Visceral perfusion deficiency detected by:
(a) Systemic hemodynamics
(b) Mixed venous O_2 saturation
(c) Gastric tonometry
(d) Lactic acid level with/without acidosis

332. Hypothermia (severe) corrected by:
(a) Extracorporeal warming by cardio-pulmonary bypass
(b) Intravenous fluid at 43°C
(c) Warm humid O_2 at 43°C
(d) CVP line IV fluid at 43°C

333. Best for hand washing in clostridium difficile colitis:
(a) Ethylene oxide
(b) Na^+ hypochlorite
(c) Chlorhexidine
(d) Alkaline glutaraldehyde

334. Etiologic factors in achalasia cardia includes:
(a) Varicella-zoster
(b) T. cruzi
(c) Neither of the above
(d) Both of the above

335. Investigation of choice for parathyroid adenoma:
(a) 99Tc-Sestamibi scan
(b) Thallium scintigraphy
(c) MRI
(d) USG

336. Ulcerative colitis – all *except*:
(a) Pyoderma gangrenosum
(b) Sacroiliitis
(c) Post-hepatic sclerosis
(d) Perivascular angiitis

337. Absorption maximum in colon:
(a) Calcium
(b) Folic acid
(c) Bile acid and Vitamin B_{12}
(d) Water and electrolyte

338. Froment's sign:
(a) Adductor pollicis longus
(b) Flexor pollicis longus
(c) Median nerve
(d) Radial nerve

339. Which one of the following doesn't cause malignancy?
(a) HPV
(b) H. pylori
(c) Schistosoma hematobium
(d) Chlamydia

340. Horner's sign – all *except*:
(a) Mydriasis (b) Ptosis
(c) Enophthalmos (d) Miosis

341. Apheresis:
(a) Separation of blood components
(b) Technology in which the blood of patient is passed through an apparatus that separates out one particular constituent and returns the remainder to the circulation
(c) It is intracorporeal therapy
(d) If separation by density is required, centrifugation is the most common method

342. DIC diagnostic is:
(a) Low fibrinogen
(b) D-dimer assay
(c) Increased PT/APTT
(d) Low platelet count

343. Carcinoma stomach ulcer–barium feature is:
(a) Extraluminal ulcer
(b) Intraluminal ulcer

(c) Radiating gastric fold from edge
(d) Large ulcer near gastric fold

344. Dilatation for anal fissure, heals fissure after:
(a) 1 month (b) 2 months
(c) 3 months (d) 4 months

345. Omega-3 fatty acid, all are true *except*:
(a) Reduced immunity
(b) Reduced LDL
(c) Reduces atherosclerosis
(d) Help in fighting against sepsis

346. Posterior-intraosseous nerve injury occurs in which condition?
(a) Fracture lower end humerus
(b) Fracture ulna
(c) Monteggia fracture/dislocation
(d) Elbow dislocation

347. In neobladder which pouch is not made?
(a) J pouch (b) S pouch
(c) W pouch (d) K pouch

348. Mondor's disease is:
(a) Thrombophlebitis of the axillary vein
(b) Thrombophlebitis of the superficial veins of chest wall
(c) Thrombophlebitis of the internal mammary vein with breast engorgement
(d) None of the above

349. After surgery 60-year-old male present with sudden dyspnea and hemoptysis, diagnosis is:
(a) Pulmonary embolism
(b) Fat embolism
(c) COPD
(d) Head injury

350. In which condition(s) does angiogenesis occur?
(a) Macular degeneration
(b) Tumor growth
(c) Healing of chronic ulcers
(d) All of the above

351. Peutz-Jeghers syndrome–all *except*:
(a) Malrotation of gut
(b) Ovarian/breast/endometrium carcinoma
(c) Multiple polyp in colon
(d) Melanosis around mouth

352. Carcinoma breast best diagnostic modality that have maximum positive predictability:
(a) FNAC
(b) USG
(c) Mammography
(d) Clinical examination

353. Sentinel lymph node biopsy true:
(a) Done by blue dye
(b) Reducing the risk of lymphedema
(c) Physician visually inspects the lymph nodes for staining and uses a gamma probe
(d) Failure to detect cancer cells in the sentinel node rules out spread of malignancy in that LN

354. In sepsis syndrome leucopenia is due to:
(a) Endotoxin
(b) Exotoxin
(c) Bone marrow suppression
(d) Idiopathic

355. False regarding spigelian (ventral) hernia:
(a) Hernia arising from aponeurotic layer between the rectus abdominis muscle medially and semilunar line laterally
(b) Almost always develop at or below the linea arcuata
(c) Do not lie below the subcutaneous fat
(d) Risk of strangulation is low

356. Hepatic artery ligation done in all *except*:
(a) Cirrhosis of liver
(b) Hemorrhage while liver biopsy
(c) Rupture of hepatic tumors
(d) Spontaneous liver rupture

357. Side effects of tamoxifen are all *except*:
(a) Endometrial carcinoma
(b) Increase in libido
(c) Increase thromboembolic phenomena
(d) Osteoporosis

358. Predisposing factor for pseudomembranous colitis all *except*:
(a) Clostridial difficile (b) Ischemic colitis
(c) Leukemia (d) DM

359. Regarding Mallory-Weiss tear which is not true?
(a) The tear involves mucosa, submucosa and muscular layer

(b) In most cases, the bleeding stops spontaneously after 24–48 hours
(c) It is often associated with alcoholism and eating disorders
(d) Tears in the mucosa at the junction of the stomach and esophagus

360. Vertebra plana is seen in all *except*:
(a) Rickets
(b) Myeloma
(c) Ewing's sarcoma
(d) Tubercular osteomyelitis

361. Which of the following is not a surgical procedure in malabsorption?
(a) Gastric bending
(b) Duodenal switch
(c) Biliary pancreatic bypass
(d) Jejunoileal bypass

362. Flow rate of Veress needle in l/min:
(a) 1.5 (b) 2
(c) 2.5 (sd) (d) 3

363. Cavitary lesions are seen in all *except*:
(a) Celiac sprue
(b) TB
(c) Lymphoma
(d) Castleman disease

364. Octreotide used in all *except*:
(a) Paraganglioma
(b) Carcinoid
(c) Pheochromocytoma
(d) Malignant lymphoma

365. Compartment syndrome all true *except*:
(a) Crush injury
(b) Closed muscle injury
(c) Intravenous drug injection
(d) Fracture of forearm bone

366. Electric burns, all *except*:
(a) Arrhythmia
(b) Muscle injury
(c) Bone fracture and dislocation
(d) Coagulation of artery and vein

367. Popliteal vein injury repair by:
(a) Contralateral saphenous graft
(b) Ipsilateral saphenous graft
(c) Ligation only
(d) Synthetic graft

368. The following are true of Zenker's diverticulum, *except*:
(a) It protrudes through the inferior constrictor muscle
(b) It protrudes anteriorly
(c) Its main symptom is dysphagia
(d) It always needs treatment

369. A gastrinoma is most likely to be associated with which of the following tumors?
(a) Breast cancer
(b) Parathyroid adenoma
(c) Small cell lung cancer
(d) Jejunal hamartomas

370. A 60-year-old patient presents with obstructive jaundice. The ultrasound shows that the gallbladder is distended, the bile duct is dilated till the terminal end and there is a mass in the head of the pancreas, indicating cancer. The most useful investigation to assess resectability is:
(a) ERCP
(b) MRCP
(c) CT scan
(d) Doppler ultrasound

371. The most common site of aortic aneurysm:
(a) Infrarenal abdominal aorta
(b) Suprarenal abdominal aorta
(c) Aortic arch
(d) Descending thoracic aorta

372. After organ transplantation, fungal infection commonly occurs:
(a) After 6 months
(b) In the first 3 months
(c) After 1 year
(d) From 6 to 12 months

373. The most common viral infection after organ transplantation is caused by:
(a) Cytomegalovirus
(b) EB virus
(c) Herpes simplex virus
(d) Varicella-zoster

374. Synovioma occurs especially in the:
(a) Knee joint
(b) Ankle joint
(c) Joints of the hand
(d) Wrist joint

375. Fractures of the clavicle are most common in:
(a) The mid shaft in males
(b) The lateral end in males
(c) The medial end in females
(d) The lateral end in females

376. ERCP in advanced HIV disease shows features similar to:
(a) Emphysematous cholecystitis
(b) Sclerosing cholangitis
(c) Choledochocele
(d) Normal

377. Among basal cell carcinomas, 85% are confined to the head and neck region. Of these, the percentage that occur in the nose are:
(a) 10% (b) 50%
(c) 26% (d) 43%

378. In esophageal cancers, one of the following statements is true:
(a) Locoregional spread is usually continuous
(b) Locoregional spread is usually discontinuous
(c) Systemic spread is mainly to the lungs
(d) Distant nodes are not involved if local nodes are free

379. Frontonasal encephaloceles are more common in:
(a) Negroid races
(b) Mongoloid races
(c) Asiatics
(d) None of the above

380. One of the most common benign tumors of the nasopharynx is:
(a) Fibroma (b) Rhabdomyoma
(c) Lipoma (d) Adenoma

381. Non-Hodgkin's lymphoma accounts for tumors of the oropharynx in the following percentage:
(a) 5 – 10 (b) 30 – 40
(c) 15 – 20 (d) 2 – 4

382. The daily requirement of iodine is:
(a) 2–3 milligrams
(b) 1–2 milligrams
(c) 0.1–0.15 milligrams
(d) 10–20 micrograms

383. Hemangiomas of the salivary glands occur more commonly in the:
(a) Parotid gland
(b) Submandibular gland
(c) Sublingual gland
(d) Glands of Blandin – Nuhn

384. A tear of the ulnar collateral ligament of the metacarpophalangeal joint of the thumb is called:
(a) Rower's thumb
(b) Carpenter's thumb
(c) Bricklayer's thumb
(d) Skier's thumb

385. 5 fluorouracil is an excellent agent for the treatment of:
(a) Cutaneous basal cell carcinoma
(b) Cutaneous squamous cell carcinoma
(c) Premalignant lesions of squamous cell carcinoma of the skin
(d) Marjolin's ulcer

386. Malignant melanoma metastasizing to the brain is:
(a) Generally treated with chemotherapy
(b) Generally treated with radiotherapy
(c) Left untreated
(d) Generally treated with interferons

387. The most common modality for the treatment of benign prostatic hypertrophy at present is:
(a) TUNA
(b) TUMT
(c) TURP
(d) Laser prostatectomy

388. Nosocomial infection in ICU is most commonly due to:
(a) Gram negative bacteria
(b) Gram positive bacteria
(c) Candida
(d) Legionella

389. The principal endogenous mediators in SIRS are:
(a) IL beta
(b) TNF beta and IL 2 beta
(c) TNF alpha, IL 1 beta and IL 6
(d) TNF alpha and IL 4

390. Direct injection, endoluminal catheter delivery and perivascular collar delivery are methods of:
(a) Endoscopic sclerotherapy
(b) Gene therapy
(c) Chemotherapy
(d) Brachytherapy

391. The Ethin Starry Silver stain is used to detect:
(a) H pylori (b) S paratyphi
(c) HINI virus (d) Acinetobacter

392. How much pancreatic function loss should happen for steatorrhoea to occur?
(a) 10% (b) 20%
(c) 80% (d) 90%

393. In the Dieulafoy's lesion, upper GI endoscopy shows:
(a) Gastric ulcer
(b) Duodenal ulcer
(c) Gastric erosions
(d) Apparently normal mucosa

394. Which type(s) of collagen is(are) deposited during the proliferative phase of wound healing?
(a) Type I (b) Type II
(c) Type III (d) Type I and II

395. Blalock Taussig, Waterson and Pott are:
(a) Operations for Fallot's tetralogy
(b) Names of double lumen endotracheal tubes
(c) Names of cardiac catheters
(d) Operations for patent ductus arteriosus

396. Following peptic ulcer surgery, reactive hypoglycemia is seen in:
(a) Early dumping
(b) Late dumping
(c) Post vagotomy diarrhea
(d) Small stomach syndrome

397. Peritoneal dissemination of gastric cancer is best detected by:
(a) Abdominal ultrasound
(b) Laparoscopy
(c) Computerised tomography
(d) Magnetic resonance imaging

398. The removal of surgical segments V, VI, VII and VIII is termed as:
(a) Right hepatectomy
(b) Extended right hepatectomy
(c) Trisegmentectomy
(d) Left hepatectomy

399. Most common site of intraperitoneal abscess is:
(a) Subphrenic
(b) Paracolic
(c) Para appendicular
(d) Pelvic

400. During surgery on the submandibular gland:
(a) Damage to the lingual nerve will cause loss of sensation to the posterior third of the tongue
(b) The submandibular gland is seen to wrap around
(c) The facial artery and vein are usually divided as they course through the deep part of the gland
(d) The hypoglossal nerve is seen to loop under the submandibular duct

401. Which agent is proven to accelerate wound healing?
(a) Vitamin A (b) Vitamin C
(c) Zinc (d) None of the above

402. A 7-year-old male child is known to have swallowed button battery. Sequential X-rays over 4 days show almost same position in the distal ileum. One should:
(a) Not worry, as it is likely to pass once it has entered the pylorus
(b) Give high roughage diet in an attempt to make it pass
(c) Give smooth muscle relaxants to dilate the ileocecal junction
(d) Consider urgent surgical removal

403. The most common site of urethral injury associated with fracture of the pelvis is:
(a) Bulbar (b) Prostatic
(c) Membranous (d) Penile

404. A 65 years old man is diagnosed to have a bladder diverticulum with a bladder stone secondary to an enlarged prostate. He should undergo:
(a) Prostatectomy first
(b) Diverticulectomy, catheterization of the bladder and prostatectomy after 6 weeks
(c) Simultaneous prostatectomy + diverticulectomy
(d) Prostatectomy and transurethral litholopaxy

405. Which of the following cancers shows the least predilection to metastasize to bone?
(a) Breast cancer (b) Prostate cancer
(c) Ovarian cancer (d) Thyroid cancer

406. A treating unit decides to hold a surgical audit of the patients treated over the previous 30 days. Which of the following will be the most important parameter for assessing their results?
(a) The diagnosis
(b) The therapeutic decision
(c) The surgical technique
(d) The outcome

407. As the first doctor at the site of a major road accident, you find a patient lying on the road. He tells you his name, but does not immediately answer more questions due to pain. The pulse appears strong, and there is no obvious large pool of blood around him. If an ambulance has also just arrived, what should next step be?
(a) Evaluate breathing with a stethoscope or by direct application of your ear to his chest
(b) Conduct a quick neurological examination for head injury
(c) Examine the back of the neck for tenderness
(d) Immediately load into the ambulance

408. A 65-year-old male on a pacemaker requires an evaluation of the thoracic spine. The appropriate investigation is:
(a) MRI, thoracic spine
(b) CT, thoracic spine
(c) Ultrasound, thoracic spine
(d) Plain X-ray, AP and lateral of the thoracic spine

409. The following is true of gout:
(a) About 90% of patients with hyperuricemia will eventually develop gout
(b) Absence of hyperuricemia during the acute attack almost rules out gout
(c) The typical first episode is a polyarticular, bilaterally symmetrical arthralgia affecting the joints of the foot
(d) Gout is usually treated by xanthine oxidase inhibitors

410. In a critically ill patient in ICU, a resident performs the "cold water" test to check for brain death. He instills 50 ml of water into the ear. What should he look for?
(a) Any movement in the body
(b) Eye movement
(c) Convulsions
(d) Gasping

411. Which of the following is an example for the true ectopic thyroid tissue?
(a) Struma ovarii
(b) Lateral aberrant thyroid
(c) Lingual thyroid
(d) Thyroglossal cyst

412. Which statement is false regarding healing of clean wounds?
(a) Tensile strength is achieved in 3 weeks and increases up to 2 years
(b) Myofibroblasts promote wound contraction at the proliferative phase
(c) Type III collagen is gradually replaced by type I for remodeling
(d) Epithelialization is complete in 12 hours by bridge formation

413. ITP not true:
(a) Normal to increased megakaryocytes
(b) Platelet count increased
(c) Splenectomy is the treatment
(d) Splenomegaly excludes the diagnosis

414. Pre-malignant condition of colon:
(a) Ulcerative colitis
(b) Diverticulitis
(c) Perianal fistula
(d) Granulomatous disorders

415. Regarding aneurysmal bone cyst, which is not correct?
(a) Malignant
(b) Occurs in long bone
(c) Occurs in flat bone
(d) On a radiograph, well-defined, expansile, lytic lesion

416. Frey's syndrome is seen in:
(a) Parotidectomy
(b) Appendicectomy
(c) Cholecystectomy
(d) Hysterectomy

417. Most common renal lesion in tuberous sclerosis:
(a) AML
(b) RCC
(c) Renal cortical cyst
(d) Oncocytoma

418. Pain sensitive structures are all *except*:
(a) Brain parenchyma
(b) Dura
(c) Blood vessels
(d) Periosteum/scalp

419. All are colloid *except*:
(a) Hypertonic saline (b) Dextran
(c) Blood (d) Gelatin

420. All can cause miosis *except*:
(a) Narcotics
(b) Pontine hemorrhage
(c) Head injury
(d) Atropine

421. Tectorial membrane is continuation of:
(a) Posterior longitudinal ligament
(b) Anterior longitudinal ligament
(c) Ligamentum flavum
(d) Denticulate ligament

422. SCIWORA common in:
(Spinal cord injury without apparent radiological abnormality)
(a) Children (b) Adult
(c) Old (d) Infant

423. Parotid tumor which spread through perineural sheath:
(a) Adenoid cystic carcinoma
(b) Pleomorphic adenoma
(c) Mucoepidermoid carcinoma
(d) Adenocarcinoma

424. Deep lobe of parotid is enlarged in:
(a) Posterior pharyngeal wall swelling
(b) Supratonsillar swelling
(c) Nasopharyngeal swelling
(d) Maxillary swelling

425. Frey's syndrome occurs due to:
(a) Auriculotemporal nerve
(b) Facial nerve
(c) Lingual nerve
(d) Maxillary nerve

426. Lateral retropharyngeal node enlarge due to:
(a) Carcinoma cheek
(b) Carcinoma larynx
(c) Carcinoma nasopharynx
(d) Carcinoma anterior 2/3rd of tongue

427. Patey's mastectomy does not remove:
(a) Skin and areola (b) Nipple
(c) Pectoralis major (d) Pectoralis minor

428. Grey Turner sign is bluish discoloration at:
(a) Loin/flank (b) Umbilicus
(c) Penis (d) Scalp

429. Gas under dome of diaphragm is seen in all *except*:
(a) Ruptured uterus
(b) Ruptured appendix
(c) Ruptured duodenal ulcer
(d) Liver abscess

430. Courvoisier's law–Enlarged gallbladder which is non-tender and with mild jaundice, the cause is unlikely to be:
(a) Gall stones
(b) Carcinoma gallbladder
(c) Carcinoma pancreas
(d) Acute cholecystitis

431. Predisposing factors for carcinoma stomach are all *except*:
(a) Previous gastric surgery
(b) Atrophic gastritis
(c) Benign ulcer
(d) Smoking

432. Maximum suppression of gastric secretion occurs in:
(a) Truncal vagotomy and antrectomy
(b) Truncal vagotomy and pyloroplasty
(c) Highly selective vagotomy
(d) Partial gastrectomy

433. Aortic aneurysm visible on plain X-ray:
(a) 10% (b) 20%
(c) 50% (d) 60%

434. Narrowest part of male urethra:
(a) External urinary meatus
(b) Membranous urethra
(c) Bladder neck
(d) Penile urethra

435. Hunterian ligature used for:
(a) Varicose vein (b) AV fistula
(c) Lymphatic fistula (d) Aneurysm

436. Most common presentation of testicular tumor:
(a) Pain
(b) Painless swelling
(c) Gynecomastia
(d) Infertility

437. Investigation of choice for upper GI bleeding:
(a) Barium meal (b) Endoscopy
(c) USG (d) Tc 99 scan

438. Choledochal cyst is mostly:
(a) Congenital (b) Traumatic
(c) Inflammatory (d) Iatrogenic

439. TPN causes all *except*:
(a) Hepatic dysfunction
(b) Renal insufficiency
(c) Cholestatic liver disease with villous hyperplasia
(d) Demineralization of bone

440. In athletes groin pain – most common cause:
(a) Musculotendinous injury
(b) Pubic symphysis injury
(c) Hip arthritis
(d) Ilioinguinal neuralgia

441. Temperature in autoclave at 15 lbs pressure at 15 minutes should be:
(a) 100°C (b) 160°C
(c) 121°C (d) 80°C

442. Investigation for gastric emptying after taking digestible solid:
(a) Scintigraphy
(b) Clearance of radiopaque dye
(c) Electrical activity
(d) Intragastric pressure monitor

443. All are true regarding CCK, *except*:
(a) Improve cholestasis after TPN
(b) Contraction of gallbladder
(c) Decreases bacterial gut translocation
(d) Improves gut mobility

444. Gut translocation all *except*:
(a) Gram positive bacteria
(b) Gram negative bacteria
(c) Anaerobic
(d) Fungi

445. Which statement is false concerning keloids and hypertrophic scars?
(a) Hypertrophic scars usually extend beyond the borders of the original wound
(b) Keloids are the result of an overgrowth of dense fibrous tissue that usually develops after healing of a skin injury
(c) Hypertrophic scars are characterized by erythematous, pruritic, raised fibrous lesions

(d) Treatment of either condition includes intralesional injections and/or excision

446. Mallory-Weiss syndrome:
(a) More common towards esophagus
(b) More common towards stomach
(c) Surgery is the main treatment
(d) Full thickness rupture

447. Posterior urethral valve 1 is situated:
(a) Above verumontanum
(b) Below verumontanum
(c) At verumontanum
(d) At bladder neck

448. Goiter with hypothyroidism:
(a) Graves' disease
(b) Hashimoto's
(c) Follicular carcinoma
(d) Medullary carcinoma

449. Central part of hyoid is removed in:
(a) Thyroid fistula
(b) Thyroglossal cyst
(c) Ranula
(d) Branchial cyst

450. Dose not to be reduced in chronic renal failure:
(a) Streptomycin (b) Cefaloridine
(c) Gentamicin (d) Aztreonam

451. Blood stain discharge from nipple is not present in:
(a) Duct ectasia (b) Duct papilloma
(c) Fibroadenoma (d) Carcinoma

452. In MRM muscle that is cut:
(a) Pectoralis major (b) Pectoralis minor
(c) Serratus anterior (d) Latissimus dorsi

453. Most common cause of death in excessive burn:
(a) Hypovolemia
(b) Infection
(c) Pulmonary edema
(d) Metabolic problem

454. Osseous metastasis most common in:
(a) Carcinoma bronchus
(b) Carcinoma pancreas
(c) Carcinoma colon
(d) Carcinoma stomach

455. Respiratory distress (chronic pulmonary insufficiency) in:
(a) Hiatus hernia (b) Pancreatitis
(c) Duodenal ulcer (d) Cholecystitis

456. Most common malignant tumor of intestine:
(a) Adenocarcinoma
(b) Lymphoma
(c) Lipoma
(d) Leiomyosarcoma

457. Dysphagia lusoria:
(a) Double aortic arch
(b) Diverticulum
(c) Aberrant right subclavian artery
(d) Aberrant left subclavian artery

458. Space of parona:
(a) Below patella
(b) Between iliopsoas
(c) Drain little finger
(d) In elbow joint

459. Cock's peculiar tumor:
(a) Infected sebaceous cyst
(b) Sebaceous horn on head
(c) Osteomyelitis of skull bone
(d) Infected lipoma

460. Most common cause of intestinal obstruction in adults:
(a) Volvulus
(b) Malignancy
(c) Internal herniation
(d) Postoperative adhesion

461. Low anterior resection is done for:
(a) Tumor located 1 cm above puborectalis muscle on DRE
(b) Tumor located 2 cm above puborectalis muscle on DRE
(c) Tumor located 3 cm above puborectalis muscle on DRE
(d) Tumor located 5 cm above puborectalis muscle on DRE

462. Retropharyngeal group of LN involved in:
(a) Larynx (b) Thyroid
(c) Nasopharynx (d) Esophagus

463. False statement about compartment syndrome is:
(a) Pain is greater than expected, unresponsive to analgesia
(b) Pain on passive stretch of muscles in the affected compartment
(c) Paresthesia is early sign
(d) Prolonged use of tourniquets promote compartment syndrome

464. Minor surgery in patients with additional risk factors is stratified as what type of risk for DVT?
(a) Mild (b) Moderate
(c) High (d) Highest

465. False statement about electrosurgical injuries during laparoscopy:
(a) Incidence is 1-2 cases per 1000 operations
(b) Occurs due to inadvertent handling of tissues during current application
(c) Direct coupling between portion of bowel and metal instrument
(d) Intraabdominal injuries present usually within 48 hours with fever and abdominal pain

466. Which amongst the following is a monofilament absorbable suture?
(a) Chronic catgut
(b) Polyglyconate
(c) Polyglactin
(d) Polyglycolic acid

467. The false statement about refeeding syndrome is:
(a) Characterized by severe fluid and electrolyte shifts in malnourished patients undergoing refeeding
(b) Common in parenteral compared to enteral nutrition
(c) Patients at risk include alcoholics and severely malnourished
(d) Calorie delivery should be rapid, vitamins and trace elements to be withheld

468. The false statement about TPN is:
(a) Peripherally inserted central venous catheter is preferred when the duration on TPN is longer than 2 weeks
(b) Hickman's line is inserted under radiological guidance preferably
(c) Hypoglycemia is common due to insulin resistance
(d) A weight change of >1 kg/day indicates fluid retention

469. Duodenal atresia treatment:
(a) Duodenoduodenostomy
(b) Duodenojejunostomy
(c) Gastrojejunostomy
(d) Gastroduodenostomy

470. Platelets have a shelf life of:
(a) 24 hours (b) 48 hours
(c) 5 days (d) 7 days

471. Complications of massive transfusion include all *except*:
(a) Coagulopathy (b) Hypocalcemia
(c) Hyperkalemia (d) Hyperthermia

472. The false statement about leprosy is:
(a) Caused by mycobacterium leprae
(b) Initial infection occurs in childhood
(c) Tuberculoid leprosy is when host resistance is poor
(d) Skin biopsy is usually confirmatory

473. The false statement about tropical chronic pancreatitis is:
(a) Cassava ingestion is regarded as etiological factor
(b) Occurs in malnutrition in developing countries
(c) Low incidence of pancreatic cancer affected by this disease
(d) Microscopically fibrosis is predominant factor with plasma cell and lymphocytic infiltration

474. Typhoid associated perforation:
(a) Usually occurs between 2 and 3 weeks of illness

(b) Perforation if occurs within a week has very poor prognosis
(c) Wound following laparotomy should be perfectly apposed
(d) Occurs mainly in jejunum

475. Qualities in malignant transformation of the cell has all the following *except*:
(a) Establish autonomous lineage
(b) Obtain immortality
(c) Presence of apoptosis
(d) Angiogenic competence

476. Tumor growth is best described by:
(a) Linear chart
(b) Area chart
(c) Gompertzian curve
(d) None of the above

477. First successful documented human blood transfusion is done by:
(a) Karl Landsteiner (b) Jame Blundell
(c) Albert Hustin (d) Richard Lower

478. What is false about perioperative red blood cell transfusion criteria?
(a) Rarely indicated with hematocrit greater than 30%
(b) Often indicated for hematocrit less than 21%
(c) For levels between 21% and 30%, clinical factors such as risk of complications from inadequate oxygenation should guide the need for transfusion
(d) None of the above

479. Correction of coagulopathy with fresh frozen plasma is necessary if the INR is:
(a) <1 (b) >1
(c) <1.25 (d) >1.5

480. Metabolic responses to starvation include all *except*:
(a) Hepatic glycogenolysis
(b) Adaptive ketogenesis
(c) Reduction in resting energy expenditure
(d) All are true

481. The general recommendation of tourniquet on the upper limb is:
(a) 50 mm Hg above the systolic pressure
(b) 100 mm Hg above the systolic pressure
(c) Twice the systolic pressure
(d) 150 mm Hg above the systolic pressure

482. In patients suffering from psychiatric disorders requiring surgical intervention all the following are true *except*:
(a) General anesthesia is preferred over local anesthesia
(b) Monoamine oxidase inhibitor can continue
(c) Tricyclic antidepressants to be withheld
(d) Two consultants signature to be obtained before proceeding for any surgery in case of adults who are deemed not competent to give consent

483. In taking informed consent, the surgeon has to inform the patient of all life and limb threatening complications and minor complications if its incidence is:
(a) >1% (b) >2%
(c) >5% (d) >10%

484. Rate of surgical site infection (SSI) in contaminated wound is:
(a) 10-15% (b) 15-20%
(c) <4% (d) >40%

485. Following is the indication for fresh frozen plasma transfusion:
(a) Volume replacement
(b) Nutritional supplement
(c) Hypoalbuminemia
(d) Correction of antithrombin III level

486. Pseudomembranous colitis treatment is:
(a) Vancomycin (b) Cephalosporin
(c) Gentamycin (d) Clindamycin

487. The stages of wound healing includes all *except*:
(a) Inflammatory (b) Infiltrative
(c) Proliferation (d) Maturation

488. In wound healing the collagen that is initially deposited is:

(a) Type I (b) Type II
(c) Type III (d) Type IV

489. Keloid scar is made of:
(a) Dense areolar tissue
(b) Dense granulomatous tissue
(c) Dense collagen tissue
(d) Dense epithelialisation

490. In recent advances in wound healing the only approved growth factor used on diabetic foot ulcer is:
(a) Platelet derived GF
(b) Epithelial derived GF
(c) Macrophage derived GF
(d) Erythrocyte derived GF

491. SIRS is defined by all *except*:
(a) Temperature >38°C
(b) Heart rate >120/min
(c) Respiratory rate >20/min
(d) White cell counts >12,000 cells/mm^3

492. Classification of cholecystectomy wound is:
(a) Clean
(b) Clean contaminated
(c) Contaminated
(d) Dirty

493. CVP increases over 15 mm in all *except*:
(a) Over infusion
(b) Pneumothorax
(c) Pulmonary embolism
(d) Deep inhalation

494. In adrenal insufficiency after infusion of 0.25 mg of cosyntropin, at 60 minutes cortisol level is:
(a) 9 μg/dl (b) 18 μg/dl
(c) 27 μg/dl (d) 36 μg/dl

495. Tangential excision is done in:
(a) Circumferential burns
(b) Full thickness burns
(c) Electrical burns
(d) Partial thickness burns

496. Superficial burn involving subcutaneous fat:
(a) 1° (b) 2°
(c) 3° (d) 4°

497. Most common cause of pancreatic pseudocyst:
(a) Infection (b) Hemorrhage
(c) Obstruction (d) Trauma

498. Child Pugh classification of liver disease includes all *except*:
(a) Bilirubin
(b) Hepatic encephalopathy
(c) Ascitis
(d) APTT

499. Most common cause of rectal bleed in child:
(a) Juvenile polyps
(b) Adenomatous polyps
(c) Intussusception
(d) Anal fissures

500. Hydrostatic enema is curative in:
(a) Meconium ileus (b) Intussusception
(c) Mega colon (d) Anal fissure

501. Which is a sympathetic ganglion?
(a) Celiac (b) Ciliary
(c) Aortic (d) Submandibular

502. TRIAGE is used in:
(a) Road traffic accidents
(b) War casualties
(c) All mass casualties
(d) Industrial accidents

503. Duodenal atresia treatment:
(a) DD (b) DJ
(c) GJ (d) GD

504. Indication for intubation are all *except*:
(a) $PaO_2 < 60$
(b) $PaCO_2 < 20$
(c) $Pa/FiO_2 < 200$
(d) Impending respiratory failure

505. RPF, not a causative agent:
(a) Somatostatin (b) Phentolamine
(c) Ergotamine (d) Hydralazine

506. Embryonic stem cell derived from:
(a) Morula (b) Blastocyst
(c) Zygote (d) Embryonic cell

507. Bare area of liver supplied by:
(a) Inferior phrenic artery
(b) Hepatic artery

(c) Right gastric artery
(d) Left gastric artery

508. Hypoxia induces vasoconstriction in:
(a) Coronary artery (b) Cerebral artery
(c) Pulmonary artery (d) Systemic artery

509. Malignant thrombophlebitis is seen in all *except*:
(a) Lung carcinoma
(b) Pancreas carcinoma
(c) Stomach carcinoma
(d) Prostate carcinoma

510. Hemopoietic stem cell:
(a) CD 18 (b) CD 22
(c) CD 34 (d) CD 15

511. Wolfe's graft is:
(a) Mesh split
(b) Thin split thickness
(c) Partial thickness
(d) Full thickness

512. Hernia least likely to strangulate:
(a) Femoral (b) Direct inguinal
(c) Indirect inguinal (d) Umbilical hernia

513. Aortic opening does not have:
(a) Azygous (b) Hemiazygos
(c) Thoracic duct (d) Aorta

514. Increase in CO_2 is seen in:
(a) Metabolic acidosis
(b) Respiratory alkalosis
(c) Diabetic ketoacidosis
(d) Metabolic alkalosis

515. External genitalia and perineum in female is supplied by:
(a) External pudendal nerve
(b) Profunda femoris nerve
(c) Femoral nerve
(d) Internal pudendal nerve

516. Regarding aprotinin which is not correct?
(a) Decreases the need of RBC transfusions in surgery
(b) Not FDA approved
(c) Anticoagulant
(d) Increase in the risk of death with Trasylol compared with tranexamic acid

517. Regarding Henoch-Schönlein purpura which statement is not correct?
(a) Purpura, arthritis and abdominal pain are known as the "classic triad"
(b) Forty percent have evidence of kidney involvement, mainly in the form of hematuria
(c) In adults, kidney involvement progresses to ESRD
(d) The findings on renal biopsy do not correlate with the severity of symptoms

518. MEN 1 all are true *except*:
(a) Wermer's syndrome
(b) Overactivity of the pituitary gland is the most common sign of this disorder
(c) Most common neoplasia in the pituitary gland is prolactinoma
(d) WDHA syndrome is due to increase in VIP

519. In AIDS which part is most commonly involved by CMV?
(a) Stomach (b) Colon
(c) Jejunum (d) Duodenum

520. Malignant hyperthermia–which ion channel is involved?
(a) Na (b) K
(c) Ca (d) Cl

521. Abdominal compartment syndrome grade 3 has how much of IAP?
(a) 10 – 15 cm H_2O (b) 16 – 25 cm H_2O
(c) 26 – 35 cm H_2O (d) 36 – 47 cm H_2O

522. Hypocalcemia includes all *except*:
(a) Perioral anesthesia
(b) Digital hyperesthesia
(c) Hypotonia
(d) Psychosis

523. Intraabdominal calcification seen in:
(a) Meconium ileus
(b) Meconium plug syndrome
(c) Meconium peritonitis
(d) Inspissated meconium

524. Lymphangioma sarcoma is a complication of:
(a) Lymphedema (b) Lymphangioma
(c) Lymphoma (d) Lymphorrhea

525. Radioiodine therapy in Graves' disease:
(a) 1-5 millicuries (b) 5-15 millicuries
(c) 15-25 millicuries (d) 40-60 millicuries

526. Indication of dialysis are all *except*:
(a) BUN >100 (b) Hyperkalemia
(c) Encephalopathy (d) Severe acidosis

527. CBD stone 2.5 cm (residual) with cholangitis, treatment is:
(a) Endoscopic removal
(b) Supraduodenal approach
(c) Transduodenal approach
(d) PTBD
(e) ESWL

528. Rectal ulcer involving muscular propria with pararectal lymph node, modified Astler Collen grading is:
(a) B2 (b) C1
(c) C2 (d) D1
(e) D2

529. Which statement is false concerning scars and scabs?
(a) A scab is a temporary crust of dried blood clot that forms to protect a damaged area of the skin
(b) Some scabs are disfiguring and warrant cosmetic repair
(c) A scar is a permanent deposition of fibrous tissue to replace damaged or lost skin
(d) Scabs will fall off on their own

530. Mandibular development occurs from how many processes?
(a) 2 (b) 3
(c) 4 (d) 5
(e) 1

531. Clear discharge from wound in Southampton scale is graded as:
(a) Ia (b) IIa
(c) IId (d) III
(e) IV

532. Which of the following is not GCT?
(a) Sertoli cell tumor
(b) Embroynal cell tumor
(c) Yolk sac tumor
(d) Seminoma
(e) Choriocarcinoma

533. Trendelenburg sign is for:
(a) Varicose veins
(b) Congenital dislocation of hip
(c) Carcinoma stomach
(d) Carcinoma liver
(e) Renal cell carcinoma

534. 1 Gray =
(a) 100 rads (b) 1 rads
(c) 10 rads (d) 1000 rads
(e) 3 rads

535. Limberg flap:
(a) Rotation (b) Axial
(c) Transposition (d) Interpolation
(e) Is a type of graft

536. In intestinal obstruction gases are:
(a) H_2S and N_2 (b) N_2 and O_2
(c) CO_2 and N_2 (d) H_2S and N_2
(e) H_2S and CO_2

537. Gene inhibiting apoptosis:
(a) BCL-2 (b) P 53
(c) RAS (d) MYC
(e) PTC

538. Most appropriate method to measure intraabdominal pressure:
(a) Foley's in bladder
(b) Catheter in IVC
(c) Catheter in portal vein
(d) NG tube in stomach
(e) Pressure transducer in peritoneal cavity

539. Dangerous layer of scalp:
(a) Skin
(b) Connective tissue
(c) Aponeurotica
(d) Loose areolar tissue
(e) Pericranium

540. Strawberry angioma best treated with:
(a) Conservative (b) Laser
(c) Cryosurgery (d) Surgery
(e) Radiation

541. Anion gap increased in all *except*:
(a) DKA
(b) Ureteroileostomy
(c) Salicylate poisoning
(d) Methanol
(e) Hypovolemic shock

542. Pneumatosis intestinalis appearance on X-ray is due to:
(a) NEC
(b) Meconium ileus
(c) Small bowel atresia
(d) Volvulus neonatorum
(e) Duodenal atresia

543. Factors involved in angiogenesis all *except*:
(a) Metalloproteinase (b) Angiotensin
(c) TGF-β (d) FGF
(e) PDGF

544. Lymph node scanning agent used is:
(a) Selenium (b) Phosphorus
(c) Sulphur (d) Gallium
(e) Gadolinium

545. Functional segment of liver include:
(a) Hepatic artery, portal vein, bile duct
(b) Hepatic artery only
(c) Portal vein only
(d) Bile duct only
(e) Hepatic artery and portal vein

546. Which statement is false on comparing surgical sutures with staplers?
(a) Staplers carry the risk of foreign body ingestion in mentally impaired patients
(b) Sutures carry the risk of needle stick
(c) Staplers provide more meticulous skin approximation
(d) Suturing requires longer training

547. Synergistic gangrene caused by all *except*:
(a) Staphylococcus
(b) Coliform
(c) Peptostreptococcus
(d) Anaerobic streptococcus
(e) Clostridia

548. Barrett's esophagus:
(a) Squamous to columnar
(b) Columnar to squamous
(c) Squamous to transitional
(d) Transitional to columnar
(e) Columnar to transitional

549. Risk of malignancy is seen in:
(a) Sclerosing adenosis
(b) Apocrine metaplasia
(c) Fibroadenosis
(d) Cystosarcoma
(e) Giant fibroadenoma

550. Most sensitive investigation in renal obstruction:
(a) Whitaker (b) Captopril
(c) IVU (d) DTPA
(e) DMSA

551. Adrenaline (1:20,000) in local anesthesia is equivalent to:
(a) 2.5 μg/ml (b) 5 μg/ml
(c) 20 μg/ml (d) 30 μg/ml
(e) 50 μg/ml

552. EMLA cream:
(a) Lignocaine 2.5% and prilocaine 2.5%
(b) Lignocaine 1% and prilocaine 1%
(c) Bupivacaine 2.5% and lignocaine 2.5%
(d) Prilocaine 2.5% and bupivacaine 2.5%
(e) Lignocaine 2% and prilocaine 1%

553. Hypokalemia is seen in all *except*:
(a) Renal failure
(b) Metabolic alkalosis
(c) Thiazide diuretics
(d) Hyperaldosteronism
(e) Addison's disease

554. Puestow's operation done for:
(a) Chronic pancreatitis
(b) CBD stones
(c) Acute appendicitis
(d) Acute cholecystitis
(e) Pancreatic stones

555. 'E' in ASA classification is:
(a) Emergency surgery
(b) Elective surgery
(c) ECG required
(d) ECT received
(e) Extra risk

556. Boerhaave syndrome caused by:
(a) Full thickness esophagus
(b) Partial thickness esophagus
(c) Full thickness stomach
(d) Partial thickness stomach
(e) None

557. Pheochromocytoma true is all *except*:
(a) Can be detected by MIBG
(b) 10% patients can be normotensive
(c) 10% can have normal epinephrine levels
(d) 10% can be malignant
(e) 10% detected in elderly

558. In pulmonary edema, drug contraindicated is:
(a) Morphine (b) Pethidine
(c) Mannitol (d) Furosemide
(e) Tramadol

559. Citation, the number of surname above which *et al.* used?
(a) 3 (b) 4
(c) 5 (d) 6
(e) 7

560. Denominator in Z score:
(a) Standard deviation (b) Mean
(c) Range (d) Median
(e) Range minus mean

561. Type II error is:
(a) False positive
(b) False negative
(c) True positive
(d) True negative
(e) Both true positive and false positive

562. The study in which the participants are not known to anybody but research and staff:
(a) Confidentiality (b) Ethics
(c) Double blind (d) Anonymous
(e) Triple blind

563. 50th percentile when numbers are arranged in order of magnitude:
(a) Mean (b) Median
(c) Mode (d) Range
(e) Standard deviation

564. Approximately what percentage of scores fall within one standard deviation of the mean in a normal distribution?
(a) 34% (b) 95%
(c) 99% (d) 68%
(e) 77%

565. Research will be qualitative if:
(a) Generalized population
(b) Standardized measure
(c) Random sampling
(d) Case control
(e) Cohort study

566. The most frequently occurring number in a set of values is called:
(a) Mean (b) Median
(c) Mode (d) Range
(e) Standard deviation

567. As a general rule, the ________ is the best measure of central tendency because it is more precise.
(a) Mean (b) Median
(c) Mode (d) Range
(e) Standard deviation

568. Second hit pancreatitis is due to:
(a) Endotoxin absorption
(b) Bacterial translocation
(c) Increased permeability
(d) Pancreatic edema
(e) Fluid sequestration

569. NICE guidelines used for:
(a) Laparoscopic inguinal hernia
(b) Laparoscopic femoral hernia
(c) Laparoscopic ventral hernia
(d) Umbilical hernia
(e) Laparoscopic recurrent hernia

570. Most common malignant tumor of intestine:
(a) Adenocarcinoma
(b) Lymphoma
(c) Lipoma
(d) Leiomyosarcoma
(e) Squamons cell carcinoma

571. Resection of prolapsed rectum and sigmoid done in:
(a) Altemeier's (b) Well's
(c) Ripstein (d) Delorme
(e) Lahauts

572. Borrmann's classification for ulcerative lesion with elevated margin and sharp border:
(a) I (b) II
(c) III (d) IV
(e) V

573. Grade III liver injuries:
(a) Parenchymal depth – 1-3 cm
(b) < 10 cm subcapsular hematoma
(c) Couinaud's segment – 1-3 involved
(d) Couinaud's segment – > 3 in single lobe involved
(e) Parenchymal depth – > 3 cm

574. Crohn's is associated with all *except*:
(a) Psoriasis
(b) Iritis
(c) Arthritis
(d) Sclerosing cholangitis

575. Following are correct about abdominal hyperplastic tuberculosis *except*:
(a) Ileocecal junction is the most common site
(b) Barium meal shows pulled up caecum
(c) ATT is to be given in all the cases
(d) Fishner and Sterling signs are characteristic

576. The prognosis of carcinoma stomach after resection depends on:
(a) The nature of margin of proximal resection
(b) Stage at presentation
(c) Amount of stomach removal
(d) Short clinical history

577. A 50 years old lady with history of not passing stools for the last 10 days. Abdominal X-ray do not show air-fluid levels. The probable diagnosis is:
(a) Intestinal pseudo-obstruction
(b) Malignancy
(c) Duodenal obstruction
(d) Paralytic ileus

578. The most common site of involvement of ischemic colitis:
(a) Ascending colon
(b) Transverse colon
(c) Splenic flexure
(d) Sigmoid colon

579. A young man presents with history of dysphagia for liquids more than solids. The investigation of choice in this case:
(a) Esophagoscopy (b) Barium swallow
(c) USG (d) CT scan

580. Which tumor is not associated with smoking?
(a) Esophageal carcinoma
(b) Hepatocellular carcinoma
(c) Laryngeal carcinoma
(d) Bronchial carcinoma

581. Which one is true about acute cholecystitis?
(a) Stone are always present to cause jaundice
(b) Should be operated after one week
(c) Leucocytosis is frequent
(d) It always leads to suppurative cholangitis

582. Treatment of choice in case of a symptomatic hydatid cyst is:
(a) Symptomatic treatment only
(b) Instillation of hypertonic saline
(c) Excision
(d) Anti-helminthic therapy

583. Following can be detected by USG in case of surgical jaundice *except*:
(a) Degree of obstruction
(b) Cause of obstruction
(c) Duration of obstruction
(d) Site of obstruction

584. Transrectal ultrasonography, frequency used is:
(a) <3.5 MHz (b) 3.5-5 MHz
(c) 7 MHz (d) >7 MHz

585. Least common site of metastasis from carcinoma lung:
(a) Liver (b) Skin
(c) Bone (d) Brain

586. Most common retroperitoneal tumor:
(a) Lipoma (b) Liposarcoma
(c) Fibrosarcoma (d) Neuroblastoma

587. Which wound closure device is preferred for mid-line laparotomy incision?
(a) Tissue adhesives (skin glue)
(b) Surgical tapes
(c) Sutures
(d) Staples

588. Dislocation of humerus results in injury to:
(a) Radial nerve (b) Median nerve
(c) Ulnar nerve (d) Axillary nerve

589. Pseudoclaudication occurs due to compression of:
(a) Cauda equina
(b) Femoral nerve
(c) Femoral artery
(d) External iliac artery

590. All are true about the chemodectoma:
(a) RT is the treatment of choice
(b) Inoperable most of the time at exploration
(c) Can be moved in horizontal plane but not upside down
(d) FNAC is diagnostic

591. Treatment of choice for carotid body tumor:
(a) Excision (b) Radiotherapy
(c) Embolization (d) Chemotherapy

592. The best cosmetic results for a large port-wine hemangioma is:
(a) Excision with sclerotherapy
(b) Excision with pedicle flap reconstruction
(c) Laser dissection
(d) Tattooing

593. Ranson's criteria all *except:*
(a) Age >70 years
(b) LDH >40
(c) Alkaline phosphatase > 80
(d) WBC > 18000

594. Acute DVT of the leg can be diagnosed by the presence of all the following *except*:
(a) Tenderness in the calf area
(b) Venography
(c) Color Doppler
(d) Presence of prominent veins in the region of saphenous system

595. Anosmia is caused by all *except*:
(a) Nasal polyp (b) HPV
(c) Head trauma (d) Cocaine abuse

596. Foamy liver is caused by:
(a) Cirrhosis (b) Hydatid cyst
(c) Gas gangrene (d) Portal pyemia

597. Quincke triad of GI bleed, jaundice and abdominal pain. Diagnosis is:
(a) Pancreatic laceration with pancreatitis
(b) Duodenal perforation
(c) Hemobilia
(d) Pyloric stenosis

598. Which of the following condition is associated with nipple discharge?
(a) Phyllodes tumor
(b) Mondor's disease
(c) Posterior pituitary tumor
(d) Intraductal papilloma

599. All of the following are indications of radiotherapy after excision of pleomorphic adenoma *except*:
(a) Histologically benign recurrence
(b) Malignant transformation
(c) Deep lobe involvement
(d) Positive margins

600. A young man presents with upper GI variceal bleed with compensated liver disease. Treatment of choice is:
(a) TIPPS
(b) Liver transplant
(c) Endoscopic sclerotherapy
(d) Propranolol

601. Ogilvie's syndrome occurs with the following:
(a) Neuroleptic drugs
(b) Malignant infiltration of celiac plexus
(c) Excess parasympathetic tone
(d) Severe metabolic illness

602. All are true about the axillary vein thrombosis *except*:
(a) Occurs after heavy exercise
(b) Low dose anti-coagulants are sufficient for treatment
(c) Embolectomy is required in all the cases
(d) Occasionally associated with cervical rib

603. Most common cause of pancreatic pseudocyst is:
(a) Trauma
(b) Acute pancreatitis
(c) Annular pancreas
(d) Iatrogenic

604. Most common type of mesenteric cyst:
(a) Enterogenous
(b) Chylolymphatic cyst
(c) Teratoma
(d) Arterial cyst

605. The following investigation is done to diagnose Meckel's diverticulum:
(a) USG (b) CT scan
(c) Barium meal (d) TC 99 scan

606. According to Nyhus classification which one is true?
(a) Type I – Direct hernia
(b) Type II – Indirect hernia with normal internal ring
(c) Type IIIa – Indirect hernia
(d) Type IIIc – Femoral hernia

607. In a young patient with tension pneumothorax and respiratory distress. The immediate management is:
(a) Intubation
(b) Insertion of needle in the intercostals space
(c) Immediate thoracotomy
(d) ICD insertion

608. The________ is often the preferred measure of central tendency if the data are severely skewed.
(a) Mean (b) Median
(c) Mode (d) Range

609. Which of the following is the formula for range?
(a) H+L (b) L×H
(c) L–H (d) H–L

610. Which is a raw score that has been transformed into standard deviation units?
(a) z score (b) SDU score
(c) t score (d) e score

611. Which of the following is not a measure of variability?
(a) Median (b) Variance
(c) Standard deviation (d) Range

612. Which of the following is not a common measure of central tendency?
(a) Mode (b) Range
(c) Median (d) Mean

613. Perforated appendix—most common organism:
(a) E. coli (b) Bacteroides
(c) Klebsiella (d) Staphylococcus

614. Full thickness burn on both upper extremity and chest, IV access by:
(a) Femoral (b) Saphenous
(c) Ante cubital (d) Scalp

615. Most common case of massive hemorrhage:
(a) Fracture femur
(b) Partial tear of artery by bone chips
(c) Open fracture tibia/fibula
(d) Crush injury foot

616. Early sign of compartment syndrome in anterior compartment of calf:
(a) Absent pulse
(b) Hypoesthesia of first web space
(c) Pain in calf muscle
(d) Foot drop

617. What is the best statement describing hair removal before surgery?
(a) Be 24 hours before surgery using electric hair clippers
(b) Be immediately before surgery using electric hair clippers
(c) Be 12 hours before surgery using a razor
(d) Be immediately before surgery using a sticky tape

618. Shock after spinal anesthesia managed by:
(a) Colloids
(b) Beta blockers
(c) Alpha agonists
(d) Mephentermine

619. Neurogenic shock is characterized by:
(a) Decreased peripheral vascular resistance
(b) Bradycardia
(c) Can lead to organ dysfunction
(d) Circulatory in nature

620. Military antishock trouser act like:
(a) Dopamine (b) Norepinephrine
(c) Whole blood (d) Atropine

621. Pectus excavatum all *except*:
(a) Shrunken appearance of stomach
(b) Most common congenital abnormality of anterior chest wall
(c) Cobbler's chest
(d) Never compromise respiratory and cardiac function

622. Pierre-Robin syndrome:
(a) Cleft lip (b) Cleft palate
(c) Micrognathia (d) Glossoptosis

623. Hypertrophic pyloric stenosis with vomiting and dehydration, most important ion to be replaced:
(a) Sodium (b) Potassium
(c) Chloride (d) Bicarbonate

624. Treatment of non-responsive metabolic alkalosis:
(a) NH_4Cl
(b) HCl
(c) Chloride
(d) Hypertonic saline

625. Pulse oximetry gives false reading in all *except*:
(a) Opaque nail polish
(b) Hyperbilirubinemia
(c) Carboxyhemoglobin
(d) Methemoglobin

626. Composite graft all *except*:
(a) High failure rate
(b) Includes skin and subcutaneous tissue
(c) Donor side should be closed with skin graft
(d) Used for correcting complex defects

627. 10 days after burn – nutrition assessment best by:
(a) Daily weight
(b) N_2 balance measurement
(c) Serum albumin
(d) Skin thickness

628. Most common complication of pulmonary artery catheterization:
(a) Injection site hematoma
(b) Dysrhythmia
(c) Knotting
(d) Pneumothorax

629. Which statement is false concerning scar contracture?
(a) It is the last phase of primary wound healing
(b) Composed of dense collagen, thin-wall blood vessels
(c) Seen commonly in 2nd or 3rd degree burns
(d) Could lead to physical deformity and functional limitations

630. Pulmonary artery pressure measured at:
(a) End expiration (b) Early expiration
(c) Mid expiration (d) Mid inspiration

631. Malignant hyperthermia:
(a) Frequently associated with succinylcholine
(b) Can be associated with intravenous narcotics
(c) Frequently associated with respiratory alkalosis
(d) Found in late phase of anesthesia

632. Postoperative pain – best management:
(a) Epidural
(b) Preoperative sedation
(c) Intraoperative analgesia
(d) Wound infiltration of local anesthesia in wound

633. Partial left colon obstruction in endometriosis:
(a) Danazol
(b) Transverse colostomy
(c) Hysterectomy and bilateral salpingo-oophorectomy
(d) Left colectomy

634. Malignancy associated with:
(a) Cell polymorphism
(b) Nuclear polymorphism
(c) Atypia
(d) Polyclonal origin

635. Management of malignant pleural effusion:
(a) Repeated thoracentesis with sclerosant injection
(b) Tube thoracotomy
(c) Radiotherapy
(d) Thoracotomy + pleurectomy

636. Verrucous carcinoma all *except*:
(a) Metastasis to distal parts of body
(b) Superficial and exophytic
(c) Low grade squamous cell carcinoma
(d) Not associated with metastasis

637. Nodular melanoma:
(a) Most malignant
(b) Smooth and convex
(c) Seen in elderly
(d) Pigmented

638. All true for giant congenital nevi *except*:
(a) Histology similar to acquired nevi
(b) In small nevi – spontaneous regression
(c) Multiple surgery with primary closure and grafting
(d) Radiotherapy is an option

639. Cosmetically useful treatment for large capillary hemangioma:
(a) Laser
(b) Surgery with grafting
(c) Cryoablation
(d) Radiotherapy

640. What happens within hours of repairing a full thickness surgical incision is:
(a) Wound contracture
(b) Primary intention wound healing
(c) Delayed primary wound healing
(d) Secondary intention wound healing

641. Most appropriate treatment for intrahepatic biliary atresia:
(a) Portoenterostomy
(b) Orthotopic liver transplant
(c) Liver transplant
(d) Wait and watch

642. After removal of 2/3rd of liver, regeneration is complete in:
(a) 4-6 months (b) 8-10 weeks
(c) 2-3 months (d) 12 months

643. Most common small bowel tumor in child <10 years:
(a) Lymphoma
(b) Leiomyosarcoma
(c) Carcinoid
(d) Carcinoma

644. The most common site for carcinoid in gastrointestinal tract:
(a) Ileum (b) Stomach
(c) Rectum (d) Colon

645. True about squamous cell carcinoma of the lip are all *except*:
(a) 90% occur in upper lip
(b) Predisposed by sum exposure
(c) Radiotherapy is the treatment of choice
(d) Radiosensitive

646. Surgical gloves were invented by:
(a) Listed (b) Halsted
(c) Hassan (d) Veress

647. All of the following are the features of malignancy on mammography *except*:
(a) Nodular calcification
(b) Irregular mass
(c) Attenuated architecture
(d) Speckled margins

648. Reactivation of Mycobacterium tuberculosis occurs in all the following conditions *except*:
(a) HIV
(b) Allergic asthma
(c) Collagen vascular disorder
(d) Immunocompromised states

649. During preoperative bowel preparation, antibiotics result in:
(a) Diarrhea
(b) Bacterial super infection
(c) Colitis
(d) Immunocompromised states

650. Thyroid storm occurs in all the following clinical situations *except*:
(a) Thyroiditis with hypothyroidism
(b) Thyroiditis with hyperthyroidism
(c) During radioiodine therapy
(d) Intercurrent illness in hyperthyroidism

651. Which one of the following is most appropriate management for a patient with gangrene?
(a) Anti-gas gangrene serum
(b) Surgical debridement
(c) Antibiotics
(d) Observation

652. Definitive factors delaying wound healing include all *except:*
(a) Hypoxia
(b) Anemia
(c) Aging
(d) Hypoalbuminemia

653. Which of the following statement is true regarding surgical site infection?
(a) Use of mechanical drain constitute clean contaminated wound
(b) Uncontrolled spillage of viscous may lead to SSI in 10–12% of cases
(c) Apparent inflammation occurs in clean contaminated wound
(d) Minimum of 48 hours antibiotic coverage is required in clean wounds

654. All are true about cystic hygroma *except:*
(a) Cystic spaces lined by endothelium
(b) 50% of them present at birth
(c) Most of them regress after waitful watching
(d) Bleomycin has been used effectively in the treatment

655. All are proinflammatory mediators *except:*
(a) IL-1 (b) IL-6
(c) IL-9 (d) TNF-alpha

656. A 48 years old man hit by truck was brought to ER in an anxious state. On examination airway was patent, BP-90/50 mm Hg, P-130 bpm, Respiratory rate-32 bpm. All of the following statements are true *except:*
(a) Patient must have lost 30–40% of total blood
(b) Crystalloid suffices the treatment
(c) Urine output is important parameter in management
(d) Pulse pressure will be low

657. All are true about blood transfusion *except:*
(a) James Blundell performs the first successful documented human transfusion
(b) Landsteiner discovers the ABO system
(c) Cryoprecipitate is rich in factor VIII and fibrinogen
(d) One pint platelet precipitate increase platelets count by 25000–30000

658. **SIRS definition contains all *except:***
(a) Temperature < 36 degree celcius
(b) Heart rate > 90
(c) BP < 90 mm of Hg
(d) Respiratory rate > 20 bpm

659. **All are true about tracheoesophageal fistula *except:***
(a) Type C is most common
(b) Male predominance
(c) 'A' in VACTERAL stands for abdominal anomalies
(d) Maternal polyhydramnios often present

660. **True about tumor markers in general are all *except:***
(a) Correlates with amount of tumor burden
(b) Prognosticate the disease
(c) Best for screening in most of the cancers
(d) Predicts the response to therapy

661. **Father of modern surgery:**
(a) Alexis Carrel (b) Ambroise Pare
(c) Theodor Kocher (d) William Halsted

662. **All are features of acute adrenal insufficiency *except:***
(a) Hyponatremia
(b) Metabolic alkalosis
(c) Hypoglycemia
(d) Hyperkalemia

663. **Surgical and anesthetic risk scores are all *except:***
(a) ASA
(b) Hinchey score
(c) POSSUM
(d) Anaerobic threshold

664. **All are signs of head injury *except:***
(a) Bilateral Raccoon eyes
(b) Battles sign
(c) CSF rhinorrhea
(d) Mobius sign

665. **Spider leg deformity in excretory urogram occurs in:**
(a) Hydronephrosis
(b) Polycystic kidney disease
(c) Ureterocele
(d) Renal agenesis

666. **Most common stone in UTI:**
(a) Phosphate (b) Urate
(c) Cysteine (d) Calcium oxalate

667. **All are true about seminoma *except:***
(a) Constitute most of the tumors in > 60 years old people
(b) Most common presentation being painless swelling or nodule in the gonad
(c) Secondary hydrocele can occur in 5–10% of cases
(d) Majority are confined to testis

668. **Best approach for surgical repair of the injury to abdominal aorta above the level of renal artery involving SMA, celiac trunk and suprarenal branch:**
(a) Right medial visceral rotation
(b) Left medial visceral rotation
(c) Right lateral visceral rotation
(d) Left lateral visceral rotation

669. **Most common complication of varicose vein stripping is:**
(a) Infection
(b) Hemorrhage
(c) Ecchymosis
(d) Thromboembolism

670. **Adverse prognostic factors for Hodgkin's lymphoma include all *except:***
(a) Male gender (b) B symptoms
(c) Raised ESR (d) Erythrocytosis

671. **Most common tumor of posterior mediastinum:**
(a) Bronchogenic cysts
(b) Thymoma
(c) Neurogenic tumors
(d) Aneurysms

672. **True about burn resuscitation is:**
(a) Colloid preferred in first 24 hours

(b) Colloid preferred if burnt area is >15% of TBSA
(c) Urine output should be maintained at 50–60 ml per hour
(d) Half of calculated fluid is given in initial 16 hours

673. Clinical triad of normal pressure hydrocephalus are all *except:*
(a) Magnetic gait (b) Dementia
(c) Urinary urgency (d) Diplopia

674. Contralateral neck lymph node (< 6 cm) in head and neck cancers is:
(a) N1 (b) N2b
(c) N2c (d) N3

675. Radical neck dissection includes all *except:*
(a) Cervical lymph nodes
(b) Sternocleidomastoid
(c) Phrenic nerves
(d) Internal jugular vein

676. Treatment of DCIS includes all *except:*
(a) Mastectomy
(b) Breast conservation surgery
(c) Endocrine therapy
(d) Radiotherapy alone

677. Contraindication for breast conservation surgery include all *except:*
(a) Diffuse suspicious calcification
(b) Inability to obtain clear margins
(c) Contraindication to radiation therapy
(d) Size of tumor 5 cm

678. BRCA1 and BRCA2 carriers have a life long rates of breast cancer between:
(a) 10–20% (b) 20–40%
(c) 50–70% (d) 90–100%

679. LD flap is based on:
(a) Pectoral branches
(b) Thoracodorsal artery
(c) Internal mammary artery
(d) Subscapular artery

680. Thyroidea ima artery is a branch of:
(a) Superior thyroid artery
(b) Inferior thyroid artery
(c) Innominate artery
(d) Brachiocephalic trunk

681. All are features of SIRS *except:*
(a) Temperature ≥ 38°C (100.4°F)
(b) Heart rate ≤ 90 beats per minute
(c) $PaCO_2$ ≤ 32 mm Hg or mechanical ventilation
(d) White blood cell count ≥ 12,000/l or ≥10% band forms

682. False about Hyperkalemia:
(a) Serum potassium concentration above 5.0 mEq/l
(b) Hyperkalemia is more common than Hypokalemia in surgical patient
(c) Caused by excessive potassium intake
(d) High peaked T waves (early), widened QRS complex, flattened P wave on ECG

683. Parenteral nutrition not indicated in:
(a) Short-bowel syndrome secondary to massive small-bowel resection
(b) High-output enterocutaneous fistulas
(c) Patients with severe metabolic derangement
(d) Critically ill patients who are hypermetabolic for > 5 days

684. Beck's triad includes all *except:*
(a) Dilated neck veins
(b) Muffled heart tones
(c) Decreased air entry in lungs
(d) Decline in arterial pressure

685. False about Pseudoxanthoma elasticum:
(a) A rare inherited disorder of connective tissue
(b) Fragmentation and calcification of the fibers
(c) ABCC6 gene is responsible
(d) First described by Antoine Marfan in 1896

686. Bell stages' refers to:
(a) Necrotizing enterocolitis
(b) Meconium ileus
(c) Intestinal atresia
(d) Hypertrophic pyloric stenosis

687. Jefferson fracture refers to:
(a) Bursting fracture of the ring of the atlas
(b) Bursting fracture of the dens of the axis
(c) Hangman's fracture
(d) Jumped facet

688. False about malignant hyperthermia:
(a) An autosomal dominant disorder
(b) Calcium channel blockers are helpful in treatment
(c) Diagnosed with the caffeine-contracture halothane test
(d) Hypermetabolic acute disorder

689. Within few hours of undergoing thyroidectomy patient presents with a swelling in the neck and respiratory distress. The immediate intervention would be:
(a) Wait and watch
(b) Firm compression over the wound
(c) Cut the sutures and decompress the wound
(d) Arrange for blood

690. First gastrectomy was performed by:
(a) William Mayo (b) Mikulicz
(c) Billroth (d) Kocher

691. Segments of liver are named after:
(a) Calot (b) Graham cole
(c) Couinaud (d) Blumgart

692. Gold standard treatment for a 7 mm radiopaque calculus in distal CBD:
(a) Laparoscopic CBD exploration
(b) Lithotripsy
(c) ERCP
(d) Open CBD exploration

693. Choice of operation in annular pancreas:
(a) Gastrojejunostomy
(b) Pancreatectomy
(c) Division of the annular pancreas
(d) Duodenoduodenostomy

694. The rectus relaxing incision in inguinal hernia repair is named after:
(a) Shouldice
(b) Lytle
(c) Halsted Tanner
(d) Lichtenstein

695. Bloody vicious cycle or deadly triad includes all *except:*
(a) Hypothermia
(b) Metabolic acidosis
(c) Hypotension
(d) Coagulopathy

696. All are premalignant oral cavity lesions *except:*
(a) Erythroplakia
(b) Leukoplakia
(c) Chronic hyperplastic candidiasis
(d) Lichen planus

697. What is the color of the glove on the intra-abdominal hand is recommended to reduce the glare during hand-assisted laparoscopic surgery?
(a) Black (b) Green
(c) Brown (d) White

698. Boutonniere deformity is seen in which of the following conditions of the hand?
(a) Pulp space infection
(b) Rheumatoid arthritis
(c) Osteoarthritis
(d) Dupuytren's contracture

699. Which of the following is not a common hernia?
(a) Paraumbilical (b) Obturator
(c) Femoral (d) Umbilical

700. All of the following make the borders of the inferior lumbar triangle of petit *except*:
(a) Crest of the ileum
(b) External oblique muscle
(c) Latissimus dorsi
(d) Erector spinae

701. Platelet shelf life:
(a) 2 days (b) 4 days
(c) 3 days (d) 5 days

702. Not a complication of blood transfusion:
(a) Air embolism
(b) Coagulopathy
(c) Hyperthermia
(d) Hyperkalemia

703. All are used in the treatment of hyperkalemia *except:*
(a) Oral ion-exchange resin
(b) Sodium bicarbonate
(c) Emergency dialysis
(d) Oral coconut water

704. Which disease is described best by the following manifestations: grand mal epilepsy,

mental retardation, hypertension, angiomyolipoma, adenoma sebaceum, bilateral enlarged kidneys and normal renal function?
(a) Autosomal dominant polycystic kidney disease
(b) Von Hippel-Lindau disease
(c) Tuberous sclerosis
(d) Sturge-Weber syndrome

705. **Which of the following conditions could happen in chronic pancreatitis and malabsorption syndrome with steatorrhea?**
(a) Hyperoxaluria
(b) Hypercalciuria
(c) Hyperuricosuria
(d) Hyperphosphaturia

706. **What is the appropriate intravenous maintenance fluid for a 16 kg girl?**
(a) 43 ml/hr of normal saline
(b) 78 ml/hr of ¼ normal saline
(c) 69 ml/hr of ½ normal saline
(d) 54 ml/hr of ¼ normal saline

707. **Which medicine(s) might enhance hypoprothrombinemic effect on oral anticoagulants?**
(a) Allopurinol
(b) Aminoglycosides
(c) Cimetidine
(d) All of the above

708. **Which of the following does not affect wound healing?**
(a) Age (b) Gender
(c) Medications (d) Anemia

709. **What does delay wound healing in diabetics?**
(a) Diabetic neuropathy
(b) Occurrence of infections
(c) Chronicity of diabetes
(d) All of the above

710. **Which wound(s) heal(s) first?**
(a) 10 cm long clean surgical wound
(b) 22 cm long clean surgical wound
(c) 4 cm infected wound
(d) (a) and (b)

711. **What is the optimal time for delayed primary wound closure?**
(a) Not before the second postoperative day
(b) Not before the third postoperative day
(c) Not before the fourth postoperative day
(d) Not before the fifth postoperative day

712. **When the bottom of a pressure sore wound turns red, that is an indicative of:**
(a) Granulation tissue formation
(b) Necrotic tissue formation
(c) Sloughed tissue accumulation
(d) Presence of infection

713. **What kind of cells initiates granulation of a lacerated wound left to heal by secondary intention?**
(a) Myofibroblasts
(b) Macrophages
(c) Neutrophils
(d) Collagens

714. **What is the proper sequence of wound healing phases?**
(a) Inflammation, hemostasis, proliferative, maturation
(b) Hemostasis, proliferative, inflammation, maturation
(c) Hemostasis, inflammation, proliferative, maturation
(d) Inflammation, proliferative, hemostasis, maturation

715. **The movement of an organism in response to a chemical stimulus is called:**
(a) Chemokinesis (b) Haptotaxis
(c) Necrotaxis (d) Chemotaxis

ANSWERS

1.	C	2.	C	3.	D	4.	C	5.	A	6.	C
7.	B	8.	C	9.	D	10.	B	11.	A	12.	D
13.	C	14.	D	15.	C	16.	D	17.	B	18.	D
19.	A	20.	D	21.	D	22.	D	23.	B	24.	D
25.	D	26.	D	27.	D	28.	B	29.	D	30.	A
31.	A	32.	B	33.	D	34.	C	35.	C	36.	D
37.	A	38.	D	39.	A	40.	D	41.	C	42.	A
43.	D	44.	A	45.	A	46.	A	47.	D	48.	C
49.	B	50.	D	51.	D	52.	D	53.	A	54.	C
55.	B	56.	A	57.	D	58.	B	59.	A	60.	A
61.	B	62.	C	63.	A	64.	A	65.	B	66.	A
67.	D	68.	D	69.	D	70.	B	71.	A	72.	B
73.	C	74.	A	75.	C	76.	A	77.	D	78.	D
79.	A	80.	D	81.	D	82.	D	83.	D	84.	D
85.	B	86.	B	87.	C	88.	D	89.	C	90.	D
91.	FTTTF	92.	TFTTT	93.	FTTTF	94.	FFFTT	95.	FTFTT	96.	TFFFT
97.	TTTTF	98.	FFFTT	99.	FTFTF	100.	TFTTF	101.	FFTTT	102.	FFTTF
103.	FTFTT	104.	FTTFT	105.	TTFTF	106.	TFTTF	107.	TFTTF	108.	TFFTT
109.	FFTFT	110.	TTFTT	111.	TFFTT	112.	FFTTT	113.	FTTFF	114.	TTTF
115.	TFTFT	116.	TTTFF	117.	D	118.	A	119.	C	120.	A
121.	A	122.	B	123.	A	124.	A	125.	C	126.	D
127.	B	128.	A	129.	D	130.	C	131.	C	132.	B
133.	C	134.	B	135.	B	136.	C	137.	A	138.	A
139.	B	140.	A	141.	B	142.	D	143.	A	144.	C
145.	A	146.	A	147.	B	148.	C	149.	C	150.	D
151.	A	152.	C	153.	A	154.	A	155.	C	156.	A
157.	B	158.	D	159.	D	160.	D	161.	C	162.	B
163.	C	164.	B	165.	D	166.	C	167.	C	168.	B
169.	D	170.	B	171.	D	172.	D	173.	A	174.	C
175.	D	176.	A	177.	D	178.	A	179.	A	180.	C
181.	A	182.	B	183.	A	184.	D	185.	A	186.	D
187.	D	188.	A	189.	C	190.	B	191.	D	192.	B
193.	A	194.	B	195.	D	196.	B	197.	D	198.	C
199.	C	200.	C	201.	A	202.	A	203.	B	204.	A
205.	D	206.	D	207.	B	208.	A	209.	A	210.	D
211.	A	212.	C	213.	B	214.	A	215.	D	216.	B
217.	A	218.	B	219.	A	220.	C	221.	D	222.	B
223.	A	224.	B	225.	C	226.	A	227.	A	228.	B
229.	A	230.	B	231.	B	232.	A	233.	B	234.	A
235.	C	236.	A	237.	A	238.	D	239.	C	240.	A

241.	C	242.	D	243.	A	244.	D	245.	A	246.	A
247.	A	248.	A	249.	A	250.	B	251.	B	252.	A
253.	C	254.	C	255.	A	256.	D	257.	A	258.	A
259.	D	260.	D	261.	C	262.	B	263.	C	264.	C
265.	B	266.	A	267.	A	268.	D	269.	C	270.	A
271.	B	272.	D	273.	C	274.	A	275.	A	276.	A
277.	C	278.	D	279.	A	280.	A	281.	D	282.	D
283.	B	284.	B	285.	C	286.	C	287.	D	288.	C
289.	C	290.	B	291.	C	292.	A	293.	D	294.	C
295.	A	296.	A	297.	A	298.	A	299.	B	300.	A
301.	B	302.	D	303.	C	304.	D	305.	D	306.	D
307.	D	308.	D	309.	B	310.	D	311.	B	312.	A
313.	A	314.	D	315.	C	316.	C	317.	A	318.	A
319.	A	320.	B	321.	A	322.	D	323.	A	324.	B
325.	B	326.	A	327.	B	328.	D	329.	D	330.	A
331.	A	332.	B	333.	B	334.	D	335.	A	336.	D
337.	D	338.	A	339.	D	340.	A	341.	C	342.	B
343.	B	344.	C	345.	A	346.	C	347.	D	348.	B
349.	A	350.	D	351.	A	352.	C	353.	D	354.	A
355.	C	356.	A	357.	B	358.	B	359.	A	360.	A
361.	A	362.	B	363.	A	364.	D	365.	B	366.	D
367.	A	368.	B	369.	C	370.	C	371.	A	372.	A
373.	C	374.	A	375.	A	376.	B	377.	D	378.	B
379.	C	380.	D	381.	C	382.	C	383.	A	384.	D
385.	A	386.	C	387.	C	388.	A	389.	C	390.	B
391.	A	392.	D	393.	D	394.	C	395.	A	396.	B
397.	B	398.	A	399.	D	400.	B	401.	D	402.	A
403.	C	404.	C	405.	C	406.	D	407.	B	408.	B
409.	C	410.	B	411.	C	412.	D	413.	B	414.	A
415.	A	416.	A	417.	A	418.	A	419.	A	420.	D
421.	A	422.	A	423.	A	424.	B	425.	A	426.	D
427.	C	428.	A	429.	A	430.	A	431.	C	432.	A
433.	C	434.	A	435.	D	436.	B	437.	B	438.	A
439.	B	440.	A	441.	C	442.	B	443.	D	444.	D
445.	A	446.	B	447.	B	448.	B	449.	B	450.	D
451.	C	452.	B	453.	B	454.	A	455.	A	456.	A
457.	C	458.	C	459.	A	460.	D	461.	B	462.	C
463.	C	464.	B	465.	D	466.	B	467.	D	468.	A
469.	A	470.	C	471.	D	472.	C	473.	C	474.	A
475.	C	476.	C	477.	D	478.	D	479.	D	480.	C
481.	B	482.	C	483.	A	484.	B	485.	D	486.	A
487.	B	488.	C	489.	B	490.	A	491.	B	492.	B
493.	D	494.	B	495.	D	496.	D	497.	A	498.	D
499.	A	500.	B	501.	A	502.	C	503.	A	504.	B

505.	D	506.	B	507.	A	508.	C	509.	D	510.	C
511.	D	512.	B	513.	B	514.	D	515.	D	516.	C
517.	D	518.	B	519.	B	520.	C	521.	B	522.	C
523.	C	524.	A	525.	B	526.	A	527.	A	528.	B
529.	B	530.	A	531.	D	532.	A	533.	B	534.	A
535.	C	536.	A	537.	A	538.	E	539.	D	540.	A
541.	B	542.	A	543.	A	544.	C	545.	A	546.	C
547.	A	548.	A	549.	D	550.	D	551.	D	552.	A
553.	E	554.	A	555.	A	556.	A	557.	D	558.	C
559.	D	560.	A	561.	A	562.	A	563.	B	564.	D
565.	E	566.	C	567.	A	568.	B	569.	A	570.	A
571.	A	572.	B	573.	E	574.	B	575.	D	576.	B
577.	A	578.	C	579.	B	580.	B	581.	C	582.	C
583.	C	584.	C	585.	B	586.	B	587.	D	588.	D
589.	A	590.	C	591.	A	592.	C	593.	C	594.	D
595.	B	596.	C	597.	C	598.	D	599.	D	600.	A
601.	C	602.	C	603.	B	604.	B	605.	D	606.	D
607.	B	608.	B	609.	D	610.	A	611.	A	612.	B
613.	A	614.	B	615.	A	616.	A	617.	B	618.	D
619.	D	620.	C	621.	D	622.	C	623.	B	624.	C
625.	A	626.	C	627.	A	628.	B	629.	A	630.	C
631.	C	632.	A	633.	C	634.	C	635.	D	636.	A
637.	A	638.	A	639.	A	640.	B	641.	A	642.	D
643.	B	644.	A	645.	A	646.	B	647.	C	648.	B
649.	C	650.	A	651.	B	652.	C	653.	C	654.	C
655.	C	656.	B	657.	D	658.	C	659.	C	660.	C
661.	D	662.	B	663.	B	664.	D	665.	B	666.	A
667.	A	668.	B	669.	A	670.	D	671.	C	672.	B
673.	D	674.	C	675.	C	676.	D	677.	D	678.	C
679.	B	680.	D	681.	B	682.	B	683.	C	684.	C
685.	D	686.	A	687.	A	688.	B	689.	C	690.	C
691.	C	692.	C	693.	D	694.	C	695.	C	696.	D
697.	A	698.	B	699.	B	700.	D	701.	D	702.	C
703.	D	704.	C	705.	A	706.	D	707.	D	708.	B
709.	D	710.	D	711.	C	712.	A	713.	B	714.	C
715.	D										

(Important MCQs)

CHAPTER 1 Anatomy

1. **Arteries arising from abdominal aorta, from above downwards is:**

   (a) Inferior phrenic artery→adrenal artery →renal artery→gonadal artery

   (b) Inferior phrenic artery→renal artery→ adrenal artery→gonadal artery

   (c) Inferior phrenic artery→gonadal artery →renal artery→adrenal artery

   (d) Inferior phrenic artery→renal artery→ gonadal artery→adrenal artery

(Answer is A) Arteries arising from abdominal aorta– From above downwards.

- Paired inferior phrenic arteries–first to arise.
- Celiac trunk.
- Adrenal arteries.
- Superior mesenteric artery.
- Renal artery (at L2 vertebrae).
- Gonadal artery.
- Inferior mesenteric artery.
- Middle sacral artery– final branch.
- Bifurcation at L4 vertebrae.

2. **Boundary of retroperitoneum are all *except:***

   (a) Sacrospinalis and quadratus lumborum muscles

   (b) Transversus abdominis muscle

   (c) Diaphragm

   (d) Rectus muscle

(Answer is D) The retroperitoneum is bounded posteriorly by the abdominal wall, which consists of the lumbodorsal fascia and the enclosed sacrospinalis and quadratus lumborum muscles. Laterally, the retroperitoneum is contiguous with the preperitoneal fat and is bounded laterally by the transversus abdominis musculature of the lateral abdominal wall. The peritoneum is the anterior limit while cranially the diaphragm.

3. **Which statement regarding lumbodorsal fascia is not correct?**

   (a) The lumbodorsal fascia originates from the spinous processes of the lumbar vertebrae

   (b) The posterior layer provides the posterior covering for the sacrospinalis muscle as well as the origin for the latissimus dorsi muscle

   (c) As it progresses upward, it separates into three layers: posterior, middle and anterior

   (d) The anterior layer of the lumbodorsal fascia forms the anterior margin of the retroperitoneum

(Answer is D) The anterior layer of the lumbodorsal fascia provides the anterior covering to the quadratus lumborum muscle and forms the posterior margin of the retroperitoneum.

4. Which statement regarding psoas muscle is not correct?

(a) Originates from 12th thoracic to 5th lumbar vertebra
(b) Insertion is at lesser trochanter of femur
(c) Action is flexion of hip
(d) Genitofemoral nerve lies posterior to psoas muscle

(Answer is D) Genitofemoral nerve lies directly atop and parallels the psoas muscle.

5. Number of muscles cut in dorsal lumbotomy incision:

(a) 0 (b) 1
(c) 2 (d) 3

(Answer is A) Dorsal lumbotomy incision allows entrance to the retroperitoneum without the violation of the musculature.

6. The limits of the pleura are:

(a) 6th rib anteriorly, the 8th rib in the midaxillary line, and the 10th rib posteriorly
(b) 10th rib anteriorly, the 1lth rib in the midaxillary line and 12th rib posteriorly
(c) 8th rib anteriorly, the 10th rib in the midaxillary line and the 12th rib posteriorly
(d) 9th rib anteriorly, the 10th rib in the midaxillary line and the 11th rib posteriorly

(Answer is C) The limits of the pleura are the 8th rib anteriorly, the 10th rib in the midaxillary line, and the 12th rib posteriorly.

7. Which one is the first branch of abdominal aorta?

(a) Superior mesenteric artery
(b) Inferior phrenic artery
(c) Lumbar artery
(d) Celiac plexus

(Answer is B) During course through the abdomen the aorta gives off a number of large branches. The paired inferior phrenic arteries are first.

8. Which one of the following is the posterior branch of abdominal aorta?

(a) Inferior mesenteric artery
(b) Testicular artery
(c) Middle sacral artery
(d) Middle adrenal artery

(Answer is C) Lumbar and middle sacral artery are posterior branches of aorta.

9. Which statement regarding origin of renal artery is correct?

(a) Originates at L2 just above the origin of superior mesenteric artery
(b) Originates at L2 just below the origin of superior mesenteric artery
(c) Originates at L1 just above the origin of superior mesenteric artery
(d) Originates at Ll just below the origin of superior mesenteric artery

(Answer is B) Overlying the 2nd lumbar vertebrae, the paired renal arteries are the next branching point of the aorta after superior mesenteric artery.

10. Relation of right gonadal artery to IVC and ureter is:

(a) Right gonadal artery crossing anterior to the IYC and then crosses over the ureter
(b) Right gonadal artery crossing anterior to the IVC and then crosses below ureter
(c) Right gonadal artery crossing posterior to IVC and then crosses over the ureter
(d) Right gonadal artery crossing posterior to the IVC and then crosses below ureter

(Answer is A) The right gonadal artery crosses anterior to the inferior vena cava. In men, the gonadal artery then crosses over the ureter.

11. Left renal vein receives:

(a) Left lumbar vein (b) Left gonadal vein
(c) Left adrenal vein (d) All of the above

(Answer is D) Typically after exiting the renal hilum,

the left renal vein receives a lumbar vein posteriorly, the left gonadal vein inferiorly, and the adrenal vein superiorly.

12. Lymphatic flow in retroperitoneum is in direction:

(a) Cranially and left to right
(b) Cranially and right to left
(c) Caudally and left to right
(d) Caudally and right to left

(Answer is B) There is flow not only cranially but also laterally, predominantly from the right to the left.

13. Confluence of common iliac veins lies in what relation to confluence of iliac arteries?

(a) Medial and anterior
(b) Lateral and anterior
(c) Medial and posterior
(d) Lateral and posterior

(Answer is C) Common iliac veins lie medial and posterior to the iliac arteries, the confluence of the iliac veins is posterior and to the right of the aortic bifurcation.

14. Which one is the first tributary of inferior vena cava?

(a) Inferior mesenteric vein
(b) Lumbar vein
(c) Middle sacral vein
(d) Lateral sacral vein

(Answer is C) The first tributary encountered along the IVC is the middle sacral vein.

15. Which one of the following statement regarding lymphatic drainage of testis is not true?

(a) Lymphatic metastases from the right testis drain primarily into the interaortocaval nodes with significant drainage to the right paracaval nodes
(b) From right testis there is a small amount of drainage to the left para-aortic nodes
(c) The left testis drains primarily to the left para-aortic nodes with significant drainage to the interaortocaval nodes
(d) There is small amount of drainage to the right paracaval nodes from left-sided tumor

(Answer is D) The left testis drains primarily to the left para-aortic nodes with significant drainage to the interaortocaval nodes. There is essentially no drainage to the right paracaval nodes from left-sided tumors.

16. Disruption of the sympathetic nerve fibers that travel through which plexuses during retroperitoneal dissection can cause loss of seminal vesicle emission?

(a) Celiac plexus
(b) Renal plexus
(c) Aortic plexus
(d) Superior hypogastric plexus

(Answer is D) At the lower extent of the abdominal aorta, much of the autonomic input to the pelvic urinary organs and genital tract travels through the superior hypogastric plexus. This plexus is contiguous bilaterally with inferior hypogastric plexuses, which extend into the pelvis. Disruption of the sympathetic nerve fibers that travel through these plexuses during retroperitoneal dissection can cause loss of seminal vesicle emission and/or failure of bladder neck closure, resulting in retrograde ejaculation.

17. Which all nerve/s passes between the transversus abdominis and the internal oblique muscle?

(a) Subcostal nerve
(b) Iliohypogastric nerve
(c) Ilioinguinal nerve
(d) All of the above

(Answer is D) The subcostal nerve is the anterior extension of the 12th thoracic nerve and extends laterally beneath the 12th rib. As one proceeds inferiorly, the iliohypogastric nerve and the ilioinguinal nerve originate together as an extension from the first lumbar spinal nerve. These three nerves cross the anterior or inner surface of the quadratus lumborum muscle before piercing the transversus abdominis muscle and continuing their course between this and the internal oblique muscle.

18. Which part of duodenum lies immediately anterior to the right renal hilum and pelvis?

(a) First part (b) Second part
(c) Third part (d) Fourth part

(Answer is B) The second (descending portion) is of most importance to the urologist because it lies immediately anterior to the right renal hilum and pelvis.

19. Which one of the following statement regarding adrenals is not true?

(a) The right gland is more superiorly located in the retroperitoneum
(b) In cases of renal ectopia, the adrenal gland is not affected
(c) The adrenal medulla is of neural crest origin and makes up approximately 90% of the adrenal mass
(d) Grossly, they are yellow-orange

(Answer is C) The adrenal cortex makes up approximately 90% of the adrenal mass.

20. Superior adrenal artery is branch of:

(a) Aorta
(b) Inferior phrenic artery
(c) Superior phrenic artery
(d) Renal artery

(Answer is B) Superiorly, branches from the inferior phrenic artery feed the adrenal, while middle branches originate directly from the aorta. Finally, branches from the ipsilateral renal artery supply the adrenal gland.

21. The adrenal cortex three layers, from external to internal are:

(a) Zona glomerulosa, zona fasciculata and zona reticularis
(b) Zona glomerulosa, zona reticularis and zona fasciculata
(c) Zona fasciculata, zona glomerulosa and zona reticularis
(d) Zona reticularis, zona fasciculata and zona glomerulosa

(Answer is A) The adrenal cortex is of mesodermal origin and makes up approximately 90% of the adrenal mass. It is composed of three layers, from external to internal, the zona glomerulosa, zona fasciculata and zona reticularis.

22. Which statement regarding dromedary hump is not correct?

(a) Focal renal parenchymal bulge along the kidney's lateral contour
(b) This is of pathologic significance
(c) It is more common on the left than the right
(d) It is believed to be caused by downward pressure from the spleen or liver

(Answer is B) Focal renal parenchymal bulge along the kidney's lateral contour, known as a dromedary hump. This is a normal variation without pathologic significance.

23. Orientation of the kidney is in what direction?

(a) Upper poles are situated more medially and posteriorly than the lower poles
(b) Upper poles are situated more laterally and posteriorly than the lower poles
(c) Upper poles are situated more medially and anteriorly than the lower poles
(d) Upper poles are situated more laterally and anteriorly than the lower poles

(Answer is A) Upper poles of kidneys are situated more medially and posteriorly than the lower, poles. Also, the medial aspect of the kidney is more anterior than the lateral aspect.

24. Gerota's fascia envelops the kidney on all aspects *except:*

(a) Medially (b) Superiorly
(c) Inferiorly (d) Laterally

(Answer is C) Gerota's fascia envelops the kidney on all aspects except inferiorly, where it is not closed but instead remains an open potential space.

25. In renal pelvis anterior to posterior is:

(a) Artery, vein and pelvis
(b) Vein, artery and pelvis
(c) Pelvis, vein and artery
(d) Pelvis, artery and vein

(Answer is B) The vein is anterior to the artery. The renal pelvis and ureter is located further posterior to these vascular structures.

26. First and most constant branch of renal artery is:

(a) Posterior (b) Apical
(c) Upper (d) Lower

(Answer is A) Generally, the first and most constant branch is the posterior segmental branch, which separates from the renal artery before it enters the renal hilum.

27. The progression of arterial supply to the kidney is as follows:

(a) Renal artery→segmental artery→ interlobar artery→arcuate artery→ interlobular artery→afferent artery
(b) Renal artery→segmental artery→ interlobular artery→arcuate artery→ interlobar artery→afferent artery
(c) Renal artery→segmental artery→ interlobar artery→interlobular artery→ arcuate artery→afferent artery
(d) Renal artery→segmental artery→ interlobular artery→ interlobar artery→ arcuate artery→afferent artery

(Answer is A) The progression of arterial supply to the kidney is as follows: renal artery→ segmental artery→interlobar artery→arcuate artery→ interlobular artery→afferent artery.

28. The correct order to reach to renal pelvis:

(a) Renal pyramid→papilla→major calyx→ minor calyx→renal pelvis
(b) Renal pyramid→papilla→minor calyx→ major calyx→renal pelvis
(c) Renal papilla→pyramid→major calyx→ minor calyx→renal pelvis
(d) Renal papilla→pyramid→minor calyx→ major calyx→renal pelvis

(Answer is B) Each renal pyramid terminates centrally in a papilla. Each papilla is cupped by a minor calyx. A group of minor calyces join to form a major calyx. The major calyces combine to form the renal pelvis.

29. The right renal vein typically receive how many veins?

(a) 0 (b) 1
(c) 2 (d) 3

(Answer is A) The right renal vein typically does not receive any vein.

30. Anatomic variations in the renal vasculature occurs in:

(a) 0% to 15% (b) 15% to 25%
(c) 25% to 40% (d) 40% to 50%

(Answer is C) Anatomic variations in the renal vasculature are common, occurring in 25% to 40% of kidneys. The most common variation is supernumerary renal arteries, with upto five arteries reported. This occurs more often on the left.

31. How many papillae are there per kidney?

(a) 5 to 7 (b) 7 to 9
(c) 9 to 11 (d) 11 to 13

(Answer is B) The renal papillae are the tip of a medullary pyramid and constitute the first gross structure of the renal collecting system. Typically, there are 7 to 9 papillae per kidney.

32. Which statement regarding compound calyces is not correct?

(a) More often encountered at middle pole
(b) These compound calyces are the result of renal pyramid fusion
(c) More likely to allow reflux into the renal parenchyma
(d) More severe scarring of the parenchyma overlying compound calyces

(Answer is A) At the upper and lower poles, compound calyces are often encountered. These compound calyces are the result of renal pyramid fusion and because of their anatomy are more likely to allow reflux into the renal parenchyma. Clinically, this can result in more severe scarring of the parenchyma overlying compound calyces.

33. Which statement regarding renal innervation is not correct?

(a) Sympathetic preganglionic nerves originate from the L2 through L4
(b) Parasympathetic fibers originate from the vagus nerve
(c) Sympathetics inducing vasoconstriction and the parasympathetics causing vasodilation
(d) Kidney functions well even without this neurologic control

(Answer is A) Sympathetic preganglionic nerves originate from the eighth thoracic through first lumbar spinal segments and then travel to the celiac and aorticorenal ganglia.

34. Blood vessels and lymphatics travel along which layer of ureter?

(a) Lamina propria
(b) Inner longitudinal layer
(c) Outer circular layer
(d) Adventitia

(Answer is D) The outermost layer is the adventitia. This thin layer surrounds the ureter and encompasses the blood vessels and lymphatics that travel along the ureter.

35. Ureter can be identified at:

(a) Bifurcation of aorta
(b) Bifurcation of common iliac artery
(c) At origin of anterior branch of internal iliac artery
(d) At origin of posterior branch of internal iliac artery

(Answer is B) As it enters the pelvis the ureter crosses anterior to the iliac vessels. This crossover point is usually at the bifurcation of the common iliac into the internal and external iliac arteries, thus making this a useful landmark for pelvic procedures.

36. Normal ureter has distinct narrowings at:

(a) Ureteropelvic junction
(b) At crossing of the iliac vessels
(c) Ureterovesical junction
(d) All of the above

(Answer is D) The normal ureter is not of uniform caliber, with three distinct narrowings classically described: the ureteropelvic junction, crossing of the iliac vessels, and the ureterovesical junction.

37. Ureter is supplied by all vessels *except:*

(a) Superior vesical artery
(b) Inferior vesical artery
(c) Superior rectal artery
(d) Middle rectal artery

(Answer is C) For the upper ureter arterial branches originate from the renal artery, gonadal artery, abdominal aorta, and common iliac artery. After entering the pelvis, additional small arterial branches to the distal ureter may arise from the internal iliac artery or its branches, especially the vesical and uterine arteries, but also from the middle rectal and vaginal arteries.

38. True physical restriction of ureter is at:

(a) Ureteropelvic junction
(b) At crossing of iliac vessels
(c) Ureterovesical junction
(d) All of the above

(Answer is C) The third site of narrowing observed in the normal ureter is the ureterovesical junction. There is a true physical restriction of the ureter as it makes the intramural passage through the bladder wall to the ureteral orifice.

39. Which statement regarding lymphatics of ureter is not correct?

(a) In the pelvis, ureteral lymphatics drain to iliac nodes
(b) In the abdomen, the interaortocaval lymph nodes are the primary drainage site for the left ureter
(c) In the abdomen, the right ureter is drained primarily to right paracaval and interaortocaval lymph nodes
(d) The lymphatic drainage of the upper ureter and renal pelvis tends to join the renal lymphatics

(Answer is B) In the abdomen, the left para-aortic lymph nodes are the primary drainage site for the left ureter whereas the abdominal portion of the right ureter is drained primarily to right paracaval and interaortocaval lymph nodes.

40. For normal ureteral peristalsis pacemaker site is located at:

(a) Renal pelvis (b) Minor calyx
(c) Major calyx (d) Renal pyramid

(Answer is B) Normal ureteral peristalsis does not require outside autonomic input but, rather, originates and is propagated from intrinsic smooth muscle pacemaker sites located in the minor calyces of the renal collecting system.

41. Which statement regarding renal innervation is not correct?

(a) Normal ureteral peristalsis requires autonomic input
(b) The ureter receives preganglionic sympathetic input from the 10th thoracic through 2nd lumbar spinal segments
(c) Postganglionic fibers arise from several ganglia in the aorticorenal, superior and inferior hypogastric autonomic plexuses
(d) Parasympathetic input is received from the 2nd through 4th sacral spinal segments

(Answer is A) Normal ureteral peristalsis does not require outside autonomic input but, rather, originates and is propagated from intrinsic smooth muscle pacemaker sites located in the minor calyces of the renal collecting system.

42. Pain caused by ureteral stone is due to all *except:*

(a) Renal pain fibers are stimulated by tension (distention) in the renal capsule
(b) Direct mucosal irritation in the upper urinary tract may also stimulate nociceptors
(c) Signals travel with the parasympathetic nerves and result in a visceral-type pain
(d) Pain and reflex muscle spasm are typically produced over the distributions of the subcostal, iliohypogastric, ilioinguinal, and/or genitofemoral nerves

(Answer is C) Signals travel with the sympathetic nerves and result in a visceral-type pain referred to the sympathetic distribution of the kidney and ureter (eighth thoracic through second lumbar).

43. Which one of the following statement regarding bony pelvis is not true?

(a) True and false pelvis are separated by the arcuate line
(b) Cooper's (pectineal) ligament overlies the pectineal line and offers a sure hold for sutures in hernia repairs
(c) The pubes is the thinnest of the pelvic bones
(d) The sacrotuberous ligament separates the greater and lesser sciatic foramina

(Answer is D) The sacrospinous ligament separates the greater and lesser sciatic foramina.

44. Which vessels can cause troublesome bleeding during placement of pelvic laparoscopic ports?

(a) Superficial circumflex iliac
(b) External pudendal
(c) Superficial inferior epigastric
(d) Superficial superior epigastric

(Answer is C) The superficial inferior epigastric vessels are encountered during inguinal incisions and can cause troublesome bleeding during placement of pelvic laparoscopic ports.

45. In rupture of penile urethra extravasation will not spread to:

(a) Scrotum
(b) Deep to dartos fascia
(c) Perineum
(d) Leg

(Answer is D) In the perineum, extravasation is limited by the fusions of Colles' fascia to the ischiopubic rami laterally and to the posterior edge of the perineal membrane; the resulting hematoma is therefore butterfly shaped. They will not extend down the leg or into the buttock, but they can freely travel up the anterior abdominal wall deep to Scarpa's fascia to the clavicles and around the flank to the back.

46. The internal inguinal ring lies at:

(a) Midway between the anterior superior iliac spine and the pubic tubercle, above the inguinal ligament
(b) Midway between the anterior superior iliac spine and the pubic tubercle, below the inguinal ligament
(c) Midway between the anterior superior iliac spine and the pubic symphysis, above the inguinal ligament
(d) Midway between the anterior superior iliac spine and the pubic symphysis, below the inguinal ligament

(Answer is A) The internal inguinal ring lies midway between the anterior superior iliac spine and the pubic tubercle, above the inguinal ligament, and 4 cm lateral to the external ring.

47. The obliterated umbilical artery serves as an important landmark:

(a) Ureter lies medial to its origin from internal iliac artery
(b) Ureter lies medial to its origin from external iliac artery
(c) Ureter lies lateral to its origin from internal iliac artery
(d) Ureter lies medial to its origin from external iliac artery

(Answer is A) The obliterated umbilical artery in the medial umbilical fold serves as an important landmark for the surgeon. It may be traced to its origin from the internal iliac artery to locate the ureter, which lies on its medial side.

48. Which structure contains the inferior epigastric vessels?

(a) The medial umbilical fold
(b) The median umbilical fold
(c) The lateral umbilical fold
(d) None of the above

(Answer is C) The lateral umbilical fold contains the inferior epigastric vessels as they ascend to supply the rectus abdominis.

49. Bifurcation of aorta and common iliac artery is at which level respectively?

(a) L3 and L5
(b) L4 and Sl
(c) L3 and sacroiliac joint
(d) L4 and sacroiliac joint

(Answer is D) The common iliac arteries arise at the level of the fourth lumbar vertebra, run anterior and lateral to their accompanying veins, and bifurcate into the external and internal iliac arteries at the SI joint.

50. Which one of the following is not the branch from posterior trunk of internal iliac artery?

(a) Accessory obturator artery
(b) Superior gluteal artery
(c) Ascending lumbar artery
(d) Lateral sacral artery

(Answer is A) In 25% of people, an accessory obturator artery arises from the inferior epigastric artery and runs medial to the femoral vein to reach the obturator canal.

51. Relative to uterine vessel, ureter is:

(a) Anteriorly (b) Posteriorly
(c) Medially (d) Laterally

(Answer is B) The uterine artery passes above and in front of the ureter ("water flows under the bridge").

52. During a psoas hitch, which nerve can get entrapped?

(a) Obturator (b) Femoral
(c) Genitofemoral (d) Pudendal

(Answer is B) During a psoas hitch, sutures should be placed in the direction of the nerve (and the psoas muscle fibers) to avoid nerve damage or entrapment. Retractor blades must not rest on the psoas muscle because they can produce a femoral nerve palsy.

53. Which statement regarding nervi erigentes is true?

(a) Originates from S2, S3 and S4 and is parasympathetic fibers from the sacral cord
(b) Originates from S1, S2 and S3 and is parasympathetic fibers from the sacral cord
(c) Originates from S2, S3 and S4 and is sympathetic fibers from the sacral cord
(d) Originates from S1, S2 and S3 and is sympathetic fibers from the sacral cord

(Answer is A) Nervi erigentes originates from S2, S3 and S4 and is parasympathetic fibers from the sacral cord.

54. During radical prostatectomy, the nerves are most vulnerable at which site?

(a) The base of the prostate, where they closely approach the prostatic capsule at the 5- and 7-O'clock positions
(b) The apex of the prostate, where they closely approach the prostatic capsule at the 5- and 7-O'clock positions
(c) The base of the prostate, where they closely approach the prostatic capsule at the 1- and 11-O'clock positions
(d) The apex of the prostate, where they closely approach the prostatic capsule at the 1- and 11-O'clock positions

(Answer is B) During radical prostatectomy, the nerves are most vulnerable at the apex of the prostate, where they closely approach the prostatic capsule at the 5- and 7-O'clock positions.

55. Ureter is divided into abdominal and pelvic portions by:

(a) Common iliac artery
(b) External iliac artery
(c) Internal iliac artery
(d) Superior vesical artery

(Answer is A) The ureter is divided into abdominal and pelvic portions by the common iliac artery.

56. The ovarian vessels cross the iliac vessels in what relation to ureter?

(a) Posterior and lateral
(b) Anterior and lateral
(c) Anterior and medial
(d) Posterior and medial

(Answer is B) The ovarian vessels (infundibulopelvic ligament) cross the iliac vessels anterior and lateral to the ureter, and dissection of the ovarian vessels at the pelvic brim is a common cause of ureteral injury. As it passes in front of the vagina, it crosses 1.5 cm anterior and lateral to the uterine cervix. The ureter may be injured at this level during hysterectomy.

57. Pelvic peritoneum should be incised in what relation to ureter?

(a) Laterally (b) Medially
(c) Anteriorly (d) Posteriorly

(Answer is B) Blood supply to the pelvic ureter enters laterally; thus, the pelvic peritoneum should be incised only medial to the ureter.

58. Which one of the following statement regarding pelvic ureter is not true?

(a) The pelvic ureter receives abundant blood supply from the common iliac artery and most branches of the internal iliac artery
(b) The pelvic ureter appears to have a low preponderance of plexiform vessels, which render it less susceptible to ischemia
(c) Pathologic enlargement of the common and internal iliac nodes can encroach on and obstruct the pelvic ureter
(d) The pelvic ureter has rich adrenergic and cholinergic autonomic innervation derived from the pelvic plexus

(Answer is B) The pelvic ureter appears to have a high preponderance of plexiform vessels, which render it more susceptible to ischemia and less suitable for ureteroureterostomy.

59. Which statement regarding female bladder neck is correct?

(a) Middle circular layer does not appear to be as robust
(b) Possess little adrenergic innervation
(c) Its sphincteric function is limited
(d) All of the above

(Answer is D) The female bladder neck differs strikingly from the male in possessing little adrenergic innervation. In addition, its sphincteric function is limited; in 50% of continent women, urine enters the proximal urethra during a cough.

60. The bulk of the lymphatic drainage of bladder passes to:

(a) External iliac lymph node
(b) Internal iliac lymph node
(c) Common iliac lymph node
(d) Obturator lymph node

(Answer is A) The bulk of the lymphatic drainage passes to the external iliac lymph nodes. Some anterior and lateral drainage may go through the obturator and internal iliac nodes, whereas portions of the bladder base and trigone may drain into the internal and common iliac groups.

61. Lymphatic drainage of prostate is primarily to:

(a) External and common iliac lymph node
(b) External and internal iliac lymph node
(c) Internal and common iliac lymph node
(d) Internal iliac lymph node and obturator lymph node

(Answer is D) Lymphatic drainage is primarily to the obturator and internal iliac nodes. A small portion of drainage may initially pass through the presacral group, or less commonly, the external iliac nodes.

62. The prostate is composed of approximately:

(a) 30% glandular elements and 70% fibromuscular stroma
(b) 70% glandular elements and 30% fibromuscular stroma
(c) 60% glandular elements and 40% fibromuscular stroma
(d) 40% glandular elements and 60% fibromuscular stroma

(Answer is B) The prostate is composed of approximately 70% glandular elements and 30% fibromuscular stroma.

63. Plicae colliculi is present in:

(a) Kidney (b) Ureter
(c) Bladder (d) Urethra

(Answer is D) Plicae colliculi is present in urethra.

64. Which one of the following statement regarding transition zone of prostate is not true?

(a) Transition zone accounts for 5% to 10% of the glandular tissue of the prostate
(b) A discrete fibromuscular band of tissue separates the transition zone from the remaining glandular compartments
(c) The transition zone commonly gives rise to benign prostatic hypertrophy
(d) 10% of adenocarcinomas of the prostate originate in this zone

(Answer is D) It is estimated that 20% of adenocarcinomas of the prostate originate in transition zone.

65. Which zone is most commonly affected by prostatic cancers and also chronic prostatitis?

(a) Posterior zone
(b) Transition zone
(c) Central zone
(d) Anterior fibromuscular stroma

(Answer is A) Seventy percent of prostatic cancers arise in posterior zone, and it is the zone most commonly affected by chronic prostatitis.

66. In BPH adenoma is supplied by:

(a) Capsular arteries
(b) Urethral arteries
(c) Superior vesical artery
(d) Obturator artery

(Answer is B) In benign prostatic hypertrophy, urethral arteries provide the principal blood supply of the adenoma.

67. Membranous urethra spans on average:

(a) 1 to 1.5 cm (b) 1.5 to 2 cm
(c) 2 to 2.5 cm (d) 2.5 to 3 cm

(Answer is C) The membranous urethra spans on average 2 to 2.5 cm (range, 1.2 to 5 cm).

68. Which statement regarding striated (external) urethral sphincter is not correct?

(a) Membranous urethra is surrounded by the striated urethral sphincter
(b) The striated sphincter is signet ring-shaped
(c) Sphincter consists only of 80% type I (slow-twitch) and 20% type II fibers
(d) Throughout its length, the posterior portion of the striated sphincter inserts into the perineal body

(Answer is C) Membranous urethra is surrounded by the striated (external) urethral sphincter, which is often incorrectly depicted as a flat sheet of muscle sandwiched between two layers of fascia. The striated sphincter is actually signet ring-shaped. In contrast to the levator ani, the sphincter consists only of fine, type I (slow-twitch) fibers.

69. Which statement regarding vas is not correct?

(a) The terminal vas is dilated and tortuous and is capable of storing spermatozoa
(b) The vas has a thick wall of outer longitudinal and inner circular smooth muscle
(c) Lined by pseudostratified columnar epithelium
(d) It has got motile stereocilia

(Answer is D) The terminal vas is dilated and tortuous (ampulla) and is capable of storing spermatozoa. The vas has a thick wall of outer longitudinal and inner circular smooth muscle and is lined by pseudostratified columnar epithelium with nonmotile stereocilia.

70. Which one of the following statement regarding seminal vesicle is not true?

(a) The seminal vesicle is a lateral outpouching of the vas
(b) Approximately 5 cm long, with a capacity of 3 to 4 ml
(c) It store sperm

(d) Contributes the largest portion of fluid to the ejaculate

(Answer is C) Despite its name, it does not store sperm but contributes the largest portion of fluid to the ejaculate.

71. Which one of the following statement regarding scrotum is not true?

(a) The anterior wall of the scrotum is supplied by the external pudendal vessels and the ilioinguinal and genitofemoral nerves
(b) The back of the scrotum is supplied by the posterior scrotal branches of the perineal vessels and nerves
(c) The anterior vessels and nerves typically run parallel to the rugae and crosses the raphe
(d) Fournier's gangrene usually does not involve testis

(Answer is C) The anterior vessels and nerves typically run parallel to the rugae and do not cross the raphe, thus, transverse or midline raphe scrotal incisions are most appropriate and they may be spared during debridement.

72. The epididymis attaches at which aspect of the testis?

(a) Posterolateral (b) Posteromedial
(c) Anterolateral (d) Anteromedial

(Answer is A) The epididymis attaches to the posterolateral aspect of the testis.

73. From which pole the biopsy should be undertaken?

(a) Lower pole for testis and upper pole for kidney
(b) Upper pole for testis and lower pole for kidney
(c) Lower pole for both testis and kidney
(d) Upper pole for both testis and kidney

(Answer is B) Testicular biopsy should be carried out in the medial or lateral surface of the upper pole, where the risk of vascular injury is minimal.

74. The mature genitourinary system develops from all of the following embryonic sources, *except:*

(a) Intermediate mesoderm
(b) Mesothelium of coelomic cavity
(c) Endoderm of the urogenital sinus
(d) Somatic ectoderm

(Answer is D) Somatic ectoderm

75. At which week of gestation do the primordial germ cells migrate to form the genital ridges?

(a) Third (b) Fourth
(c) Fifth (d) Seventh

(Answer is C) Fifth

76. All of the following develop from the mesonephric ducts, *except:*

(a) Vas deferens
(b) Seminal vesicles
(c) Appendix epididymis
(d) Appendix testis

(Answer is D) Appendix testis

77. Which period of intrauterine life does the process of organ formation (organogenesis) take place?

(a) 9 – 12 weeks (b) 12 – 15 weeks
(c) 15 – 18 weeks (d) 18 – 21 weeks

(Answer is A) 9 – 12 weeks

78. At what month of intrauterine life do testes descend into the scrotum with the aid of the intra-abdominal pressure and the gubernacula?

(a) Sixth (b) Seventh
(c) Eighth (d) Ninth

(Answer is B) Seventh

79. By which of the following structures, do the fused lower poles of horseshoe kidneys get trapped during embryologic ascent?

(a) Inferior mesenteric artery

(b) Superior mesenteric artery
(c) Celiac artery
(d) Common iliac artery

(Answer is A) Inferior mesenteric artery

80. Regarding renal ectopia, usually, the adrenals:

(a) Are cross ectopic
(b) Are at their normal position
(c) Travel with the kidneys
(d) Undergo ischemic atrophy

(Answer is B) Are at their normal position

81. How many renal papillae are there in a typical kidney?

(a) 4 to 6
(b) 7 to 9
(c) 10 to 12
(d) 13 to 14

(Answer is B) 7 to 9

82. Which innervations mediate detumescence?

(a) Cavernous nerves
(b) Dorsal nerves of the penis
(c) Sympathetic nervous system
(d) Parasympathetic nervous system

(Answer is C) Sympathetic nervous system

83. Which part of the male urethra is the narrowest?

(a) The membranous
(b) The bladder neck
(c) The bulbous
(d) The external urethral meatus

(Answer is D) The external urethral meatus

84. Which statement is true about the female urethra?

(a) Harder to catheterize when compared to the male urethra
(b) 4 inch long
(c) Opens into the vestibule below the clitoris
(d) Gets wider at the post-menopausal age

(Answer is C) Opens into the vestibule below the clitoris

85. Which structure is a part of the renal hilum?

(a) Renal pelvis
(b) Branches of the renal artery
(c) Tributaries of renal vein
(d) All of the above

(Answer is D) All of the above

86. Which artery is not a branch of the anterior division of internal iliac artery?

(a) Superior vesical artery
(b) Inferior vesical artery
(c) Superior gluteal artery
(d) Inferior gluteal artery

(Answer is C) Superior gluteal artery

87. In males, which of the following structure(s) can not be palpated during digital rectal examination?

(a) Pelvic floor muscles
(b) Seminal vesicles
(c) Anterior surface of the sacrum
(d) Median lobe of the prostate

(Answer is D) Median lobe of the prostate

88. Which of the following is not a part of the urogenital diaphragm structures?

(a) Perineal membrane
(b) Deep transverse perineal muscle
(c) Urethral sphincter
(d) Camper's fascia

(Answer is D) Camper's fascia

89. Which statement is false concerning the gubernaculum?

(a) Degenerate after birth
(b) Called the caudal genital ligaments
(c) Help guide the testes down through the inguinal canals

(d) Represent undifferentiated mesenchyme

(Answer is A) Degenerate after birth

90. Regarding multicystic kidneys, at what age does the compensatory renal growth end?

(a) At birth (b) 2 years
(c) At puberty (d) None of the above

(Answer is B) 2 years

91. What are the posterior relations of the kidneys?

(a) Quadratus lumborum and diaphragm
(b) Psoas and diaphragm
(c) Psoas and latissimus dorsi
(d) Transversus abdominus and paraspinous

(Answer is A) Quadratus lumborum and diaphragm

92. What are the abnormalities that might accompany complete ureteral duplications?

(a) Reflux to the upper pole ureter, obstruction to the lower pole ureter
(b) Reflux to the lower pole ureter, obstruction to the upper pole ureter
(c) Left ureteropelvic junction obstruction, right ureterocele
(d) Right ureteropelvic junction obstruction, left ureterocele

(Answer is B) Reflux to the lower pole ureter, obstruction to the upper pole ureter

93. Which of the following is (are) direct branch(es) of the abdominal aorta?

(a) Median sacral artery
(b) Inferior phrenic arteries
(c) Gonadal arteries
(d) All of the above

(Answer is D) All of the above

94. Which anomaly might accompany horseshoe kidneys?

(a) Ureteropelvic junction obstruction
(b) Ureterocele
(c) Ureteral reflux
(d) Ureteral atresia

(Answer is A) Ureteropelvic junction obstruction

95. Which layer lies between the superficial and deep inguinal lymph nodes?

(a) Scarpa's fascia (b) Fascia lata
(c) Dartos fascia (d) Camper's fascia

(Answer is B) Fascia lata

96. What is the narrowest part of the ureter?

(a) Uretero-pelvic junction
(b) Uretero-vesical junction
(c) Where ureters cross the pelvic brim
(d) Where ureters cross the common iliac bifurcation

(Answer is B) Uretero-vesical junction

97. Where is Santorini plexus located?

(a) At either side of the prostate
(b) In the pubo-prostatic space
(c) Anterior to the seminal vesicles
(d) Posterior to the vaso-epididymal junction

(Answer is B) In the pubo-prostatic space

98. What is false concerning renal vasculature?

(a) There are 4 surgical segments of the kidney, based on the segmental artery distribution
(b) Along the kidney convexity, there is an avascular plane
(c) There are no collaterals between segmental arteries
(d) In < 10%, the posterior branch is the first to branch off the renal artery

(Answer is D) In < 10%, the posterior branch is the first to branch off the renal artery

99. From where does the main parasympathetic efferent innervation to the pelvic plexus arise?

(a) S_1
(b) S_2-S_4
(c) T_{11}-L_2
(d) L_3-S_1

(Answer is B) S_2-S_4

100. Branches of what artery travel under the endopelvic fascia form the prostate to the sidewall of the pelvis?

(a) Obturator artery
(b) Midrectal artery
(c) Inferior vesical artery
(d) Pudendal artery

(Answer is D) Pudendal artery

101. Between which 2 fascial planes does the prostatic neurovascular bundle travel?

(a) Prostatic fascia and levator fascia
(b) Prostate capsule and prostatic fascia
(c) Denonvilliers fascia and prostate capsule
(d) Denonvilliers fascia and endopelvic fascia

(Answer is A) Prostatic fascia and levator fascia

CHAPTER

2

Clinical Decision Making

1. **Which statement regarding testicular masses is not correct:**
   (a) A firm or hard area within the testis–considered malignant until proved otherwise
   (b) Most masses arising from the testis–malignant
   (c) Most masses arising from the spermatic cord structures–benign
   (d) Pain is the most useful criterion–distinguishing torsion from epididymitis

(Answer is D) Age is the most useful criterion to distinguish torsion from epididymitis.

2. **Which of the following statement regarding genitourinary pain is not true?**
   (a) Pain arising from genitourinary tract is not related to size of stone
   (b) Inflammation of the mucosa of a hollow viscous such as the bladder or urethra usually produces severe pain
   (c) Pain associated with GU malignancies is usually a late manifestation and a sign of advanced disease
   (d) Pain due to inflammation is steady, whereas pain due to obstruction is fluctuating in intensity

(Answer is B) Inflammation of the GU tract is most severe when it involves the parenchyma of a GU organ. This is due to edema and distention of the capsule surrounding the organ. Inflammation of the mucosa of a hollow viscus such as the bladder or urethra usually produces discomfort, but the pain is not severe.

3. **Pain in the flaccid penis is usually secondary to:**
   (a) Inflammation in the bladder or urethra
   (b) Phimosis
   (c) Peyronie disease
   (d) Priapism

(Answer is A) Pain in the flaccid penis is usually secondary to inflammation in the bladder or urethra, with referred pain that is experienced maximally at the urethral meatus.

4. **How many RBC/HPF is significant?**
   (a) >1 (b) >2
   (c) >3 (d) >4

(Answer is C) Greater than three red blood cells per high-power microscopic field (HPF) is significant.

5. **All statements regarding hematuria are correct *except:***
   (a) Initial hematuria is usually secondary to inflammation in the area of kidney and bladder
   (b) Painful hematuria usually results from upper urinary tract
   (c) In patients presenting with hematuria, cystoscopy is must
   (d) Hematuria in adults should be regarded as symptoms of malignancy until proved otherwise

(Answer is A) Initial hematuria usually arises from the urethra; it occurs least commonly and is usually secondary to inflammation.

6. Regarding BPH which statement is true?

(a) BPH more commonly present with obstructive than irritative symptoms
(b) Most common presenting symptom is nocturia
(c) Post void dribbling is late presentation
(d) Most common cause of gross hematuria after 50 years of age

(Answer is B) BPH more commonly present with irritative than obstructive symptoms. Post void dribbling is early presentation and most common cause of gross hematuria after 50 years of age is bladder malignancy.

7. Which of the following is not included in AUA symptom score?

(a) Frequency, urgency, nocturia
(b) Intermittency, incomplete emptying
(c) Straining, poor stream
(d) Quality of life

(Answer is D) Quality of life is included in IPSS score and not in AUA score.

8. Which of the following is not included in IPSS?

(a) Frequency, urgency, nocturia
(b) Intermittency, incomplete emptying
(c) Incontinence
(d) Quality of life

(Answer is C) IPSS score includes urgency but not incontinence in its scoring system.

9. In IPSS moderate symptoms are scored between:

(a) 7 to 18 (b) 8 to 19
(c) 7 to 19 (d) 8 to 18

(Answer is B) The total symptom score ranges from 0 to 35 with scores of 0 to 7, 8 to 19 and 20 to 35 indicating mild, moderate and severe lower urinary tract symptoms, respectively.

10. Ectopic ureter in male can enter in all *except:*

(a) Bladder neck (b) Prostatic urethra
(c) Bulbous urethra (d) Seminal vesicles

(Answer is C) Ectopic ureters never produce urinary in continence in males because they always enter the bladder neck or prostatic urethra proximal to the external urethral sphincter.

11. Which incontinence is otherwise called as paradoxical incontinence?

(a) Continuous incontinence
(b) Stress incontinence
(c) Urge incontinence
(d) Overflow incontinence

(Answer is D) Overflow incontinence has been termed paradoxical incontinence because it can often be cured by relief of bladder outlet obstruction.

12. Children with nocturnal enuresis at which age should undergo urinary evaluation?

(a) 4 years (b) 6 years
(c) 10 years (d) 15 years

(Answer is B) All children older than age 6 years with enuresis should undergo a urologic evaluation.

13. Patients with hematospermia that persists beyond several weeks should undergo further urologic evaluation by all *except:*

(a) Genital and rectal examination
(b) Prostate-specific antigen (PSA)
(c) Urinary cytology
(d) USG scrotum

(Answer is D) A genital and rectal examination should be done to exclude the presence of tuberculosis, a prostate-specific antigen (PSA) and a rectal examination done to exclude prostatic carcinoma, and a urinary cytology done to exclude the possibility of transitional cell carcinoma of the prostate.

14. Urinary retention is side effects of all group of drugs *except:*

(a) Anticholinergics
(b) α-adrenergic antagonist
(c) Antihistamines
(d) Calcium channel blockers

(Answer is B) Urinary retention or obstructive voiding symptoms is caused by anticholinergic agents or musculotropic relaxants, anti-parkinsonian drugs, α-adrenergic agonists and antihistamines.

15. By what age phimosis is considered as normal?

(a) 1 year (b) 2 years
(c) 4 years (d) 6 years

(Answer is C) In males younger than 4 years old it is normal for the foreskin to be unretractable.

16. Peyronie's disease results in fibrosis of the:

(a) Tunica vaginalis (b) Tunica albuginea
(c) Tunica vasculosa (d) All of the above

(Answer is B) Peyronie's disease is a common condition that results in fibrosis of the tunica albuginea.

17. Incidence of testicular tumors presenting as reactive hydrocele is:

(a) 1% (b) 5%
(c) 10% (d) 20%

(Answer is C) About 10% of testicular tumors present as an associated reactive hydrocele.

18. Incidence of men with early prostate cancer who will have a normal serum PSA test is:

(a) 10% (b) 20%
(c) 30% (d) 40%

(Answer is C) 30% of men with early prostate cancer will have a normal serum PSA test.

19. Which of the following statements regarding collection of urine samples is not correct?

(a) In male patients midstream urine sample should be collected
(b) In a female, a catheterized urine sample should always be obtained
(c) In neonates suprapubic aspiration of urine sample is best
(d) Sample should be examined within 6 hours of collection

(Answer is D) Whenever possible, all urine samples should be examined within 1 hour of collection and plated for culture and sensitivity if indicated.

20. Most common cause of cloudy urine is:

(a) Dehydration (b) Chyluria
(c) Pyuria (d) Phosphaturia

(Answer is D) Cloudy urine is most commonly due to phosphaturia.

21. Urine sample should be refrigerated at what temperature?

(a) –20°C (b) 0°C
(c) 5°C (d) 20°C

(Answer is C) If urine is allowed to stand at room temperature for longer periods of time, bacterial overgrowth may occur, the pH may change, and red and white blood cell casts may disintegrate. If it is not possible to examine the urine promptly, it should be refrigerated at 5°C.

22. Conditions that decrease urine specific gravity include all *except:*

(a) Increased fluid intake
(b) Diuretics
(c) Decreased renal concentrating ability
(d) Diabetes mellitus

(Answer is D) Conditions that increase specific gravity include (1) decreased fluid intake; (2) dehydration owing to fever, sweating, vomiting and diarrhea; (3) diabetes mellitus (glucosuria); and (4) inappropriate secretion of antidiuretic hormone.

23. Urine osmolality usually vades between:

(a) 50 and 1200 mOsm/l
(b) 200 and 2000 mOsm/l

(c) 50 and 500 mOsm /l
(d) 500 and 1500 mOsm /l

(Answer is A) Osmolality is a measure of the amount of material dissolved in the urine and usually varies between 50 and 1200 mOsm/l.

24. Average urinary pH may vary from:

(a) 3.5 to 4.5 (b) 4.5 to 5.5
(c) 5.5 to 6.5 (d) 6.5 to 7.5

(Answer is C) Urinary pH may vary from 4.5 to 8; the average pH varies between 5.5 and 6.5.

25. In which condition, on microscopic examination of urine, erythrocytes will be absent and on centrifugation of blood supernatant will be pink?

(a) Hematuria (b) Hemoglobinuria
(c) Myoglobinuria (d) Porphyria

(Answer is B) In hemoglobinuria, on centrifugation of blood, the supernatant will be pink.

26. Which statement regarding hematuria is not correct?

(a) Specificity of the dipstick for hematuria compared with microscopy is lower
(b) Examining urine of first morning voided specimen, increases the likelihood of a false-negative result
(c) False-positive dipstick readings most often are due to contamination of the urine specimen
(d) The normal individual excretes about 1000 erythrocytes/ml of urine, with the upper limits of normal varying from 5000 to 8000 erythrocytes/ml

(Answer is B) Examining urine of high specific gravity, such as the first morning voided specimen, increases the likelihood of a false-positive result.

27. Ten years male child presented with hematuria, low grade fever and erythematous skin rash. Urine examination revealed dysmorphic erythrocytes and proteinuria. Diagnosis is:

(a) Buerger's disease
(b) Alport disease
(c) Goodpasture syndrome
(d) Post streptococcal glomerulonephritis

(Answer is A) Buerger's disease occurs most commonly in children and young adults, with a male predominance. Patients typically present with hematuria after an upper respiratory tract infection or exercise. Hematuria may be associated with a low-grade fever or rash, but most patients have no associated systemic symptoms.

28. (AUA) Best Practice Policy Panel for evaluation of microscopic hematuria includes all *except:*

(a) Voided urinary cytology
(b) Cystoscopy
(c) Urinary tract imaging using (USG, CT and/ or IVU)
(d) Urine culture

(Answer is D) The mainstays of evaluation, according to the panel, are voided urinary cytology, cystoscopy, and urinary tract imaging using ultrasonography, CT, and/or intravenous urography (IVU).

29. Which of the following statement regarding proteinuria is not correct?

(a) Glomerular disease is almost certain if proteinuria >3 gms/day
(b) Tubular disease is seldom if proteinuria >3 gms/day
(c) Glomerular proteinuria is the most common type of proteinuria
(d) In tubular proteinuria excreted protein is mostly albumin

(Answer is D) In tubular proteinuria, the 24-hour urine protein loss seldom exceeds 2 to 3 g and the excreted proteins are of low molecular weight rather than albumin.

30. Healthy adults excrete how much of protein in the urine daily?

(a) Nil (b) Upto 30 mg
(c) 30 to 80 mg (d) 80 to 150 mg

(Answer is D) Healthy adults excrete 80 to 150 mg of protein in the urine daily.

31. Transient proteinuria is because of all *except:*

(a) Fever
(b) Emotional stress
(c) Congestive heart failure
(d) Myocardial infarction

(Answer is D) Transient proteinuria results from fever, exercise, or emotional stress. In older patients, it may be due to congestive heart failure.

32. All are true about urine examination *except:*

(a) Dipstick test for ketones identify only acetoacetic acid
(b) Leukocyte esterase activity indicates the presence of white blood cells in the urine
(c) Nitrites are normally found in the urine
(d) The presence of nitrites in the urine is strongly suggestive of bacteriuria

(Answer is C) Nitrites are not normally found in the urine, but many species of gram-negative bacteria can convert nitrates to nitrites.

33. What levels of WBC/HPF is considered normal in men and women respectively?

(a) Any WBC/HPF is significant in both sex
(b) < 2 WBC/HPF in men and up to 5/HPF in women
(c) < 5 WBC/HPF in men and up to 2/HPF in women
(d) <5 WBC/HPF is significant in both sex

(Answer is B) It is normal to find 1 or 2 leukocytes/HPF in men and up to 5/HPF in women in whom the urine sample may be contaminated with vaginal secretions.

34. Which of the following statement regarding casts are not correct?

(a) Renal tubular cells are the least commonly observed epithelial cells in the urine and are least significant
(b) When the casts contain only mucoproteins, they are called hyaline casts and may not have any pathologic significance
(c) White blood cell casts are observed in acute glomerulonephritis
(d) Pigmented, granular muddy casts are suggestive of acute tubular necrosis

(Answer is A) Renal tubular cells are the least commonly observed epithelial cells in the urine but are most significant, because their presence in the urine is always indicative of renal pathology.

35. Crystals precipitated in acidic urine include all *except:*

(a) Calcium oxalate
(b) Uric acid
(c) Cystine
(d) Calcium phosphate

(Answer is D) Crystals precipitated in acidic urine include calcium oxalate, uric acid and cystine. Crystals precipitated in an alkaline urine include calcium phosphate and triple-phosphate (struvite) crystals.

36. Number of bacteria per HPF that correspond to colony count of 1,00,000/ml is:

(a) I (b) 3
(c) 5 (d) 10

(Answer is C) Because each HPF views between 1/20,000 and 1/50,000 ml, each bacterium seen per HPF signifies a bacterial count of more than 20,000/ml.

37. Relative osmotic load of the LOCM is how much times that of HOCM?

(a) One tenth (b) One fifth
(c) Half (d) Same

(Answer is C) LOCM do not ionize in solution, the

relative osmotic load of the agents is approximately 50% less than that of high osmolar contrast media (HOCM).

38. Which of the following dye is not a member of high osmolar contrast media (ionic)?

(a) Renografin (b) Hypaque
(c) Omnipaque (d) Conray

(Answer is C) Omnipaque is member of low osmolar contrast agent.

39. Normal bladder capacity is:

(a) (age [years] + 4) × 30
(b) (age [years] +2) × 30
(c) (age [years] + 4) × 20
(d) (age [years] + 2) × 20

(Answer is B) Normal bladder capacity is (age [years] + 2) × 30 (Koff formula).

40. Which one of the following is not a pattern of backflow while RGP?

(a) Pyelosinus (b) Pyelolymphatic
(c) Pyelovenous (d) Pyeloarterial

(Answer is D) A variety of patterns may be seen, depending on the area of extravasation. Pyelosinus backflow occurs when small tears in the collecting system allow contrast medium to enter the renal sinus. Pyelolymphatic and pyelovenous backflow occurs when extravasated media enter the lymphatic system or the venous system.

41. Investigation of choice to study anterior urethra is:

(a) MCU (b) RGU
(c) USG (d) CECT

(Answer is B) RGU is for evaluation of the anterior urethra. MCU is for evaluation of the posterior uretha.

42. Power Doppler USG all are true *except:*

(a) Based on amplitude of Doppler frequency shift instead of mean frequency shift
(b) The color sensitivity is superior
(c) Can better depict flow in the intrarenal arteries
(d) Provides more information about velocity or the direction of blood flow

(Answer is D) Power-mode Doppler imaging does not provide any information about velocity or the direction of blood flow.

43. Which statement regarding USG is not correct?

(a) The right adrenal gland may be easier to image than the left
(b) The adrenal cortex is usually more echogenic than adrenal medulla
(c) In renal USG cortex and medulla also can be differentiated, because the medullary pyramids typically are less echogenic than the cortex
(d) Corticomedullary differentiation is usually more apparent in children than adults

(Answer is B) The adrenal cortex is usually hypoechoic and the adrenal medulla is echogenic.

44. Which frequency USG probe is used to evaluate scrotal contents?

(a) 3 MHz (b) 7 MHz
(c) 10 MHz (d) 14 MHz

(Answer is C) Because the scrotal contents are superficial in location, high-frequency ultrasound probes (upto 10 MHz) may be utilized, producing excellent resolution.

45. Which one is the imaging modality of choice for evaluation of urolithiasis?

(a) Unenhanced CT (b) CECT
(c) IVU (d) USG

(Answer is A) Unenhanced CT has become the imaging modality of choice for evaluation of urolithiasis.

46. Which one of the imaging modality is not an option for evaluation of acute ureteric colic?

(a) Unenhanced CT (b) X-ray KUB
(c) IVU (d) USG

(Answer is C) IVU has no role in evaluation of acute ureteric colic as there might be no contrast uptake by the kidneys during the acute episode.

47. Which one of the following statement is not true?

(a) If the density of an adrenal mass is less than 0 HU on unenhanced CT, it may be considered an adenoma
(b) Indeterminate lesions and lesions with density less than 20 HU may represent metastases
(c) MRI is the study of choice in suspected pheochromocytoma
(d) On CT adrenal appears as inverted Y

(Answer is B) Indeterminate lesions and lesions with density greater than 20 HU may represent metastases, and a percutaneous biopsy should be considered.

48. Which statement regarding CT angiography is not true?

(a) Minimally invasive method to image the vasculature without the morbidity of direct large vessel vascular access
(b) A rapid injection rate of contrast agent is given, and a helical scan is performed during the arterial phase
(c) Oral administration of contrast agent is necessary
(d) After image acquisition, a workstation eliminates soft tissues and bone from the scan

(Answer is C) Oral administration of contrast agent is usually avoided.

49. Which one of the following statement regarding MRI is not true?

(a) Iodinated contrast media is not used
(b) The Tl-weighted images are generated by the time to return to equilibrium in the z-axis
(c) Tl-weighted images fluid is dark and fat is bright
(d) Images are created by alignment of electrons in response to an external magnet

(Answer is D) Images are created by alignment of protons in response to an external magnet.

50. Which one of the following statement regarding MRU is not true?

(a) It is a technique that seeks to image the ureters and collecting system
(b) It is useful even in pregnant women
(c) Stones generally cannot be distinguished from tumors or blood clots
(d) Lesions less than 4 mm are well visualised

(Answer is D) All lesions less than 4 mm may be difficult to image.

51. Which one of the following statement regarding Tc-MAG3 is not true?

(a) Tc-MAG3 is cleared by tubular secretion, and no glomerular filtration occurs
(b) The tracer is well suited for evaluation of renal function and diuretic scintigraphy
(c) It is an excellent tracer to evaluate renal plasma flow
(d) It is less useful in patients with renal insufficiency

(Answer is D) MAG3 is more useful in patients with renal insufficiency 99mTc-DTPA is less useful in patients with renal failure.

52. Which one of the following statement is not true?

(a) 99mTc-DTPA is primarily a glomerular filtration agent
(b) 99mTc-DTPA is also useful for evaluation of obstruction and renal function
(c) 99mTc-DMSA is cleared by both filtration and secretion, but the clearance is relatively complex and it does bind to parenchymal tissues

(d) 99mTc-DTPA is used to evaluate for cortical scars or pyelonephritis

(Answer is D) Renal cortical scintigraphy with 99mTc-DMSA is used to evaluate for cortical scars or pyelonephritis.

53. All of the following scores are related to ejaculatory dysfunction *except:*

(a) EDITS
(b) BMSFI
(c) IIEF
(d) ICIQ

(Answer is D) ICIQ score stands for international consultation on incontinence questionnaire.

54. Glitter cells:

(a) Old leukocyte
(b) Fresh leukocyte
(c) Old erythrocyte
(d) Fresh erythrocyte

(Answer is B) In fresh leukocytes cytoplasm, granules demonstrate glitter-like movement.

55. What should the management be of polytrauma patients with deteriorating hemodynamic parameters after 12 hours of initial damage control laparotomy and renal fossa packing?

(a) Reoperation
(b) Angiographic embolization of the bleeding kidney
(c) Any of the above
(d) Fresh blood transfusion and repeat contrast CT

(Answer is C) Any of the above

56. On laparotomy, for intra-abdominal hemorrhage and grade III left renal trauma, the patient is hemodynamically stable. What should the attending urologist do?

(a) Take an on-table one-shot urography and manage accordingly
(b) Explore the kidney, suture the deep parenchymal lacerations, and evacuate the hematoma
(c) Not to explore the kidney
(d) Perform damage control nephrectomy

(Answer is C) Not to explore the kidney

57. On exploring a right traumatically shattered kidney, hemorrhage is not controlled. What would be next step?

(a) Perform damage control renal packing and send the patient to the ICU with the intention to take a second look later
(b) Perform nephrectomy
(c) Insert a nephrostomy tube and close the wound under pressure
(d) Perform a full renal repair using hemostatic sutures and gauze

(Answer is B) Perform nephrectomy

58. In the setting of a seriously traumatized left kidney, renal exploration aims at all of the following, *except:*

(a) Control life-threatening bleeding
(b) Preservation of viable renal parenchyma
(c) Meticulous renal reconstruction
(d) Applying damage-control principles when necessary

(Answer is C) Meticulous renal reconstruction

59. In the setting of multiple penetrating abdominal injuries. The patient is hemodynamically unstable. On exploration, without prior imaging, the left mid ureter found half away severed. What would be the management?

(a) Insert a double J-stent over a guide wire through the tear and ensure correct positioning by fluoroscopy
(b) Perform retrograde ureteropyelography to evaluate ureteral injuries and quickly close the ureteral tear
(c) Perform temporary ureterocutaneus urinary diversion

(d) Ligate the ureter, leave a drain, and insert post op. nephrostomy

(Answer is D) Ligate the ureter, leave a drain, and insert post op. nephrostomy

60. On exploring a polytrauma patient with unstable hemodynamics, a ureteral injury was suspected. What would be the management?

(a) Leave a drain at where urine is accumulating

(b) Search the ureter and ligate it

(c) Perform retrograde ureteropyelography and manage accordingly

(d) Perform on-table urography and manage accordingly

(Answer is A) Leave a drain at where urine is accumulating

61. A 31 years man with an unstable hemodynamics presents to the casualty 3 hours after devascularization of the kidney due to hilar injury, in addition to a grade IV ipsilateral ureteral trauma. How should the ureteral injury be managed?

(a) Ligate the injured ureter and leave a drain

(b) Perform a brief ureteral repair over a stent

(c) Ligate the ureter and insert a nephrostomy tube

(d) None of the above

(Answer is D) None of the above

62. A large intraperitoneal bladder rupture associated with unstable pelvic fractures, major vessels, bleeds and grade IV anesthesia ASA classification. The patient should be managed by:

(a) Bladder packing and later repair

(b) Placing urethral and/or suprapubic tubes

(c) Emergency bladder closure

(d) None of the above

(Answer is B) Placing urethral and/or suprapubic tubes

63. A mass casualty incident is paged when:

(a) The number of injured people, before triage, is 50 or greater

(b) The sufferers have a multisystem trauma

(c) The number of the victims is significantly greater than the number of the rescuers

(d) The sufferers' conditions cannot be managed on the trauma scene

(Answer is C) The number of the victims is significantly greater than the number of the rescuers

64. In which of the following injuries the conventional management lines up with the damage control policies?

(a) Intraperitoneal bladder rupture

(b) Expanding extrarenal hematoma

(c) Posterior urethral transection

(d) Grade III mid ureteral injury

(Answer is C) Posterior urethral transection

CHAPTER

3

Basics of Urologic Surgery

1. **The Child classification assessing perioperative morbidity and mortality is based on all *except:***

(a) Bilirubin (b) Albumin

(c) Ascites (d) Clotting time

(Answer is D) The Child classification assesses perioperative morbidity and mortality and is based on:

- Bilirubin.
- Albumin.
- Prothrombin time.
- Encephalopathy.
- Ascites.

2. **Catheter sizes refer to which diameter?**

(a) Outside circumference of the catheter

(b) Inside circumference of the catheter

(c) Outside luminal diameter

(d) Inside luminal diameter

(Answer is A) Catheter sizes refer to the outside circumference of the catheter, not the luminal diameter.

3. **1 Fr =**

(a) 0.33 mm (b) 0.66 mm

(c) 1.00 mm (d) 1.33 mm

(Answer is A) Catheter size is usually referred to using the French (Fr) scale (circumference is in millimeters) in which 1 Fr = 0.33 mm in diameter.

4. **For a given outer circumference which catheter will have maximum luminal size?**

(a) Malecot

(b) 2-way foley

(c) 3-way foley

(d) All will have same diameter

(Answer is A) Catheters without a lumen for balloon inflation (e.g., Malecot) have a larger luminal size for bladder drainage than do Foley catheters of the same outer circumference. Likewise, for a given outer circumference, two-way catheters will have a larger luminal size for urinary drainage than three-way catheters.

5. **Which catheters with a curved tip are specifically designed to help bypass areas of the male urethra that are difficult to negotiate with a straight catheter?**

(a) Conical tip (b) Robinson

(c) Whistle tip (d) Coude olive tip

(Answer is D) Catheters with a curved tip (e.g., coude catheters) are specifically designed to help bypass areas of the male urethra that are difficult to negotiate with a straight catheter.

6. **Which one of the following is not the advantage of rigid endoscope over flexible endoscope for cystoscopy?**

(a) Better optics

(b) Longer working channel

(c) Ease of passing instrument over bladder neck

(d) Ease of maintaining orientation

(Answer is C) There are many advantages to the use of the rigid endoscope for cystourethroscopy: (1) better optics because of the use of a rod-lens system in rigid instruments in contrast to the fiberoptic system in flexible instruments; (2) a larger working channel that allows the urologist greater versatility in passage of accessory instruments; (3) a larger lumen for water flow, thus improving visualization; and (4) ease of manipulation and maintaining orientation during inspection within the bladder.

7. **Which statement regarding different angles of view is not correct?**
   (a) A 0-degree lens is usually used for urethroscopy
   (b) A 30-degree lens best affords visualization of the base and anterolateral aspect of the bladder
   (c) 45 to 70-degree lens is used to view the bladder dome
   (d) Angle of view greater than 90 degrees can be used to visualize the anterior bladder neck

(Answer is C) 70- to 90-degree lens is used to view the bladder dome.

8. **Which ureteric catheter is designed to occlude the ureteral orifice as contrast material is injected retrogradely?**
   (a) Whistle (b) Spiral
   (c) Olive (d) Cone

(Answer is D) The cone tip catheter is designed to occlude the ureteral orifice as contrast material is injected retrogradely, thus filling the ureter and renal collecting system at the same time.

9. **The distance from the ureteral orifice to the ureteropelvic junction is:**
   (a) Between 10 and 15 cm
   (b) Between 15 and 20 cm
   (c) Between 20 and 25 cm
   (d) Between 25 and 30 cm

(Answer is C) The distance from the ureteral orifice to the ureteropelvic junction is between 20 and 25 cm.

10. **Which statement is not true?**
   (a) Father of modern-day laparoscopy–Semm
   (b) Father of endourology–Arthur Smith
   (c) Introduce glass optics for magnification–Nitze
   (d) Introduced large, rod-shaped quartz lenses to transmit light–Veress

(Answer is D) Major advances in endoscope resolution and contrast were subsequently achieved by Hopkins, who introduced large, rod-shaped quartz lenses to transmit light in the early 1960s.

11. **Absolute contraindications to laparoscopic surgery are all *except:***
   (a) Uncorrectable coagulopathy
   (b) Intestinal obstruction, abdominal wall infection, massive hemoperitoneum and generalized peritonitis
   (c) Retroperitoneal abscess
   (d) Extensive prior abdominal surgery

(Answer is D) Absolute contraindications to laparoscopic surgery include uncorrectable coagulopathy, intestinal obstruction, abdominal wall infection, massive hemoperitoneum or pneumoretroperitoneum, generalized peritonitis or retroperitoneal abscess, and suspected malignant ascites.

12. **In lateral position pillow is placed between the legs as a cushion and also to elevate the upper leg so that it lies level with the flank, thereby obviating stretch on which nerve?**
   (a) Obturator nerve
   (b) Sciatic nerve
   (c) Femoral nerve
   (d) Lateral femoral nerve

(Answer is B) A pillow is placed between the legs as a cushion and also to elevate the upper leg so that it lies level with the flank, thereby obviating any undue stretch on the sciatic nerve.

13. Most commonly, used gas as insufflant:

(a) O_2 (b) Helium
(c) N_2O (d) CO_2

(Answer is D) Most commonly, CO_2 is used as the insufflant because it does not support combustion and is very soluble in blood.

14. In patients with COPD which gas is used for insufflation?

(a) O_2 (b) Helium
(c) N_2O (d) NO_2

(Answer is B) In patients with chronic respiratory disease, the procedure is initiated with CO_2 and then the change is made during the case to helium if necessary.

15. All are advantages for using umbilicus site of initial trocar placement *except:*

(a) Abdominal wall is thinnest
(b) Postoperative cosmesis is excellent
(c) Point of entry is fraught with the least potential for injury to a major vessel
(d) None of the above

(Answer is C) There are certain advantages to choosing the umbilical area as the site for initial trocar placement: the abdominal wall is thinnest, and postoperative cosmesis is excellent. However, this point of entry is fraught with the potential for injury to a major vessel, in particular the left common iliac, aorta, or vena cava.

16. Pneumoperitoneum pressure should never be raised above:

(a) 10 mm Hg (b) 15 mm Hg
(c) 20 mm Hg (d) 25 mm Hg

(Answer is B) The pneumoperitoneum pressure need never be raised above 15 mm Hg unless it is done so in the setting of a vascular venous injury to control bleeding.

17. Which statement regarding flo-seal is not correct?

(a) It has thrombin-soaked oxidised cellulose particles
(b) Have excellent adhesive properties on parenchymal surfaces
(c) Capable of excellent hemostatic agents in the presence of active bleeding
(d) Takes 2 minutes to prepare

(Answer is B) Thrombin-soaked oxidized cellulose particles (FloSeal) have no adhesive capability at all but are excellent hemostatic agents in the presence of active bleeding from parenchymal surfaces such as a partial nephrectomy bed, liver/spleen laceration, or in an oozing adrenal bed. This agent is also prepared by the scrub assistant and takes 2 minutes to prepare.

18. As the pnuemoperitoneum pressure increases all parameter decreases *except:*

(a) Heart rate
(b) Mean arterial pressure
(c) GFR
(d) Urine output

(Answer is B)

Effects	5mm Hg	10mm Hg	20mm Hg	40mm Hg
Heart rate	↑	↑	↑	↓
Mean arterial pressure	↑	↑	↑	↑

19. Major complication of abdominal and pelvic surgery respectively is:

(a) Vascular and bowel injury
(b) Bowel and vascular injury
(c) Liver and vascular injury
(d) Vascular and liver injury

(Answer is A) Major Complications of Transperitoneal Abdominal Surgery

Total procedures	*Abdominal*	*Pelvic*
Overall complications	13.2%	22.6%
Vascular injury	2.8%	0.5%
Bowel injury	1.1%	1.2%

20. All are signs of CO_2 gas embolus *except:*

(a) The first sign of intravascular insufflation is acute cardiovascular collapse
(b) Dysrhythmias, tachycardia, cyanosis and pulmonary edema
(c) Abrupt decrease of end-tidal CO_2 accompanied by a sudden decline in oxygen saturation
(d) "Millwheel" precordial murmur can be auscultated

(Answer is C) The diagnosis is usually made by the anesthesiologist based on an abrupt increase of end-tidal CO_2 accompanied by a sudden decline in oxygen saturation and then a marked decrease in end-tidal CO_2.

21. All are treatment options for gas embolism *except:*

(a) Immediate cessation of insufflation and prompt desufflation of the peritoneal cavity
(b) Patient is turned into a right lateral decubitus position
(c) Hyperventilate with 100% oxygen
(d) Advancement of a central venous line into the right heart with subsequent attempts to aspirate gas

(Answer is B) The treatment is immediate cessation of insufflation and prompt desufflation of the peritoneal cavity. The patient, if at all possible, is turned into a left lateral decubitus position (i.e., right side up) to minimize right ventricular outflow problems.

22. In the case of a one-wall injury of the bowel, during first port placement appropriate treatment option is:

(a) Remove port and immediately open the abdomen
(b) Remove port and place at other site
(c) Leave the port and immediately open the abdomen
(d) Leave the port and place secondary port, and repair of injured bowel can be done laparoscopically or with open technique

(Answer is D) In the case of a one-wall injury of the bowel, the surgeon can elect to leave the trocar in place and pass a second trocar in another location using an open access technique. At this time, the surgeon may elect to open and repair the bowel or, if laparoscopically skilled, may place two more ports and proceed to close the bowel using laparoscopic suturing or stapling techniques.

23. In the case of a vascular injury, during first port placement appropriate treatment option is:

(a) Remove port and immediately open the abdomen
(b) Remove port and place at other site
(c) Leave the port and immediately open the abdomen
(d) Leave the port and place secondary port, and repair of injured bowel can be done laparoscopically or with open technique

(Answer is C) If blood is coming through the trocar, then the trocar should be closed and left in place. An emergency laparotomy is done, and the trocar is followed to its point of entry into the vessel. Controlling sutures can be placed on either side of the trocar or a Satinsky clamp can be placed to isolate the area of injury, so that, as the trocar is withdrawn, the wound can be rapidly controlled.

24. The scar regains 80% of strength by:

(a) 1 week
(b) 3 weeks
(c) 3 months
(d) 3 years

(Answer is C) The scar regains strength

- 3% after 1 week.
- 20% after 3 weeks.
- 80% after 3 months.

25. In which body tissue(s) are creatine and phosphocreatine converted to creatinine?

(a) Bone marrow
(b) Skeletal muscles
(c) Brown fat
(d) Liver

(Answer is B) Skeletal muscles

26. What is the best method to evaluate calcium levels in the urine?

(a) From early morning urine sample
(b) Comparing urine and serum calcium at a given time
(c) Performing 24 hours urine collection
(d) From a mid-stream urine sample

(Answer is C) Performing 24 hours urine collection

27. On clinical examination, what accidental finding has NO connection to renal cancer?

(a) Unilateral hydrocele
(b) Bilateral varicocele
(c) Calcifications at the renal area on plain KUB film
(d) Painless hematuria

(Answer is A) Unilateral hydrocele

28. False about urodynamics:

(a) Used for evaluation of lower urinary tract dysfunction
(b) Detrusor leak point pressure is the lowest detrusor pressure at which urine leakage occurs
(c) Postvoid residual is a poor assessment of bladder emptying
(d) Uroflowmetry is a non invasive test

(Answer is C) Postvoid residual is a poor assessment of bladder emptying

29. All are urodynamic risk factors *except:*

(a) Impaired compliance
(b) Detrusor external sphincter dyssynergia
(c) Low pressure detrusor overactivity
(d) Elevated detrusor leak point pressure

(Answer is C) Low pressure detrusor overactivity

30. False about ambulatory urodynamics:

(a) Utilizes natural filling
(b) Reproduces normal everyday activities
(c) Investigation of choice for assessment of lower urinary tract dysfunction
(d) More sensitive than conventional cystometry for detecting detrusor overactivity

(Answer is C) Investigation of choice for assessment of lower urinary tract dysfunction

CHAPTER 4

Infection and Inflammation

1. **Bacteriuria without pyuria indicates:**
   (a) Tuberculosis
   (b) Stones
   (c) Cancer
   (d) Bacterial colonisation

(Answer is D) Bacteriuria without pyuria is generally indicative of bacterial colonization without infection of the urinary tract.

2. **Pyuria without bacteriuria warrants evaluation for all *except:***
   (a) Tuberculosis
   (b) Stones
   (c) Cancer
   (d) Bacterial colonisation

(Answer is D) Pyuria without bacteriuria warrants evaluation for tuberculosis, stones or cancer.

3. **Which statement is not true regarding complicated infection?**
   (a) The urinary tract is functionally or structurally abnormal
   (b) The host is compromised
   (c) Bacteria have increased virulence or antimicrobial resistance
   (d) The majority of these patients are women

(Answer is D) A complicated infection is associated with factors that increase the chance of acquiring bacteria and decrease the efficacy of therapy. The urinary tract is functionally or structurally abnormal, the host is compromised, and/or the bacteria have increased virulence or antimicrobial resistance. The majority of these patients are men.

4. **Recurrent UTI caused by the same bacteria reemerging from a focus within the urinary tract is termed as:**
   (a) Isolated infection
   (b) Unresolved
   (c) Reinfection
   (d) Persistent infection

(Answer is D) Bacterial persistence refers to a recurrent UTI caused by the same bacteria reemerging from a focus within the urinary tract, such as an infectious stone or the prostate.

5. **False about UTI is:**
   (a) UTI is more common in females than in males
   (b) In neonatal period UTI is more common in males
   (c) Prevalence of bacteriuria increases with age
   (d) With increasing age ratio of women to men with bacteriuria progressively increases

(Answer is D) The prevalence of bacteriuria in young women is 30 times more than in men. However, with increasing age, the ratio of women to men with bacteriuria progressively decreases. At least 20% of women and 10% of men older than 65 years have bacteriuria.

6. **Risk of recurrent bacteriuria decreases by which type of treatment during primary infection?**
   (a) Short-term treatment
   (b) Long-term treatment
   (c) Prophylactic treatment
   (d) Remain same irrespective of type of treatment

(Answer is D) Whether a patient receives no treatment at all, or short-term, long-term, or prophylactic antimicrobial treatment, the risk of recurrent bacteriuria remains the same; prophylactic antimicrobial therapy reduces reinfections but does not alter the underlying predisposition to recurring infection.

7. **Which statement is not true regarding UTI?**
   (a) Once a patient has an infection, he is likely to develop subsequent infection
   (b) Most reinfections occurred after 2 weeks
   (c) If antimicrobial prophylaxis is started after the second or any succeeding infection within a set, about one third of the women will be treated unnecessarily
   (d) The long-term effects of uncomplicated recurrent UTIs is renal scarring, hypertension, or progressive renal azotemia

(Answer is D) The long-term effects of uncomplicated recurrent UTIs are not completely known, but, so far, no association between recurrent infections and renal scarring, hypertension, or progressive renal azotemia has been established.

8. **Most common route of infection in UTI:**
   (a) Ascending (b) Descending
   (c) Hematogenous (d) Lymphatic

(Answer is A) Most bacteria enter the urinary tract from the bowel reservoir via ascent through the urethra into the bladder.

9. **Most common pathogen leading to community acquired and hospital acquired UTI respectively are:**
   (a) Klebsiella and E. coli
   (b) E. coli and E. coli
   (c) Proteus and E. coli
   (d) Staphylococcus and klebsiella

(Answer is B) E. coli is by far the most common cause of UTIs, accounting for 85% of community-acquired and 50% of hospital-acquired infections.

10. **Approximately 10% of symptomatic lower UTIs in young, sexually active females is caused by:**
   (a) Klebsiella
   (b) E. coli
   (c) S. saprophyticus
   (d) Proteus

(Answer is C) S. saprophyticus is now recognized as causing approximately 10% of symptomatic lower UTIs in young, sexually active females.

11. **Which statement is not true regarding type 1 pilli?**
   (a) Expressed on both nonpathogenic and pathogenic E. coli
   (b) Mediate hemagglutination of human erythrocytes
   (c) Facilitate bacterial colonization of the vaginal mucosa and bladder
   (d) Termed as mannose-sensitive hemagglutination

(Answer is B) Type I pilli are commonly expressed on both nonpathogenic and pathogenic E. coli and appear to facilitate bacterial colonization of the vaginal mucosa and bladder. These pilli mediate hemagglutination of guinea pig erythrocytes.

12. **Which HLA may be associated with increased risk of recurrent UTIs?**
   (a) A 1 (b) A 3
   (c) B3 (d) C3

(Answer is B) HLA-A3 may be associated with increased risk of recurrent UTIs.

13. **Women susceptible to recurrent UTIs has increased epithelial receptivity for E. coli on all *except:***
   (a) Introital (b) Urethral
   (c) Buccal (d) Vesical

(Answer is D) There is an increased epithelial receptivity for E. coli on the introital, urethral and buccal mucosa that is characteristic of women susceptible to recurrent UTIs and may be a genotypic trait.

14. The normal flora of the vaginal introitus, the periurethral area, and the urethra usually contain all *except* one micro-organism:

(a) Coagulase-negative staphylococci
(b) Streptococci
(c) Pneumococci
(d) Corynebacteria

(Answer is C) The normal flora of the vaginal introitus, the periurethral area, and the urethra usually contain microorganisms such as lactobacilli, coagulase-negative staphylococci, corynebacteria, and streptococci that form a barrier against uropathogenic colonization.

15. All *except* one are inhibitory factors for infection in UTI:

(a) Osmolality (b) Urea
(c) Organic acid (d) Glucose

(Answer is D) Most inhibitory factors are the osmolality urea concentration, organic acid concentration and pH. Bacterial growth is inhibited, by either very dilute urine or a high osmolality when associated with a low ph. The presence of glucose in the urine may facilitate infections.

16. Which is not the cause of renal papillary necrosis?

(a) Renal artery stenosis
(b) Urinary tract obstruction
(c) Renal transplant rejection
(d) Cirrhosis of liver

(Answer is A) Conditions associated with renal papillary necrosis are–DM, pyelonephritis, urinary tract obstruction, analgesic nephropathy, renal transplant rejection, cirrhosis of liver and renal vein thrombosis.

17. Most accurate assessment of the status of bladder urine is by:

(a) Suprapubic aspiration
(b) After per urethral catheterisation
(c) Mid stream urine
(d) After prostate massage

(Answer is A) Suprapubic aspiration of bladder urine is least likely to cause contamination of the specimen; therefore, it provides the most accurate assessment of the status of bladder urine.

18. The easiest way to prevent catheter-induced infections is:

(a) Single dose trimethoprim-sulfamethoxazole
(b) Single dose levofloxacin
(c) Single dose cephalexin
(d) Single dose nitrofurantoin

(Answer is A) The easiest way to prevent catheter-induced infections is to give a single dose of an oral antimicrobial agent, such as trimethoprim-sulfamethoxazole.

19. In dysuric patients, an appropriate threshold value for defining significant bacteriuria is:

(a) 1 CFU/ml
(b) 100 CFU/ml
(c) 1000 CFU /ml
(d) 100,000 CFU/ml

(Answer is B) In dysuric patients, an appropriate threshold value for defining significant bacteriuria is 102 CFU/ml of a known pathogen.

20. Glitter cells are:

(a) Lymphocytes
(b) Macrophages
(c) Polymorphonuclear leukocytes
(d) Platelets

(Answer is C) Fresh polymorphonuclear leukocytes (glitter cells).

21. Rapid screening method for detecting UTI should be used primarily for:

(a) Low risk asymptomatic patients

(b) Asymptomatic pregnant female
(c) Catheterized patient
(d) Pediatric age group

(Answer is A) Their main role is in screening asymptomatic patients.

22. Indications for radiologic investigation in APN include all *except:*

(a) History of stones
(b) History of genitourinary surgery
(c) DM
(d) Poor response to antimicrobial after 3 days of treatment

(Answer is D) Indications for radiologic investigation in acute clinical pyelonephritis includes poor response to appropriate antimicrobial agents after 5 to 6 days of treatment.

23. Which radionuclides scan is used to detect renal abscess?

(a) 99 mTc (b) 123 I-OH
(c) 51 Cr EDTA (d) Ga 67

(Answer is D) Gallium-67 scanning has been reported to be useful in the diagnosis of pyelonephritis and renal abscess, it is uncommonly required and may be positive in noninfectious entities.

24. Which of the following is not correctly matched?

(a) Vancomycin–inhibition of bacterial cell membrane synthesis
(b) Aminoglycosides–inhibition of ribosomal protein synthesis
(c) Quinolones–inhibition of bacterial DNA gyrase
(d) TMP-SM X–inhibition of folate metabolism

(Answer is A) Vancomycin inhibition of bacterial cell wall synthesis (at different point than β-lactams).

25. Cure of UTI is dependent on which parameter of antimicrobial?

(a) Serum level
(b) Urinary level
(c) Half life
(d) Duration of therapy

(Answer is B) Efficacy of the antimicrobial therapy is critically dependent on the antimicrobial levels in the urine and the duration that this level remains above the minimal inhibitory concentration of the infecting organism.

26. Plasmid-mediated resistance has not been reported with which drug?

(a) Fluoroquinolone (b) Aztreonam
(c) Teicoplanin (d) Nitrofurantoin

(Answer is D) All antimicrobial classes are capable of causing plasmid-mediated resistance. However, for the fluoroquinolones resistance is rarely transmitted by plasmids, and nitrofurantoin plasmid-mediated resistance has not been reported.

27. Excellent gram negative coverage can be obtained by all *except:*

(a) Third generation cephalosporin
(b) Aminoglycosides
(c) Fluoroquinolones
(d) Vancomycin

(Answer is D) Vancomycin covers all Gram positive (including MRSA) and does not cover Gram negative pathogens.

28. Which statement is not true regarding nitrofurantoin?

(a) Not effective against pseudomonas and proteus species
(b) Rapidly excreted from the urine and obtain therapeutic levels in most body tissues
(c) Not useful for upper tract and complicated infections
(d) Minimal effects on the resident bowel and vaginal flora

(Answer is B) Nitrofurantoin is rapidly excreted from

the urine but does not obtain therapeutic levels in most body tissues, including the gastrointestinal tract.

29. Even in ideal host antimicrobial prophylaxis is required in:

(a) Urethral catheterisation
(b) Urodynamics
(c) ESWL
(d) Cystoscopy

(Answer is C)

Procdure	*Ideal Host*	*Host with risk factors*	*Duration single dose*
Urethral catheterization and removal	No absolute indication	Oral fluoroquinolone	< 24 hours
Urodynamics	No absolute indication	Oral fluoroquinolone	Single dose, < 24 hours
Extracorporeal shockwave lithotripsy	Bactrim DS	If infectious stone, treat preoperatively for UTI	Single dose, < 24 hours
Urethroscopy, cystoscopy	No absolute indication	Cefazolin	Single dose <24 hours

30. Uninfected wound with controlled entry into the genital, urinary or alimentary tract is classified as:

(a) Clean
(b) Clean contaminated
(c) Contaminated
(d) Dirty

(Answer is B) *Clean contaminated:* Uninfected wound with controlled entry into the genital, urinary, or alimentary tract.

31. 7 days antimicrobial therapy in acute cystitis is prescribed for all *except:*

(a) Healthy men (b) Healthy women
(c) Pregnancy (d) Recurrent UTI

(Answer is B) Three-day therapy is the preferred regimen for uncomplicated cystitis in women.

32. Screening and treatment of asymptomatic bacteriuria is recommended for:

(a) Postmenopausal women
(b) Diabetic women
(c) Pregnant women
(d) Women with spinal cord injuries

(Answer is C)

Screening for and treatment of asymptomatic bacteriuria

Premenopausal nonpregnant women	Not recommended
Pregnant women	Recommended
Diabetic women	Not recommended
Older persons residing in the community	Not recommended
Elderly institutionalized subjects	Not recommended
Subjects with spinal cord injuries	Not recommended

33. Most common causes of unresolved bacteriuria:

(a) Rapid reinfection with a new, resistant species during initial therapy for the original susceptible organism azotemia
(b) Bacteriuria caused by two different bacterial species with mutually exclusive susceptibilities
(c) Development of resistance from initially susceptible bacteria
(d) Bacterial resistance to the drug selected for treatment

(Answer is D) Causes of unresolved bacteriuria in descending order of importance are:

1. Bacterial resistance to the drug selected for treatment.
2. Development of resistance from initially susceptible bacteria.
3. Bacteriuria caused by two different bacterial species with mutually exclusive susceptibilities.
4. Rapid reinfection with a new, resistant

species during initial therapy for the original susceptible organism azotemia.

34. Follow up of acute pyelonephritis includes all *except:*

(a) Repeat urine cultures should be performed on the fifth to the seventh day of therapy
(b) Repeat urine cultures should be performed on 10 to 14 days and 4 to 6 weeks after discontinuing antimicrobial therapy
(c) Between 10% and 30% of individuals with acute pyelonephritis relapse after a 14-day course of therapy
(d) Patients who relapse usually require a 6-week antimicrobial therapy

(Answer is D) Patients who relapse usually are cured by a second 14-day course of therapy, but occasionally a 6-week course is necessary.

35. 30-year-old male presented with acute flank pain, fever and chills. He was advised fluoroquinolones but did not respond even after 72 hours of treatment. Ideal management will be:

(a) Observation
(b) Change antibiotics
(c) USG or CT
(d) Blood culture

(Answer is C) USG or CT are commonly used to evaluate patients initially for complicated UTIs or to reevaluate patients who do not respond after 72 hours of therapy.

36. Emphysematous pyelonephritis all are correct *except:*

(a) All documented cases are found in adults
(b) Radiological hallmark is intraparenchymal gas
(c) Klebsiella and proteus are most common pathogens
(d) IVU is rarely of value

(Answer is C) E. coli is most commonly identified. Klebsiella and proteus are less common.

37. All are true regarding emphysematous pyelonephritis *except:*

(a) Obstruction is demonstrated in approximately 25% of the cases
(b) CT is the imaging procedure of choice in defining the extent of the emphysematous process and guiding management
(c) Presence of streaky or mottled gas with or without bubbly and loculated gas appears to be associated with 50% to 60% mortality rate
(d) Presence of bubbly or loculated gas or gas in the collecting system, is associated with 30% to 40% mortality rate

(Answer is D) The presence of renal or perirenal fluid, the presence of bubbly or loculated gas or gas in the collecting system, and the absence of streaky or mottled gas patterns is associated with a less than 20% mortality rate.

38. About treatment of renal abscess all are true *except:*

(a) Abscess <3 cm can be treated by IV antimicrobials
(b) Abscess >5 cm requires surgical drainage
(c) In immunocompromised host abscess should be drained percutaneously
(d) Those that do not respond to antimicrobials should be drained surgically

(Answer is D) Abscesses 3 to 5 cm in diameter and smaller abscesses in immunocompromised hosts or those that do not respond to antimicrobial therapy should be drained percutaneously.

39. Phenomenon of renal thyroidization is seen in:

(a) APN (b) CPN
(c) AGN (d) CGN

(Answer is B) In CPN some affected areas, glomeruli may be completely fibrosed and tubules atrophied. Leukocyte and hyaline casts are sometimes present in the tubules; the latter may cause resemblance to the thyroid colloid, hence the description renal thyroidization.

40. Xanthogranulomatous pyelonephritis which is true?

(a) Most cases are bilateral
(b) Xanthogranuloma cells are specific
(c) E. coli is the most common organism
(d) It is associated with renal cell carcinoma

(Answer is D) Most cases are unilateral, Xanthogranulomatous cells are not specific to xanthogranulomatous pyelonephritis but may be present anywhere inflammation or obstruction coexists Proteus to be the most common organism involved with xanthogranulomatous pyelonephritis.

41. Bear paw sign on CT is suggestive of:

(a) Chronic pyelonephritis
(b) Emphysematous pyelonephritis
(c) Xanthogranulomatous pyelonephritis
(d) Malakoplakia

(Answer is C) The Bear paw sign with areas of low-attenuation nonenhancing dilated calyces and abscesses within areas of high-attenuation enhancing renal parenchyma may be present in XPN.

42. Michaelis Gutmann bodies are seen in:

(a) Erythroplakia (b) Leukoplakia
(c) Malakoplakia (d) Interstitial cystitis

(Answer is C) It is hypothesized that bacteria or bacterial fragments form the nidus for the calcium phosphate crystals that laminate the Michaelis-Gutmann bodies.

43. Which statement regarding malacoplakia is not correct?

(a) Malacoplakia, means "soft plaque"
(b) Bacteria or bacterial fragments form the nidus for the calcium phosphate crystals that laminate the Michaelis-Gutmann bodies
(c) Lesion is characterized by large histiocytes, known as von Hansemann cells
(d) Michaelis-Gutmann bodies are necessary for the diagnosis

(Answer is D) Michaelis-Gutmann bodies may be absent in early malacoplakia and are not necessary for the diagnosis.

44. Echinococcosis is rare in which part of the world?

(a) South Africa (b) Australia
(c) New Zealand (d) United States

(Answer is D) The disease is prevalent in dogs, sheep, cattle, and humans in South Africa, Australia, New Zealand, Mediterranean countries (especially Greece), and some parts of the former Soviet Union. In the United States, the disease is rare.

45. Which statement is not true regarding echinococcosis?

(a) Hydatid cyst gradually develops at a rate of about 1 cm/year
(b) Echinococcosis cysts of the kidney are usually single and located in the cortex
(c) The laminated layer gives rise to brood capsules that increase in number, become vacuolated, and remain attached to the germinal membrane by a pedicle
(d) Complement fixation, HA, and the Casoni intradermal skin tests are less reliable but, when combined, are positive in about 90% of patients

(Answer is C) The germinal layer gives rise to brood capsules that increase in number, become vacuolated, and remain attached to the germinal membrane by a pedicle.

46. Earliest metabolic change in septicemia is:

(a) Respiratory alkalosis
(b) Respiratory acidosis
(c) Metabolic alkalosis
(d) Metabolic acidosis

(Answer is A) Earliest metabolic change in septicemia is respiratory alkalosis.

47. Which statement regarding pyelonephritis in pregnancy is not true?

(a) Pyelonephritis develops in 1% to 4% of all pregnant women

(b) Pyelonephritis develops in 20% to 40% of pregnant women with untreated bacteriuria

(c) Of the women who develop pyelonephritis during pregnancy, 60% to 75% acquire it during the third trimester

(d) The prevalence of bacteriuria increases with the occurrence of pregnancy and ranges from 20% to 30%

(Answer is D) The prevalence of bacteriuria does not change with the occurrence of pregnancy and ranges from 2% to 7%.

48. All are changes which occur in pregnancy *except:*

(a) Renal length increases

(b) Ureteral peristalsis increases

(c) GFR, RPF increases

(d) Bladder displaced anteriorly and superiorly

(Answer is B) The collecting system, especially the ureters, undergoes decreased peristalsis during pregnancy.

49. Which drug is safe to treat UTI in pregnancy?

(a) Fluoroquinolones (b) Trimethoprim

(c) Erythromycin (d) Nitrofurantoin

(Answer is D) Agents considered safe in pregnancy are pencillin, cephalosporins and nitrofurantoin.

50. Which of the following statement regarding UTI in pregnancy is not correct?

(a) Even asymptomatic bacteriuria should be treated

(b) Risk of bacteriuria increases with duration of pregnancy

(c) Screening culture should be performed in all pregnant women during the first trimester

(d) Acute pyelonephritic patients should be managed by oral antimicrobial drugs

(Answer is D) Pregnant women with acute pyelonephritis should be hospitalized and treated initially with parenteral antimicrobial agents.

51. Incidence of bacteriuria in presence of indwelling catheter is:

(a) 1% per day of catheterization

(b) 5% per day of catheterization

(c) 10% per day of catheterization

(d) 20% per day of catheterization

(Answer is C) The development of bacteriuria in the presence of an indwelling catheter is inevitable and occurs at an incidence of approximately 10% per day of catheterization.

52. Which statement regarding fungiuria is not correct?

(a) Fungal balls typically involve candida species because of their propensity to develop pseudohyphae

(b) Candida glabrata is the second most common fungus, representing 10% to 15% of positive fungal cultures

(c) The presence of pyuria does not correlate well with the presence of symptoms or the degree of funguria

(d) Only up to 25% of asymptomatic funguria will clear spontaneously

(Answer is D) The majority of patients with asymptomatic funguria do not require treatment. Up to 75% of patients will clear spontaneously.

53. Fourniers gangrene all are true *except:*

(a) Also called necrotizing fascitis of male or idiopathic gangrene of scrotum

(b) The mortality rate averages approximately 20%

(c) Extensive incision should be made going beyond the area of involvement

(d) Orchidectomy is almost always required

(Answer is D) Orchidectomy is almost never required, because the testes have their own blood supply independent of the compromised fascial and cutaneous circulation to the scrotum.

54. Classification system describing four categories of prostatitis was described by:

(a) Meares and Stamey (b) Schaeffer
(c) Drach (d) Nickel

(Answer is C) Classification system describing four categories of prostatitis was described by Drach and colleagues.

55. According to NIH classification prostatodynia is classified as:

(a) Category I (b) Category II
(c) Category IIIA (d) Category IIIB

(Answer is D)

Prostatodynia	Category IIIB (Noninflammatory CPPS)	Insignificant number of white blood cells in expressed prostatic secretions, post-prostatic massage urine sediment (VB3), or semen

56. Four glass test was performed which suggested no uropathogen but excessive leucocytosis in postprostatic massage sample. Which category of prostatitis it is?

(a) Category I (b) Category II
(c) Category IIIA (d) Category IIIB

(Answer is C) Category IIIA, or inflammatory CPPS (based on the presence of excessive leukocytes in EPSs or post-prostatic massage urine or semen.

57. The NIH-CPSI consist of how many questions?

(a) Five (b) Seven
(c) Nine (d) Eleven

(Answer is C) Index consists of nine questions that address the three most important domains of the CP experience.

58. Recommended test for men for evaluation of CPPS is:

(a) Urine cytology (b) CMG
(c) TRUS (d) PSA

(Answer is A) Recommended test

- Lower urinary tract localization test
- Symptom inventory or index (NIH-CPSI)
- Flow rate
- Residual urine determination
- Urine cytology

59. TRUS confirms a large prostatic abscess. Ideal route of drainage is:

(a) Transrectal drainage
(b) Transurethral drainage
(c) Transperineal drainage
(d) Percutaneous needle drainage

(Answer is D) More recently it has been suggested that percutaneous drainage of the abscess is the most effective and less morbid procedure.

60. Suggested algorithm for treatment of chronic inflammatory prostatitis:

(a) Surgery, prostatic massage, alfa blocker, finasteride
(b) Antibiotics, alfa blocker, prostatic massage
(c) Antibiotics, prostatic massage, alfa blocker, surgery
(d) Analgesics, muscle relaxants, perineal exercises, reassurance

(Answer is B) Antibiotics, alfa blocker, prostatic massage.

61. Chronic orchitis involves inflammation and pain in the testis, usually without swelling, persisting for more than:

(a) 2 weeks (b) 4 weeks
(c) 6 weeks (d) 8 weeks

(Answer is C) Chronic orchitis involves inflammation and pain in the testis, usually without swelling, persisting for more than 6 weeks.

62. Which is not correctly matched as most common organism causing epididymitis?

(a) Children–coliform organism

(b) Sexually active heterosexual–gonococcus. chlamydia
(c) Sexually active homosexual–gonococcus chlamydia
(d) Adults–coliform organism

(Answer is C) In homosexual men practicing anal intercourse, E. coli and Haemophilus influenzae are most commonly responsible.

63. To be diagnosed with interstitial cystitis, patients must have all *except:*

(a) Patients must have both glomerulations on cystoscopic examination and a classic Hunner ulcer
(b) An examination for glomerulations should be undertaken after distention of the bladder under anesthesia to 80 to 100 cm H_2O for 1 to 2 minutes
(c) The glomerulations must be diffuse and present in at least three quadrants of the bladder
(d) There must be at l east 10 glomerulations per quadrant

(Answer is A) To be diagnosed with interstitial cystitis, patients must have either glomerulations on cystoscopic examination or a classic Hunner ulcer, and they must have either pain associated with the bladder or urinary urgency.

64. Interstitial cystitis all are true *except:*

(a) It is diagnosis of exclusion
(b) Allergies were the most common association, with over 40% affected
(c) Duration of symptoms less than 9 months
(d) Mast cells act as a pathognomonic marker

(Answer is C) Duration of symptoms less than 9 months excludes IC.

65. Which statement regarding etiology of IC is not true?

(a) No data currently to suggest that stress initiates the chronic syndrome of IC
(b) No clear data suggesting pelvic floor dysfunction has been associated with PBS/IC
(c) No reports have ever documented a relationship to suggest that IC is a premalignant lesion
(d) No clear indication of a primary role for autoimmunity as the cause of IC has been observed

(Answer is B) Pelvic floor dysfunction has been associated with PBS/IC for many years, and uncontrolled trials suggest that treatment of the pelvic floor can be effective in ameliorating symptoms.

66. Which cell has been reported to be associated with IC, both as a pathogenetic mechanism and as a pathognomonic marker?

(a) Monocytes (b) Platelets
(c) NK cell (d) Mast cell

(Answer is D) Mast cells have frequently been reported to be associated with IC, both as a pathogenetic mechanism and as a pathognomonic marker.

67. Most accurate marker of PBS/IC is:

(a) Eosinophil cationic protein
(b) Glycosaminoglycan excretion
(c) Urinary histamine and methylhistamine
(d) APF

(Answer is D) The urine antiproliferative factor (APF) may prove to be the most accurate marker of PBS/IC when confirmed by other centers. It appears to have the highest sensitivity and specificity of the variety of possible markers tested and fits nicely into an etiologic schema.

68. What is the oral drug of choice for treatment for IC?

(a) Amitriptyline (b) Gabapentin
(c) Hydroxyzine (d) Montelukast

(Answer is A) Amitriptyline has become a staple of oral treatment for IC.

69. Montelukast is:
(a) PGE receptor inhibitor
(b) PGF receptor inhibitor
(c) LT B2 receptor inhibitor
(d) LT D4 receptor inhibitor

(Answer is D) Leukotriene D4 receptor antagonist.

70. Bladder "cocktail" used for IC include all *except:*
(a) 50 ml of 50% DMSO
(b) 10 mg of triamcinolone
(c) 1,00,000 units of BCG
(d) 44 mEq of sodium bicarbonate

(Answer is C) 50 ml of 50% DMSO as a bladder "cocktail" with 10 mg of triamcinolone, 40,000 units of heparin, and 44 mEg of sodium bicarbonate.

71. Which of the following is both a diagnostic and therapeutic modality?
(a) Urodynamics
(b) Bladder biopsy
(c) Bladder hydrodistention
(d) KCL test

(Answer is C) Hydrodistention of the bladder under anesthesia, while technically a surgical treatment, is often the first therapeutic modality employed, often as a part of the diagnostic evaluation.

72. Regarding treatment of interstitial cystitis all are true *except:*
(a) Up to 90% of cases shows spontaneous resolution
(b) Patient education is an important initial step
(c) Amitriptyline has become staple of oral treatment
(d) Mainstay of treatment is intravesical DMSO

(Answer is A) There is a 50% temporary spontaneous remission rate, with a mean duration of 8 months.

73. "Strawberry vulva" or "strawberry cervix" is characterstic of which infection?
(a) Chlamydia (b) Gonococcus
(c) Trichimoniasis (d) Herpes simplex

(Answer is C) Clinical examination in trichimoniasis, may reveal a frothy discharge and the characteristic "strawberry vulva" or "strawberry cervix.

74. 25-year-male presented with single painless, indurated ulcer at glans. Patient also has bilateral non tender inguinal lymphadenopathy. Appropriate treatment will be:
(a) Acyclovir 400 mg TDS–10 days
(b) Benzathiazide penicillin 2.4 million units IM single dose
(c) Doxycydine 100 mg BD–21 days
(d) Erythromycin 500 mg QID–21 days

(Answer is B) Benzathiazide penicillin G (2.4 million units intramuscularly as a single dose) remains the treatment of choice for primary syphilis.

75. 30-year-male presented with painful genital ulcer which is friable and bleeds easily. He also has painful inguinal lymph nodes. Diagnosis is:
(a) Granuloma inguinale
(b) LGV
(c) Chancroid
(d) Syphilis

(Answer is C) Chancroid causes a painful, non-indurated ulcer on the penis or vulvovaginal area. The ulcer has a friable base covered with a gray or yellow purulent exudate and a shaggy border.

76. Vesicles grouped on erythematous base that does not follow neural distribution is pathognomonic of:
(a) Granuloma inguinale
(b) HSV
(c) Chancroid
(d) Syphilis

(Answer is B) A group of vesicles on an erythematous

base that does not follow a neural distribution is pathognomonic of HSV infection.

77. A 40-year-male has painless vesicle ulcer and painful matted lymph nodes with fistulous tracts. Diagnosis is:

(a) Granuloma inguinale

(b) LGV

(c) Chancroid

(d) Syphilis

(Answer is B) In lymphogranuloma small, painless vesicle or papule progresses to an ulcer, white painful, atted, large nodes develop with fistulous tracts.

78. Gonococcal urethritis all are true *except:*

(a) Caused by gram negative diplococcus

(b) Incubation period is 3-14 days

(c) Usually thick curdy urethral discharge

(d) Ceftriaxone is drug of choice

(Answer is C) Candidiasis is characterised by white, thick, curdy vaginal discharge.

79. Risk of sero-conversion after needle stick injury for HIV and hepatitis B respectively is:

(a) 0.3%, 12%

(b) 3%, 1.2%

(c) 0.3%, 1.2%

(d) 3%, 12%

(Answer is A) In HIV the risk of sero-conversion after a needle stick injury appears to be approximately 0.3%. This rate can be compared with the risk of hepatitis B infection from an accidental needle stick, which is estimated at 12% per stick.

80. Which retroviral drug has renal stones as adverse effect?

(a) Zidovudine

(b) Lamivudine

(c) Nevirapine

(d) Indinavir

(Answer is D) Indinavir is a potent protease inhibitor has been associated with urolithiasis.

81. Which statement regarding HIV is not correct?

(a) Eradication of HIV is not possible with available antiviral drugs

(b) In the absence of treatment, the typical course of HIV occurs over 8 to 12 years

(c) Without antiretroviral therapy, AIDS usually leads to death in 6 to 8 years

(d) In 60% to 70% of HIV-infected patients, the median time between infection and the development of AIDS is 10 years, in the absence of therapy

(Answer is C) Without antiretroviral therapy, AIDS usually leads to death in 2 to 3 years

82. Which statement is not true regarding HIV-2 infection?

(a) There have been very few cases of HIV-2 in the developed world

(b) It is transmitted less readily than HIV-1

(c) It is more virulent than HIV-1

(d) Both HIV-1 and HIV-2 have similar modes of transmission

(Answer is C) HIV-2 is transmitted less readily than HIV-1 and the virus is less virulent.

83. Which statement is not true regarding HIV detection?

(a) HIV RNA can be detected from day 12

(b) HIV RNA assays have a sensitivity of 100% in diagnosing acute infection, but at the cost of lowered specificity (97%)

(c) The first antibodies can generally be detected on day 42

(d) The nadir in plasma HIV RNA levels is a marker for the duration of virus suppression

(Answer is C) The first antibodies can generally be detected on day 21.

84. Most patients with indinavir induced stones will require what modality of treatment?

(a) ESWL

(b) PCNL
(c) Conservative treatment
(d) Nephrectomy

(Answer is C) Conservative treatment in most cases, consisting of hydration, analgesics and temporary cessation of indinavir.

85. Regarding Kaposi sarcoma (KS) which statement is not true?

(a) The risk of KS increases 1000 fold, among HIV-infected patients
(b) KS is the most common vascular neoplasm in certain HIV-infected populations
(c) KS is associated with human herpes virus 6
(d) No specific therapy is curative

(Answer is C) KS-associated herpesvirus or human herpesvirus 8 is essential for all forms of KS.

86. Palpable lesion >0.5 cm is called as:

(a) Plaque (b) Papule
(c) Patch (d) Pustule

(Answer is A) Common descriptive terms for skin lesions include macule, a flat lesion smaller than 0.5 cm; patch, a flat lesion larger than 0.5 cm; papule, an elevated 0.5 cm lesion; nodule, a deeper-based papular lesion; plaque, a palpable lesion larger than 0.5 cm; vesicle, a fluid-filled palpable lesion smaller than 0.5 cm; pustule, a pus-filled palpable lesion; bulla or blister, a fluid-filled lesion larger than 0.5 cm.

87. Which one of the following is primary skin lesion?

(a) Scale (b) Crust
(c) Erosion (d) Vesicle

(Answer is D) Vesicle, pustule and bulla are primary skin lesion.

88. Red plaques covered with white scale is noted over glans penis. It is pruritic. Diagnosis is:

(a) Lichen planus
(b) Seborrheic dermatitis
(c) Psoriasis
(d) Reiter's syndrome

(Answer is A) In lichen planus lesions appear as red to pink plaques or patches covered with white to gray scale.

89. Thirty years old male has sharply demarcated erythematous plaque with silvery-white scales over elbow and knees. Diagnosis is:

(a) Lichen planus
(b) Seborrheic dermatitis
(c) Psoriasis
(d) Reiter's syndrome

(Answer is C) The characteristic lesion in psoriasis is a sharply demarcated erythematous plaque with silvery-white scales. Its pattern can be limited to the elbows or knees or distributed over the entire surface of the skin.

90. Reiter's syndrome includes all *except:*

(a) Urethritis (b) Arthritis
(c) Conjunctivitis (d) Pancreatitis

(Answer is D) Reiter's syndrome occurs as a triad of arthritis of at least a month's duration in association with urethritis, cervicitis, or enteritis and conjunctivitis. Iritis may also occur.

91. Which dermatological disorder is associated with squamous cell carcinoma?

(a) Lichen planus
(b) Seborrheic dermatitis
(c) Psoriasis
(d) Lichen sclerosus

(Answer is D) LS has been associated with squamous cell carcinoma of the penis, particularly those variants not associated with HPV, and may represent a premalignant condition.

92. Regarding fixed drug eruption all are true *except:*

(a) Usually 1 to 2 days after the first exposure

(b) Commonly involves the lips, face, hands, feet and genitalia
(c) After subsequent reexposure to the drug, the reaction presents in the same location, usually within 24 hours
(d) The most common medications causing this reaction are sulfonamides, nonsteroidal anti-inflammatory agents

(Answer is A) A fixed drug eruption occurs in response to oral medications, usually 1 to 2 weeks after the first exposure.

93. Which statement regarding Behcet syndrome is not correct?

(a) The genital lesions are smaller and generally less painful than the oral lesions
(b) Optic involvement occurs in 90% of cases and may lead to blindness
(c) Likely involves a genetic predisposition and an autoimmune mode of pathogenesis
(d) Individuals may also suffer from epididymitis, thrombophlebitis and aneurysms

(Answer is A) The genital lesions are larger and generally more painful than the oral lesions.

94. Verrucous carcinoma all are true *except:*

(a) Also called Buschke-Lowenstein tumor
(b) Slow growing variant of BCC
(c) Associated with HPV 6 and 11
(d) Most common location is glans penis

(Answer is B) Venucous carcinoma, or Buschke-Lowenstein tumor, is a variant of squamous cell carcinoma.

95. Langhan's giant cells are activated:

(a) Neutrophil (b) Eosinophil
(c) Lymphocyte (d) Macrophage

(Answer is D) The activated macrophages become epithelioid cells, which may form into Langhan's giant cells.

96. Regarding HIV infected patients with TB which statement is not true?

(a) TB is the most common opportunistic infection in AIDS patients
(b) The probability that an HIV-infected person who was previously infected with M. tuberculosis will develop active TB is 25% per year
(c) Normal host without HIV infection and a similar M. tuberculosis experience will have a 5% to 10 % lifetime probability of developing active TB
(d) Among patients with both TB and AIDS, almost two thirds develop TB within 6 months of developing AIDS

(Answer is B) The probability that an HIV-infected person who was previously infected with M. tuberculosis will develop active TB is 10% per year.

97. Regarding TB of kidney which statement is not true?

(a) The patient usually complains of frequent painless micturition
(b) 50% of patients do not have any leukocytes in the urine
(c) Microscopic hematuria is present in upto 50%
(d) Commonly, the symptoms are intermittent

(Answer is B) The urine is classically characterized by a sterile pyuria; however, up to 20% of patients do not have any leukocytes in the urine.

98. All about mycobacterium is true *except:*

(a) Humans is the only reservoir
(b) Strictly aerobic
(c) Slow growing with doubling time of 20 minutes
(d) AFB smear identify organism only if levels are > 10000 bacilli /ml of sputum

(Answer is C) M. tuberculosis is strictly aerobic but slow growing with a doubling time of 15 to 20 hours.

99. Which is false regarding TB genitourinary tract?

(a) Bladder and ureter TB are always secondary to renal TB
(b) Most common site affected in ureter is PUJ
(c) Renal TB is caused by activation of blood borne metastatic renal infection
(d) Earliest form of infection in urinary bladder starts around ureteric orifice

(Answer is B) Tuberculous ureteritis is always an extension of the disease from the kidney. The site most commonly affected is the ureterovesical junction.

100. All about TB epididymis is correct *except:*

(a) TB of testis is always secondary to TB epididymis
(b) Disease starts in globus minor due to increase blood supply
(c) Usual presentation is painless scrotal swelling
(d) TB epididymis can be the first and only presentation of genitourinary TB

(Answer is C) The usual presentation is a painful, inflamed scrotal swelling.

101. 5 mm of Induration in tuberculin test is considered positive in all the cases *except:*

(a) HIV-positive persons
(b) Recent contacts of tuberculosis (TB) case patients
(c) Patients with organ transplants
(d) Injection drug abusers

(Answer is D) Injection drug abusers–more than 10 mm induration is considered positive.

102. Radiological test used as standard practice for evaluation of genitourinary TB is:

(a) Plain radiograph
(b) Intravenous urogram (IVU)
(c) Retrograde pyelography (RGP)
(d) Ultrasound

(Answer is B) The introduction of the high-dose intravenous urogram has been a major advance in the investigation of renal tract abnormality and is now standard practice.

103. Which is the imaging modality of choice for the diagnosis and evaluation of genitourinary TB?

(a) Plain radiograph
(b) Intravenous urogram (IVU)
(c) CECT
(d) Ultrasound

(Answer is C) CT has become more widely available and has arguably replaced IVU as the imaging modality of choice for the diagnosis and evaluation of genitourinary TB.

104. Which statement is false regarding urine examination in TB patients?

(a) Sterile pyuria is a classical finding
(b) Preferably 3 early morning samples of urine should be cultured
(c) Secondary bacterial infection with E. coli is uncommon
(d) Microscopic hematuria is seen in up to 50% of cases

(Answer is B) At least three, but preferably five, consecutive early morning specimens of urine should be cultured. Overt hematuria is present in only 10% of patients, but microscopic hematuria is present in up to 50%.

105. Which is not the adverse affect of ATT drug?

(a) Streptomycin-ototoxic, hepatotoxic
(b) Rifampicin-renal insufficiency
(c) Pyrazinamidc-arthralgia, hyperuricemia
(d) Isoniazid-hepatotoxic, peripheral neuropathy

(Answer is B) Hepatotoxicity is the major adverse reaction to rifampicin. Liver failure requires a moderate reduction in dosage, but full doses can be given with renal insufficiency.

106. Which statement regarding mode of action of ATT is not correct?

(a) Isoniazid inhibits the synthesis of mycolic acids

(b) Rifampicin acts to inhibit bacterial RNA synthesis by interfering with RNA-directed DNA polymerase

(c) Streptomycin interferes with bacterial protein synthesis

(d) Pyrizinamide inhibits fatty acid synthetase

(Answer is B) Rifampicin acts to inhibit bacterial RNA synthesis by interfering with DNA-directed RNA polymerase.

107. A 6 months regimen of ATT is effective in which type of tuberculosis?

(a) TB meningitis

(b) TB osteomyelitis

(c) TB genitourinary tract

(d) Disseminated TB

(Answer is C) 6-month regimens are effective for most forms of TB, including genitourinary TB, with the exception of disseminated TB, TB osteomyelitis and TB meningitis.

108. Which one is the indication for partial nephrectomy?

(a) Non-functioning kidney without calcification

(b) Renal TB leading to hypertension

(c) Coexisting renal carcinoma

(d) Slowly growing area of calcification threatening whole of the kidney

(Answer is D) There are only two indications for partial nephrectomy: (1) the localized polar lesion containing calcification that has failed to respond after 6 weeks of intensive chemotherapy and (2) an area of calcification that is slowly increasing in size and is threatening to gradually destroy the whole kidney. Partial nephrectomy is difficult to justify in the absence of calcification.

109. Indications for permanent urinary diversion in patients with GUTB are all *except:*

(a) Enuresis

(b) Incontinence

(c) Psychiatric disturbance

(d) Poor renal function

(Answer is D) There are only three indications for permanent urinary diversion: (1) a history of psychiatric disturbance or obvious subnormal intelligence, (2) enuresis not related to small bladder capacity, and (3) intolerable diurnal symptoms with incontinence that has not responded to chemotherapy or bladder dilatation.

110. Not true about Schistosoma haematobium is:

(a) Human infection is acquired by exposure to fresh water that harbor infected snails

(b) Egg laying occurs in vesical and pelvic venules

(c) Laterally spined eggs in urine, feces and tissues are diagnostic

(d) In active infection all stages are seen

(Answer is C) S. haematobium eggs measure 80 to 150 mm, are ovoid, and are terminally spined, which differentiates them from laterally spined S. mansoni eggs.

111. Which statement regarding praziquantel is not correct?

(a) Praziquantel is the drug of choice for all Schistosoma species

(b) It is active against all clinical forms and stages of the disease

(c) Cure rates with praziquantel for S. haematobium infection approaches 100%

(d) Recommendation is single oral dose of 40 mg/kg in 1 day for S. haematobium

(Answer is D) The current recommendation is two oral doses of 40 mg/kg in I day for S. haematobium.

112. Which statement regarding genital filariasis is not correct?

(a) Wuchereria bancrofti accounts for 90% of cases of human lymphatic filariasis
(b) Wuchereria is an exclusively human parasite without animal reservoirs
(c) Most common urban vectors of W. bancrofti are the Culex pipiens complex
(d) Nonlymphatic filariasis is caused by Brugia malayi

(Answer is D) Nonlymphatic filariasis is caused by Onchocerca volvulus, the agent of African river blindness.

113. Which statement regarding DEC is not correct?

(a) All patients with filarial infection, symptomatic or not, should be treated with DEC
(b) Administered as 6 mg/kg/day in three divided doses for 2 weeks
(c) DEC is approved by the U.S. Food and Drug Administration
(d) No effect on adult filariae

(Answer is D) The objective of DEC therapy is to kill the adult worms and to abolish microfilaremia.

114. In ICU infections, candida species isranked:

(a) First (b) Third
(c) Fourth (d) Seventh

(Answer is C) Recent studies revealed that Candida species accounted for 10.1% of intensive care unit infections, which ranked them fourth after Pseudomonas aeruginosa (12.4%), Staphylococcus aureus (12.3%) and coagulase-negative staphylococci (10.2%).

115. Most common predisposing factors for candidemia and primary sites of infection is:

(a) Intravascular catheters
(b) Total parenteral nutrition
(c) Urinary tract
(d) Respiratory tract

(Answer is A) Predisposing factors for candidemia and primary sites of infection included intravascular catheters (65%), total parenteral nutrition (42%), urinary tract (11%), gastro-intestinal tract (8%) and respiratory tract (7%).

116. With a documented single episode of candiduria, the major associated illnesses include:

(a) DM
(b) Urinary tract disease
(c) Malignancy
(d) Malnutrition

(Answer is A) With a documented single episode of candiduria, the major associated illnesses included diabetes mellitus (39%), urinary tract disease (37.7%), malignancy (22.2%) and malnutrition (17%).

117. Treatment of vulvovaginal candidiasis is:

(a) Single dose voriconazole
(b) Single dose amphotericin
(c) Single dose itraconazole
(d) Single dose fluconazole

(Answer is D) Treatment with oral fluconazole (a single 150 mg dose) is as effective as topical intravaginal therapy in the treatment of vulvovaginal candidiasis.

118. Treatment of urinary bladder candidal infection includes all *except:*

(a) Itraconazole (b) Amphotericin
(c) Fluconazole (d) Flucytosine

(Answer is A) Itraconazole is effective in the treatment of infections caused by Aspergillus, Blastomyces, Coccidioides and Histoplasma.

119. Reservoir of cryptococcal infection in AIDS patient is:

(a) Kidney (b) Adrenal
(c) Prostate (d) Testis

(Answer is C) In AIDS patients, the prostate has been recognized as a "reservoir" for relapsing cryptococcosis, following successful treatment for cryptococcal meningitis.

120. Which one of the anti-fungal does not belong to triazole group?

(a) Itraconazole (b) Voriconazole
(c) Fluconazole (d) Ketoconazole

(Answer is D) The imidazoles include the topical drugs clotrimazole and miconazole and the oral agent ketoconazole.

121. Incubation period of LGV:

(a) < 3 days (b) 3-30 days
(c) 30-90 days (d) 90-180 days

(Answer is B) Incubation period from LGV 3-30 days.

122. What does make UTI more common in mid-aged females than in males?

(a) Short female urethra
(b) Pregnancy
(c) Vaginal colonization with enterobacteria
(d) All of the above

(Answer is D) All of the above

123. Which organism is capable of proliferation in the urine and causing urethritis?

(a) Ureaplasma urealyticum
(b) Chlamydia trachomatis
(c) E. coli
(d) Neisseria gonorrhea

(Answer is A) Ureaplasma urealyticum

124. What helps in treating Candida albicans cystitis is?

(a) Sodium bicarbonate (b) Phyto soya
(c) Ascorbic acid (d) Sol palmetto

(Answer is A) Sodium bicarbonate

125. Which agent is safe to kidneys?

(a) Amoxicillin (b) Gentamycin
(c) Diclofenac (d) Herb extract

(Answer is A) Amoxicillin

126. Which of the following carries the greatest risk of HIV transmission to health care workers?

(a) Splash of patient's blood to the eyes
(b) Splash of patient's blood to the mouth
(c) Surgical suture needle stick
(d) Hollow bore needle stick

(Answer is D) Hollow bore needle stick

127. Which antibiotic is the best to treat soft tissue infection with methicillin-resistant Staphylococcus aureus (MRSA) in hospitalized patients?

(a) Vancomycin (b) Cefotaxime
(c) Penicillin G (d) Tobramycin

(Answer is A) Vancomycin

128. Which agent is most likely to cause hemorrhagic cystitis?

(a) Cisplatin (b) Ifosfamide
(c) Phosphomycin (d) Amphotericin B

(Answer is B) Ifosfamide

129. What is the number of bacteria per high-power field microscopy that matches colony counts of 100,000/ml?

(a) 100 (b) 50
(c) 10 (d) 5

(Answer is D) 5

130. Which of the following might cause sterile pyuria?

(a) Renal tuberculosis
(b) Urinary tract stones
(c) Interstitial cystitis
(d) All of the above

(Answer is D) All of the above

131. Which microbe causes "red diaper syndrome"?

(a) Serratia marcescens
(b) Streptococcus pyogenes
(c) Clostridium difficile
(d) Staphylococcus saprophyticus

(Answer is A) Serratia marcescens

132. What type of renal tubular acidosis (RTA) does demonstrate aldosterone resistance?

(a) Type 1 (b) Type 2
(c) Type 3 (d) Type 4

(Answer is D) Type 4

133. What is false concerning coagulase splitting bacteria (Griess) test?

(a) It is a reduction reaction that converts nitrate to nitrite
(b) Nitrazine reagent papers are used to elicit the reaction
(c) It is false negative in diluted urine, on taking vitamin C, and in gram +ve bacteria
(d) The reaction takes 4 minutes to complete

(Answer is D) The reaction takes 4 minutes to complete

134. Bacterial resistance to antibiotics may occur because of:

(a) Inherited chromosomal-mediated resistance
(b) Acquired chromosomal-mediated resistance
(c) Extrachromosomal-mediated resistance
(d) All of the above

(Answer is D) All of the above

135. What class of antibiotics might cause vestibular and/or auditory impairment?

(a) Aminoglycosides
(b) α anti-pseudomonal penicillins
(c) Cephalosporins
(d) Fluoroquinolones

(Answer is A) Aminoglycosides

136. What antibiotic could result in "red man syndrome"?

(a) Vancomycin (b) Clindamycin
(c) Streptomycin (d) Tobramycin

(Answer is A) Vancomycin

137. What is false concerning fosfomycin antibiotic?

(a) Has a limited cross-resistance with most common antibacterial agents
(b) Causes injection site reactions
(c) Is active against most uropathogens
(d) Is effective as a single-dose agent

(Answer is B) Causes injection site reactions

138. What is the most appropriate antibiotic class for prophylaxis before urologic surgery?

(a) Aminoglycosides
(b) Macrolides
(c) Cephalosporins
(d) Fluoroquinolones

(Answer is C) Cephalosporins

139. What is false concerning asymptomatic bacteriuria during pregnancy?

(a) Occurs in 2 – 10% of pregnancies
(b) Commonly occurs in the first trimester
(c) Usually, associated with urinary tract abnormalities
(d) Could progress to serious complications if left untreated

(Answer is C) Usually, associated with urinary tract abnormalities

140. What is false concerning asymptomatic bacteriuria during pregnancy?

(a) Could lead to pyelonephritis, low birth weight, premature labor
(b) Pregnant women are at higher risk of UTI in weeks 6 throughout 24

(c) Antibiotics should be culture-based and given, preferably, intravenous in a single shot
(d) Screening for asymptomatic bacteriuria should begin at first antenatal visit

(Answer is C) Antibiotics should be culture-based and given, preferably, intravenous in a single shot

141. What antibiotic is safe at all stages of pregnancy?

(a) Nitrofurantoin (b) Amoxicillin
(c) Sulphonamides (d) Doxycycline

(Answer is B) Amoxicillin

142. What is true concerning urinary frequency during pregnancy?

(a) Could be a sign of UTI
(b) Occurs because the bladder capacity decreases
(c) Occurs because the renal blood flow increases
(d) All are true

(Answer is D) All are true

143. When should UTI be treated in pregnancy?

(a) When a positive urine culture is obtained
(b) Asymptomatic bacteriuria should be treated
(c) Catheterized pregnants should not be treated
(d) When UTI is recurrent

(Answer is B) Asymptomatic bacteriuria should be treated

144. What antibiotic classes are safe and effective throughout pregnancy?

(a) Aminopenicillins and cephalosporins
(b) Co-trimoxazole and nitrofurantoins
(c) Fluoroquinolones and minoglycosides
(d) Macrolides and clindamycin

(Answer is A) Aminopenicillins and cephalosporins

145. Among bacteriuria cases in pregnant women, what is the incidence of acute clinical pyelonephritis in untreated cases?

(a) 0.5 – 5% (b) 5 – 15%
(c) 15 – 25% (d) 25 – 35%

(Answer is D) 25 – 35%

146. Why could pyuria be sterile?

(a) Because standard laboratory culture specifications might not be favorable for growth of atypical organisms
(b) Because UTI could show fewer than 10 white cells/mm^3 in urine
(c) Because laboratories may not report significant growth of a defined urinary pathogen
(d) All of the above

(Answer is D) All of the above

147. Which of the following does not cause sterile pyouria?

(a) Inadequately treated UTI
(b) Renal papillary necrosis
(c) Acute emphysematous pyelonephritis
(d) Urinary tract tuberculosis

(Answer is C) Acute emphysematous pyelonephritis

148. What condition causes sterile pyuria?

(a) Urethral infection with trichomonas vaginalis
(b) Bladder infection with adenovirus
(c) Kawasaki's disease
(d) All of the above

(Answer is D) All of the above

149. What is true concerning bacterial colonization in the bladder?

(a) Always asymptomatic
(b) Shows a serological immune antibody response

(c) A common cause of sterile pyuria
(d) Typically, at this stage, the body demonstrates bacteriuria

(Answer is A) Always asymptomatic

150. The virulence of uropathogenic E. coli depends on all the following, *except*:

(a) P blood group antigen
(b) P fimbriae in descending infections
(c) Emolysins
(d) Dr family of adhesins in ascending infections

(Answer is B) P fimbriae in descending infections

151. Asymptomatic bacteriuria should be treated in the following situations:

(a) The elderly
(b) Long-term catheterized patient
(c) Pregnancy
(d) None of the above

(Answer is C) Pregnancy

152. What could cause unresolved bacteriuria?

(a) Drug resistance
(b) Non-compliance
(c) The presence of persistent pathology
(d) All of the above

(Answer is D) All of the above

153. What is the proper term to describe high bacterial count in urine without pus?

(a) Asymptomatic bacteriuria
(b) Sterile pyouria
(c) Bacterial colonization
(d) Unresolved bacteriuria

(Answer is C) Bacterial colonization

154. What is true concerning the treatment of catheter associated bacteriuria?

(a) Should be flushed frequently, but no antibiotic is advised
(b) Should be treated if febrile UTI has developed
(c) Should be treated only if urine culture is positive
(d) Should be treated once the catheter is removed

(Answer is B) Should be treated if febrile UTI has developed

155. What could not cause recurrent UTI in a 25 years woman?

(a) Bladder neck suspension surgery
(b) Chronic constipation
(c) Poor genital hygiene
(d) Contraceptive diaphragm

(Answer is A) Bladder neck suspension surgery

156. What is (are) the cause(s) of recurrent community acquired UTI in women?

(a) Uncontrolled DM
(b) Sexual activity with multiple partners
(c) High vaginal receptivity to bacterial adherence
(d) All of the above

(Answer is D) All of the above

157. What is false regarding malakoplakia?

(a) An uncommon granulomatous disease that affect the skin and/or urinary bladder
(b) Might be due to a disturbed function of B lymphocytes
(c) Characterized by the presence of basophilic inclusion structure (Michaelis-Gutmann body)
(d) Might be due to a defective phagolysosomal activity of monocytes or macrophages

(Answer is B) Might be due to a disturbed function of B lymphocytes

158. What is true concerning malakoplakia?

(a) A premalignant condition

(b) Can be locally aggressive and invades surrounding structures causing bone erosions

(c) Kidneys are the most commonly affected organs

(d) Characterized by rounded intracellular inclusions (owls-eyes) in large eosinophilic histocytes

(Answer is B) Can be locally aggressive and invades surrounding structures causing bone erosions

159. What is (are) the prominent clinical finding(s) in the diagnosis of acute pyelonephritis?

(a) Fever, chills, abdominal pain

(b) Costovertebral angle tenderness

(c) Hypogastric and loin pain

(d) Flank pain, dysuria

(Answer is B) Costovertebral angle tenderness

160. What is false concerning acute pyelonephritis?

(a) CBC reveals leucocytosis with predominance of neutrophils

(b) Contrast CT reveals one or more focal wedge-like swollen regions of the kidney parenchyma, sparing the cortex, and demonstrating reduced enhancement "rim sign"

(c) Children, recurrent acute pyelonephritis might lead to renal scarring

(d) Pregnancy, recurrent acute pyelonephritis might lead to preterm labor

(Answer is B) Contrast CT reveals one or more focal wedge-like swollen regions of the kidney parenchyma, sparing the cortex, and demonstrating reduced enhancement "rim sign"

161. What is true regarding acute pyelonephritis?

(a) A cause of obstruction should be sought

(b) PCN is placed to decompress the kidney and preserve renal function

(c) Bloodborn staphylococci are commoner than ascending E.coli infections

(d) Blood and urine cultures must dictate the antibiotic choice from day 1

(Answer is A) A cause of obstruction should be sought

162. What is false concerning peri-renal abscess?

(a) Could result from intrarenal abscess of ascending infection

(b) Urine culture might be negative

(c) Plain KUB X-ray has no value in the diagnosis

(d) Surgical drainage is the proper treatment

(Answer is C) Plain KUB X-ray has no value in the diagnosis

163. What is true regarding contrast CT imaging for a renal abscess?

(a) Abscess appears as a low attenuation cystic cavity containing gas

(b) Renal parenchyma around the abscess cavity may show hypo enhancement in nephrogram phase

(c) Associated fascial and septal thickening are seen with obliteration of perinephric fat

(d) All of the above

(Answer is D) All of the above

164. What is false concerning genitourinary TB?

(a) The most common extrapulmonary site of infection

(b) Bladder TB is secondary to renal TB, and usually begins at the ureteral orifices

(c) The kidneys, TB is typically bilateral, cortical, and adjacent to the glomeruli; they may remain dormant for ages

(d) Epididymal TB might occur by

hematogenous or direct spread from the urinary tract

(Answer is A) The most common extrapulmonary site of infection

165. What is true regarding genitourinary TB?

(a) Commonly, TB enters the urinary tract via intravesical instillation of attenuated live BCG to treat bladder cancer
(b) CT urography may show infundibular stricture with or without hydrocalicosis
(c) Renal ultrasonography reveals calyceal erosions "moth-eaten calyx"
(d) TB of the vas appears, clinically, as a thin hard strictured tube

(Answer is B) CT urography may show infundibular stricture with or without hydrocalicosis

166. What is false concerning the management of genitourinary TB?

(a) Prostatic TB is better drained per rectum before initiating the medications
(b) Renal TB may require nephroureterectomy
(c) Peripheral neuritis is a known side effect of isoniazid
(d) Moxifloxacin might result in tendon rupture

(Answer is A) Prostatic TB is better drained per rectum before initiating the medications

167. All of the following etiologies for interstitial cystitis have been theorized, *except*:

(a) Allergic, type I hypersensitivity response
(b) Pelvic floor dysfunction
(c) Up-regulation of histaminergic and muscarinic neuro-receptors
(d) Neural hypersensitivity

(Answer is A) Allergic, type I hypersensitivity response

168. Which of the following conditions is not associated with interstitial cystitis?

(a) Inflammatory bowel disease
(b) Rheumatoid arthritis
(c) Systemic lupus erythematosus
(d) Fibromyalgia

(Answer is B) Rheumatoid arthritis

169. What is false concerning the cystoscopic findings of interstitial cystitis?

(a) Hunner's ulcers are multiple ulcerative patches surrounded by mucosal congestion on the dome or lateral walls
(b) Ulcers might get distorted after over-distention, because discrete areas of mucosal scarring rupture during the procedure
(c) Non-ulcerative type, overdistention demonstrates glomerulations on the dome and lateral walls
(d) Overdistention results in mucosal tears and submucosal hemorrhage

(Answer is B) Ulcers might get distorted after overdistention, because discrete areas of mucosal scarring rupture during the procedure

170. What is false regarding biopsy-taking from interstitial cystitis bladder?

(a) Pathognomonic histology for interstitial cystitis
(b) Basically, biopsies are performed to exclude carcinomas and other varieties of cystitis
(c) Diagnostic biopsies include the presence of discrete micro-ulcers and increased numbers of mast cells in the detrusor muscle or submucosa
(d) None of the above

(Answer is C) Diagnostic biopsies include the presence of discrete micro-ulcers and increased numbers of mast cells in the detrusor muscle or submucosa

171. How should a proper routine urine specimen be collected?

(a) Early morning sample, after cleansing the perineum and meatus
(b) Urethral catheterization under strict aseptic technique
(c) A clean catch of midstream voided urine
(d) Suprapubic aspiration, as urine is sterile

(Answer is C) A clean catch of midstream voided urine

172. What is true regarding honeymoon cystitis?

(a) A self-limiting infection where antibiotics are not required
(b) Exclusively for UTI experienced by a girl after sexual intercourse on her wedding night
(c) Post-coital voiding has no value in the occurrence of the infection
(d) Self-initiated medication helps control the infection

(Answer is D) Self-initiated medication helps control the infection

173. What does not predispose to acute epididymitis?

(a) TUR ejaculatory duct
(b) Prolonged urethral catheterization
(c) Prostatic biopsy
(d) Vas ligation

(Answer is C) Prostatic biopsy

174. What are the most common organisms causing acute epididymitis in males younger than 35 years?

(a) N. gonorrhea and C. trachomatis
(b) E. coli and Pseudomonas species
(c) Mycoplasma genitalium and Ureaplasma species
(d) Trichomonas vaginalis and Gardnerella vaginalis

(Answer is A) N. gonorrhea and C. trachomatis

175. Management of acute epididymo-orchitis in hospitalized patients includes all of the following, *except*:

(a) Scrotal support and elevation
(b) Ice packs
(c) Non-steroidal anti-inflammatory agents
(d) Urethral catheterization

(Answer is D) Urethral catheterization

176. What is false concerning epididymitis?

(a) Should be distinguished from testicular torsion in the emergency setting
(b) Viral epididymitis is common in the elderly
(c) Chronic epididymitis might complicate BPH
(d) Chronic epididymitis might require epididymectomy

(Answer is B) Viral epididymitis is common in the elderly

177. What is not a complication of mumps orchitis?

(a) Infertility
(b) Hypogonadotropic hypogonadism
(c) Non seminomatous germ cell tumor
(d) Chronic orchalgia

(Answer is C) Non seminomatous germ cell tumor

178. What is true regarding chronic epididymitis symptomatology?

(a) Pain is dull aching in the scrotum, perineum, inner thighs and lower abdomen
(b) Dysuria, frequency, and/or urgency
(c) Long-standing (> 6 weeks) history of scrotal pain and tenderness
(d) Low grade fever, malaise and urethral discharge

(Answer is C) Long-standing (> 6 weeks) history of scrotal pain and tenderness

179. What is true concerning scrotal abscesses?

(a) Could be a complication of chronic epididymitis and orchalgia
(b) Testicular torsion must be excluded
(c) Infected hair follicles and scrotal lacerations are predisposing factors

(d) Urethral discharge is not uncommon presentation

(Answer is C) Infected hair follicles and scrotal lacerations are predisposing factors

180. What is false regarding Fournier's gangrene?

(a) Defined as a polymicrobial chronic infection of the perineal, perianal, or genital areas
(b) The disease progresses, branches from the inferior epigastric, deep circumflex iliac, and external pudendal arteries get thrombosed
(c) Presents as a dark skinned–scrotum, subcutaneous crepitation, and foul smell
(d) Surgical debridement often spares the testes

(Answer is A) Defined as a polymicrobial chronic infection of the perineal, perianal, or genital areas

181. Histologically, the pathognomonic finding of Fournier gangrene include:

(a) Necrosis of the superficial and deep fascial planes
(b) Fibrinoid thrombosis of the nutrient arterioles
(c) Polymorphonuclear cell infiltration
(d) All of the above

(Answer is D) All of the above

182. What is the likelihood of contracting gonorrheal disease following a single intercourse with an infected woman?

(a) 1.7% (b) 7%
(c) 17% (d) 71%

(Answer is C) 17%

183. What is false concerning Chlamydia trachomatis urethritis in males?

(a) Produces yellow whitish, scanty, frothy urethral discharge
(b) Shows gram (+), extracellular diplococcic
(c) Infection could be contracted from the spouse's eyes
(d) Responds fairly to azithromycin

(Answer is B) Shows gram (+), extracellular diplococcic

184. What is false regarding Gonorrheal STD in women?

(a) Nucleic acid amplification tests are the preferred to diagnose Gonococcal and Chlamydial infections
(b) Shows dark yellow, purulent, thick urethral discharge
(c) The most common site of the infection is the endocervix
(d) The incubation period is 2 – 3 weeks

(Answer is D) The incubation period is 2 – 3 weeks

185. What is false in the treatment and prevention of STDs?

(a) Antibiotic therapy is recommended for affected individuals with documented trichomonal infection and sexual partners even if asymptomatic
(b) Empirical treatment for gonococcal urethritis should cover chlamydia trachomatis
(c) Consistent and proper usage of condoms is estimated to prevent HIV transmission by approximately 80 to 95%
(d) Vaccinations are available for the prevention of human papillomavirus, N. gonorrhea, chlamydia trachomatis

(Answer is D) Vaccinations are available for the prevention of human papillomavirus, N. gonorrhea, chlamydia trachomatis

186. What is (are) the complication(s) of sexually transmitted infections?

(a) Pelvic inflammatory disease
(b) Lymphogranuloma venereum
(c) Infertility
(d) All of the above

(Answer is D) All of the above

187. What is false regarding Herpes simplex (HSV) infection?

(a) Characterized by neurovirulence
(b) The incubation period of primary genital herpes is 2 – 3 weeks
(c) HSV can be isolated in the urine
(d) HSV-1 infection causes urethritis more often than HSV-2 does

(Answer is B) The incubation period of primary genital herpes is 2 – 3 weeks

188. What is true concerning the definition of UTI in women, based on culture results from a suprapubic aspirate of urine?

(a) Any amount of uropathogen grown in culture indicates UTI
(b) For cystitis, more than 1000 CFU/ml indicates UTI
(c) For pyelonephritis, more than 10,000 CFU/ml indicates UTI
(d) For asymptomatic bacteriuria, more than 100,000 CFU/ml indicates UTI

(Answer is A) Any amount of uropathogen grown in culture indicates UTI

189. Which of the following is not a first-choice antimicrobial agent for uncomplicated acute cystitis in women?

(a) Nitrofurantoin monohydrate/macrocrystals
(b) Trimethoprim-sulfamethoxazole
(c) Ampicillin
(d) Fosfomycin

(Answer is C) Ampicillin

190. What is false concerning urinary catheter-associated UTI (CAUTI)?

(a) Once a catheter is placed, the daily incidence of bacteriuria is 3-10%
(b) Long-term catheterization, over 90% of patients develop bacteriuria
(c) The practice of using urinary catheters to control incontinence in bed-ridden patients should be discouraged
(d) Urine bags should be placed on the floor to enhance gravity drainage

(Answer is D) Urine bags should be placed on the floor to enhance gravity drainage

191. What is not a poor clinical practice on caring for urethral catheters?

(a) Taking urine samples by draining the urine bag
(b) Daily cleansing the external meatus
(c) Placing the urine bag on the floor
(d) Changing the urine bag once it is full

(Answer is B) Daily cleansing the external meatus

192. What is true regarding urinary catheter-associated UTI (CAUTI)?

(a) Indwelling catheter insertion must be under sterile condition
(b) Systemic antibiotics help best in preventing bacteriuria
(c) Greater than 90% of nosocomial UTIs are related to urethral catheters
(d) Intermittent catheterization carries the incidence of 1-3% of developing bacteriuria per insertion

(Answer is D) Intermittent catheterization carries the incidence of 1-3% of developing bacteriuria per insertion

193. What is false about urinary catheters?

(a) Condom catheters carry less risk of UTI if compared to urethral
(b) Suprapubic catheters carry less risk of UTI if compared to urethral
(c) Latex catheters carry less risk of UTI if compared to silicon
(d) Intermittent catheterization carry less risk of UTI if compared to indwelling catheters

(Answer is C) Latex catheters carry less risk of UTI if compared to silicon

194. What is false concerning eosinophilic cystitis?

(a) Probably due to antibody/antigen reaction
(b) Has no diagnostic findings on cystoscopy
(c) Has no specific medical therapy
(d) Histology, Von Brunn's nests appear invaginating the urothelium into the lamina propria

(Answer is D) Histology, Von Brunn's nests appear invaginating the urothelium into the lamina propria

195. What is false concerning cystitis glandularis?

(a) Rarely, the urothelial cell nests show a central lumen lined by glandular epithelium
(b) In some cases, it may form polypoid masses that mimic urothelial neoplasms
(c) It might appear as multinodular exophytic mass seen on cystoscopy
(d) Cystitis cystica and cystitis glandularis frequently coexist in the same specimen

(Answer is A) Rarely, the urothelial cell nests show a central lumen lined by glandular epithelium

196. What is false regarding cystitis cystica?

(a) Most cysts appear as filling defects on cystography
(b) Most often found in the trigone area
(c) The cyst lumens contain eosinophilic secretions that may have a few inflammatory cells
(d) Cystitis cystica and cystitis glandularis are reactive urothelial changes

(Answer is A) Most cysts appear as filling defects on cystography

197. What is false concerning emphysematous cystitis?

(a) The hallmark in the diagnosis is the cystoscopic findings
(b) Risk factors include transplant recipients
(c) CT shows intramural and/or intraluminal gas in the bladder
(d) Requires surgical debridement and probably cystectomy

(Answer is A) The hallmark in the diagnosis is the cystoscopic findings

198. What is false regarding viral cystitis?

(a) Pediatrics, adenovirus types 11 and 21 could result in hemorrhagic cystitis
(b) Immunosuppressed children are especially susceptible to Cytomegalovirus and Adenoviruses 7, 21 and 35
(c) Pediatrics, acute viral cystitis might present as acute retention of urine
(d) Classically, treatment should be culture-specific

(Answer is D) Classically, treatment should be culture-specific

199. What is false regarding schistosomal cystitis?

(a) Eosinophilic immune reaction is generated in response to the eggs
(b) Chronic schistosomiasis can eventually result in small bladder and the development of cancers
(c) Schistosoma mansoni often causes urinary tract infections
(d) Could cause inflammatory polys and recurrent hematuria

(Answer is C) Schistosoma mansoni often causes urinary tract infections

200. What kind of non-infectious cystitis, do patients with systemic lupus erythematosus (SLE), likely to develop?

(a) Cystitis glandularis
(b) Cystitis cystica
(c) Eosinophilic cystitis
(d) Cystitis follicularis

(Answer is C) Eosinophilic cystitis

201. Ureteral dilation in schistosomiasis could be due to:

(a) Vesicoureteral reflux
(b) Stenosis of the lower ureter
(c) Edematous ureteral wall causing deficient peristalsis
(d) Any of the above

(Answer is D) Any of the above

202. What condition(s) could occur in schistosomal ureter?

(a) Beading of the lower ureteral segment
(b) Ureteral fibrosis and calcifications of the distal ureter
(c) Stricture at the uretero-vesical junction
(d) All of the above

(Answer is D) All of the above

203. What is false concerning "foreign body" cystitis?

(a) Most commonly due to indwelling catheters
(b) The areas of inflammation are usually confined to the lateral walls or the dome of the bladder
(c) Radiographic changes are nonspecific or present as bullous edema
(d) Indwelling catheters are associated with squamous cell carcinoma of the bladder

(Answer is B) The areas of inflammation are usually confined to the lateral walls or the dome of the bladder

204. What kind of cystitis does not progress to malignancy?

(a) Foreign-body cystitis due to vesical calculi
(b) Von Brunn's nests of cystitis cystica and cystitis glandularis
(c) Schistosomiasis cystitis
(d) Inverted papilloma of the bladder

(Answer is B) Von Brunn's nests of cystitis cystica and cystitis glandularis

205. What could cause scrotal sinus?

(a) Improperly drained hair follicle scrotal abscess
(b) Syphilitic orchitis
(c) Tuberculous epididymitis
(d) All of the above

(Answer is D) All of the above

206. In which segmented voided bladder (VB) specimen, the diagnosis of chronic prostatitis is confirmed?

(a) VB_1 and VB_3
(b) Prostatic secretions and the VB_3
(c) Prostatic secretions and the VB_2
(d) Prostatic secretions and the VB_1

(Answer is B) Prostatic secretions and the VB_3

207. What type of scrotal ulcers is painless, punched out, with yellowish grey floor?

(a) Tuberculous ulcer (b) Malignant ulcer
(c) Gummatous ulcers (d) Traumatic ulcer

(Answer is C) Gummatous ulcers

208. What condition does not present as an acute loin pain with fever and marked flank tenderness?

(a) Ascending UTI causing acute lobar nephroma
(b) Acute pyelonephritis in a transplanted kidney
(c) Infected renal subscapular hematoma
(d) Perinephric abscess causing septicemia

(Answer is B) Acute pyelonephritis in a transplanted kidney

209. What is the most common cause of relapsing UTI in males?

(a) Chronic epididymitis
(b) Epididymo-orchitis
(c) Chronic bacterial prostatitis

(d) Venereal cysto-urethritis

(Answer is C) Chronic bacterial prostatitis

210. Irritative LUTS and dyspareunia in postmenopausal women are most likely to be due to:

(a) Giggle incontinence
(b) Estrogen deficiency
(c) Cystitis glandularis
(d) Cystitis cystica

(Answer is B) Estrogen deficiency

211. What is false regarding "urethral syndrome" in postmenopausal women?

(a) Of vaginal secretions increases after menopause
(b) Estrogen deficiency manifests as trophic urethritis and atrophic vaginitis
(c) Topical conjugated estrogen replacement carries a significant risk of breast and endometrial cancers
(d) Manifestations might include obstructive symptoms and non-infectious cystitis

(Answer is C) Topical conjugated estrogen replacement carries a significant risk of breast and endometrial cancers

212. What is false concerning acute glomerulonephritis?

(a) Manifested as a sudden onset of hematuria, proteinuria, oliguria, edema, hypertension, and RBC casts in the urine
(b) Post-streptococcus GN has an incubation period of 1-3 weeks with specific strains of group A beta-hemolytic streptococcus
(c) The triad of sinusitis, pulmonary infiltrates and nephritis, suggests Wegener's granulomatosis
(d) C_3, C_4, ESR and antistreptolysin O titer are increased

(Answer is D) C_3, C_4, ESR and antistreptolysin O titer are increased

213. What is false concerning Xanthogranulomatous Pyelonephritis?

(a) Most commonly associated with Proteus or E. coli infection
(b) Characterized by lipid-laden foamy macrophages
(c) The overall prognosis is poor
(d) Might involve adjacent structures or organs

(Answer is C) The overall prognosis is poor

214. What is true regarding Xanthogranulomatous Pyelonephritis?

(a) CT shows the characteristic "bear paw" sign
(b) Is an infected, obstructed, poorly functioning kidney containing stones
(c) Nephrectomy is the treatment
(d) All of the above

(Answer is D) All of the above

215. When comparing nosocomial to community-acquired UTI, the latter is:

(a) 45% are caused by E. coli
(b) Related to an indwelling urinary catheter in approximately 40% of cases
(c) Responds fairly to oral antibiotics
(d) Tends to report higher antibiotic resistance

(Answer is C) Responds fairly to oral antibiotics

216. What is false concerning UTI in long-term care facilities?

(a) Catheterized individuals, entry of bacteria into the bladder is facilitated by the bacterial glycocalyx biofilm
(b) Infection cannot be reliably distinguished from bacteriuria by lab tests
(c) Co-trimoxazole is the preferred antibiotic for empiric therapy
(d) Symptomatic UTI may be a diagnosis of exclusion

(Answer is C) Co-trimoxazole is the preferred antibiotic for empiric therapy

217. What is false concerning post UTI renal scarring in pediatrics?

(a) The incidence of scarring following a single episode of febrile UTI is 4.5%
(b) Intrarenal reflux is common in convex papillae
(c) Scarring and chronic pyelonephritis lead to hypertension in 10-20%
(d) Scarring is best detected and followed up by DMSA

(Answer is B) Intrarenal reflux is common in convex papillae

218. What is false regarding pediatric renal parenchyma scarring?

(a) Chronic pyelonephritis and HTN lead to ESRD in 10% of the cases
(b) Neonatal symptoms of UTI are vague and non-specific, that delay the diagnosis and end in more scarring
(c) Despite adequate treatment, scarring continues after an attack of pyelonephritis as a chronic immune reaction against renal tubules
(d) Neonates have low intrarenal pelvic pressure, that predisposes to ascending infections

(Answer is D) Neonates have low intrarenal pelvic pressure, that predisposes to ascending infections

219. What is true concerning "ovarian vein syndrome"?

(a) Manifests as recurrent renal colics due to ureteral obstruction
(b) Treatment is surgical mobilization of ureter and ligation of the vein
(c) Commonly, occurs at the left side
(d) The pain worsens on sitting upright and during pregnancy

(Answer is B) Treatment is surgical mobilization of ureter and ligation of the vein

220. What is false concerning "chronic orchialgia syndrome"?

(a) Is a constant or intermittent pain of testes for more than 3 months
(b) Could be due to appendix testis torsion-detorsion
(c) Could be due to radiculitis resulting from a degenerative lesion in the thoracolumbar vertebrae
(d) Could be a result of entrapment neuropathy of ilioinguinal or genitofemoral nerve

(Answer is B) Could be due to appendix testis torsion-detorsion

221. What is false regarding the etiology and treatment of orchialgia syndrome?

(a) Small indirect inguinal hernia may irritate the genital branch of genitofemoral nerve causing orchialgia
(b) Might respond to a selective nerve block
(c) The recommended treatment is orchiectomy with implantation of a testicular prosthesis
(d) Psychotherapy and stress management might alleviate the pain

(Answer is C) The recommended treatment is orchiectomy with implantation of a testicular prosthesis

222. What is true regarding balanoposthitis?

(a) Best diagnosed by ascending urethrography
(b) Occurs mostly in diabetic and immunosuppressed patients
(c) Could be due to maceration injury, irritant dermatitis, or Candida
(d) Commonly presents with deep inguinal lymphadenopathy

(Answer is C) Could be due to maceration injury, irritant dermatitis, or Candida

223. What are the sequelae of recurrent uncomplicated UTI in young women?

(a) Minimal
(b) Chronic persistent infections
(c) Chronic relapsing infections
(d) Bouts of chronic pyelonephritis

(Answer is A) Minimal

224. What is the percentage of occurrence of Staphylococcus saprophyticus in symptomatic lower UTIs in young sexually active females?

(a) 5% (b) 10%
(c) 15% (d) 20%

(Answer is B) 10%

225. What is the least important measure in indwelling catheter care?

(a) Cleansing the urethral meatus with aseptic agent
(b) Careful aseptic insertion of the catheter
(c) Maintenance of a closed drainage system
(d) Maintaining a dependent drainage system

(Answer is A) Cleansing the urethral meatus with aseptic agent

226. What is the most virulent factor for bacterial adherence?

(a) P blood group (b) Fimbria
(c) Pili (d) hemolysin

(Answer is C) Pili

227. What is the most significant biological difference in women susceptibility to UTI?

(a) Adherence of bacteria to vaginal cells
(b) Vaginal dryness
(c) O serogroup
(d) Vaginal pH

(Answer is A) Adherence of bacteria to vaginal cells

228. What is the bladder's first-line defense against infections?

(a) Natural sloughing of bladder mucosa
(b) Voiding
(c) Urine osmolarity
(d) Urine pH

(Answer is B) Voiding

229. What is the most significant complication of papillary necrosis?

(a) Ureteral obstruction
(b) Proteinuria
(c) Stone formation
(d) Renal scarring

(Answer is A) Ureteral obstruction

230. Screening for bacteriuria is mostly indicated for:

(a) Seniors' house residents
(b) ICU patients with indwelling urinary catheters
(c) Pregnant women
(d) Neurogenic bladder patients on CIC

(Answer is C) Pregnant women

231. No need for radiologic studies for recurrent UTI in:

(a) Children (b) The elderly
(c) Men (d) Women

(Answer is D) Women

232. What is the most important pharmacokinetic property of a drug to cure UTI?

(a) Mode of administration
(b) Level in the serum
(c) Level in the urine
(d) Dosage

(Answer is C) Level in the urine

233. What is the mortality rate of emphysematous pyelonephritis?

(a) 43% (b) 53%
(c) 63% (d) 73%

(Answer is A) 43%

234. What are the most indicative symptoms of chronic pyelonephritis?

(a) Fever and chills
(b) Suprapubic pain and pyuria
(c) Flank pain and tenderness
(d) None of the above

(Answer is D) None of the above

235. What is the earliest clinical finding of urosepsis?

(a) Elevated body temperature
(b) Dropped blood pressure
(c) Elevated heart rate
(d) Reduced urine output

(Answer is C) Elevated heart rate

236. A 44 years male presents with recurrent left pyelonephritis and Proteus infection. His kidney is dilated and contains a stone. A renal biopsy showed foamy macrophages with neutrophils and cellular debris. What is the treatment?

(a) PCNL after treating the infection
(b) Cystoscopy and placing a retrograde ureteral stent followed by ESWL
(c) Perc. nephrostomy and placing antegrade ureteral stent
(d) Nephrectomy

(Answer is D) Nephrectomy

237. A 48 years woman presents with recurrent cystitis. Cystoscopy showed a raised bladder lesion. Biopsies from the lesion reveals Von Hansemann histiocytes, and Michaelis-Gutmann bodies. What is the treatment?

(a) Sulfonamide for several months
(b) TUR of the bladder lesion followed by proper staging
(c) Radical cystectomy and urinary diversion
(d) Intravesical installation of mitomycin without irradiation

(Answer is A) Sulfonamide for several months

238. What is the ideal antibiotic class for self-start therapy on treating recurrent cystitis in a 32 years married woman?

(a) Aminopenicillins
(b) Fluoroquinolones
(c) Aminoglycosides
(d) Nitrofurantoins

(Answer is B) Fluoroquinolones

239. What antimicrobial agent treats UTI and does NOT alter the gut flora?

(a) Trimethoprim-sulfamethoxazole
(b) Fluoroquinolones
(c) Aminoglycosides
(d) Nitrofurantoins

(Answer is D) Nitrofurantoins

240. What group of patients should be treated for UTI only when symptomatic?

(a) Patients with indwelling catheters
(b) Neurogenic bladder patients on CIC
(c) Pregnant women
(d) Children under 5 years

(Answer is A) Patients with indwelling catheters

241. As per NIH classification of prostatitis, which type requires no treatment?

(a) Type I (b) Type II
(c) Type III (d) Type IV

(Answer is D) Type IV

242. A 60 years man underwent TURP for, only, obstructive LUTS. Histology of prostate chips reveals prostatitis. What NIH type of prostatitis would it be?

(a) Type I (b) Type II
(c) Type III (d) Type IV

(Answer is D) Type IV

243. Directed physiotherapy could be of value in treating what NIH type of prostatitis?

(a) Type II (b) Type III-a
(c) Type III-b (d) Type IV

(Answer is C) Type III-b

244. What is true concerning granulomatous inflammation of the prostate?

(a) A common cause of elevated PSA level
(b) Might follow BCG treatment
(c) Sequelae of untreated type III-b prostatitis
(d) Shows homogenous enhancement following Gd-DTPA on prostate MRI

(Answer is B) Might follow BCG treatment

245. What is the laboratory differentiation between type III-a and type III-b prostatitis?

(a) The cytological examination of the urine and/or EPS
(b) Transrectal ultrasonographic examination
(c) The presence of $\geq$10 WBCs/HPF in the urine with negative culture in type III-b
(d) The positive urine culture, and negative EPS support type III-a

(Answer is A) The cytological examination of the urine and/or EPS

246. What is false concerning the presentation of prostatitis syndrome?

(a) Type I could harbor prostate abscess
(b) Type II presents as intermittent urinary tract infections
(c) Type III-a presentation might include psychological complaints
(d) Between 10-15% of men with type IV, have pus cells in their semen but no symptoms

(Answer is C) Type III-a presentation might include psychological complaints

247. Which of the following has NO role in bacterial colonization in the prostate?

(a) Intraprostatic ductal reflux
(b) Paraphimosis
(c) Specific blood groups
(d) Unprotected anal intercourse

(Answer is B) Paraphimosis

248. What factor(s) increase(s) the risk of bacterial colonization in the prostate?

(a) Acute epididymitis
(b) Indwelling urethral catheters
(c) Transurethral surgery
(d) All of the above

(Answer is D) All of the above

249. UPOINT system for phenotype categorization:

(a) Categorizes CP-CPPS, IC, and painful bladder syndrome based on 5 etiological principles
(b) Meant to classify CP-CPPS and IC patients into 6 domains
(c) Helps establish a reliable diagnosis of CP/CPPS or IC
(d) The diagnostic scores of UPOINT depend on cystoscopy, TRUS, urine analysis and culture of uncommon microbes

(Answer is B) Meant to classify CP-CPPS and IC patients into 6 domains

250. Which treatment modality has NO proven efficacy in CP/CPPS?

(a) Selective nerve block
(b) Balloon dilation
(c) Botulinum A toxin injection
(d) ESWL

(Answer is B) Balloon dilation

251. What is false concerning Brucellosis epididymitis?

(a) Commonly presents with scrotal pain, swelling, fever and leucocytosis

(b) Epididymo-orchitis is the most frequent genitourinary complication of brucellosis
(c) Epididymo-orchitis occurs in 10-15% of male patients with brucellosis
(d) Treatment includes doxycycline and rifampicin for 6-8 weeks

(Answer is A) Commonly presents with scrotal pain, swelling, fever and leucocytosis

252. What is the most commonly affected organ by genitourinary brucellosis?

(a) Kidneys (b) Bladder
(c) Prostate (d) Epididymis

(Answer is D) Epididymis

253. What are the most commonly affected organs by genitourinary schistosomiasis?

(a) Kidneys and adrenals
(b) Bladder and ureters
(c) Prostate and vasa
(d) Testes and epididymis

(Answer is B) Bladder and ureters

254. What are the most commonly affected organs by genitourinary tuberculosis?

(a) Kidneys, prostate and epididymis
(b) Bladder, ureters and renal pelvis
(c) Vasa, scrotum and adrenals
(d) Testes, bladder neck and seminal vesicles

(Answer is A) Kidneys, prostate and epididymis

255. What is false regarding prostatic abscesses?

(a) Clinically, cannot be differentiated from acute bacterial prostatitis
(b) Medical management is often unsuccessful
(c) Harbors prostate cancer in approximately 4.3% of cases
(d) Management include suprapubic urinary diversion

(Answer is C) Harbors prostate cancer in approximately 4.3% of cases

256. Using low-dose prophylactic or suppressive antimicrobials might be an option in treating the following type of prostatitis:

(a) Acute bacterial prostatitis presenting with abscess formation
(b) Recurrent or refractory chronic bacterial prostatitis
(c) Asymptomatic prostatitis with pyuria resistant to common antimicrobials
(d) Curiously, chronic inflammatory prostatitis could respond to low-dose suppressive antibiotic

(Answer is B) Recurrent or refractory chronic bacterial prostatitis

257. What is false concerning corpora amylacea of the prostate?

(a) Are premalignant, and found in 1-6% of prostate biopsies
(b) Are small hyaline masses of unknown significance found in the prostate gland
(c) They are degenerate cells or thickened secretions in the prostate ducts
(d) Might appear as prostate calcifications on X-ray KUB

(Answer is A) Are premalignant, and found in 1-6% of prostate biopsies

258. What is essential on diagnosing bladder pain syndrome BPS/IC?

(a) Sterile pyuria on 3 consecutive cultures
(b) The presence of glomerulations and/or Hunner's ulcer on endoscopy
(c) Pain and discomfort related to the bladder
(d) Urgency and frequency with no documented infection

(Answer is C) Pain and discomfort related to the bladder

259. What is the best statement that describes the action of antiproliferative factor?

(a) Inhibits bladder epithelial cell proliferation
(b) Inhibits the bladder proliferative growth factors
(c) Stimulates the proliferation inhibitory factors
(d) None of the above

(Answer is A) Inhibits bladder epithelial cell proliferation

260. What type of bladder cells secretes antiproliferative factor?

(a) Bladder epithelial cells
(b) Type C nerve endings in the bladder
(c) Type A delta nerve endings in the bladder
(d) The innermost longitudinal fibres of detrusor muscle

(Answer is A) Bladder epithelial cells

261. What is the average age of onset of BPS/IC patients?

(a) 30 (b) 40
(c) 50 (d) 60

(Answer is B) 40

262. What is the preferred antibiotic for BPS/IC cases?

(a) Rifampicin (b) Doxycycline
(c) Azithromycin (d) None of the above

(Answer is D) None of the above

263. What type of cells is implicated most in the pathogenesis of BPS/IC?

(a) Histocytes (b) T lymphocytes
(c) Mast cells (d) B lymphocytes

(Answer is C) Mast cells

264. What is true concerning BPS/IC?

(a) The onset of symptoms is insidious
(b) The lesion has no proven relation to bladder cancer
(c) Left untreated, the bladder will turn small, contracted, with submucosal calcifications
(d) A single positive urine culture refutes the diagnosis

(Answer is B) The lesion has no proven relation to bladder cancer

265. What are the diagnostic findings on cystometrogram for BPS/IC?

(a) Discomfort on placing urethral catheter and pain on bladder filling
(b) Difficulty in zeroing the pressure and diminished response to first cough
(c) Low filling pressure but high voiding pressure
(d) Uninhibited bladder contractions with a relative bladder hypotonia

(Answer is A) Discomfort on placing urethral catheter and pain on bladder filling

266. Which of the following is not a treatment option for BPS/IC?

(a) Substitution cystoplasty and continent diversion
(b) Fulguration of a Hunner's ulcer or hydrodistention
(c) Intravesical installation of silver nitrate or dimethyl sulfoxide
(d) Low dose external beam irradiation

(Answer is D) Low dose external beam irradiation

267. What is false concerning HIV infection?

(a) AIDS patients in active infection show low CD_4 + T-cell count
(b) The diagnosis is confirmed by positive anti-HIV-1, anti-HIV-2 antibodies
(c) Patients receiving antiviral therapy could still be infectious

(d) Herpes simplex virus increases HIV replication in infected persons

(Answer is B) The diagnosis is confirmed by positive anti-HIV-1, anti-HIV-2 antibodies

268. What is true concerning HIV infection?

(a) HIV is a retrovirus that infects B-cells and dendritic cells
(b) Circumcised men are at lower risk for HIV infection
(c) HPV infection increases the risk for cancers in HIV patients by 6.3 times
(d) Plasma HIV RNA load is a predictor of disease remission

(Answer is B) Circumcised men are at lower risk for HIV infection

269. What is the most common intrascrotal pathology in AIDS patients?

(a) Beaded vas deferens
(b) Testicular microlithiasis
(c) Testicular atrophy
(d) Epididymal granuloma

(Answer is C) Testicular atrophy

270. What type of human herpes virus is implicated in all forms of Kaposi sarcoma?

(a) 2 (b) 6
(c) 7 (d) 8

(Answer is D) 8

271. What is the estimated risk of untreated Chlamydial infections in producing pelvic inflammatory disease?

(a) 1 – 2.7% (b) 5 – 9%
(c) 10 – 27% (d) 30 – 47%

(Answer is C) 10 – 27%

272. What is false concerning antiretroviral medications?

(a) Multiple antiretroviral drugs can be combined into a single pill
(b) Might cause radiolucent renal stones
(c) Can lead to a significant rise in the serum level of PDE5 inhibitors, if taken simultaneously
(d) Have the advantage of "structured treatment interruptions" (drug holidays)

(Answer is D) Have the advantage of "structured treatment interruptions" (drug holidays)

273. HIV infection increases the incidence of the following cancers, *except*:

(a) Kaposi sarcoma
(b) Hodgkin's lymphoma
(c) Non-Hodgkin's lymphoma
(d) Cervical cancer

(Answer is B) Hodgkin's lymphoma

274. In males, HIV infection increases the incidence of the following genitourinary tumors:

(a) Testicular (b) Renal
(c) Penile (d) All of the above

(Answer is D) All of the above

275. What is the most common serotype of HPV associated with squamous cell carcinoma of the penis?

(a) 16 (b) 18
(c) 22 (d) 12

(Answer is A) 16

276. Epididymal cysts are common in the following conditions, *except*:

(a) Von Hippel-Lindau disease
(b) Tuberous sclerosis
(c) Cystic fibrosis
(d) Autosomal dominant polycystic kidney disease

(Answer is B) Tuberous sclerosis

277. During the initial 3-month period of HIV infection, what would be the best diagnostic lab test?

(a) Viral load assay
(b) Western blot analysis
(c) Southern blot analysis
(d) HIV-1/HIV-2 serology assay

(Answer is A) Viral load assay

278. What are the target immune cells for HIV?

(a) Phagocytes (b) CD_4 T cells
(c) B lymphocytes (d) Natural killer cells

(Answer is B) CD_4 T cells

279. The relative risk of prostate cancer in men with HIV compared to uninfected individuals is:

(a) Greater than 8-fold (b) Greater than 6-fold
(c) Greater than 4-fold (d) Comparable

(Answer is D) Comparable

280. What virus(s) could cause orchitis?

(a) Coxsackie B (b) Epstein-Barr
(c) Varicella (d) All of the above

(Answer is D) All of the above

281. What condition is associated with renal papillary necrosis?

(a) Nephrotic syndrome
(b) Hypertension
(c) Sickle cell hemoglobinopathy
(d) Sarcoidosis

(Answer is C) Sickle cell hemoglobinopathy

282. Which of the following conditions does not cause bacterial persistence?

(a) Perivesical abscess with fistula to bladder
(b) Acute tubular necrosis
(c) Renal papillary necrosis
(d) Xanthogranulomatous pyelonephritis

(Answer is C) Renal papillary necrosis

283. What host's factors do not increase the risk of developing infections?

(a) Advanced age
(b) Anatomical anomalies
(c) Poor drug compliance
(d) Smoking

(Answer is C) Poor drug compliance

284. Which of the following factors increases the risk of UTI due to promotion of microbial colonization?

(a) Neurogenic bladder
(b) The use of spermicide
(c) Urinary catheterization
(d) Fecal incontinence

(Answer is B) The use of spermicide

285. Which of the following factors increases the risk of UTI due to facilitation of microbial ascent?

(a) Sexual activity
(b) The use of spermicide
(c) Estrogen depletion
(d) Fecal incontinence

(Answer is D) Fecal incontinence

286. Which of the following does not cause unresolved bacteriuria?

(a) Giant staghorn stone
(b) Perivesical abscess with fistula to the bladder
(c) Bacterial resistance
(d) Self-inflicted infection

(Answer is B) Perivesical abscess with fistula to the bladder

287. Which statement best defines "reinfection"?

(a) A new episode of UTI caused by different species or occurring at long intervals
(b) Recurrent UTIs caused by the same organism in each instance, classically, at close intervals
(c) Recurrent UTIs due to failure of medical therapy to eradicate the infection

(d) Recurrent UTIs due to a persistent pathology that is obstinate to surgery

(Answer is A) A new episode of UTI caused by different species or occurring at long intervals

288. What is false concerning renal hydatid cysts?

(a) Might rupture into the collecting system causing (hydatiduria) and renal colic

(b) Are formed by the eggs of the tapeworm Echinococcus granulosus

(c) Most cysts are asymptomatic but might manifest as flank mass, dull pain, or hematuria

(d) The most reliable diagnostic test uses partially purified hydatid arc 5 antigens in a double-diffusion test

(Answer is B) Are formed by the eggs of the tapeworm Echinococcus granulosus

289. What is false concerning "sepsis syndrome"?

(a) Poor tissue perfusion manifests as hyperlactemia and decreased capillary refill

(b) Acute oliguria indicates an organ dysfunction and circulatory collapse

(c) Septic shock is an extreme form of sepsis when hypotension persists despite adequate fluid resuscitation

(d) Hypotension is a sign of hyperdynamic circulation at an early septic shock

(Answer is D) Hypotension is a sign of hyperdynamic circulation at an early septic shock

290. What is the preferred antimicrobial prophylaxis for transrectal prostate biopsy?

(a) Aminoglycoside

(b) Fluoroquinolone

(c) 2nd generation cephalosporin

(d) Doxycycline

(Answer is B) Fluoroquinolone

291. Under which surgical wound classification, does diagnostic cystoscopy under sterile technique fit?

(a) Dirty – infected

(b) Contaminated

(c) Clean – contaminated

(d) Clean

(Answer is C) Clean – contaminated

292. A 40 years man presents with clinical acute pyelonephritis, on intravenous antibiotics for 4 days, CT shows a renal abscess. What is next in the treatment?

(a) Carry on the full antibiotic course, and then repeat CT

(b) Incision and drainage of the renal abscess with/without nephrectomy

(c) The abscess size dictates management

(d) Perc. drainage of the renal abscess

(Answer is C) The abscess size dictates management

293. Factors associated with higher rates of HPV infection are all *except*:

(a) Presence of foreskin

(b) Increased number of sexual partners

(c) Lack of condom use

(d) Obesity

(Answer is D) Obesity

294. True about HPV infection are all *except*:

(a) HPV 6 and 11 associated with condyloma and low grade dysplasia

(b) HPV 42, 43, 44 are associated with penile carcinoma

(c) 47% of all carcinoma penis is caused by HPV

(d) Koilocyte in histopathology is pathognomonic for HPV infection

(Answer is B) HPV 42, 43, 44 are associated with penile carcinoma

295. False about genital warts is:

(a) Subclinical disease may be detected by the application of 5% acetic acid solution to the penis, followed by inspection with a magnifying glass
(b) Topical treatment of choice is podophyllotoxin 0.5%
(c) CO_2 laser can be used
(d) A 1% gel preparation of cidofovir is the new broad spectrum antiviral agent used

(Answer is B) Topical treatment of choice is podophyllotoxin 0.5%

296. In a patient with presumed UTI, a urine pH > 7.5 most commonly suggest infection with:

(a) Proteus (b) E. coli
(c) TB (d) Schistosomiasis

(Answer is A) Proteus

297. All are features of glomerular hematuria *except*:

(a) Absence of RBC cast
(b) Dysmorphic RBCs
(c) Proteinuria
(d) Cola colored urine

(Answer is A) Absence of RBC cast

298. False about proteinuria:

(a) Protein concentration in urine seldom exeeds 20 mg/dl
(b) Glomerular proteinuria is the most common type of proteinuria
(c) Normal excretion of proteins is 80-150 mg/day
(d) Most common cause of overflow proteinuria is IgA nephropathy

(Answer is D) Most common cause of overflow proteinuria is IgA nephropathy

299. False about retroperitoneal fibrosis:

(a) Most commonly affects 40-60 years age group
(b) Fibrotic mass centres around L4-L5 level
(c) Typically presents with colicky pain
(d) May present as DVT

(Answer is C) Typically presents with colicky pain

300. The antigen initiating inflammatory response in RPF is:

(a) Steroid
(b) Ceroid
(c) Bicunin
(d) Uroplakin

(Answer is B) Ceroid

301. Most common malignancy associated with retroperitoneal fibrosis is:

(a) Lymphoma
(b) RCC
(c) Testicular tumor
(d) Retroperitoneal sarcoma

(Answer is A) Lymphoma

302. All are typical imaging findings of retroperitoneal fibrosis *except*:

(a) Hydronephrosis
(b) Medial deviation of proximal and mid ureter
(c) Low signal intensity on T1 weighted MRI
(d) MRI is the most sensitive imaging for assessing disease activity

(Answer is D) MRI is the most sensitive imaging for assessing disease activity

303. False about management of retroperitoneal fibrosis:

(a) Ureteral stent placement is not difficult in ureteral obstruction caused by RPF
(b) Primary medical management is beta blockers
(c) Tamoxifen is useful
(d) Mycophenolate mofetil is used

(Answer is B) Primary medical management is beta blockers

304. False about surgery for retroperitoneal fibrosis:

(a) Standard surgical management is laparoscopic ureterolysis

(b) Omental wrapping of the ureter may be needed

(c) Intraperitonealization of the ureter may be done

(d) Bilateral ureterolysis is required most of the time

(Answer is A) Standard surgical management is laparoscopic ureterolysis

305. All are true about presentation of GUTB *except*:

(a) Fever, weight loss, malaise and night sweats are seen only in 20% of patients

(b) 50% has only dysuria on presentation

(c) Typical lab findings are sterile pyuria and/or hematuria

(d) The typical sites of hematogenous seeding are bladder and prostate

(Answer is D) The typical sites of hematogenous seeding are bladder and prostate

306. False about renal TB4:

(a) 80% of GUTB occurs in kidney

(b) Miliary TB usually do not affect renal function

(c) Autonephrectomy occurs in 3% cases

(d) Risk for squamous cell carcinoma

(Answer is C) Autonephrectomy occurs in 3% cases

307. Gold standard for diagnosis of GUTB is:

(a) Urine AFB culture

(b) Urine TB PCR

(c) Urine AFB staining

(d) CB NAAT of epididymal biopsy

(Answer is A) Urine AFB culture

308. False about CB NAAT for diagnosis of GUTB:

(a) Provides results in 1-2 days

(b) Gene Xpert provides molecular detection of Rifampicin resistanace

(c) Sensitivity of Gene Xpert in urine sample is around 80-95%

(d) CB NAAT can be used to monitor response to treatment

(Answer is D) CB NAAT can be used to monitor response to treatment

309. All are true about radiography findings of GUTB *except*:

(a) Calcification is seen in > 50% cases

(b) Trinagular ring like calcification in collecting system implies papillary necrosis

(c) Mural calcification of ureter is a typical finding

(d) Seminal vesicle calcification may be seen

(Answer is C) Mural calcification of ureter is a typical finding

310. Gold standard imaging for early renal TB is:

(a) IV Urography

(b) Ultrasonography

(c) X-ray KUB

(d) DMSA scan

(Answer is A) IV Urography

311. In GUTB CT has more sensitivity than IVU for:

(a) Subtle papillary necrosis

(b) Minimal urothelial thickening

(c) Calcification

(d) All of the above

(Answer is C) Calcification

312. Type of ureteric orifice in GUTB:

(a) Cone (b) Horseshoe

(c) Stadium (d) Golf hole

(Answer is D) Golf hole

313. First new drug developed specifically for TB is:

(a) Bedaquiline
(b) Linezolid
(c) Prulifloxacin
(d) Trovafloxacin

(Answer is A) Bedaquiline

314. Elsberg syndrome occurs due to:

(a) Diabetes mellitus
(b) Anogenital herpes
(c) Polio
(d) Tethered spinal cord

(Answer is B) Anogenital herpes

CHAPTER 5

Molecular and Cellular Biology

1. **Chemoattractant complement is:**
   (a) C3a (b) C3b
   (c) C5a (d) C5b

(Answer is C)

Complement	
Phagocytosis	C3b
Most critical component	C3
Membrane attack complex	C5b+ C6 –9
Anaphylatoxins	C3a, C5a
Chemoattractant	C5a

2. **Most critical component in the complement pathway is:**
   (a) C 1 (b) C 2
   (c) C 3 (d) C 4

(Answer is C) The most critical component is C3, which has a molecular weight of about 195 kD.

3. **Which complement acts as opsonin and anaphylatoxin respectively?**
   (a) C2a and C2b, C3b respectively
   (b) C3a and C2b, C3b respectively
   (c) C3b and C3a, C5a respectively
   (d) C2b and C3a, C5a respectively

(Answer is C) Some bind directly to the cell membrane and act as an opsonin for phagocytes such as neutrophils and macrophages that have receptors for C3b. In addition, fragments C3a and C5a serve as powerful anaphylatoxins.

4. **Which one of the following is primary lymphoid tissue?**
   (a) Thymus
   (b) Spleen
   (c) Lymph node
   (d) Unencapsulated tissue lining urogenital tract

(Answer is A) The primary lymphoid organ is the thymus, which is responsible for the selection and education of T cells, and the bone marrow itself, which is responsible for the education of B cells. Secondary or peripheral lymphoid tissue includes the spleen, lymph nodes, and unencapsulated tissue lining the alimentary, respiratory and urogenital tracts.

5. **Which CD is considered pan 8 cell marker?**
   (a) CD 16 (b) CD 18
   (c) CD 19 (d) CD 25

(Answer is C) CD19

6. **Which CD is considered pan T cell marker?**
   (a) CD 1 (b) CD 2
   (c) CD 3 (d) CD 4

(Answer is C) CD 3

7. **Which CD is IL2 receptor, also called as Tac?**
   (a) CD 16 (b) CD 18
   (c) CD 19 (d) CD 25

(Answer is D) CD-25, IL 2-receptor, also called Tac.

8. **Which statement regarding NK cells is not correct?**
   (a) NK cells are large granular lymphocytes that can destroy various nucleated cells, including tumors and virus-infected cells

(b) They are an important component of innate immunity and do not require prior contact with antigen
(c) They are MHC restricted
(d) They also participate in antibody-dependent cell-mediated cytotoxicity

(Answer is C) NK cells are not MHC restricted.

9. Which one of the following is not the antigen presenting cell?

(a) Macrophages
(b) B cells
(c) Neutrophils
(d) Vascular endothelium

(Answer is C) Macrophages, monocytes, some B cells, Langerhans cells of the skin, dendritic reticulum cells, and vascular endothelium can process and present antigen.

10. Which statement is not true regarding major histocompatibility complex?

(a) The MHC describes a region of genes located on chromosome 6
(b) Virtually all nucleated cells express HLA class I antigens
(c) The cell surface MHC markers are called HLA because they were first identified on white blood cells
(d) Each individual inherits three class I and one class II antigen from each parent

(Answer is D) Each individual inherits two class I and one class II antigen from each parent, so six HLA antigens constitute an individual's tissue type (three from each parent).

11. Which statement is not true regarding activation of intracellular calcium?

(a) Phosphorylation of the enzyme PLC-g is a critical event in transmitting the activation signal from the membrane downstream
(b) Once activated, PLC-g cleaves membrane-bound PIP2 into two active components, inositol triphosphate (IP3) and diacylglycerol (DAG)
(c) IP3 induces the release of Ca2+ into the cytosol from storage sites within the endoplasmic reticulum, which raises the intracellular levels of Ca2+
(d) Above event leads to the closing of the Ca2+ channels in the plasma membrane, which decreases Ca2+ levels

(Answer is D) IP3 induces the release of Ca2+ into the cytosol from storage sites within the endoplasmic reticulum, which raises the intracellular levels of Ca2+. This event also leads to the opening of the Ca2+ channels in the plasma membrane, which further increases Ca2+ levels.

12. Which IL is responsible for activation of acute phase proteins?

(a) IL 2 (b) IL 4
(c) IL 6 (d) IL 8

(Answer is C) IL 6–Source–Type 2 CD4+ T cells, macrophages. Function-Stimulation of acute phase proteins, activation of lymphocytes.

13. Protein responsible for apoptosis:

(a) Caspase (b) Collagenase
(c) Telomerase (d) Gangliosides

(Answer is A) The proteins responsible for executing the suicide program, the caspases, are essentially common to all the stimuli and pathways and mediate the nuclear and cytoplasmic alterations characteristic of apoptotic cell death.

14. Which one of the following is not a tumor specific antigen?

(a) MAGE (b) BAGE
(c) RAGE (d) LAGE

(Answer is D) Antigens appear to be relatively tumor specific and are encoded by a family of genes referred to as MAGE-l , MAGE-2, BAGE and RAGE.

15. DNA is fusion of all *except:*

(a) Adenine and guanine
(b) Cytosine and thymine
(c) Ribose sugar
(d) Phosphate and hydrogen bond

(Answer is C) In a rudimentary form, DNA is the fusion of three different elements: A base (either a pyrimidine or a purine), a sugar (in the case of DNA called 2-dioxyribose, for RNA called ribose), and a phosphate (which links individual nucleotides together).

16. Which statement regarding DNA expression is not correct?

(a) Protein synthesis occurs in nucleus
(b) Transcription–linear DNA is converted into linear RNA
(c) Translation–linear RNA is converted into linear amino acid
(d) Transfection–addition of DNA sequences to a cell

(Answer is A) Physical locations of the genetic code (DNA) and the manifestation of that code (protein synthesis) are separate. DNA is in the nucleus and protein synthesis is cytoplasmic.

17. Which enzyme is responsible for synthesis of first copy of RNA?

(a) DNA polymerase I
(b) DNA polymerase II
(c) RNA polymerase I
(d) RNA polymerase II

(Answer is D) The enzyme RNA polymerase II is responsible for synthesizing the first copy of RNA, which is a complementary replica of the template DNA.

18. Which one of the following is the Initiation codon?

(a) AUG (b) UAA
(c) UAG (d) UGA

(Answer is A) Three codons, UAA, UAG and UGA, do not encode for any amino acids but instead function as STOP codons, they signal for chain termination. The initiation codon is AUG.

19. Which constitutes the maximum RNA?

(a) t RNA (b) r RNA
(c) m RNA (d) d RNA

(Answer is B) Ribosomal RNA (r RNA), which constitutes about 80% of the RNA within a cell, makes up part of the ribosome, the cytoplasmic structure integral in protein synthesis.

20. Not true about oncogenes are:

(a) Mutated form of proto-oncogenes
(b) Proto-oncogenes can be converted to oncogenes by gene amplification and chromosomal translocation
(c) Oncogenes act as a dominant accelerator for tumor growth
(d) To be active both allele need to be expressed

(Answer is D) Unlike oncogenes, which can be active with only one allele expressed, classically both copies of tumor suppressor genes need to be inactivated to permit carcinogenesis.

21. Regarding hypermethylation which statement is not correct?

(a) It is an example of epigenetic change
(b) Methylation occurs exclusively on dinucleotide sequence AT
(c) Methylation of normally unmethylated genes can supress gene expression
(d) Loss of methylation of normally methylated genes can increase gene expression

(Answer is B) DNA methylation occurs exclusively on cytosine nucleotides in the dinucleotide sequence CG.

22. Hereditary papillary renal cell carcinoma is associated with which chromosome?

(a) Chromosome 3 (b) Chromosome 7
(c) Chromosome 9 (d) Chromosome 13

(Answer is B) Hereditary papillary renal cell carcinoma is associated with 7q31.

23. Birt-Hogg Dube syndrome is associated with all *except:*

(a) Oncocytoma
(b) Chromophobe RCC
(c) Papillary RCC
(d) Chromophilic RCC

(Answer is D) Families have been described with oncocytomas, chromophobe renal carcinomas and papillary renal carcinomas.

24. Heriditary prostate cancer is described as all *except:*

(a) Cluster of three affected relatives within a nuclear family
(b) Occurrence of prostate cancer in three generations
(c) Two affected relatives who both developed prostate cancer when younger than 55 years of age
(d) Three affected relatives who both developed prostate cancer when younger than 45 years of age

(Answer is D) HPC has been defined as either a cluster of three affected relatives within a nuclear family or the occurrence of prostate cancer in three generations or two affected relatives who both developed prostate cancer when younger than 55 years of age.

25. Check points of control in cell cycle are at:

(a) G1S only
(b) G2S only
(c) G1S and G2M both
(d) SG2 only

(Answer is C) The two main points of control are the G1S and G2M checkpoints.

26. Regarding TP53 in urologic malignancies which statement is not true?

(a) TP53 plays important role in DNA repair, cell cycle arrest and apoptosis
(b) It is the second most common mutated gene in human tumors, first being RB gene
(c) TP53 status in primary tumors may predict likelihood of recurrence
(d) TP53 status also predicts response to BCG or to chemotherapy

(Answer is B) TP53 is most commonly mutated gene in human tumors, including genitourinary malignancies. Close to 50% of all tumors have TP53 mutations.

27. At G1S checkpoint expression of which cyclin is important?

(a) Cyclin A (b) Cyclin B
(c) Cyclin C (d) Cyclin D

(Answer is D) Cyclin D expression is critical at the GIS checkpoint.

28. G2M check point responds to:

(a) Hypoxia
(b) DNA damage
(c) Nutrient poor environment
(d) Cytokines

(Answer is B) Unlike the G1S checkpoint, which responds to a variety of extracellular signals in addition to DNA damage, G2M appears to be similar to S-phase arrest and respond only to DNA damage.

29. RB clear association is not demonstrated with which malignancy?

(a) Prostate (b) Lung
(c) Bladder (d) Renal

(Answer is D) RB is rarely inactivated in renal carcinoma cell lines or tumors, and analysis of clinical specimens has not demonstrated a clear association between prognosis and RB expression.

30. Nucleotide excision repair is major defense against:

(a) UV radiation and chemical exposure
(b) Oxidative stress and replication errors
(c) Errors made by DNA polymerase
(d) Chemotherapeutic agents

(Answer is A) NER is a major defense against DNA damage caused by ultraviolet radiation and chemical exposure.

31. p53 induced apoptosis is mediated by which mechanism?

(a) Increase nuclear membrane permeability
(b) Decrease nuclear membrane permeability
(c) Increase mitochondria membrane permeability
(d) Increase cytoplamic membrane permeability

(Answer is C) TP53-induced apoptosis is mediated through BCL2 family members. Whereas each pro-apoptotic BCL2 family member responds to different stimuli, the principal mechanism by which they induce cell death is by increasing mitochondrial membrane permeability.

32. Which is the most well studied BCL2 family proapoptotic and antiapoptotic factor respectively?

(a) BCL2 and BAX
(b) BAX and BCL2
(c) BAD and BCLW
(d) BCLW and BAD

(Answer is B) BAX is the most well studied pro-apoptotic BCL2 family member. BCL2 is the best studied anti-apoptotic BCL2 family member.

33. Loss of heterozygosity (LOH) on which chromosome is the earliest and the most common genetic abnormality in prostate cancer?

(a) 2 (b) 4
(c) 6 (d) 8

(Answer is D) LOH on chromosome 8p is the earliest and most common genetic abnormality in prostate cancer.

34. Role of TGF-β are all *except:*

(a) Increase angiogenesis
(b) Immuno-stimulant
(c) Stimulate production of extracellular matrix
(d) Physical and invasive support for malignant growth

(Answer is B) TGF-β is a positive regulator of stromal cell growth, stimulates extracellular matrix production, simultaneously induces cell cycle arrest in epithelial and hematopoietic cell populations, and is a potent immuno-suppressant.

35. Which is responsible for cell-cell adhesion and tissue integrity?

(a) Integrins (b) Cadherins
(c) Fibronectin (d) Caveolin

(Answer is B) The integrins primarily mediate adhesion and interactions with the extracellular matrix, the cadherins are responsible for cell-cell adhesion and tissue integrity.

36. HIV is caused by:

(a) HTLV1 (b) HTLV2
(c) HTLV3 (d) HTLV4

(Answer is C) HTLV 3, more commonly known as human immunodeficiency virus (HIV 1), has been linked to an increased risk of malignancy.

37. Most dominant subtype that has been identified in HPV-positive lesions is:

(a) HPV 16 (b) HPV 18
(c) HPV 31 (d) HPV 33

(Answer is A) HPV 16 appears to be the dominant subtype and has been identified in up to 90% of HPV-positive lesions.

38. Regarding angiogenesis which statement is not correct?

(a) In normal adult tissues inducer of angiogenesis predominates
(b) Two best studied angiogenetic factors are FGF-2 and VEGF
(c) Hyperthermia and interferons inhibit angiogenesis
(d) Chemotherapic agents like bleomycin and vincristine are inhibitor of angiogenesis

(Answer is A) In normal adult tissues, the inhibitors of angiogenesis predominate, but in developing tissues, in wound healing, and in cancer, inducers of angiogenesis gain the upper hand and new vessels are formed.

39. α-methylacyl-coenzyme-A racemase (AMACR) helps in identification of:

(a) Carcinoma kidney
(b) Carcinoma bladder
(c) Carcinoma prostate
(d) Carcinoma testis

(Answer is C) α-methylacyl-coenzyme-A racemase (AMACR) in identification of small foci of prostate carcinoma in the prostate. AMACR mRNA expression in malignant prostate specimens is approximately nine-fold higher than in normal prostate tissues and by immunohistochemical staining is overexpressed in prostate cancer and HGPIN.

40. 12p chromosome is hallmark for which malignancy?

(a) Ca kidney (b) Ca bladder
(c) Ca prostate (d) Ca testis

(Answer is D) 12p isochromosome was first identified in testis tumors in the 1980s, and experimentally this cytogenetic hallmark of testicular tumors has diagnostic and prognostic value.

41. Which is the most common type of synthetic prostheses for urologic use?

(a) Teflon (b) Silicone
(c) Polyglycolic acid (d) Polylactic acid

(Answer is B) The most common type of synthetic prostheses for urologic use are made of silicone.

42. A limiting factor for the engineering of tissues is that cells cannot be implanted in volumes exceeding:

(a) 1 mm^3 (b) 2 mm^3
(c) 3 mm^3 (d) 4 mm^3

(Answer is C) A limiting factor for the engineering of tissues is that cells cannot be implanted in volumes exceeding 3 mm^3.

43. Which statement regarding stem cell is not correct?

(a) Embryonic stem cells has the ability to proliferate in an undifferentiated but pluripotent state
(b) Adult stem cells do not transdifferentiate spontaneously to a malignant phenotype
(c) Fetal cells are multipotent and are able to differentiate into all three germ layers
(d) Fetal cells spontaneously transdifferentiate to a malignant phenotype

(Answer is D) Fetal stem cells derived from amniotic fluid and placentas have been described and represent a novel source of stem cells. The cells express markers consistent with human embryonic stem cells but do not form teratomas and do not spontaneously transdifferentiate to a malignant phenotype.

44. Death receptor is:

(a) CD35 (b) CD45
(c) CD85 (d) CD95

(Answer is D) Death receptor is CD95, or FAS, which appears to play an important role in cancer immunosurveillance.

45. At which type of renal tubular acidosis (RTA), typically, potassium levels increase?

(a) Type 1 (b) Type 2
(c) Type 3 (d) Type 4

(Answer is D) Type 4

46. Which type of renal tubular acidosis (RTA) is more likely to form renal stones?

(a) Type 1 (b) Type 2
(c) Type 3 (d) Type 4

(Answer is A) Type 1

47. At which condition is alpha-fetoprotein most frequently elevated?

(a) Infiltrating ductal carcinoma of the breast
(b) Seminoma
(c) Hepatocellular carcinoma
(d) Malignant melanoma

(Answer is C) Hepatocellular carcinoma

48. What is the half-life of β-HCG?

(a) 5 – 7 days (b) 24 – 36 hours
(c) 2 – 3 days (d) 12 – 24 hours

(Answer is B) 24 – 36 hours

49. What causes Cushing's disease is?

(a) Bilateral adrenal hyperplasia
(b) Pituitary over secretion of ACTH
(c) Exogenous administration of glucocorticoids
(d) Immune-mediated disease

(Answer is B) Pituitary over secretion of ACTH

50. Where is the gene "sex-determining region" (SRY) located at?

(a) Long arm of X chromosome
(b) Long arm of Y chromosome
(c) Short arm of Y chromosome
(d) Short arm of X chromosome

(Answer is C) Short arm of Y chromosome

51. What is the nature of the prostate-specific antigen?

(a) Protease (b) Lyase
(c) Carboxylase (d) Hydrolase

(Answer is A) Protease

52. What does apoptosis mean?

(a) Programmed cell death
(b) New vascular formation
(c) Uninhibited neural stimulation
(d) Premature muscular contraction

(Answer is A) Programmed cell death

CHAPTER 6

Reproductive and Sexual Function

1. **Which statement is not true regarding steroid hormones?**
   (a) Derived from cholesterol
   (b) Usually bound to carrier proteins
   (c) Cell membrane permeable
   (d) Stored in secretory granules

(Answer is D) Steroid hormones

- Derived from cholesterol.
- They are not stored in secretory granules.
- In plasma, these hormones are usually bound to carrier proteins.
- Steroid hormones are cell membrane-permeable.
- Examples of steroid hormones are testosterone and estradiol.

2. **Neurohypophysis secretes which hormone?**
   (a) ADH (b) LH
   (c) FSH (d) GH

(Answer is A) The posterior lobe, or neurohypophysis, is formed during development as a ventral outpocket of hypothalamus. The secretion of the two neurohypophysial hormones, oxytocin and vasopressin, is driven by neural stimuli.

3. **The first identifiable step separating the ovarian and testicular pathways of differentiation occurs at about which weeks after conception?**
   (a) 5 (b) 7
   (c) 9 (d) 11

(Answer is B) The first identifiable step separating the ovarian and testicular pathways of differentiation is the movement of primordial germ cells into the medullary cords, at about 7 weeks after conception.

4. **Inner to outer layer of testis is in following order:**
   (a) Tunica vaginalis, tunica albuginea, tunica vasculosa
   (b) Tunica vasculosa, tunica albuginea, tunica vaginalis
   (c) Tunica albuginea, tunica vasculosa, tunica vaginalis
   (d) Tunica albuginea, tunica vaginalis, tunica vasculosa

(Answer is B) The testicular parenchyma is surrounded by a capsule made up of three layers: the outer visceral layer of the tunica vaginalis, the tunica albuginea, and the innermost layer of the tunica vasculosa.

5. **In human testis, interstitial tissue takes up how much of the total testicular up how much of the total testicular?**
   (a) 0% to 10% (b) 10% to 20%
   (c) 20% to 30% (d) 30% to 40%

(Answer is C) In humans, interstitial tissue takes up 20% to 30% of the total testicular volume.

6. **The correct order of flow of fluid and spermatozoa toward the epididymis:**
   (a) Seminiferous tubules, rete testis, ductuli efferentes, caput epididymis
   (b) Rete testis, seminiferous tubules, ductuli efferentes, caput epididymis
   (c) Seminiferous tubules, ductuli efferentes, rete testis, caput epididymis

(d) Seminiferous tubules, ductuli efferentes, caput epididymis, rete testis

(Answer is A) The seminiferous tubules are long, highly coiled and looped, both ends of which usually terminate in the rete testis. The rete testis coalesces to form the 6 to 12 ductuli efferentes, which act as conduits to carry testicular fluid and spermatozoa into the caput epididymis.

7. **Which one of the following statement regarding testis is not correct?**
   (a) The testis has rich somatic and autonomic innervations
   (b) The arterial supply to the human testis and epididymis is derived from three sources
   (c) The veins within the testis are unusual in that they do not run with the corresponding intratesticular arteries
   (d) There are prominent lymphatic ducts in the spermatic cord of the human testis

(Answer is A) The testis has no somatic innervation but receives autonomic innervation.

8. **Incidence of single artery entering testis is:**
   (a) 20-30% (b) 30-40%
   (c) 40-50% (d) 50-60%

(Answer is D) A single artery enters the testis in 56% of cases; two branches enter in 31% of cases; and three or more branches enter in 13% of cases.

9. **Peak of testosterone occurs in the blood at all ages *except:***
   (a) 12 and 18 weeks of gestation
   (b) At 2 weeks of birth
   (c) At 2 months of age
   (d) At second decade

(Answer is B) Peak of testosterone occurs in the blood of the human fetus between 12 and 18 weeks of gestation. Another testosterone peak occurs at approximately 2 months of age. Testosterone reaches a maximal concentration during the second or third decade of life, then reaches a plateau, and declines thereafter.

10. **Which one of the following statement regarding blood testis barrier is correct?**
   (a) Spermatogonia and young spermatocytes are outside the blood-testis barrier in the adluminal compartment
   (b) Mature spermatocytes and spermatids are sequestered above the barrier in the basal compartment
   (c) The presence of germ cells is not necessary for the development of the barrier
   (d) Testicular insult, such as biopsy, torsion, or trauma, will induce antisperm antibodies if the insult occurs before puberty

(Answer is C) Spermatogonia and young spermatocytes are outside the blood-testis barrier in the basal compartment, whereas mature spermatocytes and spermatids are sequestered above the barrier in the adluminal compartment. Testicular insult, such as biopsy, torsion, or trauma, will not induce antisperm antibodies if the insult occurs before puberty.

11. **Correct order for formation of mature spermatozoa is:**
   (a) Spermatogonia, spermatids, spermatozoa, spermatocytes
   (b) Spermatogonia, spermatocytes, spermatids, spermatozoa
   (c) Spermatogonia, spermatids, spermatocytes, spermatozoa
   (d) Spermatogonia, spermatozoa, spermatocytes, spermatids

(Answer is B) It involves a proliferative phase during which spermatogonia divide either to replace their number (stem cell renewal) or to produce daughter cells committed to become spermatocytes, a meiotic phase when spermatocytes undergo reduction division, resulting in haploid spermatids; and a spermiogenic phase when spermatids undergo a dramatic metamorphosis in size and shape to form mature spermatozoa.

12. **During spermiogenesis which change does not occur?**
    (a) Loss of cytoplasm
    (b) Formation of the acrosome
    (c) Migration of cytoplasmic organelles
    (d) Loss of the flagellum

(Answer is D) Changes include loss of cytoplasm, formation of the acrosome, formation of the flagellum, and migration of cytoplasmic organelles to positions characteristic of the mature spermatozoon.

13. **The correct order from proceeding from least to most differentiated is:**
    (a) Leptotene primary spermatocytes; preleptotene primary spermatocytes; zygotene primary spermatocytes; pachytene primary spermatocytes
    (b) Preleptotene primary spermatocytes; leptotene primary spermatocytes; zygotene primary spermatocytes; pachytene primary spermatocytes
    (c) Preleptotene primary spermatocytes; leptotene primary spermatocytes; pachytene primary spermatocytes; zygotene primary spermatocytes
    (d) Leptotene primary spermatocytes; preleptotene primary spermatocytes; pachytene primary spermatocytes; zygotene primary spermatocytes

(Answer is B) Proceeding from the least to the most differentiated, they were named dark type A spermatogonia (Ad); pale type A spermatogonia (Ap); type B spermatogonia (B); preleptotene primary spermatocytes (R); leptotene primary spermatocytes (L); zygotene primary spermatocytes (z); pachytene primary spermatocytes (p); secondary spermatocytes (II); and Sa, Sb1, Sb2, Sc, Sd1 and Sd2 spermatids.

14. **The entire spermatogenic process in humans requires how many days?**
    (a) 32 (b) 64
    (c) 128 (d) 256

(Answer is B) The entire spermatogenic process in humans requires approximately 64 days.

15. **Which hormone will initiate and qualitatively maintain spermatogenesis in humans?**
    (a) Estradiol (b) Testosterone
    (c) FSH (d) LH

(Answer is B) Testosterone will initiate and qualitatively maintain spermatogenesis in humans.

16. **DAZ is localized at which chromosome?**
    (a) Long arm of Y chromosome
    (b) Short arm of Y chromosome
    (c) Long arm of X chromosome
    (d) Short arm of X chromosome

(Answer is A) One gene localized on the long arm of the Y chromosome in a region referred to as AZFc (Azoospermic Factor) is DAZ (deleted in azoospermia).

17. **In humans, half of the total number of epididymal spermatozoa are stored in:**
    (a) Caput
    (b) Corpus
    (c) Cauda
    (d) Same number in all three parts

(Answer is C) In humans, approximately half of the total number of epididymal spermatozoa are stored in the caudal region.

18. **Sperm fertility maturation in humans is, in most part, achieved at the level of:**
    (a) Proximal caput epididymis
    (b) Distal caput or proximal corpus epididymis
    (c) Distal corpus or proximal cauda epididymis
    (d) Distal cauda epididymis

(Answer is C) Sperm fertility maturation in humans is, in most part, achieved at the level of the distal corpus or proximal cauda epididymis.

19. Which part of sperm provides necessary for motility?

(a) Acrosome (b) Nucleus
(c) Mitochondria (d) Di-sulphide bonds

(Answer is D) The outer dense fibers, rich in disulfide bonds, are thought to provide the sperm tail with the rigidity necessary for progressive motility.

20. Which statement regarding spermatozoa structure is not true?

(a) The oval sperm head, consists principally of a nucleus, which contains the highly compacted chromatin material
(b) Head consist of acrosome, a membrane-bound organelle that contains the enzymes required for penetration
(c) Head consist of helically arranged mitochondria
(d) The outer dense fibers, rich in disulfide bonds, are thought to provide sperm tail

(Answer is C) The middle piece of the spermatozoa is a highly organized segment consisting of helically arranged mitochondria surrounding a set of outer dense fibers and the characteristic 9 + 2 microtubular structure of the sperm axoneme.

21. Which structure has the greatest muscle-lumen ratio of any hollow viscus in the human body?

(a) Epididymis (b) Seminal vesicle
(c) Ductus deferens (d) Fallopian tube

(Answer is C) Ductus deferens has the greatest muscle-lumen ratio (~10:1) of any hollow viscus in the human body.

22. Which statement regarding fertility is not correct?

(a) The chance of a normal couple conceiving is 90% by 1 year
(b) Approximately 40% of cases of infertility are due entirely to a male factor
(c) Approximately 30% to 40% of cases of infertility involve both male and female factors
(d) Baseline pregnancy rate is 1% to 3% per month for infertile couples

(Answer is B) Approximately 20% of cases of infertility are due entirely to a male factor.

23. Average number of days of viability of sperm and ova respectively is:

(a) 3 days and 1 day (b) 5 days and 1 day
(c) 1 day and 5 days (d) 1 day and 3 days

(Answer is B) Studies have shown that conception may occur when sexual relations take place up to 5 days before ovulation but, owing to the short life span of oocytes, will not occur if sexual relations are performed the day after ovulation.

24. Lubricants that impair *in vitro* sperm motility include:

(a) Vegetable oil (b) Raw egg white
(c) Peanut oil (d) Saliva

(Answer is D) Lubricants, such as astroglide, lubafax, K-Y jelly, Keri lotion, surgilube and saliva, adversely affect sperm motility. Lubricants that do not impair *in vitro* sperm motility include peanut oil, safflower oil, vegetable oil, and raw egg white.

25. After a febrile illness, spermatogenesis may be impaired for:

(a) 1 month (b) 2 months
(c) 3 months (d) 4 months

(Answer is C) After a febrile illness, spermatogenesis may be impaired for up to 3 months.

26. Which one of the following statement regarding ejaculation is not correct?

(a) Before the ejaculation of the major portion of the ejaculate comes from the glands of Littre and the bulbourethral glands is secreted

(b) The last fraction of the ejaculate consists of seminal vesicle secretions

(c) The secretions from Cowper's glands account for only 0.1 to 0.2 ml

(d) Major amount of contribution in ejaculate is from prostate

(Answer is D) The secretions from Cowper's glands account for 0.1 to 0.2 ml, prostatic secretions account for 0.5 ml, and the secretions from the seminal vesicles account for 1.5 to 2.0 ml.

27. Patients with obstructed seminal vesicles is usually associated with all *except:*

(a) Azoospermia

(b) Alkaline semen

(c) Fructose negative semen

(d) Semen does not coagulate

(Answer is B) Patients with obstructed seminal vesicles or congenital absence of the seminal vesicles, which is usually associated with bilateral absence of the vas deferens, demonstrate azoospermic, acidic, fructose-negative semen that does not coagulate. In addition, their ejaculate volume is low (<1.0 ml).

28. The World Health Organization reference values are all *except:*

(a) Total sperm number: 20×10^6 or more spermatozoa per ejaculate

(b) Motility: 50% or more with grade "a + b" motility

(c) Morphology: 15% or more by strict criteria

(d) Viability: 75% or more of sperm viable

(Answer is A) Volume: 2.0 ml or more

pH: 7.2 or more

Sperm concentration: 20×10^6 or more spermatozoa/ml

Total sperm number: 40×10^6 or more spermatozoa per ejaculate

Motility: 50% or more with grade "a + b" motility or 25% or more with grade "a" motility

Morphology: 15% or more by strict criteria

Viability: 75% or more of sperm viable

WBCs: Less than 1 million/ml.

29. Incidence of primary hormonal etiology in infertile men is:

(a) 1% (b) 3%

(c) 7% (d) 10%

(Answer is B) Although male reproductive function is critically dependent on endocrinologic control, less than 3% of infertile men have a primary hormonal etiology.

30. Patients with complete testicular failure will have:

(a) Elevated FSH, normal LH and testosterone

(b) Elevated FSH and LH and decreased testosterone

(c) Low FSH and LH and high testosterone

(d) Low FSH, LH and testosterone

(Answer is B) Patients with complete testicular failure have inadequate Leydig and Sertoli cell function that results in elevated gonadotropin levels associated with normal or low testosterone levels.

31. Men at what sperm level should get serum FSH and morning testosterone levels evaluated?

(a) 5 million/ml (b) 10 million/ml

(c) 15 million/ml (d) 20 million/ml

(Answer is B) All men with an indication in the history or physical examination or a sperm density less than 10 million/ml should have serum FSH and morning testosterone levels measured because endocrine abnormalities are rarely present when the sperm concentration is greater than 10 million/ml.

32. The most common cause of ejaculatory failure is:

(a) Medication (b) Diabetes mellitus
(c) Multiple sclerosis (d) Spinal cord injury

(Answer is D) The most common cause of ejaculatory failure is spinal cord injury. Other neurologic disorders such as diabetes mellitus and multiple sclerosis are frequent causes.

33. In a patient with low volume ejaculate, post ejaculation urinalysis was done, it was negative for sperm, next step will be:

(a) Sympathomimetics
(b) Electroejaculation
(c) TRUS
(d) Seminal vesicle aspiration

(Answer is C) If post ejaculation urinalysis is negative for sperm, TRUS is done if it is abnormal seminal vesicle aspiration is done and if it is normal sympathomimetics are administered.

34. In azoospermic patient with normal palpable vas and testis with normal FSH level, next step will be:

(a) TRUS (b) Vasography
(c) Testicular biopsy (d) Cranial MRI

(Answer is C) Patients with vas present, normal testicular volume, and normal serum FSH require testicular biopsy to differentiate between spermatogenic abnormalities and ductal obstruction.

35. Oligospermia refers to sperm densities of less than:

(a) 05 million sperm/ml
(b) 10 million sperm/ml
(c) 15 million sperm/ml
(d) 20 million sperm/ml

(Answer is D) Oligospermia refers to sperm densities of less than 20 million sperm/ml.

36. Patient with semen parameters-antisperm antibody +, low motility but high viability sperm should be evaluated with:

(a) TRUS
(b) Electron microscopy
(c) Seminal vesicle aspiration
(d) Testicular biopsy

(Answer is B) The finding of a high fraction of viable sperm in the presence of low or absent sperm motility suggests an ultrastructural abnormality, such as that found in primary ciliary dyskinesia and Kartagener's syndrome.

37. Antisperm antibodies can be detected in:

(a) 60% of patients after vasectomy and one third after CBAVD
(b) 40% of patients after vasectomy and one third after CBAVD
(c) 60% of patients after vasectomy and two third after CBAVD
(d) 40% of patients after vasectomy and two third after CBAVD

(Answer is A) Approximately 60% of men after vasectomy develop antisperm antibodies whereas approximately one third of patients with CBAVD are found to have antisperm antibodies.

38. Incidence of ASA in infertile and fertile patients is:

(a) 5% and 1% (b) 10% and 2%
(c) 15% and 3% (d) 20% and 4%

(Answer is B) Antisperm antibodies are detected in approximately 10% of males presenting with infertility as opposed to 2% or less of fertile men.

39. Round cells are:

(a) Mature germ cells and leukocytes
(b) Immature germ cells and leukocytes
(c) Mature germ cells and monocytes
(d) Immature germ cells and monocytes

(Answer is B) Both immature germ cells (spermatocytes) and leukocytes appear similar under wet mount microscopy and are known as round cells.

40. WBC staining is recommended for:

(a) More than 10 to 15 round cells/HPF or more than 1 million round cells/ml
(b) More than 5 round cells/HPF or more than 1 million round cells/ml
(c) More than 10 to 15 round cells/HPF or more than 0.1 million round cells/ml
(d) More than 5 round cells/HPF or more than 0.1 million round cells/ml

(Answer is A) WBC staining of semen in patients with more than 10 to 15 round cells/HPF or more than 1 million round cells/ml.

41. Routine genital tract bacterial cultures are indicated in all *except:*

(a) All cases of infertility
(b) In symptomatic patients
(c) In patients with documented pyospermia
(d) In patients with symptoms and documented pyospermia

(Answer is A) Routine genital tract bacterial cultures are not indicated in the absence of clinical symptoms or documented pyospermia.

42. Which one of the following statement is not true?

(a) Less than 3% of infertile men have a primary hormonal etiology
(b) Antisperm antibodies are detected in approximately 10% of males presenting with infertility
(c) Approximately 6% of infertile men are found to have chromosome abnormalities detected by karyotype analysis
(d) Microdeletions of sections of the long arm of the Y chromosome have been identified in approximately 3% -7% of azoospermic men

(Answer is D) Microdeletions of sections of the long arm of the Y chromosome have been identified in approximately 13% of azoospermic men and 3% to 7% of oligospermic men.

43. Men with unilateral absence of the vas deferens is associated with which anomaly?

(a) Kidney agenesis (b) Ureter agenesis
(c) Adrenal agenesis (d) Prostate agenesis

(Answer is A) Ipsilateral renal anomalies are present in up to 80% of men with unilateral absence of the vas deferens, with the most common anomaly being renal agenesis.

44. Which statement is not true regarding Sertoli cell–only syndrome?

(a) Also called as germ cell aplasia
(b) Testicular histology reveals seminiferous tubules containing Sertoli cells with a complete absence of all germ cells
(c) Have normal-sized testes associated with normal levels of FSH
(d) Normal spermatogenesis

(Answer is D) Many patients with a Sertoli cell–only pattern on a diagnostic biopsy have low levels of spermatogenesis in other areas of the testis.

45. Which one of the following statement regarding Kallman syndrome is not true?

(a) The presence of midline defects may help in the prepubertal diagnosis
(b) A delay in pubertal development is the hallmark
(c) It is a genetically heterogeneous disorder that may be inherited in an X-linked, AD or AR pattern
(d) Gonadotropin therapy is contraindicated

(Answer is D) GnRH therapy is contraindicated in patients with acquired hypogonadotropic hypogonadism due to pituitary tumors, pituitary surgery, or head trauma.

46. Which is the most common cause of endogenous androgen excess?

(a) Turner's syndróme
(b) Congenital adrenal hyperplasia
(c) Klinefelter's syndrome
(d) Kallman syndrome

(Answer is B) Congenital adrenal hyperplasia is the most common cause of endogenous androgen excess.

47. Androgen receptor gene is located at:

(a) Short arm of chromosome X
(b) Long arm of chromosome X
(c) Short arm of chromosome Y
(d) Long arm of chromosome Y

(Answer is B) Androgen receptor gene is located on the X chromosome at Xq 11-12, this syndrome is inherited as an X-linked recessive trait.

48. Which one of the following statement regarding Klinefelter's syndrome is not true?

(a) Patient with mosaic Klinefelter's syndrome and severe oligospermia, ICSI combined with IVF is a possibility
(b) A phenotypic male with small firm testes, gynecomastia, and elevated gonadotropins
(c) 50% of the patients may have normal testosterone concentrations
(d) Normal sperm count is present in 50% of the patients

(Answer is D) Azoospermia is typically present in Klinefelter's syndrome.

49. Which one of the following statement regarding varicocele is not true?

(a) Majority of men with varicoceles are fertile
(b) Improvement in seminal parameters is demonstrated in approximately 70% of patients after surgical varicocele repair
(c) Improvements in morphology is most common after varicocele repair
(d) The varicocele is the most common correctable cause of male infertility

(Answer is C) Improvements in motility are most common, occurring in 70% of patients, with improved sperm densities in 51% and improved morphology in 44% of patients, after surgical varicocele repair.

50. Chemotherapeutic agents adversely affect spermatogenesis in the following ways *except:*

(a) Cells most susceptible to the adverse effects of chemotherapy are those most actively dividing and consist of spermatogonia and spermatocytes
(b) Majority will recover spermatogenesis within 4 years
(c) There appears to be increased risk of birth defects in children born to patients after chemotherapy
(d) Contraception should be used during and for a period of time (6 to 24 months) after chemotherapy

(Answer is C) There appears to be no increased risk of birth defects in children born to patients after chemotherapy.

51. Radiotherapy adversely affect spermatogenesis in the following ways *except:*

(a) Germinal epithelium is very radiosensitive
(b) Spermatids are more resistant than spermatogonia or spermatocytes
(c) Leydig cells are reasonably radioresistant; therefore, testosterone levels usually remain normal after radiation exposure
(d) Semen quality will usually return to baseline within 4 years after radiation therapy for seminoma

(Answer is D) Semen quality will usually return to baseline within 2 years after radiation therapy for seminoma. Approximately one fourth of patients may become permanently infertile from such radiation treatment. After radiation therapy most patients are advised to avoid conception for a minimum of 6 to 24 months.

52. Which statement regarding idiopathic infertility is not correct?

(a) Up to 25% of patients exhibit abnormal semen analyses for which no cause can be identified

(b) Vast majority of these patients have abnormalities of all semen parameters

(c) Pregnancy rate for untreated couples is less than 5%

(d) If empirical pharmacologic therapy is going to be used, it should be administered for a minimum of a 3 to 6 months period

(Answer is C) There is a significant background pregnancy rate (26%) for untreated couples with abnormal semen parameters independent of treatment.

53. Which one of the following statement regarding penile vibratory stimulation is not true?

(a) Penile vibratory stimulation results in ejaculation in approximately 70% of spinal cord–injured men

(b) This approach works best in patients with upper motor neuron lesions such as spinal cord injuries above T10

(c) This approach should be attempted in only those patients who have failed to respond to electroejaculation

(d) Pretreatment of these patients includes 20 mg of sublingual nifedipine

(Answer is C) Electroejaculation should be attempted in only those patients who are not candidates for or have failed to respond to penile vibratory stimulation.

54. Which statement regarding ART is not correct?

(a) Varicocele repair has been more cost effective than IVF with ICSI

(b) Repeat vasectomy reversal has been more cost effective than IVF with ICSI

(c) Patients with epididymal obstruction, vasoepididymostomy has been more cost effective than IVF with ICSI

(d) IVF as an initial treatment for infertile couples in general is more cost effective than IUI

(Answer is D) IVF as an initial treatment for infertile couples in general is less cost effective than more standard approaches such as IUI.

55. Regarding sperm retrival which statement is not true?

(a) For obstructive azoospermia, there appears to be no significant difference in pregnancy rates regardless of the sperm retrieval technique employed

(b) MESA is commonly employed to retrieve sperm out of the ductal system in cases with CBAVD

(c) In patients with nonobstructive azoospermia, open surgical testicular sperm extraction techniques retrieve sperm in a greater percent of patients and yield higher numbers of sperm than percutaneous techniques

(d) In men with obstructive azoospermia, pregnancy rates by ICSI by fresh epididymal sperm is more than frozen sperm

(Answer is D) In men with obstructive azoospermia, there is no difference in pregnancy rates by ICSI between frozen and fresh epididymal sperm.

56. Regarding testicular biopsy which statement is not true?

(a) Results of a single biopsy of one testis indicates spermatogenic process in the remainder of that testis or the contralateral testis

(b) Multiple biopsies or microscopic sperm extraction from both testes should be performed in patients with nonobstructive azoospermia

(c) If there is a discrepancy in size, biopsy of the larger, more normal testis should be performed first

(d) Least vascular site for biopsy is, upper medial portion of the testis

(Answer is A) Results of a single biopsy of one testis may not be indicative of the spermatogenic process in the remainder of that testis or the contralateral testis.

57. Most common complication of testicular biopsy is:

(a) Bleeding
(b) Infection
(c) Testicular atrophy
(d) Inadvertent biopsy of the epididymis

(Answer is A) The most common complications after testis biopsy are bleeding and formation of hematomas.

58. Varicoceles are present in:

(a) 15% of the normal male population
(b) 25% of patients with male infertility
(c) 70% of patients with secondary infertility
(d) 25% of men with abnormal semen parameters compared with 11% of men with normal semen

(Answer is A) Varicoceles are present in 15% of the normal male population and in up to 40% of patients with male infertility.

59. USG examination demonstrating veins larger than what diameter, is consistent with the diagnosis of a varicocele?

(a) 2.0mm (b) 2.5mm
(c) 3.0mm (d) 3.5mm

(Answer is D) USG examination demonstrating veins 3.5 mm or larger in diameter, with reversal of venous flow after the Valsalva maneuver, is consistent with the diagnosis of a varicocele.

60. Indication for varicocelectomy are all *except:*

(a) Varicocele is palpable on physical examination, corroborated by ultrasound examination with abnormal semen analysis
(b) Adult men with a varicocele and abnormal semen parameters who may wish to conceive in the future
(c) Adolescent men with varicoceles with reduction in volume of the ipsilateral testis
(d) Varicocele detected on ultrasound only

(Answer is D) Studies have demonstrated that subclinical varicoceles have no impact on fertility and that repair of subclinical varicoceles does not improve fertility rates.

61. Factors predicting successful repair of varicocelectomy are all *except:*

(a) Lack of testicular atrophy
(b) Sperm density greater than 50 million per ejaculate
(c) Sperm motility of 60% or more
(d) Serum FSH values more than 300 ng/ml

(Answer is D) Preoperative factors associated with an increased likelihood of postoperative pregnancy are lack of testicular atrophy, sperm density greater than 50 million per ejaculate, sperm motility of 60% or more, and serum FSH values less than 300 ng/ml.

62. Which one of the following statement regarding complication associated with varicocele repairs is not true?

(a) Testicular artery is generally preserved in radiographic and laparoscopic approach
(b) Least recurrence rates is seen in microscopic and laparoscopic approach
(c) Occurrence of hydrocele is least in microscopic and laparoscopic approach
(d) Maximum recurrence rates is seen in conventional and retroperitoneal approach

(Answer is C)

Complication rates associated with different varicocele repairs

Technique	*Artery Preserved*	*Hydrocele (%)*	*Recurrence (%)*
Retroperitoneal	No	7	11-15
Conventional inguinal	No	3-39	9-16
Laparoscopic	Yes	5-8	<2
Radiographic	Yes	0	4-11
Microscopic inguinal or subinguinal	Yes	0	<2

63. The most common complication after non-microsurgical varicocelectomy is:

(a) Testicular atrophy
(b) Recurrence
(c) Epididymal injury
(d) Hydrocele

(Answer is D) The most common complication after non-microsurgical varicocelectomy is hydrocele formation, occurring in 3% to 39% of cases.

64. A semen analysis should be performed after how many months of varicocele repair?

(a) 1 month (b) 2 months
(c) 3 months (d) 4 months

(Answer is D) A semen analysis should be performed 4 months after varicocele repair.

65. Vasovasostomy should be considered in the following instance:

(a) Material coming from proximal vas lumen is thick, pasty and devoid of sperm
(b) Fluid is creamy, containing only debris
(c) Fluid is clear and copious with no visible sperm
(d) If there is no fluid whatsoever when the vas is milked toward the cut end

(Answer is C) If there are sperm or sperm parts (sperm heads, sperm with partial tails) in large numbers or the fluid is clear and copious with no visible sperm, vasovasostomy is generally indicated. If the fluid is thick, pasty and devoid of sperm or contains only a few sperm heads, vasoepididymostomy should be considered.

66. Patency and pregnancy rates after microsurgical vasovasostomy respectively is:

(a) 35% to 45% and 20% to 40%
(b) 55% to 65% and 30% to 55%
(c) 65% to 75% and 40% to 60%
(d) 75% to 85% and 45% to 70%

(Answer is D) Most studies with large number of patients have generally found patency rates of 75% to 85% and pregnancy rates of 45% to 70%.

67. Most common karyotypic abnormality associated with non-obstructive azoospermia is:

(a) XXY (b) XYY
(c) Turner's syndrome (d) Down syndrome

(Answer is A) Approximately 12% of non-obstructive azoospermic men will have an abnormal karyotype. The most common karyotypic abnormality is an extra X chromosome (47, XXY), a condition commonly known as Klinefelter's syndrome.

68. IVF with ICSI is indicated in following *except:*

(a) Congenital bilateral absence of the vas deferens
(b) Men with few viable sperm in the ejaculate
(c) Azoospermic men with varicoceles
(d) Men with obstructive azoospermia

(Answer is D) IVF is indicated in men with non-obstructive azoospermia.

69. Which one of the following statement regarding IVF and ICSI is not true?

(a) Fertilization rates are in the range of 70%, and delivery rates per retrieval are 50%
(b) The incidence of major fetal abnonnalities is 3.2% compared with 1.6% in natural conception
(c) Embryos that cleave and continue to

develop are transferred to the uterus transvaginally 5 to 7 days after fertilization

(d) IVF with ICSI is now the treatment of choice for severe uncorrectable male factor infertility

(Answer is C) Embryos that cleave and continue to develop are transferred to the uterus transvaginally 3 to 5 days after fertilization.

70. Prosthesis tends to extrude at:

(a) Between the 11 and 1 O'clock

(b) Between the 5 and 7 O'clock

(c) Between the 2 and 5 O'clock

(d) Between the 7 and 11 O'clock

(Answer is B) The strength and thickness of the tunica correlate in a statistically significant fashion with location. The most vulnerable area is located on the ventral groove (between the 5 and 7 O'clock positions), where the longitudinal outer layer is absent; most prostheses tend to extrude here.

71. Branches of the penile artery are all *except:*

(a) Dorsal (b) Bulbourethral

(c) Cavernous (d) Circumflex

(Answer is D) The three branches of the penile artery are the dorsal, bulbourethral and cavernous.

72. Which artery is responsible for engorgement of the glans during erection?

(a) Dorsal (b) Bulbourethral

(c) Cavernous (d) Circumflex

(Answer is A) The dorsal artery is responsible for engorgement of the glans during erection.

73. Mechanism of erection include all the following *except:*

(a) Dilation of the arterioles and arteries by increased blood flow in both the diastolic and systolic phases

(b) Compression of the subtunical venous plexuses between the tunica albuginea and the peripheral sinusoids, reducing venous outflow

(c) Relaxation of emissary veins between the inner circular and outer longitudinal layers

(d) Increase in PO_2 and intracavernous pressure

(Answer is C) Mechanism of erection includes stretching of the tunica to its capacity, which occludes the emissary veins between the inner circular and outer longitudinal layers and further decreases venous outflow to a minimum.

74. Tunica is thick, thin and absent in following order:

(a) Corpora cavernosa, corpora spongiosum, glans

(b) Corpora cavernosa, glans, corpora spongiosum

(c) Glans, corpora spongiosum, corpora cavernosa

(d) Corpora spongiosum, corpora cavernosa, glans

(Answer is A) Pressure in the corpus spongiosum and glans is only one third to one half that in the corpora cavernosa because the tunical covering, which is thin over the corpus spongiosum and virtually absent over the glans.

75. Regarding penile neuroanatomy origin of sympathetic and parasympathetic pathways are from:

(a) T11 to L2 and S2 to S4 spinal segments respectively

(b) T10 to L1 and S2 to S4 spinal segments respectively

(c) S2 to S4 and T11 to L2 spinal segments respectively

(d) S2 to S4 and T10 to L2 spinal segments respectively

(Answer is A) The sympathetic pathway originates from the 11th thoracic to the 2nd lumbar spinal segments and passes through the white rami to the sympathetic chain ganglia. The para-sympathetic pathway arises from neurons in the intermediolateral cell columns of the second, third, and fourth sacral spinal cord segments.

76. Brain center involved in visually evoked sexual stimulation:

(a) Medial amygdala
(b) Pyriform cortex
(c) Hippocampus
(d) Inferior frontal cortex

(Answer is D) Right insula and inferior frontal cortex.

77. All the following are mediator for detumescence *except:*

(a) Endothelin
(b) Prostaglandin 12 (PG12)
(c) Angiotensin II
(d) NO

(Answer is D) NO released from nonadrenergic, non-cholinergic neurotransmission and from the endothelium is the principal neurotransmitter mediating penile erection.

78. Neurotransmitters implicated in promotion of sexual function include all *except:*

(a) Dopaminergic
(b) Adrenergic
(c) 5-HTI A receptor agonists
(d) 5-HT2 C receptor agonists

(Answer is C) 5-HT1 A receptor agonists inhibit erectile activity but facilitate ejaculation; stimulation of 5-HT2 C receptors causes erection.

79. Which statement regarding NO is not correct:

(a) Synthesis of NO is catalyzed by NOS, which converts larginine and oxygen to L-citrulline and NO
(b) iNOS in virtually expressed in all cell types
(c) iNOS and nNOS being considered responsible for initiating and sustaining erection, respectively
(d) The most physiologically relevant receptor for NO is sGC

(Answer is C) nNOS and eNOS being considered responsible for initiating and sustaining erection, respectively.

80. Regarding physiology of erection which statement is not true?

(a) NO released by nNOS contained in the terminals of the cavernous nerve initiates the erection process
(b) Upon entering the smooth muscle cells, NO stimulates the production of cGMP
(c) Cyclic GMP activates protein kinase G, which in turn opens calcium channels and closes potassium channels
(d) The smooth muscle regains its tone when cGMP is degraded by phosphodiesterase

(Answer is C) Cyclic GMP activates protein kinase G, which in turn opens potassium channels and closes calcium channels.

81. Which PDEs have not been identified in the corpus cavernosum?

(a) PDE 8 (b) PDE 6
(c) PDE 4 (d) PDE 3

(Answer is B) With the exception of PDE 6, which is specifically expressed in photoreceptor cells, all PDEs have been identified in the corpus cavernosum.

82. Which is the principal PDE for the termination of cavernous cGMP signaling?

(a) PDE 2 (b) PDE 4
(c) PDE 5 (d) PDE 6

(Answer is C) There is ample evidence that PDE 5 is by far the principal PDE for the termination of cavernous cGMP signaling.

83. MMAS and NHSLS studies were done for:

(a) Carcinoma prostate (b) ED
(c) BPH (d) Carcinoma testis

(Answer is B) Modern probability sampling techniques were used by two surveys obtaining prevalence data of ED in the United States: the Massachusetts Male Aging Study (MMAS) and the National Health and Social Life Survey (NHSLS).

84. Impotence after radical prostatectomy is due to injury of:

(a) Cavernosal nerve (b) Dorsal nerve
(c) Capsular arteries (d) Uretral atteries

(Answer is A) Because of the close relationship between the cavernous nerves and the pelvic organs, the incidence of iatrogenic impotence resulting from various pelvic surgical procedures is reportedly high: radical prostatectomy, 43% to 100%.

85. Testosterone enhances all *except:*

(a) Sexual interest
(b) Frequency of sexual acts
(c) Frequency of nocturnal erections
(d) Fantasy-induced or visually stimulated erections

(Answer is D) Testosterone (1) enhances sexual interest, (2) increases the frequency of sexual acts, and (3) increases the frequency of nocturnal erections but has little or no effect on fantasy-induced or visually stimulated erections.

86. Which antihypertensive does not result in ED?

(a) Diuretics
(b) β blocker (nonselective)
(c) α2 blocker
(d) ACE inhibitor

(Answer is D) ACE inhibitors lack any easily appreciated peripheral or central effect that would interfere with sexual function.

87. Regarding International Index of Erectile Function (IIEF) which statement is not true?

(a) It has 15 items
(b) It quantify five domains
(c) Minimum score is 0
(d) Maximum score is 25

(Answer is C) ED severity is classified into five categories based on the IIEF-5: severe (5 to 7), moderate (8 to 11), mild to moderate (12 to 16), mild (17 to 21) and no ED (22 to 25).

88. All are IIEF domain *except:*

(a) Erectile function
(b) Orgasmic function
(c) Sexual desire
(d) Ejaculation volume

(Answer is D) The IIEF is the most widely used SAQ, and it is statistically validated in many languages. Its 15 items address and quantify five domains: erectile function, orgasmic function, sexual desire, intercourse satisfaction and overall satisfaction.

89. All *except* one is the feature of organic ED:

(a) Gradual in onset
(b) Varying course
(c) Global circumstances
(d) Non-coital erection is poor

(Answer is B)

Differentiation between Psychogenic and Organic ED

Characteristic	*Organic*	*Psychogenic*
Onset	Gradual	Acute
Circumstances	Global	Situational
Course	Constant	Varying
Noncoital erection	Poor	Rigid

90. A body of evidence including high-quality systematic reviews of case-control or cohort studies directly applicable to the target population and demonstrating overall consistency of results is which level of recommendation?

(a) A (b) B
(c) C (d) D

(Answer is B) A body of evidence including high-quality systematic reviews of case-control or cohort studies directly applicable to the target population and demonstrating overall consistency of results.

91. All are B grade recommendation for ED *except:*

(a) DICC
(b) ICI
(c) CT angiography
(d) NPTR

(Answer is C) CT angiography is grade D recommendation.

92. Regarding combined intracavernous injection and stimulation which statement is not true?

(a) This screening test is the most commonly performed diagnostic procedure for ED
(b) It allows to bypass neurologic influences
(c) It allows to bypass hormonal influences
(d) It allows to bypass vascular influences

(Answer is D) This screening test is the most commonly performed diagnostic procedure for ED. It allows the clinician to bypass neurologic and hormonal influences and to evaluate the vascular status of the penis directly and objectively.

93. In a patient after performing ICI test penis did not return to flaccid state. This patient should be managed with phenylephrine in dose of:

(a) 500 mg/ml, given 1 ml every 3 to 5 minutes until detumescence
(b) 1000 mg/ml, given 1 ml every 3 to 5 minutes until detumescence
(c) 500 mg/ml, given 1 ml every minute until detumescence
(d) 1000 mg/ml, given 1 ml every minute until detumescence

(Answer is A) Patient should not leave the office until the penis becomes flaccid spontaneously or by injection of a diluted phenylephrine solution (500 mg/ml, given 1 ml every 3 to 5 minutes until detumescence).

94. Which in the following is the most reliable and least invasive evidence-based assessment of ED?

(a) CIS and blood flow measurement by duplex ultrasound
(b) Dynamic infusion cavernosometry and cavernosography (DICC)
(c) CT angiography
(d) MRI

(Answer is A) The penile blood flow study, which consists of CIS and blood flow measurement by duplex ultrasound, is the most reliable and least invasive evidence-based assessment of ED.

95. Below what value PSV can be considered as indicator for cavernous arterial insufficiency?

(a) 25 cm/s (b) 35 cm/s
(c) 45 cm/s (d) 55 cm/s

(Answer is A) PSV less than 25 cm/s after intracavernous injection and sexual stimulation has a 100% sensitivity and 95% specificity in selecting patients with abnormal penile arteriography, because it reflects severe cavernous arterial insufficiency.

96. In a patient in whom doppler spectral waveform continues to exhibit high systolic flow (>25 cm/s PSV) and EDV (>5 cm/s) accompanied by quick detumescence after self-stimulation. Diagnosis is:

(a) Arteriogenic impotence
(b) Venogenic impotence
(c) Neurogenic impotence
(d) Psychogenic impotence

(Answer is B) When the Doppler spectral waveform continues to exhibit high systolic flow (>25 cm/s PSV) and persistent end-diastolic flow velocity

(EDV) (>5 cm /s) accompanied by quick detumescence after self-stimulation, the patient is considered to have venogenic impotence.

97. Resistive index is defined as:

(a) RI = PSY - EDV/PSV
(b) RI = EDV - PSV/PSV
(c) RI = PSV - EDV/EDV
(d) RI = EDV - PSV/EDV

(Answer is A) RI = PSV - EDV/PSV. RI greater than 0.9 was associated with normal results during DICC in 90% of their series and an RI less than 0.75 was associated with venous leakage in 95%.

98. Normal NPTR criteria includes all *except:*

(a) Four to five erectile episodes per night
(b) Mean duration longer than 30 minutes
(c) An increase in circumference of more than 3 cm at the base and more than 2 cm at the tip
(d) Maximal rigidity above 70% at base and 50% at tip

(Answer is D) Normal NPTR criteria: Four to five erectile episodes per night; mean duration longer than 30 minutes; an increase in circumference of more than 3 cm at the base and more than 2 cm at the tip; and maximal rigidity above 70% at both base and tip.

99. To diagnose hypogonadism testosterone levels should be less than:

(a) 200 ng/dl (b) 350 ng/dl
(c) 500 ng/dl (d) 1000 ng/dl

(Answer is B) Morning testosterone values below 350 ng/dl in a young man with chronically elevated gonadotropins make a clear diagnosis of hypogonadism.

100. For measuring testosterone level, blood should be drawn at:

(a) 8:00 AM and 11:00 AM
(b) 11:00 AM and 2:00 PM
(c) 2:00 PM and 5:00 PM
(d) 8:00 PM and 11:00 PM

(Answer is A) Circadian rhythm of testosterone levels should be considered in measuring serum testosterone; blood should be drawn between 8:00AM and 11:00 AM.

101. Absolute contraindication to androgen supplementation is:

(a) Hepatocellular carcinoma
(b) Lung cancer
(c) Breast cancer
(d) Bladder cancer

(Answer is C) The presence of prostate or breast cancer is an absolute contraindication to androgen supplementation.

102. Regarding PDE-5 inhibitor which statement is true?

(a) Increases NO level
(b) Without sexual stimulation and NO release, these inhibitors are ineffective
(c) Side effects include slight increase in BP
(d) Patient with stroke in previous 1 year should be warned for taking PDE-5 inhibitors

(Answer is B) PDE-5 inhibitors do not increase the nitric oxide level, but they potentiate nitric oxide's effect to enhance erection. Side effects includes– headaches, flushing, slight lowering of blood pressure, dyspepsia.

103. Regarding PDE-5 which is not true?

(a) Tadalafil is the only PDE-5 inhibitor with a cardiac conduction precaution
(b) Visual side effects are seen more commonly with sildenafil than with vardenafil and tadalafil
(c) Half life of tadalafil is 18 hours compare to 4 hours of sildenafil and vardenafil
(d) Bachache and myalgia are more common with tadalafil

(Answer is A) Vardenafil is the only PDE-5 inhibitor with a cardiac conduction precaution.

104. ED patients in high risk category includes *except:*

(a) Uncontrolled hypertension
(b) Congestive heart failure (NYHA class III or IV)
(c) Recent myocardial infarction (>2 wk,<6 wk)
(d) Obstructive hypertrophic cardiomyopathy

(Answer is C) High risk group includes Unstable or refractory angina pectoris, Uncontrolled hypertension, Congestive heart failure (NYHA class III or IV), Recent myocardial infarction (<2 wk), High-risk arrhythmia, Obstructive hypertrophic cardiomyopathy and Moderate-to-severe valve disease, particularly aortic stenosis.

105. All *except* one is true about papaverine:

(a) Require refrigeration
(b) Incidence of fibrosis is up to 33%
(c) Incidence of priapism is up to 35%
(d) Elevation of liver enzymes

(Answer is A) The advantages are its low cost and stability at room temperature. The major disadvantages are the incidences of priapism (up to 35%) and corporeal fibrosis (1% to 33%), thought to be a result of low acidity (pH, 3 to 4).

106. Regarding action of papaverine which statement is not true?

(a) Increases cyclic AMP
(b) Increases cyclic GMP
(c) Opens voltage-dependent calcium channels
(d) Impair calcium-activated potassium and chloride currents

(Answer is C) Papaverine, an alkaloid isolated from the opium poppy, exerts an inhibitory effect on POE, leading to increased cyclic AMP and cyclic GMP in penile erectile tissue. Papaverine also blocks voltage-dependent calcium channels, thus impairing calcium influx, and it may also impair calcium-activated potassium and chloride currents.

107. All *except* one is true about alprostadil:

(a) High incidence of painful erection
(b) High incidence of prolonged erection
(c) Low incidence of fibrosis
(d) Require refrigeration

(Answer is B) Its advantages are lower incidences of prolonged erection, systemic side effects, and fibrosis. The disadvantages include a higher incidence of painful erection and higher cost, and, once reconstituted into liquid from powder, it has a shortened half-life if not refrigerated.

108. Only pharmacologic agent with FDA approval for ED management by both intracavernous and intraurethral routes:

(a) Papaverine (b) Phentolamine
(c) Alprostadil (d) Moxisylyte

(Answer is C) Alprostadil, the synthetic formulation of PGE1, is the only pharmacologic agent with FDA approval for ED management by both intracavernous and intraurethral routes.

109. Which statement regarding vacuum constriction device is not true?

(a) Patients taking aspirin should exercise caution when using these devices
(b) To avoid injury, the ring should not be left in place for longer than 30 minutes
(c) The erection produced by a vacuum device is different from a physiologic erection or one produced by intracavernous injection
(d) The device cannot be used successfully by men with a malfunctioning penile prosthesis in place

(Answer is D) The device can be used successfully by men with a malfunctioning penile prosthesis in place.

110. According to DSM-IV-R definition latencies less than how many seconds is consistent with the diagnosis of premature ejaculation?

(a) 15 seconds (b) 30 seconds
(c) 60 seconds (d) 2 minutes

(Answer is A) The DSM-IV-R definition indicates that latencies of 15 seconds or less are consistent with the diagnosis.

111. Which drug exerts the strongest ejaculation delay?

(a) Sertraline (b) Clomipramine
(c) Fluoxetine (d) Paroxetine

(Answer is D) Meta-analysis of drug treatment studies has demonstrated that paroxetine exerts the strongest ejaculation delay.

112. Which one of the following is not a level A recommendation for treatment for premature ejaculation?

(a) SSRI
(b) Topical local anesthetics
(c) PDE-5 inhibitors
(d) All the above are level A recommendation

(Answer is C) Based on the level of evidence rating of the studies reviewed, treatment of PE with PDE-5 inhibitors has a grade C recommendation.

113. First, second and third line therapy for ED is:

(a) PDE inhibitors, intracavernous injection, vacuum constriction device
(b) PDE inhibitors, vacuum constriction device, intracavernous injection
(c) Intracavernous injection, vacuum constriction device, PDE inhibitors
(d) Intracavernous injection, PDE inhibitors, vacuum constriction device

(Answer is B)

First-line therapy	PDE-5 inhibitors
Second-line therapy	VCDs, IUD
Third-line therapy	ICI
Fourth-line therapy	Prosthesis implantation

114. Malleable devices all are true *except:*

(a) High mechanical failure
(b) Easy to use
(c) Constant penile rigidity
(d) Increase risk of erosion

(Answer is A) Malleable devices have the advantage of very low mechanical failure rates and ease of use. Disadvantages include constant penile rigidity and an increased risk of erosion.

115. Which one of the following is not the three piece inflatable penile prosthesis?

(a) AMS Ultrex
(b) AMS Ambicor
(c) AMS 700 CX
(d) AMS 700 CXR

(Answer is B)

Two-piece inflatable	AMS Ambicor
Three-piece inflatable	AMS 700 CX
	AMS 700 CXM
	AMS 700 CXR
	AMS 700 Ultrex

116. Compare to normal penile erection, prosthetic implantation does not provide:

(a) Normal girth expansion
(b) Normal rigidity
(c) Normal length
(d) Normal sensation

(Answer is C) The glans penis is not included in the erection, and for most men the erection is shorter than their normal erection.

117. Advantage of penoscrotal approach over infrapubic approach in penile prosthesis implantation is all *except:*

(a) Better corporeal exposure

(b) No dorsal nerve injury
(c) Pump fixation possible
(d) Reservoir placement under direct vision

(Answer is D)

Comparison of Infrapubic and Penoscrotal Implant Approaches

	Infrapubic approach	*Penoscrotal approach*
Advantages	Reservoir placement under direct vision	Better corporeal exposure No dorsal nerve injury Pump fixation possible
Disadvantages	Limited corporeal exposure Possible dorsal nerve injury Inability to anchor pump	Blind reservoir placement

118. Infections occurring after penile prosthesis implantation in early (in the first few weeks following implantation) and late (6 months to 1 or 2 years after implantation) phase are:

(a) Gram positive in both phases
(b) Gram negative in both phases
(c) Gram positive in early phase and gram negative in late phase
(d) Gram negative in early phase and gram positive in late phase

(Answer is D) Infections occurring after penile prosthesis implantation are either early (in the first few weeks following implantation) or late (6 months to 1 or 2 years after implantation). The former are often associated with gram-negative bacteria, whereas the later are usually associated with gram-positive bacteria such as Staphylococcus epidermidis.

119. When should penile prosthesis reimplantation be done after device removal for infection?

(a) Immediately after incisions have healed and postoperative edema has resolved
(b) After 2-3 months
(c) After 6-9 months
(d) Should not be ever done

(Answer is A) To minimize loss of penile size and to facilitate corporeal dilation, prosthesis reimplantation is performed as soon as possible after device removal for infection. When all incisions have healed and postoperative edema has resolved (usually 2 to 3 months after device removal), reimplantation is advised.

120. Which group of antibiotics decreases penile prosthesis infection rate?

(a) Vancomycin, gentamycin, cefuroxime
(b) Rifampin, minocycline, polyvinyl-pyrrolidone
(c) Rifampin, gentamycin, vancomycin
(d) Gentamycin, cefuroxime, PVP

(Answer is B) Rifampin, minocycline, polyvinyl-pyrrolidone (PVP), reduces the infection rate.

121. If urethral perforation occurs, the implant procedure should be:

(a) Urethra repaired and implantation procedure continued
(b) Abandon implant, urethra repaired and suprapubic catheter placed and implantation done after 10 days
(c) Abandon implant, urethral catheter should be left in for 7 to 10 days
(d) Abandon implant, urethra repaired and perurethral catheter placed and implantation done after 10 days

(Answer is C) If urethral perforation occurs, the implant procedure should be abandoned and a urethral catheter should be left in for 7 to 10 days.

122. In the case of erosion of one cylinder of an inflatable device:

(a) Remove the infected cylinder only
(b) Remove the infected cylinder and replace it with new cylinder
(c) Remove the whole prosthesis
(d) Repair the eroded area of cylinder

(Answer is A) In the case of erosion of one cylinder of an inflatable device into the meatus or through the glans, this cylinder should be removed as soon as possible to avoid spread of bacteria along the cylinder to its tubing and thus to the rest of the prosthesis. Many men are able to have coitus with only one inflatable cylinder; thus, a later procedure to reimplant the second cylinder is not always necessary.

123. Best candidate for penile revascularization procedures is:

(a) Fifty-year-old men with long standing DM
(b) Twenty-five-year old men with generalized arterial disease
(c) Thirty-year-old men with pelvic fracture
(d) Twenty-year-old men with Peyronie's plaques

(Answer is C) Those patients with discrete focal arterial lesions found on selective pudendal arteriography, particularly younger patients who have a history of trauma (pelvic fracture or perineal blunt trauma), who do not have diabetes or neurologic disease and who are not currently users of tobacco, are the best candidates for penile revascularization procedures.

124. Study necessary to demonstrate the adequacy of the proposed donor artery and for planning the exact nature of the surgery is:

(a) CDUS (b) DICC
(c) Arteriogram (d) MRI

(Answer is C) A common iliac arteriogram and a selective internal pudendal arteriogram are necessary to demonstrate the adequacy of the proposed donor artery. The selective internal pudendal study also is necessary for planning the exact nature of the surgery.

125. Which statement regarding penile revascularization is not correct?

(a) The most common donor artery for penile revascularization is the inferior epigastric artery
(b) Complications of penile vascular surgery are penile numbness and hypoesthesia
(c) Veno-occlusive surgery should be considered in a patient who complaint of short-duration erections only with sexual stimulation
(d) Late results of penile veno-occlusive surgery are much better than early results

(Answer is D) Early results of penile veno-occlusive surgery are much better than long-term results after 2 years.

126. Alternative donor vessel for penile revascularization apart from inferior epigastric artery is:

(a) Superior epigastric artery
(b) Saphenous vein
(c) Deep dorsal vein
(d) Dorsal artery

(Answer is B) Alternative donor vessel for the inferior epigastric artery is the reverse saphenous vein graft.

127. All statements regarding Peyronie's disease are correct *except:*

(a) Thirty to 40% of men with Peyronie's disease will also have Dupuytren's contracture
(b) In most patients, reassurance is sufficient
(c) Most patients with Peyronie's disease demonstrate lesions ventrally
(d) Most likely begins with buckling trauma that causes injury to the septal insertion of the tunica albuginea

(Answer is C) Most patients with Peyronie's disease demonstrate lesions dorsally. Because the tunica albuginea is bilaminar on the dorsum, it is possible that these layers might delaminate with buckling trauma.

128. Which investigation has least role in evaluation of Peyronie's disease?

(a) Plain radiography (b) USG
(c) CT (d) MRI

(Answer is C) Computed tomographic scanning has no place in the examination of the penis. However, magnetic resonance imaging (MRI), which does not effectively demonstrate plaque calcification, does image the plaque well.

129. Which is not tried for the treatment of Peyronie's disease?

(a) Vitamin D (b) Interferon alfa-2b
(c) Colchicine (d) Verapamil

(Answer is A) Vitamin E and not Vitamin D is tried for Peyronie.

130. Only indication of surgery in Peyronie's disease is:

(a) Penile pain
(b) Erectile dysfunction that precludes intercourse
(c) Shortening of penis
(d) Penile deformity

(Answer is B) Most investigators consider curvature or erectile dysfunction that precludes intercourse the indication for surgery.

131. Interval after which definite erectile tissue functional damage occurs in ischemic priapism is?

(a) 2 hours (b) 4 hours
(c) 6 hours (d) 8 hours

(Answer is B) 4-hour duration of ischemic priapism is relevant as an interval after which definite erectile tissue functional damage occurs.

132. Nonischemic priapism, all statements are true *except:*

(a) Also termed as venous or low-flow priapism
(b) Penile or perineal trauma is most frequently associated
(c) The corpora cavernosa are not usually fully rigid or painful
(d) Cavernous blood gas values do not reveal hypoxia or acidosis

(Answer is A) Nonischemic priapism, also termed arterial or high-flow priapism, features elevated vascular flow through the corpora cavernosa.

133. Recurrent priapism can be observed in:

(a) Leukemia
(b) Sickle cell anemia
(c) Penile trauma
(d) Heavy alcohol intake

(Answer is B) Frequent recurrent episodes of priapism is observed in sickle cell patients.

134. Which one is the first line treatment for ischemic priapism?

(a) Aspiration of blood
(b) Proximal shunt
(c) Distal shunt
(d) Observation

(Answer is A) Definitive first-line treatment consists of evacuation of blood and irrigation of the corpora cavernosa along with intracavernous injection of an α-adrenergic sympathomimetic agent.

135. Which is the most effective shunt procedure for priapism?

(a) Winter shunt (b) EI-Ghorab shunt
(c) Quackels (d) Grayhack shunt

(Answer is B) The EI-Ghorab procedure is regarded as the most effective distal shunt, although it is more invasive and thus commonly performed secondarily.

136. Anastomosis of the saphenous vein to one of the corpora cavernosa is named as:

(a) Winter shunt (b) EI-Ghorab shunt
(c) Quackels (d) Grayhack shunt

(Answer is D) Anastomosis of the saphenous vein to one of the corpora cavernosa (Grayhack shunt).

137. Which one is the initial management for non-ischemic priapism?

(a) Aspiration of blood
(b) Proximal shunt
(c) Distal shunt
(d) Observation

(Answer is D) The initial management of nonischemic priapism should be observation. The recommendation is based on the finding that spontaneous resolution is the outcome of untreated nonischemic priapism in up to 62% of reported cases.

138. Episodes of recurrent priapism can be readily treated by all *except:*

(a) Baclofen (b) Digoxin
(c) Terbutaline (d) Alprostadil

(Answer is D) Systemic therapies including hormonal agents–baclofen, digoxin and terbutaline have been proposed, the most consistently successful treatment and is supported as a primary recommendation.

139. Which in the following is the diagnosis of high-flow priapism and localization of a ruptured artery?

(a) CIS and blood flow measurement by duplex ultrasound
(b) Dynamic infusion cavernosometry and cavernosography (DICC)
(c) CT angiography
(d) MRI

(Answer is A) CIS and blood flow measurement by duplex ultrasound are best tool available for the diagnosis of high-flow priapism and localization of a ruptured artery.

140. All the following decrease with aging *except:*

(a) Hematocrit (b) Muscle mass
(c) Bone mass (d) Fat mass

(Answer is D) Muscle mass and bone mass decreases with age while fat mass increases with age.

141. With testosterone therapy which factor does not increase?

(a) Sexual desire (b) Hematocrit
(c) Bone mass (d) Fat mass

(Answer is D) With testosterone fat mass decreases and bone mass and muscle mass increases.

142. In patients at risk for or suspected of having hypogonadism, if T levels are below or at the lower limit of the accepted normal values, next step is:

(a) Confirm with a second determination together with assessment of LH and FSH
(b) Confirm with a second determination together with assessment of LH and prolactin
(c) Assess LH and FSH
(d) Assess LH and prolactin

(Answer is B) In patients at risk for or suspected of having hypogonadism, if T levels are below or at the lower limit of the accepted normal values, it is prudent to confirm the results with a second determination together with assessment of gonadotropins (LH) and prolactin.

143. Contraindication of testosterone therapy are all *except:*

(a) Prostate cancer
(b) Breast cancer
(c) Hepatocellular cancer
(d) Polycythemia

(Answer is C) The presence of prostate or breast carcinoma is an absolute contraindication for T treatment. T therapy in older men can often result in a significant increase in red blood cell mass and hemoglobin levels. This may lead to termination of therapy, a decrease of dose, or a switch to a different formulation of T.

144. Which is not true regarding MUSE?

(a) This technique relies on the absorption of medication through the mucosal lining into the surrounding corpus spongiosum
(b) Synthetic formulation of prostaglandin E1
(c) Responder rate is approximately 50%
(d) Most common side effects is minor urethral bleeding

(Answer is D) The most common side effects include local urogenital pain (approximately one third of patients) and minor urethral bleeding (5%).

145. Which of the following hormones, primarily, controls spermatogenesis?

(a) GnRH (b) Testosterone
(c) LH (d) FSH

(Answer is B) Testosterone

146. How many days does spermatogenesis take in the man?

(a) 16 (b) 32
(c) 64 (d) 90

(Answer is C) 64

147. In which organelle in Leydig cell does testosterone synthesis take place?

(a) Ribosome
(b) Mitochondria
(c) Golgi apparatus
(d) Endoplasmic reticulum

(Answer is D) Endoplasmic reticulum

148. Which part of the prostate prevents the seminal fluid from entering the bladder during ejaculation?

(a) Central zone
(b) Peripheral zone
(c) Preprostatic tissue
(d) Anterior fibromuscular stroma

(Answer is C) Preprostatic tissue

149. Which lab results indicate poor prognosis of male infertility?

(a) Azoospermia; normal FSH; increase LH
(b) Azoospermia; decrease FSH; normal LH
(c) Oligospermia; increase FSH; normal LH
(d) Oligospermia; normal FSH; decrease LH

(Answer is C) Oligospermia; increase FSH; normal LH

150. Which of the following explains infertility in liver cirrhosis male patients?

(a) Decrease plasma estradiol levels
(b) Increase plasma testosterone-estradiol-binding globulin levels
(c) Suppression of suprarenal androgens
(d) Exaggerated pituitary response to feedback hormones

(Answer is B) Increase plasma testosterone-estradiol-binding globulin levels

151. Which of the following diabetes mellitus treatments causes erectile dysfunction?

(a) Long-acting insulin (b) Metformin
(c) Sulfonylurea (d) None of the above

(Answer is D) None of the above

152. Which class of the following diuretics could cause erectile dysfunction?

(a) Loop diuretics
(b) Thiazide diuretics
(c) Potassium sparing diuretics
(d) Osmotic diuretics

(Answer is B) Thiazide diuretics

153. What is the most likely diagnosis of an erectile dysfunction patient with low plasma testosterone and high prolactin levels?

(a) Pituitary adenoma
(b) Adrenal adenoma
(c) Kallmann syndrome
(d) Klinefelter syndrome

(Answer is A) Pituitary adenoma

154. Which statement is false concerning capacitation of spermatozoa?

(a) Occurs after acrosome reaction
(b) Entails removal of a glycoprotein layer
(c) It is a biochemical event of sperm maturation
(d) Changes occur in the female genital tract

(Answer is A) Occurs after acrosome reaction

155. All of the following conditions are related to obesity syndrome, *except*:

(a) Super fertility
(b) Increase aromatization reaction
(c) Increase resistance to circulating insulin
(d) Sleep apnea

(Answer is A) Super fertility

156. Which statement is false concerning smegma?

(a) It is the white secretion produced under the foreskin in males
(b) It has a crucial role in penile cancer development
(c) It contains lysozymes, chymotrypsin, neutrophil elastase and cytokines
(d) Female smegma can be found between the labia

(Answer is B) It has a crucial role in penile cancer development

157. Which organ contributes most to the seminal fluid volume?

(a) Testes
(b) Prostate
(c) Seminal vesicles
(d) Bulbourethral glands

(Answer is C) Seminal vesicles

158. Which of the following is NOT a component of the normal semen?

(a) Zinc
(b) Fructose
(c) Prostate-specific antigen
(d) Alkaline phosphatase

(Answer is D) Alkaline phosphatase

159. Which statement is NOT related to Klinefelter syndrome?

(a) Sterility is the rule
(b) Has a considerable short life span
(c) Treatment requires testicular microdissection and sperm extraction
(d) 47 XXY karyotype

(Answer is B) Has a considerable short life span

160. How does estrogen prevent lower UTI in postmenopausal women?

(a) Increasing vaginal secretions
(b) Decreasing vaginal pH
(c) Increasing normal vaginal flora
(d) Decreasing bacterial adherence

(Answer is B) Decreasing vaginal pH

161. Where is the centre of "reflex erection" located at?

(a) The brain cortex
(b) The sacral cord
(c) The lumbar cord
(d) The hypothalamus

(Answer is B) The sacral cord

162. Which hormone measures testicular germ cell function best?

(a) LH
(b) FSH
(c) HCG
(d) None of the above

(Answer is B) FSH

163. What is the earliest clinical sign of puberty in boys?

(a) Hoarseness of voice

(b) Enlargement of testes
(c) Appearance of axillary hair
(d) Change in body odor

(Answer is B) Enlargement of testes

164. What causes pure testicular feminization is:

(a) Over estrogen synthesis
(b) Defective end-organ androgen response
(c) Extra X chromosome (XXY)
(d) Failure of genital ridge regression

(Answer is B) Defective end-organ androgen response

165. Which class of the following agents does not impair spermatogenesis?

(a) Alkylating agents (b) Phenothiazines
(c) Antiandrogens (d) Prostaglandins

(Answer is B) Phenothiazines

166. What is true regarding hematospermia?

(a) Should be investigated thoroughly like hematuria
(b) Is rarely associated with significant urologic pathology
(c) Carries a risk of infertility
(d) Mandates testicular biopsy

(Answer is B) Is rarely associated with significant urologic pathology

167. The majority of circulating testosterone is:

(a) Bound to sex hormone-binding globulin
(b) Free
(c) Bound to α1-antichymotrypsin
(d) Bound to albumin

(Answer is A) Bound to sex hormone-binding globulin

168. Serum testosterone should be measured:

(a) At mid-day
(b) At the hour of sleep
(c) In the morning
(d) Late afternoon

(Answer is C) In the morning

169. How long post bilateral orchiectomy, will patients be functionally castrated?

(a) Immediately (b) After 2 hours
(c) After 12 hours (d) After 24 hours

(Answer is B) After 2 hours

170. What degrades semenogelin and determines the consistency of the seminal coagulum is:

(a) Spermine
(b) Acid phosphatase
(c) PSA
(d) Semenoglobulin

(Answer is D) Semenoglobulin

171. Which of the following contributes second to the seminal fluid by volume?

(a) Seminal vesicles
(b) The prostate
(c) Testes
(d) Bulbourethral glands

(Answer is B) The prostate

172. In which of the following conditions testosterone supplementation is not indicated?

(a) Delayed puberty
(b) Idiopathic infertility
(c) Symptomatic hypogonadism
(d) Testicular dysgenesis

(Answer is B) Idiopathic infertility

173. Which statement is false concerning testosterone deficiency in older men?

(a) Age advances, free testosterone declines more than total testosterone does
(b) Sex hormone-binding globulin increases gradually with age
(c) The diurnal rhythm of serum testosterone fluctuates sharply with age and manifests as changes in mood and cognitive function

(d) Consensus on testosterone replacement in this group of patients

(Answer is C) The diurnal rhythm of serum testosterone fluctuates sharply with age and manifests as changes in mood and cognitive function

174. What could not result of testosterone administration to men with late-onset hypogonadism?

(a) Decrease in fat-free mass and increase in fat mass
(b) Increase in lean muscle mass and decrease in BMI and waist size
(c) Improvement in sexual function in men with low libido
(d) Improvement in glycaemic control and lipid profile

(Answer is A) Decrease in fat-free mass and increase in fat mass

175. What is (are) the clinical manifestation(s) suggestive of androgen deficiency in older men?

(a) Changes in mood, fatigue and anger
(b) Sleep disturbances
(c) Decreased body hair
(d) All of the above

(Answer is D) All of the above

176. All of the following are clinical manifestations of androgen deficiency in middle-age men, *except*:

(a) Erectile dysfunction
(b) Gynecomastia
(c) Insulin deficiency
(d) Visceral obesity

(Answer is C) Insulin deficiency

177. All of the following manifestations suggest prepubertal-onset hypogonadism, *except*:

(a) Sarcopenia
(b) Short stature
(c) Unclosed epiphyses
(d) High-pitched voice

(Answer is B) Short stature

178. The followings are indications for testosterone treatment, *except*:

(a) Hypopituitarism
(b) Sexual dysfunction and low testosterone in a 40 years old man
(c) Asymptomatic 65 years old man with significantly low total and free testosterone
(d) Low bone mass in a hypogonad man aging 35 years

(Answer is C) Asymptomatic 65 years old man with significantly low total and free testosterone

179. Which of the following is (are) contraindication(s) for testosterone treatment?

(a) Haematocrit > 0.54%
(b) Severe obstructive sleep apnoea
(c) Infertile man wishing to have children
(d) All of the above

(Answer is D) All of the above

180. In a 55 years man newly started on testosterone replacement therapy, which of the following timely changes are false?

(a) Improvement in erectile function and ejaculation may require up to 6 months
(b) Sexual interest may improve after 3 weeks of treatment, and reach a plateau in 6 weeks
(c) Erythropoiesis may become evident at 2 months and peaks at 4 months
(d) Mild increase in PSA and prostate volume, plateauing at 12 months

(Answer is C) Erythropoiesis may become evident at 2 months and peaks at 4 months

181. Which of the following urologic conditions is (are) related to metabolic syndrome?

(a) Nephrolithiasis
(b) Prostate cancer
(c) Erectile dysfunction
(d) All of the above

(Answer is D) All of the above

182. Which of the following is false concerning abdominal adiposity and urologic conditions?

(a) Obesity is associated with an increased risk of liposarcoma of the bladder
(b) Obese women, weight loss may improve stress urinary incontinence
(c) Obesity is associated with an increased risk of prostate enlargement
(d) Obese men, weight loss significantly improves erectile function

(Answer is A) Obesity is associated with an increased risk of liposarcoma of the bladder

183. Which of the following is true regarding obesity and urologic conditions?

(a) Obesity has been linked to an increased risk of subfertility in males
(b) Losing weight has not been hypothesized to explain floating kidneys
(c) Weight loss may improve urge incontinence in obese women
(d) Boys, weight loss gives a false impression of micropenis

(Answer is A) Obesity has been linked to an increased risk of subfertility in males

184. Metabolism of serum testosterone occurs in all of the following body tissues, *except*:

(a) The liver
(b) The kidneys
(c) The prostate
(d) The skin

(Answer is B) The kidneys

185. As men age, which of the following hormones increase?

(a) Dehydroepiandrosterone
(b) Melatonin
(c) Thyroxin
(d) Leptin

(Answer is D) Leptin

186. Which of the following is an absolute contra-indication for testosterone replacement therapy?

(a) The presence of prostate or breast cancer
(b) Hematocrit > 0.55%
(c) Severe LUTS due to BPH
(d) Obstructive sleep apnoea

(Answer is A) The presence of prostate or breast cancer

187. Which of the following ailments is (are) linked with erectile dysfunction?

(a) Smoking
(b) Insulin resistance
(c) Hypertension
(d) All of the above

(Answer is D) All of the above

188. What does not take place during full erection?

(a) Increased blood flow into the corpora cavernosa and glans
(b) Accommodating the incoming blood by relaxation of sinusoidal smooth muscles
(c) Contraction of the ischiocavernosus muscles reduces the venous outflow
(d) Increase in intracavernous pressure and PO_2

(Answer is C) Contraction of the ischiocavernosus muscles reduces the venous outflow

189. Which of the following statements is false regarding the role of nitrous oxide (NO) in erection?

(a) Is the chief mediator of penile erection
(b) Stimulates the production of cGMP

(c) NO released from eNOS contributes to the cessation of erection
(d) NO released from nNOS contributes to the initiation of erection

(Answer is C) NO released from eNOS contributes to the cessation of erection

190. Regarding physiologic erection, "Latch state" refers to:

(a) A period of smooth muscle relaxation after prolonged contraction
(b) A state of skeletal rigidity when the intracorporal pressure exceeds the systolic
(c) The period between latching emissary veins till detumescence
(d) The state when no more blood can enter the corpora nor it can leak out

(Answer is A) A period of smooth muscle relaxation after prolonged contraction

191. All of the following statements regarding erectile dysfunction (ED) are true, *except*:

(a) Primary ED refers to a lifelong dysfunction of unknown etiology
(b) Primary psychological ED is usually related to personality traits
(c) Psychological ED is the most common form of ED for men under 40
(d) Aging is the single most important factor to ED

(Answer is B) Primary psychological ED is usually related to personality traits

192. At the flaccid state, the penis has the following criterion:

(a) The penile venous plexus is contracted
(b) The trabecular smooth muscles are relaxed
(c) Venous leak is evident
(d) Cavernosal spaces are widened

(Answer is C) Venous leak is evident

193. What causes the intracorporal smooth muscles to contract at the flaccid state?

(a) Intrinsic myogenic activity
(b) Adrenergic neurotransmission
(c) Endothelium-derived contracting factors
(d) All of the above

(Answer is D) All of the above

194. What neural transmitter controls detumescence?

(a) Dopamine (b) Norepinephrine
(c) Serotonin (d) Acetylcholine

(Answer is B) Norepinephrine

195. In what percentage of patients do LH-RH agonists result in a reduction of sexual desire?

(a) 10% (b) 30%
(c) 50% (d) 70%

(Answer is D) 70%

196. Sexual dysfunction is expected after:

(a) Intracorporal injection of epinephrine
(b) The induction of antiretroviral therapy
(c) Ablating urethral tumors at the membranous level
(d) Correction surgery of penile fracture

(Answer is B) The induction of antiretroviral therapy

197. What is true regarding erectile dysfunction after renal transplantation?

(a) About half of the patients continue to have ED
(b) The vast majority of patients will end up having ED
(c) The operation will help improve ED symptoms in > 65% of cases
(d) None of the above

(Answer is A) About half of the patients continue to have ED

198. Endothelial dysfunction could explain ED in patients with:

(a) Hyperlipidemia
(b) Diabetes mellitus
(c) Chronic renal failure-related hypertension
(d) All of the above

(Answer is D) All of the above

199. In males, testosterone does not:

(a) Boosts sexual desire
(b) Increases the frequency of sexual attempts
(c) Increases the number of nocturnal erections per night
(d) Augments the visually erotic stimuli

(Answer is D) Augments the visually erotic stimuli

200. Risk factors for erectile dysfunction do not include:

(a) Passive cigarette smoking
(b) Stroke
(c) Penile fracture
(d) Priapism

(Answer is C) Penile fracture

201. In contrast to psychological ED, organic ED is characterized by the following:

(a) Abrupt onset
(b) Stable symptoms
(c) Normal nocturnal erection
(d) Favorable response to PDE inhibitors

(Answer is D) Favorable response to PDE inhibitors

202. What is false concerning the IIEF-5 questionnaire (SHIM) for ED?

(a) 5 questions with 5 scores in each
(b) A sum of 7 indicates mild ED requiring no treatment
(c) Questions the patient over the past 6 months
(d) Covers the aspects of erection initiation, maintenance and satisfaction

(Answer is B) A sum of 7 indicates mild ED requiring no treatment

203. What is false concerning erectile dysfunction questionnaires?

(a) Are self-administered
(b) Enquire patient's complaints as well as patient's satisfaction
(c) Help follow-up patients on treatment including those with penile implants
(d) Are subjectively reliable

(Answer is C) Help follow-up patients on treatment including those with penile implants

204. What is the most compelling pre op. test for a 55 years ED patient going for penile arterial revascularization?

(a) Penile angiography
(b) Penile duplex ultrasonography combined with pharmaco-stimulation
(c) Dynamic infusion cavernosometry and cavernosography
(d) All are comparable

(Answer is A) Penile angiography

205. Self-administered intracavernosal pharmacotherapy for ED is indicated most for patients with:

(a) History of priapism
(b) Poor manual dexterity
(c) Severe coagulopathy
(d) Arteriogenic ED

(Answer is D) Arteriogenic ED

206. Endocrine conditions that may be associated with erectile dysfunction include all of the following, *except*:

(a) Hypogonadism
(b) Pheochromocytoma
(c) Hyperthyroidism
(d) Diabetes mellitus

(Answer is B) Pheochromocytoma

207. What is the likelihood that a man with cavernous arterial peak systolic velocity of ≥ 40 cm/sec presents with arteriogenic ED?

(a) Never
(b) Unlikely
(c) Likely
(d) Always

(Answer is A) Never

208. Fill the space, "men with ED are 45% more likely than controls to suffer from a cardiac event within ... of ED diagnosis".

(a) 3 months (b) 5 months
(c) 3 years (d) 5 years

(Answer is D) 5 years

209. What is the absolute contraindication for using PDE-5 inhibitors?

(a) Uncontrolled hypertension
(b) Concomitant use of nitrate
(c) Uncontrolled coagulopathy
(d) Concomitant use of intracavernosal vasodilators

(Answer is B) Concomitant use of nitrate

210. Which of the following conditions is associated with high-flow priapism?

(a) Sickle cell disease
(b) Falling astride on a ladder
(c) The presence of metastasizing tumor thrombus
(d) Using pharmacologic erection therapy

(Answer is B) Falling astride on a ladder

211. Which of the following is not associated with low-flow priapism?

(a) Chronic hemolysis
(b) Vascular occlusion
(c) Coital trauma to the penis
(d) Tissue ischemia

(Answer is C) Coital trauma to the penis

212. What is the most common cause of priapism in men over 50?

(a) Sickle cell disease
(b) Falling astride on a ladder
(c) Metastasizing tumor thrombus
(d) Pharmacologic erection therapy

(Answer is D) Pharmacologic erection therapy

213. Which of the following mechanisms best explain the development of high-flow priapism?

(a) Traumatic force could result in a laceration of the cavernous artery within the corpora cavernosa
(b) Penile injury, especially penetrating, could result in an iatrogenic arterial-venous shunt
(c) Traumatic injury to emissary veins by the needle of intracavernosal pharmacotherapy could impair the cavernosal outflow
(d) Blunt trauma to the penis could ruin the sinusoidal ability to contract

(Answer is A) Traumatic force could result in a laceration of the cavernous artery within the corpora cavernosa

214. What is false concerning low-flow priapism?

(a) There is decreased or absent cavernosal artery inflow
(b) Aspirated cavernosal blood is dark, anoxic, acidotic and hypercarbic
(c) Penile arteriography helps differentiate low from high-flow type
(d) Pain is related to soft tissue ischemia

(Answer is C) Penile arteriography helps differentiate low from high-flow type

215. What is the duration of an ischemic episode of priapism, after which spontaneous erection has not been reported?

(a) 6 hours (b) 12 hours
(c) 24 hours (d) 36 hours

(Answer is D) 36 hours

216. Which surgical procedure is indicated to treat low-flow priapism?

(a) Angio-embolization
(b) Percutaneous distal penile shunt
(c) Arterial revascularization
(d) Surgical ligation

(Answer is B) Percutaneous distal penile shunt

217. What is false concerning priapism?

(a) Low-flow type causes harder erection than high-flow does
(b) The majority of low-flow type is of unknown etiology
(c) High-flow type causes no pain
(d) Stuttering priapism is recurrent painful erections that occurs usually with sickle cell disease

(Answer is C) High-flow type causes no pain

218. What is true concerning high-flow priapism?

(a) Blood aspirate is dark red
(b) Treated by selective embolization of the feeding artery
(c) Corporal blood gas shows pH < 7.25, $PO_2 < 30$, $PCO_2 > 60$
(d) 60% of cases are idiopathic

(Answer is B) Treated by selective embolization of the feeding artery

219. What is false concerning stuttering priapism?

(a) Erection resolution could occur spontaneously or after aspiration and phenylephrine injection
(b) Commoner in sicklers
(c) Treatment entails monthly injection of LH-RH antagonist
(d) Could respond to self-administered intracorporal injection of sympathomimetic amine

(Answer is C) Treatment entails monthly injection of LH-RH antagonist

220. What is false regarding priapism treatment?

(a) Sicklers presenting with ischemic priapism can be treated by packed RBC transfusion or exchange transfusion
(b) An emergency measure, using tru-cut needle to create a glans-cavernous shunt helps relieve painful erection
(c) Emergency management of painful, hard priapism is intracorporal injection of phenylephrine in a dose of 3-5 ml of (1 ml of 10 mg in 100 of saline), exchange and repeat every 10 min
(d) Cavernosa-saphenous end-to-side anastomosis adequately treats stuttering type

(Answer is D) Cavernosa-saphenous end-to-side anastomosis adequately treats stuttering type

221. All of the following statements about priapism are true, *except*:

(a) High-flow and stuttering priapism are the result of nitrous oxide imbalance
(b) Spontaneous resolution of high-flow priapism occurs in 2/3 of cases
(c) Ischemic priapism, aspiration alone will be curative in 1/3 of cases
(d) Phenylephrine, 200 µg/ml given in 0.5 ml aliquots, not exceeding a total dose of 1 mg, is used to treat ischemic priapism

(Answer is A) High-flow and stuttering priapism are the result of nitrous oxide imbalance

222. Which of the following neurotransmitters has a facilitatory role in the seminal ejaculation process?

(a) GABA
(b) Dopamine
(c) Serotonin
(d) Acetylcholine

(Answer is B) Dopamine

223. What is false concerning seminal ejaculation?

(a) Involves pulsatile contractions of the bulbocavernosus and pelvic floor muscles
(b) Involves relaxation of the internal urinary sphincter
(c) Mediated by sympathetic spinal cord reflexes and somatic nerves S_2 - S_4
(d) Has a restricted voluntary control

(Answer is B) Involves relaxation of the internal urinary sphincter

224. What is false concerning seminal emission?

(a) Involves expulsion of the seminal fluid into the posterior urethra
(b) Involves contractions of seminal vesicles and the prostate
(c) Mediated by androgens and sympathetic nerves T_{10} - L_2
(d) Followed by the feeling of tension relief

(Answer is D) Followed by the feeling of tension relief

225. All of the following etiologies explain the occurrence of life-long premature ejaculation, *except:*

(a) Hyposensitivity of the 5-HT_2C and/or hypersensitivity of the 5-HT_1A receptor
(b) Hyperthyroidism and practicing masturbation in profusion
(c) Nonspecific neurobiologic and genetic variations
(d) Undefined psychological and environmental factors

(Answer is B) Hyperthyroidism and practicing masturbation in profusion

226. Which of the following does not cause delayed ejaculation?

(a) Hyperthyroidism
(b) Psychological factors
(c) Degeneration of penile afferent nerves
(d) Treatment with SSRIs

(Answer is A) Hyperthyroidism

227. What could not cause retrograde ejaculation?

(a) Treatment with pseudoephedrine
(b) Treatment with tamsulosin
(c) TUIP
(d) Long standing DM

(Answer is A) Treatment with pseudoephedrine

228. What is false concerning premature ejaculation (PE)?

(a) Delayed ejaculation commonly alternates with PE
(b) Treatment includes topical anesthetics, SSRI and tramadol
(c) The acquired type could be due to prostatitis or hyperthyroidism
(d) The prevalence is 4 - 40% in men's population

(Answer is A) Delayed ejaculation commonly alternates with PE

229. How common is the association between psychological disturbances and ejaculation disorders?

(a) Uncommon
(b) Not uncommon
(c) Common
(d) Exceedingly common

(Answer is D) Exceedingly common

230. Positioning the penis upright after malleable prosthesis implantation surgery helps:

(a) Reduce the risk of infection
(b) Lessen edema and pain
(c) Expedite wound healing
(d) Avoid sutures disruption

(Answer is B) Lessen edema and pain

231. What is the preferred space for placing the reservoir of inflatable penile prosthesis?

(a) The scrotum
(b) The retropubic space
(c) The suprapubic space
(d) Caudal to the umbilicus

(Answer is B) The retropubic space

232. What is the treatment of infected inflatable penile prosthesis?

(a) High dose, culture-based IV antibiotic
(b) Removing the infected part
(c) Removing all prosthetic parts
(d) Exchanging the infected part

(Answer is C) Removing all prosthetic parts

233. How to manage the failure of one cylinder of inflatable penile prosthesis?

(a) Changing the failed cylinder
(b) Removing the failed cylinder
(c) Removing the entire prosthetic parts
(d) Reassurance

(Answer is D) Reassurance

234. Which ED medication acts on both D_1 and D_2-like receptors?

(a) Alprostadil, urethral suppository
(b) Apomorphine, sublingual
(c) Sildenafil, swallowable
(d) Papaverine intracorporal injection

(Answer is B) Apomorphine, sublingual

235. Regarding female sexual health, which statement is false?

(a) Similar to males, female sexual health requires physical, emotional and mental well-being
(b) Urinary incontinence has a negative impact on sexual arousal
(c) Estrogen, progesterone and testosterone levels decline sharply after menopause
(d) Hormonal contraception decreases bioavailable testosterone

(Answer is C) Estrogen, progesterone and testosterone levels decline sharply after menopause

236. Which statement is false concerning erectile dysfunction?

(a) The cardiovascular risk of sexual activity can be estimated from patient's level of exercise tolerance
(b) Lifestyle modifications like regular exercising and optimizing body fitness can improve erectile function
(c) Has been found in 15 - 25% of men post radical prostatectomy
(d) Shares common risk factors with ischemic heart disease

(Answer is C) Has been found in 15 - 25% of men post radical prostatectomy

237. What is false concerning avanafil?

(a) Administered around 15 - 30 minutes before sexual activity
(b) Its dosage is adapted according to efficacy and tolerability
(c) Its efficacy has been shown in difficult-to-treat cases like diabetics
(d) Can be taken with or without food

(Answer is C) Its efficacy has been shown in difficult-to-treat cases like diabetics

238. What is true regarding the half-life of PDE5Is?

(a) For sildenafil and vardenafil is about 4 hours
(b) For tadalafil is 17 – 36 hours
(c) For avanafil is 6 – 17 hours
(d) All of the above

(Answer is D) All of the above

239. Which of the following PDE5Is can be taken safely with organic nitrate?

(a) Vardenafil (b) Tadalafil
(c) Avanafil (d) None of the above

(Answer is D) None of the above

240. What is false concerning PDE5Is non-respondents?

(a) Most commonly due to waiting too long after taking the medication, before attempting sex
(b) Could be a result of incorrect drug dosing
(c) Using PDE5Is without sexual stimulation leads to "no-response"
(d) The management of non-respondents relies largely on the underlying cause

(Answer is A) Most commonly due to waiting too long after taking the medication, before attempting sex

241. All of the following are intracavernosal injection therapy for ED, *except*:

(a) Alprostadil (b) Phenylephrine
(c) Phentolamine (d) Papaverine

(Answer is B) Phenylephrine

242. Which of the following impair(s) erectile function least?

(a) The anti-triglyceride fenofibrate
(b) The antipsychotic risperidone
(c) Testosterone and anabolic steroids
(d) The anti-diabetes metformin

(Answer is D) The anti-diabetes metformin

243. Studying an ED case includes the following, *except*:

(a) Intracorporal injection of prostaglandin E_1
(b) Intracorporal aspiration for analysis
(c) Biothesiometry
(d) Nocturnal penile tumescence (rigidity scanner)

(Answer is B) Intracorporal aspiration for analysis

244. What is the least blood test recommended to investigate a 52 years obese man who has diabetes type II and complains of erectile dysfunction?

(a) Cholesterol (b) TSH
(c) Hb A_1C (d) Testosterone

(Answer is B) TSH

245. The proposed mechanism for treating ED patients with penile low-intensity shock wave therapy is:

(a) Neovascularization
(b) Accelerating blood inflow
(c) Breaking down atheromatous plaques
(d) Anti-fibrosis

(Answer is A) Neovascularization

246. What is the single most commonly used agent for intracavernosal injection to treat ED?

(a) Verapamil (b) Papaverine
(c) Alprostadil (d) Phentolamine

(Answer is C) Alprostadil

247. The most common drawback of intraurethral prostaglandin E_1 pellets is:

(a) Pellet expulsion (b) Pellet migration
(c) Prolonged erection (d) Urethral burning

(Answer is D) Urethral burning

248. Nocturnal erections are explained as a result of:

(a) Sexual fantasy during sleep
(b) Reflex response to a full bladder
(c) The physiology of rapid eye movement phase of sleep
(d) Uninhibited reflexes triggered by tactile stimuli to the penis by the underwear

(Answer is C) The physiology of rapid eye movement phase of sleep

249. Erection in spinal cord injury patients is explained as:

(a) Reflexogenic erection activated by tactile stimuli to the genital area mediated through a reflex arc at S_2 to S_4 levels

(b) Psychogenic erections are activated by neural impulses originating from the external genitalia and mediated by spinal cord neural centre located at T_{11} to L_2 levels

(c) Primarily a vascular phenomenon, activated by neurologic signals from anywhere below the injury level and expedited in the appropriate hormonal milieu and erotic atmosphere

(d) Basically a hormonal response triggered by visual sexual stimuli in the presence of adequate serum testosterone along with enhanced libido and fantastic mindset

(Answer is A) Reflexogenic erection activated by tactile stimuli to the genital area mediated through a reflex arc at S_2 to S_4 levels

250. What is the most common form of sexual dysfunction in women?

(a) Sexual interest/arousal disorder

(b) Orgasmic disorder

(c) Genito-pelvic pain/penetration disorder

(d) Substance/medication-induced sexual dysfunction

(Answer is A) Sexual interest/arousal disorder

251. What is false concerning hyper-sexuality?

(a) Might be a side effect of Parkinson's disease medications

(b) Could be a type of obsessive compulsive disorder

(c) Could result from biochemical changes accompanying dementia

(d) Divided into satyriasis for females and nymphomania for males

(Answer is D) Divided into satyriasis for females and nymphomania for males

252. The testicular interstitium contains all of the following cells, *except*:

(a) Leydig cells (b) Sertoli cells

(c) Mast cells (d) Macrophages

(Answer is B) Sertoli cells

253. Both ends of the seminiferous tubules end in the:

(a) Rete testis (b) Straight tubules

(c) Efferent ductules (d) Epididymis

(Answer is A) Rete testis

254. The blood-testis barrier is constructed of the following cell types:

(a) Sertoli - Sertoli cells

(b) Myoid - Leydig cells

(c) Spermatogonia - Endothelial cells

(d) Spermatogonia - Leydig cells

(Answer is A) Sertoli - Sertoli cells

255. What is false concerning the function of the epididymis?

(a) Thermally and hormonally dependent

(b) Entails sperm transportation, storage and motility maturation

(c) Motility maturation is achieved at late caput or early corpus

(d) Neutral α-glucosidase activity is an indicator of epididymal function

(Answer is C) Motility maturation is achieved at late caput or early corpus

256. Testosterone peaks at the following intervals of male's life, *except*:

(a) Early gestation

(b) Late gestation

(c) 2 months after delivery

(d) Puberty

(Answer is B) Late gestation

257. What is false concerning chemotherapy-related infertility?

(a) DNA damage can be detected up to 2 years following chemotherapy
(b) Is toxic to actively dividing cells especially up to the preleptotene stage
(c) Treatment for Hodgkin disease leads to infertility in > 80% of patients
(d) The agents mostly associated with infertility are the anthracyclines such as doxorubicin

(Answer is D) The agents mostly associated with infertility are the anthracyclines such as doxorubicin

258. What is false concerning semen analysis for infertility cases?

(a) Should be provided after at least 3 to 4 days of abstinence
(b) Should be processed within 1 hour of ejaculation
(c) Should be provided in 2 to 3 samples, at a minimum of 2 to 3 days apart
(d) Fertility boosters must be withheld 90 days before analysis

(Answer is D) Fertility boosters must be withheld 90 days before analysis

259. What is false concerning seminal volume in fertility issues?

(a) Per the WHO-2010 criteria, the lower reference limit is 1.5 ml
(b) Low volume could be due to an improper collection or retrograde ejaculation
(c) High volume could be due to hypergonadotropism and after relieving ductal obstruction
(d) Each day of abstinence is associated with an increase in semen volume of 0.4 ml, up to 7 days

(Answer is C) High volume could be due to hypergonadotropism and after relieving ductal obstruction

260. What is false concerning seminal density in fertility issues?

(a) Per the WHO-2010 criterion for density, the lower reference limit is 15 million sperm per ml, or > 50-60 million total sperm
(b) Each day of abstinence is associated with an increase in sperm density by 10-15 million sperm/ml, up to 7 days
(c) Oligospermia could be due to improper collection or retrograde ejaculation
(d) Severe oligospermia is when sperms count is < 5 million/ml

(Answer is C) Oligospermia could be due to improper collection or retrograde ejaculation

261. What is false concerning sperm motility in fertility issues?

(a) As per the WHO-2010 criterion for normal motility, the lower reference limit is 40%
(b) In sperm motility testing, grade 3 is movement in a straight line
(c) Abnormal motility could be due to sperm ultra-structural abnormalities or partial ductal obstruction
(d) Motility is basically an acrosomal function

(Answer is D) Motility is basically an acrosomal function

262. What is false concerning sperm morphology in fertility issues?

(a) Per the WHO-2010 criterion for normal morphology, the lower reference limit is 4%
(b) Per Kruger strict criteria, any shortage in the sperm's density or motion is enough to consider the semen abnormal
(c) Stress pattern of abnormal semen includes teratospermia
(d) Teratospermia could be due to smoking, varicocele, or endocrinopathy

(Answer is B) Per Kruger strict criteria, any shortage in the sperm's density or motion is enough to consider the semen abnormal

263. What is the lower radiation dose that could render the subject infertile when his testes are exposed to?

(a) 7.5 Gy (b) 11.5 Gy
(c) 15.5 Gy (d) 19.5 Gy

(Answer is A) 7.5 Gy

264. Scrotal temperature is physiologically lower than body temperature by:

(a) 0° to 0.5°C (b) 1° to 2°C
(c) 2° to 4°C (d) 4° to 6°C

(Answer is C) 2° to 4°C

265. Which of the following conditions could cause brownish semen?

(a) Using doxorubicin chemotherapy
(b) Spinal cord injury
(c) The first few ejaculates after relieving ductal obstruction
(d) Fungal UTI

(Answer is B) Spinal cord injury

266. What is the lower limit of testicular diameter under which impaired spermatogenesis is expected?

(a) 3.1 cm (b) 3.6 cm
(c) 4.1 cm (d) 4.6 cm

(Answer is D) 4.6 cm

267. What is false in obesity-related infertility?

(a) BMI increases, SHBG, estrogen and testosterone decrease
(b) The odds of infertility increase by 10% for every 9 kg (20 pounds) a man is overweight
(c) Sleep fragmentation has been proposed as the mechanism by which sleep apnea disrupts nocturnal testosterone rhythm resulting in hypotestosteronemia
(d) Men reporting symptoms of ED, increased weight is found in 80% of subjects

(Answer is A) BMI increases, SHBG, estrogen and testosterone decrease

268. What is false concerning obstructive azoospermia (OA)?

(a) Defined as the absence of spermatozoa and spermatogenetic cells in semen and post-ejaculate urine due to obstruction
(b) The most common cause of acquired OA is vasal obstruction
(c) Congenital forms of epididymal obstruction include chronic Young's syndrome
(d) Cystic obstructions of ejaculatory ducts are usually congenital and are typically paramedian

(Answer is D) Cystic obstructions of ejaculatory ducts are usually congenital and are typically paramedian

269. What is true regarding obstructive azoospermia (OA)?

(a) Usually seminal vesicles are dilated when A-P diameter is > 7 mm
(b) Functional obstruction of the distal seminal ducts might be attributed to local neuropathy or using SSRI medications
(c) Non-OA is less common than OA occurring in 20% of men with azoospermia
(d) Post-inflammatory obstructions causing OA are most commonly due to chlamydial epididymitis

(Answer is B) Functional obstruction of the distal seminal ducts might be attributed to local neuropathy or using SSRI medications

270. Which of the following clinical findings has NO relation to male infertility?

(a) The volume of left testis is 18 ml, while the right is 20 ml
(b) Enlarged and hardened epididymis

(c) Absent, nodular or beaded vas
(d) Palpable seminal vesicle per rectum

(Answer is A) The volume of left testis is 18 ml, while the right is 20 ml

271. What is false concerning sperm DNA fragmentation?

(a) Associated with high chances of miscarriages
(b) DNA fragmentation index of $\geq 2\%$ seriously reduces the success rates after ICSI
(c) Detected by the sperm chromatin dispersion test and TUNEL assay
(d) Commonly caused by diabetes mellitus

(Answer is B) DNA fragmentation index of $\geq 2\%$ seriously reduces the success rates after ICSI

272. What is false concerning testicular biopsy for fertility issues?

(a) Should be combined with extraction of testicular sperms for fertilization and/or cryopreservation
(b) Selected cases of azoospermia, it is indicated to exclude obstruction
(c) The technique of choice in obstructive azoospermia is TESE
(d) Spermatogenic pockets may be patchy, thereby, biopsies might miss areas of sperm population

(Answer is C) The technique of choice in obstructive azoospermia is TESE

273. What is false concerning the role of Y-chromosome microdeletions in male infertility?

(a) AZF-c deletions are the most common
(b) Deletions are rare with a sperm concentration > 5 million/ml
(c) Removal of the AZF-b region is associated with Sertoli-cell-only syndrome
(d) Total AZF deletions do not impose a risk for cryptorchidism or testicular cancer

(Answer is C) Removal of the AZF-b region is associated with Sertoli-cell-only syndrome

274. The highest recurrence rate after testicular varicocele repair has been reported post:

(a) Laparoscopic repair
(b) High ligation
(c) Retrograde embolization
(d) Inguinal approach

(Answer is B) High ligation

275. What is false concerning male contraception?

(a) A combination of progesterone with LH-RH antagonists result in complete suppression of spermatogenesis
(b) Prevent early recanalization after vasectomy, cauterization and fascial interposition are advised
(c) The shorter the interval is from vasectomy to reversal, the higher the pregnancy rate will be
(d) Periodic abstinence has a failure rate of 20%

(Answer is A) A combination of progesterone with LH-RH antagonists result in complete suppression of spermatogenesis

276. What is false concerning treating male infertility?

(a) Clomiphene citrate and tamoxifen have been widely used in idiopathic oligoastheno-teratospermia
(b) Hormonal replacement therapy in male infertility has been approved for hypo-gonadotropic hypogonadism cases
(c) Is recommended to use testosterone supplement for treating unexplained male infertility
(d) Is advised to operate on men with a clinical varicocele, oligospermia and/or unexplained infertility

(Answer is C) Is recommended to use testosterone

supplement for treating unexplained male infertility

277. Which of the following modalities of testicular varicocele repair could be complicated by right shoulder pain?

(a) Antegrade sclerotherapy
(b) Retrograde embolization
(c) Microsurgical inguinal or subinguinal with delivery of the testis
(d) Laparoscopy

(Answer is D) Laparoscopy

278. During vasectomy reversal, the absence of spermatozoa in vas deferens fluid suggests the presence of:

(a) Secondary epididymal obstruction
(b) Distal vas deferens obstruction
(c) Ejaculatory duct obstruction
(d) Primary testicular failure

(Answer is A) Secondary epididymal obstruction

279. A 24 years man complains of secondary infertility. Physical examination reveals enlarged bilateral epididymi. Repeated semen analyses show azoospermia with positive fructose, volumes of 2.5, 1.9 and 2.7 ml, and no sperms identified in the post-ejaculation urinalysis. FSH is 3.2 IU/l. Semen α-glucosidase is 8.1 mU ml^{-1}. Transrectal ultrasound reveals seminal vesicles of 0.8 and 1.3 cm in largest diameters, with no midline cyst. The procedure of choice is:

(a) TESE/ICSI
(b) PESA/IVF
(c) IUI
(d) None of the above, just reassurance

(Answer is B) PESA/IVF

280. A 32 years diabetic man has secondary infertility. Physical examination is normal. Repeated semen analyses show azoospermia with positive fructose and volumes of 0.5, 1.0 and 0.7 ml. Post-ejaculation urinalysis shows sperms in abundance. FSH is 7.8 IU/l. The procedure of choice is:

(a) TESE/ICSI
(b) PESA/IVF
(c) IUI
(d) None of the above, just reassurance

(Answer is C) IUI

281. A 20 years man has secondary infertility. Physical examination is normal. Repeated semen analyses show azoospermia with negative fructose and volumes of 0.5, 1.0 and 0.7 ml. No sperms are identified in the post-ejaculation urinalysis. FSH is 7.8 IU/l. Semen α-glucosidase is 9.6 mU ml^{-1}. Transrectal ultrasound reveals seminal vesicles of 2.8 and 1.9 cm in largest diameters with no midline cyst. The procedure of choice is:

(a) TESE/ICSI
(b) TURED
(c) IUI
(d) None of the above, just reassurance

(Answer is B) TURED

282. What is the likelihood that an infertile man with FSH $\leq$ 7.6 IU/l and the testis long axis is > 4.6 cm, has an obstruction?

(a) Never (b) Unlikely
(c) Likely (d) Always

(Answer is D) Always

283. What is the threshold of sperm concentration above which intrauterine insemination success is favorable?

(a) 31.0 million/ml (b) 37.0 million/ml
(c) 42.0 million/ml (d) 48.0 million/ml

(Answer is D) 48.0 million/mL

284. Under light microscopy, leukocytes and immature germ cells in a semen sample look

similar. What additional test is required to distinguish between the two types of cells?

(a) Papanicolaou stain
(b) TUNEL assay
(c) Sperm chromatin configuration test
(d) Indicator

(Answer is A) Papanicolaou stain

285. Male infertility associated with androgen receptor insensitivity is characterized by:

(a) High testosterone, high estradiol
(b) Low testosterone, low estradiol
(c) High testosterone, low estradiol
(d) Low testosterone, high estradiol

(Answer is A) High testosterone, high estradiol

286. Patients with bilateral absence of the vas should be evaluated for:

(a) Klinefelter syndrome
(b) Cystic fibrosis gene mutation
(c) Supernumerary X chromosome
(d) Partial AZF–a region deletion

(Answer is B) Cystic fibrosis gene mutation

287. In the domain of male infertility, what is true concerning post coital test?

(a) Abnormal in 10% of infertile couples
(b) Indicated in semen hyperviscosity and unexplained infertility
(c) A normal result, sperm function tests should be considered
(d) All of the above

(Answer is D) All of the above

288. All of the following causes of male infertility can be treated by medical means, *except*:

(a) Klinefelter syndrome
(b) Endocrinopathy
(c) Antisperm antibodies
(d) Retrograde ejaculation

(Answer is A) Klinefelter syndrome

289. What is false concerning gonadotropin-releasing hormone (GnRH)?

(a) Secreted by the hypothalamus
(b) Released in a pulsatile manner around every 70-90 minutes
(c) Secretion is stimulated by melatonin from the pineal gland and inhibited by testosterone
(d) The half-life is 20-50 minutes

(Answer is D) The half-life is 20-50 minutes

290. What is false concerning spermatocytes?

(a) Primary spermatocytes pass through the preleptotene, leptotene, zygotene, and pachytene stages to become secondary spermatocytes
(b) During meiosis cells cross from the basal to the adluminal compartments
(c) Secondary spermatocytes undergo a reduction division (mitosis) to become spermatids
(d) Secondary spermatocytes contain small nuclei with fine chromatin

(Answer is C) Secondary spermatocytes undergo a reduction division (mitosis) to become spermatids

291. Which process of germ cell development involves the formation of the acrosome and flagella?

(a) First meiosis (b) Second meiosis
(c) Spermiogenesis (d) Mitosis

(Answer is C) Spermiogenesis

292. A 36 years man having Klinefelter syndrome underwent unsuccessful TESE/ICSI. Which of the following treatment options is not reasonable to consider?

(a) Additional ICSI (b) IUI
(c) Adoption (d) Donated sperms

(Answer is B) IUI

293. Which of the following coital lubricants is not spermicidal?

(a) Vegetable oil (b) Surgilube
(c) K-Y jelly (d) Saliva

(Answer is A) Vegetable oil

294. What is true regarding the effects of the following drugs on fertility potentials?

(a) Cyproterone, cimetidine and ketoconazole have antiandrogen properties
(b) Sulfasalazine and doxorubicin decrease testosterone levels by 42%
(c) Nitrofurantoin and tetracycline depress spermatogenesis
(d) Spironolactone results in irreversible oligoasthenospermia

(Answer is A) Cyproterone, cimetidine and ketoconazole have antiandrogen properties

295. Sertoli-cell-only syndrome is characterized by all of the following, *except*:

(a) Small to normal-sized testes and azoospermia
(b) Normal LH, low testosterone, high FSH
(c) Normal secondary sex characteristics
(d) Histology reveals normal Sertoli and Leydig cells

(Answer is B) Normal LH, low testosterone, high FSH

296. What is the most common cause of acquired testicular failure in adults?

(a) Infections (b) Trauma
(c) Radiation exposure (d) Drug induced

(Answer is A) Infections

297. All of the following viruses could cause orchitis, *except*:

(a) Mumps virus (b) Echovirus
(c) Retrovirus (d) Group B arbovirus

(Answer is C) Retrovirus

298. All of the following are true regarding "vanishing testes syndrome", *except*:

(a) Patients have normal male karyotype 46 XY and normal SRY gene
(b) Cryopreservation is advised for future ART
(c) Causes might be related to infection, vascular disease or torsion
(d) Affected individuals cannot have biological children

(Answer is B) Cryopreservation is advised for future ART

299. In an infertile man, a testicular biopsy that shows normal Sertoli cells and Leydig cells, normal-sized seminiferous tubules, and normal tunica propria points to the following condition:

(a) Sertoli-cell-only syndrome
(b) Maturation arrest
(c) Hypospermatogenesis
(d) Cryptorchid testes

(Answer is B) Maturation arrest

300. On working up a case of infertility, testicular biopsy shows decreased number of spermatogonia, germ cell hypoplasia, Sertoli cell atrophy, tubular hyalinization, hyperplastic Leydig cells, and deformed tubules. What would be the proper diagnosis?

(a) Cryptorchid testes
(b) Klinefelter syndrome
(c) Post-testicular obstruction
(d) Immunogenic infertility

(Answer is B) Klinefelter syndrome

301. What is false concerning immunogenic male infertility?

(a) Patients with antisperm antibody > 1:32 might respond to immunosuppression cyclic steroids
(b) The emergence of antisperm antibodies after vasectomy is uncommon

(c) The presence of antisperm antibodies might appear as abnormal clumping, agglutination or an abnormal postcoital test result
(d) Radioimmunoassay and immunobead test help detect antisperm antibodies

(Answer is B) The emergence of antisperm antibodies after vasectomy is uncommon

302. Which statement is false regarding male infertility in spinal cord injury patients?

(a) Analysis might reveal disruptions in nuclear maturity and DNA composition of spermatozoa with neutrophil infiltration
(b) The main issue is an ejaculation that can be managed by electroejaculation or sperm retrieval techniques
(c) Sperm aspirated from the vas deferens are of better quality if compared to ejaculated sperms
(d) Treated by immunosuppression using cyclic steroids for 6 months

(Answer is D) Treated by immunosuppression using cyclic steroids for 6 months

303. Conditions associated with increased sex hormone binding globulin are all *except*:

(a) Hepatitis
(b) Hyperthyroidism
(c) Estrogen therapy
(d) Diabetes mellitus

(Answer is D) Diabetes mellitus

304. False about Klinefelter's syndrome:

(a) Increased height >95%
(b) >95% have azoospermia
(c) Most common genetic cause for male infertility
(d) Early age at diagnosis gives offer a more favourable prognosis

(Answer is A) Increased height >95%

305. Urolift false is:

(a) Used in BPH
(b) Deployed cystoscopically
(c) Can be done as office procedure
(d) Can lead to sexual dysfunction

(Answer is D) Can lead to sexual dysfunction

CHAPTER

7

Male Genitalia

1. Which is not true regarding spermatocytic seminoma?

(a) No documented cases of metastatic disease
(b) Does not express PLAP or i(12p)
(c) Does not arise from CIS
(d) Only seen in patients with a history of cryptorchidism or bilaterality

(Answer is D) Spermatocytic seminoma

- Prognosis is favorable.
- No documented cases of metastatic disease.
- Not associated with a history of cryptorchidism or bilaterality.
- Does not express PLAP or i(12p).
- Does not occur as part of mixed GCTs.
- Does not arise from CIS.

2. Which is the most common malignancy in men in the 15- to 35-year age group?

(a) Carcinoma testis
(b) Carcinoma oral cavity
(c) Carcinoma lung
(d) Leukemia

(Answer is A) Testicular cancer, although relatively rare, is the most common malignancy in men in the 15- to 35-year age group.

3. β-hCG production is seen in how many patients with seminoma testis?

(a) Nil (b) 10%
(c) 50% (d) 100%

(Answer is B) Syncytiotrophoblastic elements occur in 10% to 15%, and lymphocytic infiltration occurs in approximately 20%. The incidence of syncytiotrophoblastic elements corresponds to the frequency of β-hCG production.

4. Which statement is not true regarding anaplastic seminoma?

(a) More aggressive and more lethal than typical seminoma
(b) Increased mitotic activity
(c) Increased invasion and metastatic spread
(d) Decreased tumor marker (hCG) production

(Answer is D) A number of features suggest that anaplastic seminoma is a more aggressive and potentially more lethal variant of typical seminoma. These characteristics include (1) greater mitotic activity, (2) higher rate of local invasion, (3) increased rate of metastatic spread, and (4) higher rate of tumor marker (β-hCG) production.

5. Cryptorchidism does not predispose to:

(a) Embryonal carcinoma
(b) Choriocarcinoma
(c) Spermatocytic seminoma
(d) Teratoma

(Answer is C) None case of spermatocytic seminoma has occurred in conjunction with cryptorchidism.

6. In which variant of carcinoma testis cut surface reveals a variegated, grayish white, fleshy tumor, often with areas of necrosis or hemorrhage and a poorly defined capsule?

(a) Embryonal carcinoma
(b) Choriocarcinoma

(c) Spermatocytic seminoma
(d) Teratoma

(Answer is A) Embryonal carcinoma is generally discovered as a small, rounded, but irregular mass invading the tunica vaginalis testis and not infrequently involving contiguous cord structures. The cut surface reveals a variegated, grayish white, fleshy tumor, often with areas of necrosis or hemorrhage and a poorly defined capsule.

7. Which is the most common testicular tumor of infants and children?

(a) Embryonal carcinoma
(b) Choriocarcinoma
(c) Yolk sac tumor
(d) Teratoma

(Answer is C) Yolk sac tumor is the most common testis tumor of infants and children.

8. Embryoid bodies is present in:

(a) Embryonal carcinoma
(b) Choriocarcinoma
(c) Yolk sac tumor
(d) Teratoma

(Answer is C) Embryoid bodies, a common finding in yolk sac tumors, resemble 1- to 2-week-old embryos.

9. Not true about yolk sac tumor is:

(a) It is the most common tumor of infancy
(b) Embryoid bodies is a common finding
(c) It is also called as juvenile embryonal carcinoma and orchioblastoma
(d) It is primarily responsible for hCG production

(Answer is D) α-Fetoprotein elevated in >90%.

10. Schiller-Duval bodies are present in:

(a) Embryonal carcinoma
(b) Choriocarcinoma
(c) Seminoma
(d) Endodermal sinus tumor

(Answer is D) Endodermal sinus tumor.

11. Which tumor is also called as endodermal sinus tumor ?

(a) Yolk sac tumor
(b) Anaplastic seminoma
(c) Embryonal carcinoma
(d) Teratoma

(Answer is C) The terms endodermal sinus tumor, adenocarcinoma of the infantile testis, juvenile embryonal carcinoma, and orchioblastoma are all used synonymously.

12. Which tumor markers does seminoma and embryonal tumor express respectively?

(a) PLAP, CD 117 and Keratin, CD 30
(b) PLAP, CD 30 and Keratin, CD 117
(c) Keratin, C D 117 and PLAP, CD 30
(d) Keratin, CD 30 and PLAP, CD 117

(Answer is A) Most seminomas express PLAP and do not stain with antibodies to keratin. The reverse applies to embryonal tumors. In addition, most seminomas express CD 117 (c- *kit* proto-oncogene protein) and not CD30 (transmembrane glycoprotein), whereas most embryonal cell carcinomas are CD30 positive and CD117 negative.

13. Most common GCT after 65 years of age is:

(a) Classic seminoma
(b) Anaplastic seminoma
(c) Spermatocytic seminoma
(d) Teratoma

(Answer is C) Spermatocytic seminoma: comprises 9% of seminomas, occurs most frequently in men > 40 years of age. In men > 65years this tumor is the most common germ cell tumor.

14. In patients with testicular cancer, risk of developing a GCT in the contralateral testis is:

(a) 2% (b) 5%
(c) 10% (d) 20%

(Answer is B) Patients with testicular cancer, the cumulative risk of developing a GCT in the contralateral testis was found to be 5.2%, which is similar to the prevalence of CIS in the contralateral testis.

15. Which condition has maximum risk for development of testicular CIS?

(a) History of testicular carcinoma
(b) EGCT
(c) Cryptorchidism
(d) Contralateral testis with unilateral testicular cancer

(Answer is B) Risk factors for the development of testicular CIS include a history of testicular carcinoma (5% to 6%), EGCT (40%), cryptorchidism (3%), contralateral testis with unilateral testicular cancer (5% to 6%), atrophic contralateral testis with unilateral testicular cancer (30%), somatosexual ambiguity (25% to 100%) and infertility (0.4% to 1.1%).

16. Best treatment option for CIS:

(a) Orchidectomy (b) Radiation
(c) Chemotherapy (d) Observation

(Answer is D) Despite the argument that early diagnosis and therapy for CIS allows preservation of the testis, whereas development of a second GCT usually results in anorchia, we nevertheless believe that a conservative approach is warranted in view of the low risks involved.

17. Peak incidence of seminoma is in:

(a) < 10 years (b) 15-20 years
(c) 25-30 years (d) 35-40 years

(Answer is D) Seminoma is rare before age 10 years and after age 60 years, but it is the most common histologic type overall, with a peak incidence between 35 and 39 years.

18. What is the incidence of malignancy in a contralateral, normally descended gonad in a patient with history of cryptorchidism?

(a) 0% (b) 0% to 5%
(c) 5% to 10% (d) 10% to 20%

(Answer is C) Between 5% and 10% of patients with a history of cryptorchidism develop malignancy in the contralateral, normally descended gonad.

19. Which is predominant tumor in men older than 50 years age?

(a) Seminoma (b) Yolk sac tumor
(c) Lymphoma (d) Choriocarcinoma

(Answer is C) Malignant testicular lymphomas are predominantly tumors of men older than 50 years age.

20. Malignant transformation in non GCT and late recurrence is feature of:

(a) Yolk sac tumor
(b) Teratoma
(c) Embryonal carcinoma
(d) Choriocarcinoma

(Answer is B) Risk of malignant transformation, that is, the development of non-germ cell malignant elements (such as sarcoma or carcinoma) and late recurrence, is associated with teratoma.

21. The primary drainage of the right testis is usually located at:

(a) Interaortocaval
(b) Para-aortic region
(c) Para-caval region
(d) Superior mesenteric

(Answer is A) The primary drainage of the right testis is usually located within the group of lymph nodes in the interaortocaval region at the level of the second vertebral body.

22. The primary drainage of the left testis is usually located at:

(a) Interaortocaval
(b) Para-aortic region
(c) Para-caval region
(d) Superior mesenteric

(Answer is B) The first echelon of nodes draining the left testis is located in the para-aortic region.

23. Inguinal node metastasis may result from all *except:*

(a) Scrotal involvement
(b) Prior inguinal surgery
(c) Retrograde lymphatic spread secondary to massive retroperitoneal lymph node deposits
(d) Epididymis

(Answer is D) Inguinal node metastasis may result from scrotal involvement by the primary tumor, prior inguinal or scrotal surgery, or retrograde lymphatic spread secondary to massive retroperitoneal lymph node deposits.

24. Doubling of GCT is:

(a) < 10 days (b) 10-30 days
(c) 6 months (d) 12 months

(Answer is B) Doubling times calculated on the basis of serial chest radiographs usually range from 10 to 30 days.

25. The usual presentation of a testicular tumor is:

(a) Pain
(b) Swelling
(c) Respiratory symptoms, such as cough or dyspnea
(d) Gastrointestinal disturbances, such as anorexia, nausea, vomiting

(Answer is B) The usual presentation of a testicular tumor is a nodule or painless swelling of one gonad.

26. Which statement regarding AFP is not true?

(a) It is a single-chain glycoprotein
(b) Molecular weight: 38,000 daltons
(c) The highest concentrations noted during the 12th to 14th weeks of gestation
(d) The metabolic half-life of AFP in humans is between 5 and 7 days

(Answer is B) AFP is a single-chain glycoprotein (MW: ~ 70,000 daltons). hCG has a molecular weight of 38,000 daltons.

27. AFP may be produced by all *except:*

(a) Pure embryonal carcinoma
(b) Teratocarcinoma
(c) Yolk sac tumor
(d) Pure choriocarcinoma

(Answer is D) AFP may be produced by pure embryonal carcinoma, teratocarcinoma, yolk sac tumor, or combined tumors but not by pure choriocarcinoma or pure seminoma.

28. Which statement regarding hCG is not true?

(a) The β subunit of hCG is distinct from that pituitary hormones
(b) Molecular weight: 38,000 daltons
(c) Elevated hCG levels may be demonstrated in malignancies (liver, pancreas, stomach, lung, breast, kidney, bladder)
(d) The serum half-life of hCG is between 5 to 7 days.

(Answer is D) This glycoprotein (molecular weight: 38,000 daltons) is composed of a and b polypeptide chains and is normally produced by trophoblastic tissue. The β subunit of hCG is structurally and antigenically distinct from that of the pituitary hormones. Elevated hCG levels may also be demonstrated in patients with various other malignancies (liver, pancreas, stomach, lung, breast, kidney, bladder) and, perhaps, in marijuana smokers. The serum half-life of hCG is 24 and 36 hours.

29. What is the incidence of patients with NSGCTs with normal marker levels even at advanced stages of disease?

(a) 0 to 5% (b) 10% to 15%
(c) 20% to 25% (d) 30% to 35%

(Answer is B) 10% to 15% of patients with NSGCTs can be expected to have normal marker levels even at advanced stages of disease.

30. Incidence of seminoma clinically confined to the testis:

(a) 15% to 25% (b) 25% to 45%
(c) 45% to 65% (d) 65% to 85%

(Answer is D) Between 65% and 85% of all seminomas are clinically confined to the testis.

31. In a patient, with testicular biopsy suggestive of pure seminoma and CT abdomen shows 4 cm RPLN, CT chest is normal. Best treatment option is:

(a) RPLND
(b) RT, 25 Gy involving para-aortic area only
(c) RT, 35 Gy involving ipsilateral external iliac, the bilateral common iliac, the paracaval and the para-aortic nodes superiorly, including coverage of the cisterna chyli
(d) 3 BEP

(Answer is C) This patient has stage IIB disease. Stage II (N1-N2) disease generally responds well to radiation therapy alone.

32. In patients with stage III (Tl-T4 N0-N3 Ml-M2 S0-S3) disease complete response to chemotherapy alone can be achieved in:

(a) Less than 50% (b) 50% to 70%
(c) 70% to 90% (d) More than 90%

(Answer is D) More than 90% of patients who present with stage III (T1-T4 N0-N3 M 1-M2 S0-S3) disease achieve a complete response to chemotherapy alone.

33. Surgical resection of post-chemotherapy residual mass is advised in seminoma if mass is:

(a) Diffuse and more than 3 cm
(b) Diffuse and less than 3 cm
(c) Discrete and less than 3 cm
(d) Discrete and more than 3 cm

(Answer is D) With residual mass, close, careful observation is favoured, as opposed to consolidation with radiation therapy or surgical excision, unless the mass is well defined, larger than 3 cm in diameter, and surgically amenable to resection.

34. Regarding protocol for surveillance in Stage I Seminoma and Nonseminomatous germ cell tumor, CT should be done at what interval during first 2 years?

(a) 1 month (b) 4 months
(c) 6 months (d) 12 months

(Answer is B) CT should be done at 4 monthly interval for first 2 years, 6 monthly for next 2 years and than annually from 5th year.

35. Poor prognosis is NSGCT include all *except:*

(a) Mediastinal primary
(b) Pulmonary visceral metastases
(c) AFP > 10,000 ng/ml
(d) hCG > 50,000 IU/l

(Answer is B) International germ cell consensus prognostic classification system for testicular cancer

Poor prognosis
Nonseminoma only
Any of the following criteria: Mediastinal primary Nonpulmonary visceral metastases AFP > 10,000 ng/ ml; hCG > 50,000 IU/l, or LDH > 10 times upper limit of normal

36. Postchemotherapy RPLND, should be considered for all *except:*

(a) 5% residual mass after primary chemotherapy with normal tumor markers
(b) Residual mass irrespective of serum tumor markers after salvage chemotherapy
(c) Recurrent resectable mass after salvage chemotherapy
(d) Resectable chemorefractory NSGCT with or without elevated serum tumor markers

(Answer is A) Postchemotherapy RPLND should be considered for the following subsets of patients:

- Residual mass and normal serum tumor markers after primary chemotherapy. Within this subset of patients, RPLND can be excluded in those patients with greater than 90% chemotherapy-induced reduction in tumor volume, and the absence of teratoma in the primary tumor.
- Residual mass irrespective of serum tumor markers after salvage chemotherapy.
- Recurrent resectable mass after salvage chemotherapy.
- Resectable chemorefractory NSGCT with or without elevated serum tumor markers.

37. Development of secondary leukemia is associated with which chemotherapy drug?

(a) Bleomycin (b) Etoposide
(c) Cisplatin (d) Ifosfamide

(Answer is B) The relationship between etoposide and the development of leukemia has been well described in patients treated for germ cell neoplasms.

38. Which statement regarding bleomycin induced pulmonary toxicity is not true?

(a) Perioperative oxygen restriction in patients treated with bleomycin is necessary
(b) Histopathologic changes include destruction of types I and II pneumocytes
(c) The median time from the start of bleomycin to lung toxicity is 4.2 months
(d) Increased risk of BPT includes age older than 40 years

(Answer is A) Perioperative oxygen restriction in patients treated with bleomycin is not necessary. Intravenous fluid management, including transfusion,was the most significant factor affecting postoperative pulmonary morbidity.

39. The most common sites of origin of EGCT is:

(a) Mediastinum
(b) Retroperitoneum
(c) Sacrococcygeal region
(d) Pineal gland

(Answer is A) The most common sites of origin in decreasing order of frequency, mediastinum, retroperitoneum, sacrococcygeal region, and pineal gland.

40. Reinke's crystals found in which testicular tumors?

(a) Seminoma (b) Gonadoblastoma
(c) Sertoli's cell tumor (d) Leydig cell tumor

(Answer is D) Homogeneous well-circumscribed tumor, characterized by hexagonal cells with pathognomonic cigar-shaped crystals in the cytoplasm (Reinke's crystals) found in 40% of tumors.

41. Which statement regarding Ieydig cell tumor is not correct?

(a) Most common non germ cell tumor of testis
(b) Radical inguinal orchiectomy is the initial treatment of choice
(c) Associated with cryptochordism
(d) 10% of tumor is malignant

(Answer is C) The etiology of Leydig's cell tumors is unknown. In contrast to GCTs, there appears to be no association with cryptorchidism.

42. Call-Exner-like bodies are seen in:

(a) Seminoma (b) Gonadoblastoma
(c) Sertoli'scell tumor (d) Leydigcell tumor

(Answer is C) Secretory materials forming Call-Exner-like bodies are occasionally seen within tubules, the morphologic appearance resembling that of granulosa cell tumors.

43. In Sertoli and Leydig cell tumor designation of malignancy can be made with certainty only in the presence of:

(a) Large size
(b) Invasion of adjacent structures

(c) Blood vessel and lymphatic invasion
(d) Metastasis

(Answer is D) Although large size, poor tumor demarcation, invasion of adjacent structures, blood vessel and lymphatic invasion, and increased mitotic activity are all suggestive of malignant potential, as with Leydig's cell tumors, the designation of malignancy can be made with certainty only in the presence of metastasis.

44. Which statement regarding gonadoblastoma is not correct?

(a) Occur almost exclusively in patients with some form of gonadal dysgenesis
(b) High incidence of bilaterality (50%)
(c) Approximately four fifths of patients with gonadoblastoma are phenotypic males
(d) Treatment is radical inguinal orchidectomy and contralateral orchidectomy when gonadal dysgenesis is present on that side

(Answer is C) Approximately four fifths of patients with gonadoblastoma are phenotypic females, usually presenting with primary amenorrhea and sometimes with a lower abdominal mass.

45. Which of the following statement regarding testicular tumor is not correct?

(a) Lymphoma is most common testicular tumor over >50 years of age
(b) Seminoma is most common secondary testicular tumor
(c) Yolk sac is most common testicular tumor of infancy
(d) Most common site of metastasis from testicular tumor is prostate

(Answer is B) Lymphoma constitute the most common secondary neoplasms of the testis and the most frequent of all testicular tumors in patients older than 50 years.

46. Most common site for relapse in ALL is:

(a) Kidney (b) Urinary bladder
(c) Prostate (d) Testis

(Answer is D) The testis appears to be a prime initial site of relapse in boys with acute lymphocytic leukemia.

47. Most common tumors of the paratesticular tissues:

(a) Malignant melanoma
(b) Lymphoma
(c) Adenomatoid tumor
(d) Rhabdomyosarcoma

(Answer is C) Adenomatoid tumors are the most common tumors of the paratesticular tissues, accounting for approximately 30% of all paratesticular tumors.

48. Most common location for tumor in testicular adnexal is:

(a) Globus major (b) Globus minor
(c) Spermatic cord (d) Tunica vaginalis

(Answer is B) Epididymis is most frequent location: Within the epididymis the globus minor is the most frequent site.

49. Incidence of permanent azoospermia after chemotherapy for testicular tumor is:

(a) 0% (b) 25%
(c) 50% (d) 75%

(Answer is B) Fifty percent of patients who receive chemotherapy experience return of normal sperm counts by 2 years, whereas 25% continue to remain azoospermic after chemotherapy.

50. To identify solid intratesticular lesions, by scrotal USG, sensitivity and specificity is:

(a) 50%-60% (b) 60%-70%
(c) 80%-90% (d) More than 95%

(Answer is D) Scrotal sonography is extremely accurate in identifying solid intratesticular lesions, with greater than 95% sensitivity and specificity.

51. If scrotal violation in patients with low-stage NSGCT has occurred, treatment is:

(a) Surveillance
(b) Scrotal scar should be widely excised with radiotherapy
(c) Scrotal scar should be widely excised with chemotherapy
(d) Scrotal scar should be widely excised with RPLND

(Answer is D) In patients with NSGCT, the scrotal scar should be widely excised with the spermatic cord remnant at the time of RPLND.

52. In testicular carcinoma CT understages retroperitoneum in how many patients?

(a) 0% to 15%
(b) 15% to 40%
(c) 40% to 55%
(d) 55% to 70%

(Answer is B) Radiologic imaging such as CT, understages 15% to 40% of patients, particularly in the retroperitoneum.

53. Most common site of late recurrence of both teratoma and viable GCT:

(a) Mediastinum
(b) Retroperitoneum
(c) Sacrococcygeal region
(d) Pineal gland

(Answer is B) The most common site of late recurrence of both teratoma and viable GCT is the retroperitoneum.

54. All are preserved in nerve-sparing RPLND *except:*

(a) Sympathetic chains bilaterally
(b) Postganglionic sympathetic nerves
(c) Hypogastric plexus
(d) Aortic plexus

(Answer is D) The most important aspect in performing nerve-sparing RPLND is the prospective identification and preservation of relevant sympathetic nerves, specifically (1) the sympathetic chains bilaterally; (2) the postganglionic sympathetic nerves arising from the sympathetic chains; and (3) the hypogastric plexus, which is the anastomosing network of nerve fibers anterior to the lower aorta.

55. All statement regarding antegrade ejaculation is correct *except:*

(a) Sympathetic fibers that mediate seminal emission originate from T12-L3 of spinal cord
(b) Sympathetic fibers from hypogastric plexus innervate seminal vesicles, vas deferens, prostate and urinary bladder
(c) Parasympathetic fibers tighten the bladder neck
(d) Pudendal somatic innervation from S2-S4 causes relaxation of external urethral sphincter

(Answer is C) Sympathetic fibers tighten the bladder neck.

56. About modified RPLND which statement is correct?

(a) Ipsilateral dissection below IMA is minimized
(b) Ipsilateral dissection above IMA is minimized
(c) Contralateral dissection above IMA is minimized
(d) Contralateral dissection below IMA is minimized

(Answer is D) In an effort to avoid disrupting the sympathetic nerves and the hypogastric plexus, all modified templates share several goals: (1) to thoroughly resect all interaortocaval and ipsilateral lymph nodes between the level of the renal vessels and the bifurcation of the common iliac artery and (2) to minimize contralateral dissection, particularly below the level of the IMA.

57. Thirty-year-old man with 6 cm para-aortic mass and testicular biopsy suggestive of NSGCT. He underwent chemotherapy. Mass has regressed but markers are still elevated. Next step is:

(a) Second line chemotherapy
(b) Radiation tharapy
(c) Observation and repeat markers after 6 months
(d) Bilateral RPLND

(Answer is A) Increased serum concentrations of AFP and β-hCG after primary cisplatin-based chemotherapy are often characterized by unresectable, viable GCT; and second-line "salvage" chemotherapy is usually recommended for these non-responders.

58. Post-chemotherapy pathologic findings in patients with advanced NSGCT after induction therapy are:

(a) Necrosis, 50%; teratoma, 40%; viable carcinoma, 10%
(b) Necrosis, 10%; teratoma, 50%; viable carcinorna 40%
(c) Necrosis, 40%; teratoma, 10%; viable carcinoma, 50%
(d) Necrosis, 50%; teratoma, 10%; viable carcinoma, 40%

(Answer is A) Post-chemotherapy pathologic findings in patients with advanced NSGCT after induction therapy are approximately as follows: necrosis, 50%; teratoma, 40%; viable carcinoma, 10%.

59. FDT PET scan should be done for:

(a) Seminoma with residual masses smaller than 3 cm after chemotherapy
(b) Seminoma with residual masses larger than 3 cm after chemotherapy
(c) Nonseminoma with residual masses smaller than 3 cm after chemotherapy
(d) Nonseminoma with residual masses larger than 3 cm after chemotherapy

(Answer is B) Patients with residual masses smaller than 3 cm after chemotherapy may be observed. An FDT PET scan should be done for masses 3 cm or larger. A negative PET scan usually implies freedom from disease, whereas a positive PET scan is often associated with residual viable seminoma and additional therapy should be considered.

60. Most common adjunctive procedure, performed after post-chemotherapy RPLND:

(a) Right nephrectomy
(b) Left nephrectomy
(c) Splenectomy
(d) Left hemicolectomy

(Answer is B) To ensure complete surgical resection of residual retroperitoneal masses, adjunctive procedures are sometimes necessary. En bloc nephrectomy is the most common adjunctive procedure. with almost a 20% rate in the Indiana post-chemotherapy experience. These are predominantly left-sided primary tumors with large-volume residual disease densely adherent to the left renal vessels and/or hilum.

61. Post-chemotherapy pathologic findings in patients with advanced NSGCT after salvage therapy are:

(a) Necrosis, 50%; teratoma, 40%; viable carcinoma, 10%
(b) Necrosis, 10%; teratoma, 40%; viable carcinoma, 50%
(c) Necrosis, 40%; teratoma, 40%; viable carcinoma, 50%
(d) Necrosis, 50%; teratoma, 10%; viable carcinoma, 40%

(Answer is B) Post-chemotherapy pathologic findings in patients with advanced NSGCT following salvage therapy are approximately as follows: necrosis, 10%; teratoma, 40%; viable carcinoma, 50%.

62. Which one of the following is a premalignant condition?

(a) Pearly penile papules
(b) Hirsute papillomas

(c) Coronal papillae
(d) Cutaneous horn

(Answer is D) Pearly penile papules, hirsute papillomas, and coronal papillae are normal and commonly encountered lesions of the glans penis.

63. All are true about BXO *except:*

(a) Hypertrophy of the rete pegs
(b) Homogenization of collagen on the upper third of the dermis
(c) Whitish patch on the prepuce or glans
(d) Atrophic epidermis

(Answer is A) Show atrophic epidermis with loss of the rete pegs and homogenization of collagen on the upper third of the dermis combined with a zone of lymphocytic and histiocytic infiltration. Whitish patch on the prepuce or glans, often involving the meatus and sometimes extending into the fossa navicularis.

64. Which statement regarding histological examination of leukoplakia is not correct?

(a) Hyperkeratosis
(b) Parakeratosis
(c) Atrophy of rete pegs
(d) Dermal edema and lymphocytic infiltration

(Answer is C) On histologic examination, there is hyperkeratosis, parakeratosis, and hypertrophy of the rete pegs with dermal edema and lymphocytic infiltration.

65. Kaposi sarcoma is associated with which herpes virus?

(a) HHV 3 (b) HHV 6
(c) HHV 8 (d) HHV 10

(Answer is C) Human herpesvirus 8, also known as Kaposi's sarcoma-associated herpesvirus, is strongly suspected of being the etiologic agent of epidemic (AIDS-related) Kaposi's sarcoma.

66. Which statement regarding condylomata acuminata is not correct?

(a) Koilocyte–a cell characterized by an empty cavity surrounding an atypical nucleus–is pathognomonic for HIV infection
(b) Approximately 5% of patients will demonstrate urethral involvement
(c) Treatment of these lesions with podophyllin may induce histologic changes suggestive of carcinoma
(d) Subclinical disease may be detected by the application of 5% acetic acid solution to the penis

(Answer is A) Koilocyte–a cell characterized by an empty cavity surrounding an atypical nucleus–is pathognomonic for HPV infection.

67. Which HPV is associated with low grade dysplasia?

(a) HPV 42 and 44 (b) HPV 16 and 18
(c) HPV 31 and 33 (d) HPV 35 and 39

(Answer is A) Virus types 6, 11 and 42 to 44 are associated with gross condylomata and low-grade dysplasia. Types 16, 18, 31, 33, 35 and 39 have a higher association with malignant disease.

68. Most frequently detected HPV in primary carcinomas, bowenoid papulosis and also in metastatic lesions:

(a) HPV 6 (b) HPV 11
(c) HPV 16 (d) HPV 18

(Answer is C) HPV 16 appears to be the most frequently detected type in primary carcinomas and has also been detected in metastatic lesions.

69. Buschke-Löwenstein tumor differs from condyloma acuminatum in:

(a) Condylomata always invades
(b) Condylomata always remain superficial
(c) Condylomata of large size invades
(d) Condylomata of large size can metastasise

(Answer is B) The Buschke-Löwenstein tumor differs from condyloma acuminatum in that condylomata, regardless of size, always remain superficial and never invade adjacent tissue.

70. Carcinoma in situ (Tis) of the penis is called erythroplasia of Queyrat at all sites *except:*

(a) Glans penis
(b) Prepuce
(c) Penile shaft
(d) Perianal region

(Answer is D) Carcinoma in situ (Tis) of the penis is called erythroplasia of Queyrat by urologists and dermatologists if it involves the glans penis, prepuce, or penile shaft and Bowen's disease if it involves the remainder of the genitalia or perineal region.

71. Risk factors for the development of squamous penile cancer are all *except:*

(a) Heavy alcohol use
(b) Smoking
(c) Penile tears and rashes
(d) HPV infection

(Answer is A) Greater than three-fold risk of penile cancer in men with penile tears and rashes. No convincing evidence has been found linking penile cancer to other factors such as occupation, other venereal diseases (gonorrhea, syphilis, herpes), marijuana use, or alcohol intake.

72. Preventing strategies for penile cancer are all *except:*

(a) Good hygiene to prevent occurrence of phimosis
(b) Avoidance of tobbaco products
(c) Post pubertal circumcision
(d) Avoiding sexual promiscuity

(Answer is C) Critical period of exposure to certain etiologic agents may have already occurred at puberty, and certainly by adulthood, rendering later circumcision relatively ineffective as a prophylactic tool for penile cancer.

73. Not true about lymphatic drainage of penis is:

(a) Lymphatics of prepuce drain external to fascia lata
(b) Lymphatics of glans drain by the way of superficial inguinal lymph nodes to deep inguinal lymph nodes
(c) Skip drainage is also possible
(d) Multiple criss-cross exists at any levels of drainage

(Answer is C) Penile lymphangiogram studies demonstrate a consistent pattern of drainage that proceeds from superficial inguinal to deep inguinal to pelvic node sites without evidence of "skip" drainage.

74. Most common site of penile tumor is:

(a) Glans penis (b) Prepuce
(c) Coronal sulcus (d) Shaft

(Answer is A) Penile tumors may present anywhere on the penis but occur most commonly on the glans (48%) and prepuce (21%). Other tumors involve the glans and prepuce (9%), the coronal sulcus (6%), or the shaft (<2%).

75. Which statement regarding role of imaging studies in penile cancer is not correct?

(a) CT scan offers no additional advantage over clinical examination in patients with no palpable lymphadenopathy
(b) CT scan does play role in examination of inguinal region of obese patient and patients with prior inguinal surgery
(c) CT scan is useful for imaging extent of primary tumor
(d) For small volume glandular lesion, imaging studies add little information to palpation

(Answer is C) CT scan has poor soft tissue resolution and is not useful in its present form for imaging the extent of the primary tumor.

76. Penile cancer invading prostate is staged as:

(a) T1 (b) T2
(c) T3 (d) T4

(Answer is C)

Ta Noninvasive verrucous carcinoma
T1 Tumor invades subepithelial connective tissue
T2 Tumor invades corpus spongiosum or cavernosum
T3 Tumor invades urethra or prostate
T4 Tumor invades other adjacent structures

77. According to AJCC staging of penile carcinoma which is not correct?

(a) Ta–non invasive verrucous carcinoma
(b) Tl–invasion of sub epithelial connective tissue
(c) N2–multiple or bilateral superficial inguinal L.N.
(d) N3–fixed inguinal L.N.

(Answer is D)

N1 Metastasis in a single regional lymph node
N2 Metastases in multiple or bilateral superficial inguinal lymph nodes
N3 Metastases in deep inguinal or pelvic lymph nodes; unilateral or bilateral

78. Most important prognostic factor for squamous penile cancer is:

(a) Tumor grade
(b) Gross appearance of tumor
(c) Morphological or microscopic pattern of tumor
(d) Presence and extent of metastasis to inguinal region

(Answer is D) The presence and the extent of metastasis to the inguinal region are the most important prognostic factors for survival in patients with squamous penile cancer.

79. Which one of the following patient can have 5-year survival of >80% after attempting curative surgery?

(a) 3 inguinal L.N. involved
(b) Bilateral involvement
(c) Involvement of pelvic nodes
(d) Inguinal L.N. of 4 cm

(Answer is D) Pathologic criteria associated with long-term survival after attempted curative surgical resection of inguinal metastases (i.e., 80% 5-year survival) include minimal nodal disease (up to two involved nodes in most series), unilateral involvement, no evidence of extranodal extension of cancer, and absence of pelvic nodal metastases.

80. All *except* which group of patients are considered for neoadjuvant therapy?

(a) 3 inguinal L.N. involved
(b) Fixed nodal metastasis
(c) Involvement of pelvic nodal metastasis
(d) Inguinal L.N. of 5 cm

(Answer is A) Fixed nodal metastasis, involvement of pelvic nodal metastasis and inguinal L.N. of more than 4 cm is indication of neoadjuvant chemotherapy.

81. Which can be categorized as a low risk in patient with penile cancer?

(a) T2 without vascular invasion
(b) T1 with vascular invasion
(c) T1 grade 3
(d) T1 grade 2

(Answer is D) Patients with stage T1, grade 1 and grade 2 tumors exhibit less than a 10% incidence of inguinal metastasis and thus considered as low risk patients.

82. Patients who present with unilateral lymphadenopathy some time after the initial presentation and treatment of the primary tumor, should be managed as:

(a) No need for bilateral inguinal lymphadenectomy in any case
(b) Bilateral inguinal lymphadenectomy in all cases
(c) Bilateral inguinal lymphadenectomy in

selected cases such as those who present with more than two LN or bulky LN

(d) Bilateral inguinal lymphadenectomy in selected cases such as those who present with two LN

(Answer is C) In patients with two or more unilateral metastases, those contralateral occult metastases were noted in 30% of cases. Thus, in patients with a bulky unilateral recurrence, a contralateral inguinal staging procedure should be considered.

83. What should be the management of patient with T1 grade 1 penile lesion with no vascular invasion, also having 2 superficial mobile right inguinal L.N. of 3 cm?

(a) 4 weeks of antibiotics, reassessment and plan accordingly

(b) Ilioinguinal dissection on right side and superficial inguinal dissection on left side

(c) Neoadjuvant chemotherapy and then ilioinguinal dissection on right side

(d) Ilioinguinal dissection on right side and then adjuvant therapy

(Answer is A) This is in low risk category patients with low-grade stage T1 lesions that lack vascular invasion should be treated with antibiotics for 4 to 6 weeks.

84. What should be the management of patient with T2 grade 1 penile lesion, also having 2 superficial mobile right inguinal L.N. of 3 cm?

(a) 4 weeks of antibiotics, reassessment and plan according to FNAC

(b) Ilioinguinal dissection on right side and superficial inguinal dissection on left side

(c) Neoadjuvant chemotherapy and then ilioinguinal dissection on right side

(d) Ilioinguinal dissection on right side and then adjuvant therapy

(Answer is B) This is in high risk category. Minimum is superficial or modified inguinal LN dissection and on the side of LN involvement, ilioinguinal dissection is must.

85. Radiation therapy may be considered in a following group of patients with penile cancer *except:*

(a) Young individuals presenting with small, superficial, exophytic lesion

(b) 2 to 4 cm invasive lesion

(c) Patients refusing surgery as an initial form of treatment

(d) Patients with inoperable tumor or distant metastases who require local therapy

(Answer is B) Radiation therapy may be considered in a select group of patients: (1) young individuals presenting with small (2 to 4 cm), superficial, exophytic, noninvasive lesions on the glans or coronal sulcus; (2) patients refusing surgery as an initial form of treatment; and (3) patients with inoperable tumor or distant metastases who require local therapy for the primary tumor but who express a desire to retain the penis.

86. Chemotherapy drugs used for carcinoma penis is:

(a) BEP (b) MVAC

(c) CMF (d) VBM

(Answer is D) Combination vincristine, bleomycin, and methotrexate therapy is administered in 8-12 weekly courses.

87. The most frequent sign of penile metastasis is:

(a) Priapism (b) Penile swelling

(c) Nodularity (d) Ulceration

(Answer is A) The most frequent sign of penile metastasis is priapism.

88. LASER therapy in penile carcinoma can be used for all the following staging of penile carcinoma *except:*

(a) Carcinoma in situ

(b) Bowenoid papulosis

(c) T1

(d) T2

(Answer is D) Laser therapy has gained popularity for the treatment of premalignant lesions and CIS (Bowen's disease, erythroplasia of Queyrat, bowenoid papulosis) as well as some stage Ta and T1 penile cancers.

89. The laser most commonly reported in the treatment of squamous cell carcinoma of penis is:

(a) CO_2 (b) Nd YAG
(c) KTP (d) Holmium

(Answer is B) The laser most commonly reported in the treatment of squamous cell carcinoma has been the Nd:YAG laser.

90. Which statement regarding partial penectomy is not true?

(a) Successful local control is accomplished in the patients by amputation of the penis at least 2 cm proximal to the tumor
(b) The urethra is dissected for a distance of 1 to 1.5 cm proximal to the corpora and then transected
(c) A ventral urethrostomy is constructed by approximating the urethra to the adjacent penile skin
(d) The local recurrence rate after partial penectomy has ranged from 0% to 8%

(Answer is B) The urethra is dissected for a distance of 1 to 1.5 cm distal to the proximal corpora and then transected.

91. Regarding boundaries of dissection in modified groin lymphadenectomy, all are true *except:*

(a) Inguinal ligament superiorly
(b) Sartorius muscle laterally
(c) Adductor medius medially
(d) The floor of the triangle is composed of the pectineus muscle and iliopsoas

(Answer is C) The femoral triangle is bounded by the inguinal ligament superiorly, the sartorius muscle laterally, and the adductor longus medially. The floor of the triangle is composed of the pectineus muscle medially and the iliopsoas laterally.

92. Regarding boundaries of dissection in modified groin lymphadenectomy, all are true *except:*

(a) Medially–adductor longus muscle
(b) Laterally–femoral artery
(c) Superiorly–spermatic cord
(d) Inferiorly–base of femoral triangle

(Answer is D) The boundaries of the dissection are the adductor longus muscle medially, the femoral artery laterally, the spermatic cord superiorly, and the fossa ovalis inferiorly.

93. Modified inguinofemoral lymphadenectomy all are true *except:*

(a) Shorter skin incision
(b) Limitation of the dissection by excluding the area lateral to the femoral artery
(c) Preservation of the saphenous vein
(d) Need to transpose the sartorius muscle

(Answer is D) Key aspects of the procedure are (1) shorter skin incision, (2) limitation of the dissection by excluding the area lateral to the femoral artery and caudal to the fossa ovalis, (3) preservation of the saphenous vein, and (4) elimination of the need to transpose the sartorius muscle.

94. Pelvic lymphadenectomy for carcinoma penis should include all *except:*

(a) Distal common iliac LN
(b) Proximal iliac LN
(c) External iliac LN
(d) Obturator LN

(Answer is B) Pelvic lymphadenectomy should include the distal common iliac, external iliac, and obturator nodes. No further benefit is gained from proximal iliac or para-aortic dissection.

95. Most common location of tumor in male urethra is:

(a) Penile urethra

(b) Prostatic urethra
(c) Urethral meatus
(d) Bulbomembranous urethra

(Answer is D) The bulbomembranous urethra is involved most frequently, accounting for 60% of tumors, followed by the penile urethra (30%) and the prostatic urethra (10%).

96. Most common histological variant of tumor in male urethra:

(a) Squamous cell carcinoma
(b) Adenocarcinoma
(c) Lymphoma
(d) Melanoma

(Answer is A) Overall, 80% of male urethral cancers are squamous cell carcinoma; 15% are transitional cell carcinoma; and 5% are adenocarcinoma, melanoma, lymphoma, paraganglioma, sarcoma, or undifferentiated tumor.

97. Male urethral cancer invading into prostate is staged as:

(a) T1 (b) T2
(c) T3 (d) T4

(Answer is B)

T1 Tumor invades subepithelial connective tissue.
T2 Tumor invades any of the following: corpus spongiosum, prostate, periurethral muscle.
T3 Tumor invades any of the following: corpus cavernosum, beyond prostatic capsule, anterior vagina, bladder neck.
T4 Tumor invades other adjacent organs.

98. Which statement regarding management of male urethral cancer is not true?

(a) Anterior urethral carcinoma prognosis is better than that of posterior urethral carcinoma
(b) Benefit from prophylactic inguinal lymph node dissection has also been demonstrated in urethral cancer
(c) Partial penectomy with a 2 cm negative margin is the treatment of choice for tumors infiltrating the corpus spongiosum and localized to the distal half of the penis
(d) For carcinoma of the bulbomembranous urethra radical cystoprostatectomy, pelvic lymphadenectomy, and total penectomy are usually required

(Answer is B) As opposed to penile carcinoma, benefit from prophylactic inguinal lymph node dissection has not been demonstrated in urethral cancer.

99. Which urological malignancy is more common in females?

(a) Kidney (b) Ureter
(c) Bladder (d) Urethra

(Answer is D) The ratio of female to male predominance is reported as 4:1, and female urethral carcinoma is the only urologic malignant neoplasm that is more common in women than in men.

100. Most common histological variant of tumor in female urethra:

(a) Squamous cell carcinoma
(b) Adenocarcinoma
(c) Lymphoma
(d) Melanoma

(Answer is A) Squamous cell carcinoma is the most common histologic type, accounting for 50% to 70% of all cases.

101. Most significant prognostic factor for local control and survival in female urethral carcinoma is:

(a) Histological variant
(b) Anatomical location and extent of tumor
(c) Presence of hematuria and pain
(d) Age at presentation

(Answer is B) Compared with proximal urethral cancers, distal lesions are associated with improved survival.

102. Time taken for imbibition and inosculation is:

(a) 24 hours each
(b) 24 and 48 hours respectively
(c) 48 and 24 hours respectively
(d) 48 hours each

(Answer is D) The initial phase, imbibition, takes about 48 hours. The second phase, inosculation, also requires about 48 hours and is the phase in which true microcirculation is re-established in the graft.

103. The full-thickness skin graft has all the following features *except:*

(a) More fastidious vascular characteristics
(b) Contract more
(c) More durable
(d) More lymphatics

(Answer is B) The full-thickness skin graft tends to have more fastidious vascular characteristics, but it does not contract as much and is more durable when mature.

104. All are true regarding buccal mucosal graft *except:*

(a) It has a panlaminar plexus
(b) It can be thinned somewhat while preserving the physical characteristics and not adversely affecting the vascular characteristics
(c) It is thought to have optimal vascular characteristics
(d) Graft has a "dry epithelial" surface which is thought to be a favorable for urethral reconstructive surgery

(Answer is D) Graft has a "wet epithelial" surface which is thought to be a favorable characteristic for many cases of urethral reconstructive surgery.

105. In which flap vascular continuity and the cutaneous continuity in the flap base are intact?

(a) Island flap
(b) Peninsula flap
(c) Free microvascular flap
(d) Random flap

(Answer is B) Peninsula flap: The vascular continuity and the cutaneous continuity in the flap base are intact.

106. The pendulous urethra is lined with:

(a) Simple squamous epithelium
(b) Stratified squamous epithelium
(c) Cuboidal epithelium
(d) Transitional epithelium

(Answer is A) The pendulous urethra is lined with simple squamous epithelium.

107. The membranous urethra is lined with:

(a) Simple squamous epithelium
(b) Stratified squamous epithelium
(c) Cuboidal epithelium
(d) Transitional epithelium

(Answer is D) The membranous urethra is lined with transitional epithelium.

108. Which segment of the urethra is unattached to fixed structures?

(a) Pendulous urethra
(b) Bulbous urethra
(c) Membranous urethra
(d) Prostatic urethra

(Answer is C) Membranous urethra: This segment of the urethra is unattached to fixed structures, has the distinction of being the only portion of the male urethra that is not invested by another structure.

109. Blood is supplied to the skin of the dorsal penis by:

(a) Superficial external pudendal vessels
(b) Deep external pudendal vessels
(c) Superficial internal pudendal vessels
(d) Deep internal pudendal vessels

(Answer is A) Blood is supplied to the skin of the penis by the left and right superficial external pudendal vessels.

110. The blood supply to the scrotal wall and ventral penile skin is:

(a) Superficial external pudendal vessels
(b) Deep external pudendal vessels
(c) Superficial internal pudendal vessels
(d) Deep internal pudendal vessels

(Answer is D) The blood supply to the scrotal wall and ventral penile skin is based on the posterior scrotal artery, a superficial vessel from the deep internal pudendal artery.

111. The deep drainage venous system of penis consists of:

(a) Superficial dorsal vein and saphenous veins
(b) Deep dorsal and circumflex veins
(c) Crural and cavernosal veins
(d) Superficial and deep dorsal veins

(Answer is C) The deep drainage system consists of the crural and cavernosal veins.

112. BXO has been associated with:

(a) Treponema pallidum
(b) Hemophilus ducreyi
(c) Borrelia burgdorferi
(d) Chlamydia trichomatis

(Answer is C) Several reports have suggested the association with chronic infection by a spirochete, Borrelia burgdorferi.

113. All *except* one investigation has been used for the evaluation of urethral stricture:

(a) Urethrography (b) Urethroscopy
(c) USG (d) MRI

(Answer is D) The use of magnetic resonance for routine strictures or pelvic fracture urethral distraction defects is not beneficial.

114. Internal urethrotomy is usually done by making a single incision at:

(a) 3 and 9 O'clock position
(b) 5 and 7 O'clock position
(c) 6 O'clock position
(d) 12 O'clock position

(Answer is D) Internal urethrotomy is done by making a single incision at the 12 O'clock position.

115. The most common complication of internal urethrotomy is:

(a) Recurrence
(b) Bleeding
(c) Extravasation of fluid
(d) Erectile dysfunction

(Answer is A) The most common complication of internal urethrotomy is recurrence of stricture.

116. Factors that contribute to success of internal urethrotomy are all *except:*

(a) Strictures of the bulbous urethra
(b) Stricture should be less than 1.5 cm in length
(c) Stricture should not be associated with dense deep spongiofibrosis
(d) Traumatic stricture

(Answer is D) The factors that contribute to success of internal urethrotomy have been defined as follows: Internal urethrotomy should be reserved for strictures of the bulbous urethra; the stricture should be less than 1.5 cm in length; and the stricture should not be associated with dense deep spongiofibrosis.

117. Ideal treatment for 2 cm bulbar urethral stricture is:

(a) Urethral dilation
(b) Internal urethrotomy
(c) Buccal urethroplasty
(d) Primary End-End anastomosis

(Answer is D) It has now been demonstrated with certainty that the most dependable technique of anterior urethral reconstruction is the complete excision of the area of fibrosis, with a primary reanastomosis of the normal ends of the anterior urethra.

118. Which statement regarding grafts and flaps is true?

(a) Onlay procedures are attended with a higher success rate than tubularized procedures and among tubularised procedures flaps are better than grafts
(b) Onlay procedures are attended with a lower success rate than tubularized procedures and among tubularised procedures flaps are better than grafts
(c) Onlay procedures are attended with a higher success rate than tubularized procedures and among tubularised procedures grafts are better than flaps
(d) Onlay procedures are attended with a lower success rate than tubularized procedures and among tubularised procedures grafts are better than flaps

(Answer is A) Onlay procedures (graft or flap) are attended with a higher success rate than tubularized grafts or tubularized skin islands. Tubularized flaps provide better results than tubularized grafts.

119. Which statement regarding distraction injury of urethra is not true?

(a) Urethral distraction injuries are the result of blunt pelvic trauma and accompany about 10% of pelvic fracture injuries
(b) Distraction injuries are for all intents unique to the membranous urethra
(c) In injuries, in which a strip of epithelium is left intact, the placement of an aligning catheter may allow the urethra to heal virtually unscarred
(d) In the prepubescent male, the injury seldom involves the prostatic urethra

(Answer is D) In the prepubescent male, in whom the prostatic urethra is more fragile, the injury can extend into that area.

120. In which type of congenital curvature, corpus spongiosum, and Buck's fascia are all normally developed and ventrally fused but however, there is a short area of inelastic tissue in the dartos layer of the penis that causes a relatively sharp bend?

(a) Type I (b) Type III
(c) Type IV (d) Type V

(Answer is B) In type III, the urethra, corpus spongiosum, and Buck's fascia are all normally developed and ventrally fused. However, there is a short area of inelastic tissue in the dartos layer of the penis that causes a relatively sharp bend.

121. Which type of congenital curvature is also known as the congenital short urethra?

(a) Type I (b) Type III
(c) Type IV (d) Type V

(Answer is D) Type V congenital curvature is also known as the congenital short urethra.

122. Penile reconstruction is most often done using which material?

(a) Abdominal tube graft
(b) Upper thigh graft
(c) Radial forearm graft
(d) Inflatable penile prosthesis

(Answer is C) Forearm flaps are the most commonly employed method for total phallic construction and penile reconstruction.

123. External spermatic artery is a branch of:

(a) Directly from aorta
(b) Inferior epigastric artery
(c) Inferior vesical artery
(d) Internal iliac artery

(Answer is B) Cremasteric (external spermatic) artery is a branch of inferior epigastric artery.

124. Regarding non scalpel vasectomy which statement is not true?

(a) Less incidence of infection and hematoma
(b) Less time consuming
(c) Less pain
(d) Higher rate of reversibility

(Answer is D) No-scalpel technique results in a significantly reduced incidence of hematoma, infection and pain. In addition, the no-scalpel vasectomy is performed in about 40% less time.

125. Most common complication following vasectomy is:

(a) Infection (b) Pain
(c) Sperm granuloma (d) Hematoma

(Answer is D) Hematoma is the most common complication of vasectomy with an average incidence of 2%.

126. Vasectomy disrupts the blood-testis barrier, resulting in detectable levels of serum antisperm antibodies in:

(a) 20% to 40% (b) 40% to 60%
(c) 60% to 80% (d) 80% to 100%

(Answer is C) Vasectomy disrupts the blood-testis barrier, resulting in detectable levels of serum antisperm antibodies in 60% to 80% of men.

127. Regarding spermatocele which statement is not true?

(a) More common in the caput region
(b) Frequency decreases with age
(c) Intervention for spermatocele is rarely indicated
(d) Resection of the spermatocele may cause epididymal obstruction

(Answer is B) The frequency increases with age.

128. An adult with bilateral UDT. Best management is:

(a) Bilateral orchidectomy
(b) Bilateral orchiopexy
(c) Observation
(d) Hormone replacement therapy

(Answer is B) Bilateral orchiopexy in adults can result in induction of spermatogenesis and pregnancy. It also preserves testicular hormonal function.

129. An adult with unilateral UDT and contralateral normal descended testis with fertility no longer an issue, maximal age of orchidectomy compared with observation is:

(a) Postpuberty (b) 25 years
(c) 32 years (d) 50 years

(Answer is D) When fetility is no longer an issue, some authors recommend orchidectomy. In the past, the maximal age at which orchidectomy was performed, compared with observation, was typically 32 years. However, with improvements in the outcome of patients with testicular cancer as well as a decline in perioper ative mortality, the current recommendation is now 50 years of age.

130. Regarding retractile testes in adult which statement is not true?

(a) Retractile testes in adult is usually not repaired
(b) A subset of men with retractile testes will be infertile
(c) Scrotal orchiopexy can improve the semen quality and fertility of some of these men
(d) When scrotal orchiopexy is performed for retractile testis, a dartos pouch operation should be performed

(Answer is A) It is likely that these testes will suffer from impaired temperature regulation and impaired spermatogenesis. Scrotal orchiopexy can improve the semen quality and fertility of some of these men.

131. Regarding seminal vesicle which statement is not true?

(a) The seminal vesicle, a strictly male organ (no female homolog)

(b) Develops from distal mesonephric duct at approximately 12 fetal weeks
(c) Secretions from seminal vesicle contribute 20% to 50% of the ejaculate volume
(d) Size of seminal vesicle decreases with advancing age

(Answer is C) Secretions from seminal vesicle contribute 50% to 80% of the ejaculate volume.

132. Patients with a suspected seminal vesicle abnormality or mass should be first investigated with:

(a) TRUS (b) CT
(c) MRI (d) Vasography

(Answer is A) Patients with a suspected seminal vesicle abnormality or mass felt on rectal examination should first have TRUS.

133. Absence of seminal vesicle is most commonly associated with:

(a) Ureteral agenesis (b) Renal agenesis
(c) Midline defects (d) Penile hypoplasia

(Answer is B) 79% of patients with absence of a seminal vesicle or vas deferens have ipsilateral renal agenesis, 12% have ipsilateral renal abnormalities, and only 9% have normal kidneys bilaterally.

134. Which statement regarding seminal vesicle mass is not correct?

(a) Tumors of the seminal vesicles are extremely rare
(b) Most masses within the seminal vesicles are not neoplastic
(c) Unless these cystic lesions are symptomatic, treatment is not usually necessary
(d) Most common neoplasm is primary adenocarcinoma

(Answer is D) It is more common for carcinoma of the bladder, adenocarcinoma of the prostate, lymphoma, or rectal carcinoma to secondarily involve the seminal vesicle.

135. Where do Cowper's gland ducts drain into?

(a) Ejaculatory ducts
(b) Prostatic urethra
(c) Membranous urethra
(d) Bulbous urethra

(Answer is D) Bulbous urethra

136. What is the most significant innervation of the vas deferens?

(a) Sympathetic nervous system
(b) Parasympathetic nervous system
(c) Somatic nervous system
(d) None of the above

(Answer is A) Sympathetic nervous system

137. Which statement is false concerning the epididymis?

(a) Each epididymis can be palpable at the posterolateral surface of the testis
(b) Has 3 parts: head, body and tail
(c) New batches of sperms stay in the epididymis around 2 days for maturation
(d) Shares the same blood supply of the testis

(Answer is C) New batches of sperms stay in the epididymis around 2 days for maturation

138. Which group(s) of lymph nodes drain(s) the glans penis?

(a) Internal and external iliac
(b) Superficial inguinal
(c) Deep inguinal
(d) Superficial and deep inguinal

(Answer is A) Internal and external iliac

139. What increases blood volume and pressure in corpora cavernosa during erection is:

(a) Increase in sympathetic discharge

(b) Contraction of ischiocavernosa and bulbocavernosa muscles
(c) Increase arterial flow and closure of emissary veins
(d) Shunting of blood from the dorsal to the central cavernosal artery

(Answer is C) Increase arterial flow and closure of emissary veins

140. Which area in the nervous system is tested by bulbocavernosus reflex?

(a) Brainstem (b) C_2-C_4
(c) S_2 - S_4 (d) L_2 - L_4

(Answer is C) S_2 - S_4

141. Which of the following is not a sex accessory tissue?

(a) The prostate gland
(b) Seminal vesicles
(c) Epididymis
(d) Bulbourethral glands

(Answer is C) Epididymis

142. In utero, which hormone stimulates the development of Wolffian ducts?

(a) Estradiol (b) DHT
(c) FSH (d) Testosterone

(Answer is D) Testosterone

143. What is the most common presentation of testicular cancers?

(a) Unilateral hydrocele
(b) Dull ache or heavy sensation in the lower abdomen
(c) Painless swelling or a nodule in the testicle
(d) Incidental finding on scrotal ultrasonography

(Answer is C) Painless swelling or a nodule in the testicle

144. What is the percentage of germ cell tumors among all testicular cancers?

(a) Greater than 90% (b) Lesser than 40%
(c) Greater than 70% (d) Lesser than 20%

(Answer is A) Greater than 90%

145. Seminoma is rare in patients:

(a) Younger than 10 years
(b) Older than 50 years
(c) Between 20 and 27 years
(d) Between 28 and 35 years

(Answer is A) Younger than 10 years

146. What is the 5-year survival rate for a localized testicular cancer?

(a) Over 80% (b) Over 85%
(c) Over 90% (d) Over 95%

(Answer is D) Over 95%

147. Which of the following is not a risk factor for developing testicular cancers?

(a) Environmental conditions exposing the testes to high temperature
(b) 47XXY genotype
(c) Prior testicular cancers
(d) Cryptorchidism

(Answer is A) Environmental conditions exposing the testes to high temperature

148. What is false regarding testicular cancer and cryptorchidism?

(a) The risk of developing germ cell tumor when an undescended testis is in the abdomen is greater than when it is in the inguinal canal
(b) Orchiopexy for boys younger than 6 years lowers the risk of cancer development
(c) A normally descended testis carries 5-20% risk of developing cancer when its mate is undescended

(d) The risk of cancer increases in cryptorchid patients over 33 years of age

(Answer is D) The risk of cancer increases in cryptorchid patients over 33 years of age

149. Clinically, what does not mimic testicular cancer?

(a) Epididymo-orchitis
(b) Indirect inguinal hernia
(c) Testicular microlithiasis
(d) Syphilitic gumma

(Answer is C) Testicular microlithiasis

150. What is true regarding radical inguinal orchiectomy for testicular cancer?

(a) Considered based on a histologic evidence
(b) Should not be performed through a scrotal incision
(c) Preoperative biopsy is required for histologic examination
(d) Entails early clamping of the cord at the external inguinal ring level

(Answer is B) Should not be performed through a scrotal incision

151. What is false concerning tumor markers of seminoma?

(a) Pure seminoma α-FP is normal
(b) Syncytiotrophoblastic giant cells are present, β-hCG may be elevated
(c) Spermatocytic seminomas rarely metastasize without sarcomatous differentiation
(d) Pure seminoma constitutes approximately 90% of pure germ cell tumors

(Answer is D) Pure seminoma constitutes approximately 90% of pure germ cell tumors

152. What is false regarding spermatocytic seminoma?

(a) Occurs in men over 60 years
(b) Does not contain an isochromosome 12p
(c) Constitutes a considerable part of mixed germ cell tumors
(d) Rarely metastasizes without sarcomatous differentiation

(Answer is C) Constitutes a considerable part of mixed germ cell tumors

153. Testicular germ cell tumors that produce only α-FP are:

(a) Yolk cell tumors
(b) Choriocarcinomas
(c) Embryonal carcinomas
(d) Pure seminomas

(Answer is A) Yolk cell tumors

154. In testicular cancer patients with residual disease after chemotherapy, what type is found in approximately 45% of resected specimens?

(a) Polyembryoma
(b) Teratoma
(c) Embryonal carcinoma
(d) Mixed germ cell tumor

(Answer is B) Teratoma

155. Seminomas are classified as "good risk" when which of the following is (are) present:

(a) Stem from the periphery of the testis
(b) Non-pulmonary visceral metastases
(c) Normal α-FP, β-hCG and LDH markers
(d) All of the above

(Answer is D) All of the above

156. What is true regarding biological markers of testicular cancers?

(a) High levels of α-FP are found only in non-seminomas
(b) High levels of α-FP may result from marijuana use
(c) β-hCG levels above 10,000 mIU/ml are seen only in germ cell tumors and hepatocellular carcinoma

(d) LDH is a useful marker for surveillance after tumor extirpation

(Answer is A) High levels of α-FP are found only in non-seminomas

157. Which of the following statements is false concerning testicular tumor markers?

(a) α-FP and/or β-hCG are elevated in approximately 80% to 85% of patients with non-seminomatous germ cell tumors
(b) β-hCG increases in either seminoma or non-seminoma
(c) LDH increases in 30% to 80% of pure seminoma patients and in 60% of non-seminoma patients
(d) High levels of α-FP might induce nipple tenderness or gynecomastia

(Answer is D) High levels of α-FP might induce nipple tenderness or gynecomastia

158. What is false concerning testicular tumor markers?

(a) Elevation of only α-FP indicates pure non-seminoma
(b) Elevation of α-FP might occur in chronic liver disease, hepatitis and alcohol abuse
(c) Elevation of LDH indicates tumor burden and growth rate
(d) Elevation of β-hCG above 10,000 mIU/ml is seen only in germ cell tumors

(Answer is A) Elevation of only α-FP indicates pure non-seminoma

159. What is false concerning post orchiectomy in clinical stage I seminoma?

(a) Active surveillance is recommended for patients with horseshoe kidney
(b) Adjuvant chemotherapy with a single dose of carboplatin is recommended as an alternative to radiation therapy
(c) The number of positive nodes dissected dictates the number of chemotherapy cycles to be given
(d) Cure is possible after radical orchiectomy alone

(Answer is C) The number of positive nodes dissected dictates the number of chemotherapy cycles to be given

160. What is false concerning surgical care for testicular cancer patients?

(a) Patients in whom retroperitoneal LN dissection (RPLND) reveals viable cancer cells after chemotherapy, subsequent chemotherapy is recommended
(b) Surgical resection is recommended for patients with residual disease after chemotherapy
(c) Open nerve-sparing RPLND might lead to premature ejaculation
(d) Non-seminoma patients stage I-A, I-B, 1S on long-term surveillance, relapses are expected in 80% of cases within the first year after orchiectomy

(Answer is C) Open nerve-sparing RPLND might lead to premature ejaculation

161. What is false concerning medical care for testicular cancer patients?

(a) Approximately 60% of patients, post-chemotherapy residual masses are either viable cancer cells or teratoma
(b) Nearly one half will be azoospermic after 2 years of therapy
(c) Seminoma stage II-B, primary chemotherapy with 3 cycles of bleomycin, etoposide and cisplatin (BEP), and 4 cycles of chemotherapy with etoposide and cisplatin (EP) are recommended
(d) Seminoma stage II-B, II-C, III after primary treatment with chemotherapy, surveillance is recommended for residual masses of 3 cm or less detected by PET scan

(Answer is C) Seminoma stage II-B, primary chemotherapy with 3 cycles of bleomycin, etoposide and cisplatin (BEP), and 4 cycles of chemotherapy with etoposide and cisplatin (EP) are recommended

162. What is false concerning intratubular germ cell neoplasia (ITGCN) of the testes?

(a) Adult choriocarcinoma arise from ITGCN
(b) Spermatocytic seminoma arises from ITGCN
(c) Typically, pediatric germ cell tumors (GCT) do not arise from ITGCN
(d) ITGCN is the common precursor for most of adult male GCT

(Answer is B) Spermatocytic seminoma arises from ITGCN

163. With regard to pure subtypes of testicular tumors, which statement is false?

(a) Pure embryonal carcinoma may increase serum α-FP and hCG levels
(b) Pure seminoma increases serum hCG levels in 15% of cases but not α-FP
(c) Typically, endodermal sinus tumors don't increase any tumor marker
(d) Pure choriocarcinoma is associated with high hCG levels but not α-FP

(Answer is C) Typically, endodermal sinus tumors don't increase any tumor marker

164. On managing testicular tumors, testis-sparing surgery is not indicated in:

(a) Suspected germ cell tumor (GCT) with a normal contralateral testis
(b) Case of bilateral synchronous testicular GCT
(c) Suspected benign testicular lesions
(d) Suspected GCT of < 2 cm tumor size in a solitary testis

(Answer is A) Suspected germ cell tumor (GCT) with a normal contralateral testis

165. What is true regarding brain metastases of testicular cancers?

(a) Should be suspected in any patient with a very high hCG level on diagnosis
(b) The most common subtype that causes brain metastases is choriocarcinoma
(c) These patients should receive 4 cycles of bleomycin-etoposide-cisplatin as first-line chemotherapy
(d) Early initiation of chemotherapy ensures a good prognosis

(Answer is B) The most common subtype that causes brain metastases is choriocarcinoma

166. What is false concerning teratoma of the testis?

(a) There is no clinical distinction between mature and immature teratoma
(b) Has no biological markers
(c) Sensitive to chemotherapy
(d) When large in size can be infiltrative and difficult to resect

(Answer is C) Sensitive to chemotherapy

167. Late toxicity of chemotherapy for testicular cancers might result in all of the following, *except*:

(a) Peripheral neuropathy
(b) Renal failure
(c) Raynaud phenomenon
(d) Hypogonadism

(Answer is B) Renal failure

168. What is the most common testicular neoplasm in men over 50?

(a) Lymphoma
(b) Spermatocytic seminoma
(c) Adenocarcinoma
(d) Cystadenoma

(Answer is A) Lymphoma

169. Leydig cell tumors and Sertoli cell tumors are benign in:

(a) 60%
(b) 70%
(c) 80%
(d) 90%

(Answer is D) 90%

170. What epididymal lesion is associated with von Hippel-Lindau syndrome?

(a) Mature teratoma
(b) Immature teratoma
(c) Cystadenoma
(d) Adenomatoid tumor

(Answer is C) Cystadenoma

171. What is the most common para-testicular tumor in adults?

(a) Rhabdomyosarcoma
(b) Liposarcoma
(c) Sarcomatoid tumor
(d) Angiosarcoma

(Answer is B) Liposarcoma

172. Which subtype of germ cell tumors has the highest propensity for hematogenous spread?

(a) Yolk cell tumors
(b) Spermatocytic seminoma
(c) Choriocarcinoma
(d) Embryonal carcinoma

(Answer is C) Choriocarcinoma

173. In seminomas, the risk factor(s) for metastases (is) are:

(a) Rete testis involvement
(b) Tumor size greater than 4 cm
(c) All of the above
(d) β-hCG of $\geq 10{,}000$ mIU/ml on diagnosis

(Answer is C) All of the above

174. Testicular cancer patients with bulky retroperitoneal lymph node disease greater than 3 cm should:

(a) Undergo laparoscopic lymph node sampling
(b) Receive induction chemotherapy
(c) Undergo extensive retroperitoneal lymph node dissection
(d) For palliative therapy

(Answer is B) Receive induction chemotherapy

175. What is true regarding retroperitoneal lymph nodes involvement in testicular cancers?

(a) Left testicular tumors spread to the periaortic lymph nodes
(b) Right testicular tumors spread to the interaortocaval lymph nodes
(c) The fashion of further spread in the retroperitoneum is from right to left
(d) All of the above

(Answer is D) All of the above

176. What is false concerning testicular germ cell tumors (GCT)?

(a) A patient with a history of GCTs, the finding of testicular microlithiasis on ultrasonography poses a higher risk of intratubular germ cell neoplasia
(b) Occur bilaterally approximately 2% of cases
(c) Are extragonadal in 1-5%
(d) Are more likely to contain embryonal tumor cells than tumors arising in the testis

(Answer is D) Are more likely to contain embryonal tumor cells than tumors arising in the testis

177. On presentation, what is the percentage of infertility among testicular germ cell tumor patients?

(a) 10 - 20%
(b) 20 - 60%
(c) 60 - 80%
(d) 80 - 90%

(Answer is B) 20 - 60%

178. What is the role of positron emission tomography (PET) in testicular cancer patients?

(a) Evaluates post chemotherapy residual masses in pure seminoma cases
(b) Helps stage non-seminomatous germ cell tumors
(c) All of the above
(d) Used for active surveillance in non-operable cases

(Answer is A) Evaluates post chemotherapy residual masses in pure seminoma cases

179. After chemotherapy for testicular cancers, how long does it take for spermatogenesis to return to the norm?

(a) 3 months
(b) 3 spermatogenic cycles
(c) 3 years
(d) Damage is permanent

(Answer is C) 3 years

180. What is the most common site of cancer occurrence in the male urethra?

(a) Fossa navicularis
(b) Bulbomembranous urethra
(c) Prostatic urethra
(d) External urethral meatus

(Answer is B) Bulbomembranous urethra

181. Anatomically, where is the weakest area in the corpora cavernosa?

(a) The glans
(b) The dorsal side
(c) The ventral side
(d) The root where the crura are

(Answer is C) The ventral side

182. The mature plaque in Peyronie disease stems from:

(a) The corpora cavernosa
(b) Buck's fascia
(c) The tunica albuginea
(d) The corpus spongiosum

(Answer is C) The tunica albuginea

183. How common could Peyronie disease lead to emotional distress?

(a) Uncommon
(b) Not uncommon
(c) Common
(d) Exceedingly common

(Answer is D) Exceedingly common

184. What is false concerning penile calcification in Peyronie disease (PD)?

(a) An indicative of a stable, mature disease
(b) Does not indicate the need for surgery
(c) Tunica albuginea calcifications are difficult to identify on MRI
(d) Around 35% of PD patients will have plaque calcification

(Answer is A) An indicative of a stable, mature disease

185. What is false concerning Peyronie disease?

(a) Affects men aged 40-70 years
(b) The initial inflammatory response of the tunica albuginea is chronic lymphocytic with plasma cell infiltration
(c) The natural history is to progress to fibrous, calcified plaque with penile angulation. Spontaneous resolution is uncommon
(d) Intralesional injection of verapamil helps improve pain, impotence, but not the curvature

(Answer is D) Intralesional injection of verapamil helps improve pain, impotence, but not the curvature

186. Which of the following is not a risk factor for Peyronie disease?

(a) Obesity
(b) Smoking
(c) Hypertension
(d) Diabetes mellitus

(Answer is C) Hypertension

187. What is an absolute contraindication to performing a graft procedure for a Peyronie disease patient with calcified plaque?

(a) Curvature > 70 degrees
(b) Weak erection
(c) Unstable penis with an indentation or hinge effect
(d) Short penis

(Answer is B) Weak erection

188. Which of the listed Peyronie disease medications has the property of being a nonspecific phosphodiesterase inhibitor with combined anti-inflammatory and antifibrogenic actions?

(a) PABA (b) Colchicine
(c) Pentoxifylline (d) Vitamin E

(Answer is C) Pentoxifylline

189. All of the following treatment modalities have been tried to treat Peyronie disease, *except*:

(a) Extracorporeal shockwave therapy
(b) External vacuum
(c) Low-dose chemotherapy
(d) Electromotive administration

(Answer is C) Low-dose chemotherapy

190. All of the following conditions have associations with Peyronie disease, *except*:

(a) Vitamin E deficiency
(b) Ingestion of calcium channel-blocking agents
(c) Elevations of serotonin levels
(d) Dupuytren contractures

(Answer is B) Ingestion of calcium channel-blocking agents

191. What is the most common manifestation of metastatic tumor spread to the penis?

(a) Penile swelling (eggplant sign)
(b) Discrete penile shaft nodules
(c) Penile pain of unknown origin
(d) Low-flow or stuttering priapism

(Answer is D) Low-flow or stuttering priapism

192. True about premalignant lesions of penis:

(a) Bowen's disease affects prepuce
(b) Erythroplasia of Queyrat affects shaft of penis
(c) Bowenoid papulosis is a penile intra-epithelial neoplasia but runs a benign course
(d) HPV is associated with cis in 33% cases

(Answer is C) Bowenoid papulosis is a penile intraepithelial neoplasia but runs a benign course

193. All are risk factors for Ca penis *except*:

(a) Alcohol (b) Phimosis
(c) BXO (d) Tobacco chewing

(Answer is A) Alcohol

194. Carcinoma penis type associated with HPV and having worst prognosis:

(a) Basaloid type
(b) Verrucous type
(c) Carcinoma cuniculatum
(d) Pseudoglandular type

(Answer is A) Basaloid type

195. All are true about clinical features of Ca penis *except*:

(a) Most commonly seen in glans
(b) Pain doesn't develop in proportion to the local destructive process
(c) Distant metastasis occur late in the course of the disease
(d) Compared to ulcerative type the papillary type has a tendency to early nodal metastasis and poorer 5-year survival

(Answer is D) Compared to ulcerative type the papillary type has a tendency to early nodal metastasis and poorer 5-year survival

196. What is the T status of carcinoma penis invading corpus cavernosum according to latest AJCC staging (2016)?

(a) T1
(b) T2
(c) T3
(d) T4

(Answer is C) T3

197. Organ preservation strategy for carcinoma penis is not favoured in:

(a) T1 grade 1
(b) >4 cm lesion
(c) Involvement of glans
(d) Ta Grade 2

(Answer is B) >4 cm lesion

198. Most important prognostic factor for survival in patients with squamous cell carcinoma penis is:

(a) Nodal status
(b) Tumor grade
(c) Morphological pattern
(d) Microscopic pattern

(Answer is A) Nodal status

199. Indication of ilioingional node dissection in carcinoma penis all *except*:

(a) T2 shaft of penis
(b) T2 glans
(c) Well differentiated with vascular invasion
(d) Moderately differentiated in prepuce

(Answer is D) Moderately differentiated in prepuce

200. False about LHRH antagonists:

(a) Flare up phenomenon can occur
(b) Reduces LH concentration by 84% in 24 hours
(c) Severe allergic reactions can occur with abarelix
(d) Degarelix has no knowm systemic allergic reactions

(Answer is A) Flare up phenomenon can occur

CHAPTER

8

Renal Physiology and Pathophysiology

1. **Which statement regarding creatinine is not true?**
   (a) Creatinine production is constant within an individual from day to day
   (b) Marked variation in production rates between individuals
   (c) The absolute rate depends upon muscle mass
   (d) As GFR falls, tubular secretion of creatinine also decreases

(Answer is D) Creatinine

- Creatinine production is constant within an individual from day to day.
- Marked variation in production rates between individuals.
- The absolute rate depends upon muscle mass, which in turn is influenced by age, sex and body mass.
- Every 50% reduction in GFR results in a doubling of PCr.
- As GFR falls, tubular secretion of creatinine increases; so, PCr may not change noticeably.
- Creatinine clearance may overestimate GFR as renal function slowly declines when measured in the "steady state".
- Creatinine production may increase in states of increased muscle breakdown or increased dietary protein intake.
- Creatinine production may decrease with liver cirrhosis.

2. **Under normal resting conditions, RBF is how much of total cardiac output?**
   (a) 10% (b) 20%
   (c) 30% (d) 40%

(Answer is B) Under normal resting conditions, RBF is 20% of total cardiac output.

3. **Correct pattern of renal blood flow is:**
   (a) Flow in outer cortex is 3 times of inner cortex, which in turn is 3 times of medulla
   (b) Flow in inner cortex is 3 times of outer cortex, which in turn is 3 times of medulla
   (c) Flow in outer cortex is 3 times of medulla, which in turn is 3 times of inner cortex
   (d) Flow in inner cortex is 3 times of medulla, which in turn is 3 times of outer cortex

(Answer is A) Flow to the outer cortex is two to three times greater than that to the inner cortex, which in turn is two to four times greater than that to the medulla.

4. **Autoregulation of intra-glomerular capillary pressure is effective to an MAP of about:**
   (a) 50 mm Hg (b) 70 mm Hg
   (c) 90 mm Hg (d) 100 mm Hg

(Answer is B) Autoregulation of IGP is effective to an MAP of about 70 mm Hg; below that, reductions in MAP lead to similar reductions in GFR, and below an MAP of 40 mm Hg, filtration ceases.

5. **Which ion delivery triggers a response through macula densa that ultimately regulates the renal plasma flow?**
   (a) Na (b) Cl
   (c) K (d) H

(Answer is B) Increased Cl^- delivery triggers a response through the macula densa that ultimately leads to an increase in afferent arteriolar tone and subsequent decrease in RPF, thus returning SN-GFR (and tubular flow) back to baseline.

6. **Which is considered to be the best measure of GFR?**

(a) DTPA (b) Creatinine
(c) Inulin (d) Urea

(Answer is C) Inulin is a fructose polysaccharide that meets the requirements, and inulin clearance is thought to be the best measure of GFR.

7. **Which is the most potent vasoconstrictor yet identified?**

(a) Vasopressin (b) Angiotensin
(c) Norepinephrine (d) Endothelin

(Answer is D) Endothelin is the most potent vasoconstrictor yet identified.

8. **Effects of angiotensin II mediated by AT2 receptor is:**

(a) Vasoconstriction
(b) Aldosterone release
(c) Sodium retention
(d) Intrarenal dilation

(Answer is D) The classical effects of angiotensin II (vasoconstriction, aldosterone release, sodium retention) are mediated by the AT1 receptor. The AT2 receptor, however, may cause intrarenal dilation and be protective against renal ischemic injury.

9. **ET-1 release is stimulated by all *except:***

(a) Angiotensin II (b) ADH
(c) Thrombin (d) NO

(Answer is D) ET-1 release is stimulated by angiotensin II, antidiuretic hormone, thrombin, cytokines, reactive oxygen species, and shearing forces acting on the vascular endothelium. ET-1 release is inhibited by nitric oxide as well as by prostacyclin and ANP.

10. **Which statement regarding ANP is not true?**

(a) ANP can increase GFR with increase in RBF
(b) ANP dilates vessels that have been preconstricted by norepinephrine, angiotensin II, or vasopressin
(c) ANP production increases during bilateral obstructive uropathy, which is one mechanism of preserving GFR
(d) ANP increases natriuresis through increased GFR, decreased renin, and decreased aldosterone production

(Answer is A) ANP can increase GFR without a change in RBF.

11. **Which statement regarding erythropoiesis is not true?**

(a) Mature RBCs are produced from multipotent progenitor cells, which in turn are derived from the fetal liver
(b) The earliest committed cell is the erythroid burst-forming unit
(c) The kidney is responsible for the majority of EPO production (90%), and the liver may contribute a smaller amount (10%)
(d) In states of anemia and chronic inflammation, erythropoiesis is increased

(Answer is D) In states of chronic inflammation, erythropoiesis is decreased.

12. **Main actions for Vitamin D activity are all *except:***

(a) Intestine (increases intestinal absorption of calcium and, to a lesser extent, phosphorus)
(b) Bones (regulates osteoblast activity)
(c) Kidney (increases reabsorption of calcium)
(d) Parathyroid gland (stimulates PTH release)

(Answer is D) The four main target organs are the intestine (increases intestinal absorption of calcium and, to a lesser extent, phosphorus), the bones (regulates osteoblast activity and, in combination with PTH, allows osteoclast activation and bone resorption), the kidney (increases reabsorption of calcium), and the parathyroid gland (suppresses PTH release).

13. Calcitriol production occurs in which organ and by which hydroxylation?

(a) Liver and 1 α-hydroxylase
(b) Kidney and 1 α-hydroxylase
(c) Liver and 25 α-hydroxylase
(d) Kidney and 25 α-hydroxylase

(Answer is B) A second hydroxylation occurs within the tubular cell. Because these cells contain both 1 α-hydroxylase and 24 α-hydroxylase, hydroxylation produces either inactive 24, 25-dihydroxycholecalciferol or 1, 25-dihydroxycholecalciferol (calcitriol), which is the biologically active form and 100 times more potent than calcidiol.

14. The renal effects of PTH are all *except:*

(a) It increases active calcium reabsorption at the level of the distal tubule
(b) It decreases phosphate reabsorption in the proximal convoluted tubule
(c) It stimulates calcitriol production by increasing 1 α-hydoxylase levels
(d) It stimulates calcitriol production by increasing 24 α-hydoxylase levels also

(Answer is D) It stimulates calcitriol production by increasing 1 α-hydoxylase levels while decreasing 24 α-hydroxylase levels.

15. All are action of ADH *except:*

(a) It increases the passive reabsorption of water at the level of the collecting duct
(b) Through interaction with the V2 receptor, it facilitates the insertion of preformed water channels AQP-2 into the luminal membrane of the principal cells
(c) Increases sodium reabsorption and potassium excretion, increases prostaglandin synthesis, increases ACTH secretion (through V3 receptors)
(d) It increases systemic vascular resistance through interaction with the V2 receptor

(Answer is D) ADH increases systemic vascular resistance through interaction with the VI receptor.

16. Factors stimulating the release of antidiuretic hormone are all *except:*

(a) Hyperosmolarity (b) Hypovolemia
(c) Pregnancy (d) Ethanol

(Answer is D) Stimuli are: Hyperosmolarity, hypovolemia, stress, nausea, pregnancy, hypoglycemia, nicotine and morphine.

17. PCT is responsible for reabsorption of how much of glomerular filtrate?

(a) 60% (b) 70%
(c) 80% (d) 90%

(Answer is A) PCT is responsible for reabsorption of 60% of the glomerular filtrate.

18. Which segment of nephron is critical to the formation of the interstitial concentration gradient?

(a) Thin ascending LOH
(b) Thick ascending LOH
(c) Cortical collecting duct
(d) Medullary collecting duct

(Answer is B) Sodium reabsorption along the Thick assending LOH, in the absence of water reabsorption, is critical to the formation of the interstitial concentration gradient.

19. Which statement regarding cortical collecting duct is not true?

(a) Condition that leads to decreased luminal flow rates, or increased aldosterone production, can lead to reduced potassium excretion

(b) The water permeability of the CCT can be greatly increased due to the insertion of preformed AQP-5 water channels into the luminal membrane

(c) Type A intercalated cells, involved mostly with H + secretion

(d) Type 8 intercalated cells. involved mostly with bicarbonate secretion

(Answer is B) The water permeability of the CCT is low in the basal state. However, it can be greatly increased in the presence ofADH. This is due to the insertion of preformed AQP-2 water channels into the luminal membrane.

20. A high UNa of greater than 20 would indicate to:

(a) Renal failure (b) Heart failure

(c) Cirrhosis (d) Nephrotic failure

(Answer is A) A high UNa of greater than 20 would indicate to renal failure. A low UNa of less than 20 would suggest heart failure, cirrhosis, or nephrotic syndrome.

21. Therapy for hyponatremia includes all *except:*

(a) Fluid restriction plus administration of hypertonic (3%) saline (about I ml/kg/hr)

(b) The serum sodium concentration should be raised no more than 25 mEq/l in the first 48 hours

(c) Target goal should be 120 to125 mEq/l

(d) If the hyponatremia is severe but chronic, the rate of correction is 2 mEq /l/hr

(Answer is D) If the hyponatremia is severe but chronic, the rate of correction should not exceed 8 to 12 mmol/l/day, or a cerebral demyelination syndrome may occur. Therefore, the rate of correction should be slower (0.5 to 1 mEq/l/hr).

22. The sodium deficit can be calculated as:

(a) 0.5 × body weight (kg) × (125 - plasma [Na])

(b) 0.5 × body weight (kg) × (145 - plasma [Na])

(c) Body weight (kg) × (125 - plasma [Na])

(d) Body weight (kg) × (145 - plasma [Na])

(Answer is A) Total sodium deficit to reach this point can be calculated as (Volume of distribution) × body weight (kg) × (125 - plasma [Na]) where volume of distribution is 0.5 for men.

23. The water deficit can be calculated as:

(a) Body weight (kg) × ((plasma [140]/1Na)-1)

(b) Body weight (kg) × ((plasma [Nal]/125)-1)

(c) 0.5 × body weight (kg) × ((plasma [Na]/125) - 1)

(d) 0.5 × body weight (kg) × ((plasma [Na]/140) - 1)

(Answer is D) The water deficit can be calculated as (Volume of distribution) × body weight (kg) × ((plasma [Na]/140) -I) where again the volume of distribution i s 0.5 for men.

24. Potassium is driven into the cells by all *except:*

(a) Insulin (b) Bicarbonate

(c) β-agonists (d) ACE inhibitors

(Answer is D) Potassium is driven into the cells by insulin, bicarbonate and β-agonists.

25. Type IV RTA all are correct *except:*

(a) It is due to impairment of cation exchange in the proximal tubule w ith reduced secretion of both H+ and K+

(b) It is due to aldosterone deficiency or resistance

(c) Patients are able to decrease urine pH to less than 5.5 in response to the acidosis

(d) Renal stones do not form

(Answer is A) Type 4 RTA is due to impairment of cation exchange in the distal tubule with reduced secretion of both H + and K+.

26. Which RTA is associated with renal stones?

(a) RTA I (b) RTA II

(c) RTA III (d) RTA IV

(Answer is A) Type I RTA (distal) is the only type associated with renal stones.

27. Which is the most common type of fibrous lesion?

(a) Intimal fibroplasia
(b) Medial fibroplasia
(c) True fibromuscular hyperplasia
(d) Perimedial fibroplasia

(Answer is B) Medial fibroplasia is the most common of the fibrous lesions, constituting 75% to 80% of the total number.

28. "String of beads" appearance is angiographically seen in which type of fibrous lesion?

(a) Intimal fibroplasia
(b) Medial fibroplasia
(c) True fibromuscular hyperplasia
(d) Perimedial fibroplasia

(Answer is B) Angiographically, medial fibroplasia demonstrates a typical "string of beads" appearance involving the distal two thirds of the main renal artery and branches.

29. Which fibrous lesion is called as girlie disease?

(a) Intimal fibroplasia
(b) Medial fibroplasia
(c) True fibromuscular hyperplasia
(d) Perimedial fibroplasia

(Answer is D) Perimedial fibroplasia occurs predominantly in young women between the ages of 15 and 30 years and has therefore been referred to, rather crudely, as girlie disease.

30. Which is only renal arterial disease in which true hyperplasia of the smooth muscle cells is present?

(a) Intimal fibroplasia
(b) Medial fibroplasia
(c) Fibromuscular hyperplasia
(d) Perimedial fibroplasia

(Answer is C) Fibromuscular hyperplasia is an extremely rare disease, constituting only 2% to 3% of fibrous lesions, and tends to occur in children and young adults. This is the only renal arterial disease in which true hyperplasia of the smooth muscle cells is present.

31. Primary site of synthesis of angiotensinogen and renin is:

(a) Both in kidney
(b) Both in liver
(c) Angiotensinogen in kidney and renin in liver
(d) Angiotensinogen kidney in liver and renin in kidney

(Answer is D) The liver is the primary site of synthesis of angiotensinogen, which is not stored but secreted directly after production. The kidney is the major site of renin production.

32. Renin is secreted from:

(a) JG cell of afferent arteriole
(b) JG cell of efferent arteriole
(c) Macula densa
(d) Principle cell of afferent arteriole

(Answer is A) Renin is a single-polypeptide-chain aspartyl protease that is secreted from the juxtaglomerular cells of the afferent arteriole.

33. Macula densa cells are present at which part of nephron?

(a) Distal tubule
(b) Descending thin LOH
(c) Ascending thin LOH
(d) Ascending thick LOH

(Answer is D) The macula densa region of the thick ascending loop of Henle comes in close proximity to the juxtaglomerular cells and influences renin release.

34. All *except* one leads to increased renin secretion:

(a) Increased cell stretch as a result of renal hyperperfusion
(b) Stimulation of the β-adrenergic nerves
(c) Prostaglandin E2 and I2 (prostacyclin) as well as exogenously administered arachidonic acid
(d) Agents that increase adenylate cyclase activity

(Answer is A) Diminished cell stretch as a result of renal hypoperfusion hyperpolarizes the juxtaglomerular cells, resulting in decreased intracellular calcium and increased renin release.

35. Major site of ACE activity for the systemic RAAS is:

(a) Liver (b) Lung
(c) Kidney (d) Adrenal

(Answer is B) Pulmonary endothelial ACE is presumed to be the major site of ACE activity for the systemic RAAS.

36. Renal autoregulation fails to maintain the GFR when the luminal diameter of the renal artery is stenosed by more than:

(a) 50% (b) 60%
(c) 70% (d) 80%

(Answer is C) Renal autoregulation fails to maintain the GFR when renal perfusion decreases below 70 to 80 mm Hg. This occurs when the luminal diameter of the renal artery is stenosed by more than 70% of the original size.

37. Cholesterol embolism occurs most commonly in:

(a) Kidney (b) Urinary bladder
(c) Adrenal (d) Urethra

(Answer is A) The organs most commonly affected by atheroembolism are the kidney, spleen, pancreas and gastrointestinal tract.

38. All are true about renovascular hypertension *except:*

(a) The onset of hypertension before the age of 30 years or after the age of 55 years
(b) Longer duration of hypertension
(c) Hypertension that is difficult to control with two or three medications
(d) Accelerated, malignant hypertension or hypertensive crises are more frequently associated with RVH

(Answer is B) Sudden onset and shorter duration of hypertension are usually associated with RVH; they may also be associated with a better chance of cure after treatment.

39. Risk factors as strongly predictive of significant ARAS are all *except:*

(a) Higher age (b) CAD
(c) Male gender (d) History of CHF

(Answer is C) A multivariate logistic-regression analysis identified the following five risk factors as strongly predictive of significant ARAS: higher age, coronary artery disease, a history of congestive heart failure, female gender, and peripheral vascular disease.

40. In captopril test which drug need not be discontinued before the test?

(a) β blockers
(b) Diuretics
(c) ACE inhibitors
(d) Ca channel blocker

(Answer is A) Patients may continue to take β blockers, but all diuretics and ACE inhibitors need to be discontinued for at least 1 week before the test.

41. All are true about captopril test *except:*

(a) This is only functional test of RVH that does not provide anatomic information
(b) The test is not reliable in patients who are azotemic, nor is it sufficiently accurate for use in children
(c) Suitable for use as a general screening test for RVH

(d) Administration of captopril in patients with RVH show a higher reactionary rise of PRA than patients with essential hypertension

(Answer is C) The low sensitivity of the captopril test makes it not suitable for use as a general screemng test for RVH.

42. Best results for captopril renography, especially in patients with impaired renal function is by:

(a) OIH (b) 99^{m}Tc-MAG3
(c) 99^{m}Tc DTPA (d) EC

(Answer is B) 99^{m}Tc-MAG3 has shown the best results for captopril renography, especially in patients with impaired renal function.

43. Which test remains the gold standard for diagnosing renal arterial disease?

(a) Duplex USG
(b) CT angiography
(c) Intra-arterial angiography
(d) MR angiography

(Answer is C) Intra-arterial angiography remains the gold standard for diagnosing renal artery disease, and it is the test against which the results of other tests are compared.

44. Patients with low or moderate suspicion of RVH, which investigation is performed as preliminary test?

(a) Plasma renin activity
(b) Renal angiography
(c) Captopril test
(d) Captopril renography

(Answer is D) Patients with low or moderate suspicion of RVH are more problematic. In these cases, it is probably reasonable to perform captopril renography as a preliminary test. A positive test should be followed by further testing, preferably definitive diagnosis through angiography.

45. In which renal artery disease initial medical management is preferred?

(a) Intimal fibroplasia
(b) Medial fibroplasia
(c) True fibromuscular hyperplasia
(d) Perimedial fibroplasia

(Answer is B) Medical management of hypertension is the preferred initial treatment for patients with medial fibroplasia because loss of renal function from progressive obstruction is uncommon with this disease.

46. Clinical clues suggesting renal salvability by renal revascularization includes all *except:*

(a) Angiographic demonstration of retrograde filling of the distal renal arterial tree
(b) A renal biopsy showing well-preserved glomeruli
(c) Kidney size less than 9 cm
(d) Function of the involved kidney on isotope renography

(Answer is C) Helpful clinical clues suggesting renal salvability include: (1) angiographic demonstration of retrograde filling ofthe distal renal arterial tree by collateral vessels on the side of total arterial occlusion (2) a renal biopsy showing well-preserved glomeruli (3) kidney size greater than 9 cm, and (4) function of the involved kidney on isotope renography or IV pyelography.

47. Revascularization to preserve renal function is generally not worthwhile in patients with serum creatinine more than:

(a) 2 (b) 3
(c) 4 (d) 5

(Answer is C) Revascularization to preserve renal function is generally not worthwhile in patients with severe azotemia (serum creatinine level >4 mg/dl).

48. Histological finding that indicates irreversible ischemic renal injury that obviates any benefit from relief of renal arterial obstruction:

(a) Tubular atrophy

(b) Interstitial fibrosis
(c) Arteriolar sclerosis
(d) Glomerular hyalinization

(Answer is D) Histologic findings of tubular atrophy, interstitial fibrosis, and arteriolar sclerosis are of lesser importance and do not necessarily preclude recovery of renal function; these findings may merely reflect the histologic changes of chronic reversible renal ischemia. However, the finding of widespread glomerular hyalinization indicates irreversible ischemic renal injury that obviates any benefit from relief of renal arterial obstruction.

49. Technical success of PTA for FD and atherosclerotic renal artery disease respectively is:

(a) 90% and 15%
(b) 50% for both diseases
(c) 70% and 30%
(d) 15% and 90%

(Answer is A) In cases of FD without stent placement, technical success has been more than 90%. In cases of RVH secondary to ASO, the cure rate is lower than that for FD, commonly around 15%.

50. Higher success of PTA with stenting is seen in treating patients with:

(a) Ostial renal artery atherosclerotic stenosis
(b) Branch renal artery atherosclerotic stenosis
(c) Main renal artery fibrous stenosis
(d) Branch renal artery fibrous stenosis

(Answer is A) Overall higher success of PTA with stenting is seen in treating ostial ASO when compared with PTA alone.

51. Which is most common type of renal artery aneurysms?

(a) Saccular aneurysms
(b) Fusiform aneurysms
(c) Dissecting aneurysms
(d) Cribiform aneurysms

(Answer is A) Saccular aneurysms are the most common type and constitute about 75% of renal artery aneurysms. They generally occur at the bifurcation of the renal artery.

52. Factors that appear to predispose to aneurysmal rupture include all *except:*

(a) Presence of calcification
(b) Size greater than 2 cm
(c) Hypertension
(d) Pregnancy

(Answer is A) Factors that appear to predispose to aneurysmal rupture include absent or incomplete calcification, aneurysmal size greater than 2 cm in diameter, coexisting hypertension and pregnancy.

53. Which is most common type of renal arteriovenous fistulas?

(a) Congenital
(b) Acquired resulting from needle biopsy
(c) Acquired resulting from renal trauma
(d) Idiopathic

(Answer is B) Acquired fistulas are the most common type, accounting for 70% to 75% of all renal arteriovenous fistulas. On angiography they appear as solitary communications between an artery and a vein. By far the most common cause is iatrogenic trauma resulting from needle biopsy of the kidney.

54. Fistulas occurring after needle biopsy of the kidney close spontaneously within:

(a) Generally heals in 2 hours
(b) Generally heals in 2 days
(c) Generally heals in 2 months
(d) Generally heals in 2 years

(Answer is D) Approximately 70% of fistulas occurring after needle biopsy of the kidney close spontaneously within 18 months.

55. Site of renal artery thrombosis and embolism respectively is:

(a) Proximal third of renal artery and peripheral arterial branches
(b) Distal third of renal artery and peripheral arterial branches
(c) Peripheral arterial branches and distal third of renal artery
(d) Peripheral arterial branches and proximal third of renal artery

(Answer is A) Renal arterial thrombosis commonly involves the proximal or middle third of the main renal artery, whereas renal arterial embolization generally involves peripheral arterial branches.

56. Page's kidney all are true *except:*

(a) Kidney compressed by a subcapsular or perirenal process causing renal ischemia
(b) Bilateral hypersecretion of renin
(c) Causes include blunt trauma, closed renal biopsy, anticoagulation, and hemorrhage from a tumor
(d) A hematoma may reabsorb, relieving the parenchymal compression without forming an adhesive fibrotic pseudocapsule

(Answer is B) The clinical equivalent of this hypertensive model is the kidney compressed by a subcapsular or perirenal process causing renal ischemia, inducing unilateral hypersecretion of renin and contralateral suppression.

57. RAS in children is caused by all *except:*

(a) Takayasu arteritis
(b) Middle aortic syndrome
(c) Neurofibromatosis
(d) PAN

(Answer is D) RAS in children is caused by:

- Takayasu arteritis.
- Fibrous dysplasia.
- Middle aortic syndrome.
- Neurofibromatosis.

58. Which of the following mediates calcium reabsorption in the distal renal tubules?

(a) Aldosterone
(b) Hypocalcemia
(c) Parathyroid hormone
(d) Vitamin D

(Answer is C) Parathyroid hormone

59. Beside renal excretion of sodium, what does atrial natriuretic hormone cause?

(a) Constriction of renal afferent arterioles
(b) Renin inhibition
(c) Aldosterone stimulation
(d) Rise in systemic blood pressure

(Answer is B) Renin inhibition

60. What is the prime effect of antidiuretic hormone on kidneys?

(a) Increase collecting duct permeability
(b) Increase medullary blood flow
(c) Decrease cortical blood flow
(d) Decrease potassium secretion

(Answer is A) Increase collecting duct permeability

61. What is the best initial therapy for hyponatremic dehydration?

(a) Administration of hypertonic saline
(b) Administration of crystalloid
(c) Administration of normal saline
(d) Administration of ringer lactate

(Answer is C) Administration of normal saline

62. What do the specialized cells, at the juxta-glomerular apparatus, produce?

(a) Erythropoietin (b) Renin
(c) Angiotensin I (d) Angiotensinogen

(Answer is B) Renin

63. Renal blood flow is autoregulated by:

(a) Sympathetic nervous system
(b) Parasympathetic nervous system
(c) Urinary output

(d) Afferent arteriolar resistance

(Answer is D) Afferent arteriolar resistance

64. Which of the renal artery occlusive conditions, commonly, do not affect renal function?

(a) Intimal fibroplasia
(b) Medial fibroplasia
(c) Medial hyperplasia
(d) Serosal hyperplasia

(Answer is B) Medial fibroplasia

65. What is the creatinine clearance in ml/min for a 70 kg man aging 50 years with 1.1 mg/dl serum creatinine?

(a) 79.54 (b) 44.19
(c) 84.15 (d) 94.25

(Answer is A) 79.54

66. Which of the following lab results indicates prerenal failure?

(a) Serum BUN: creatinine > 20
(b) Urine [Na] < 30 mEq/l
(c) Na excretion fraction < 1
(d) All of the above

(Answer is C) Na excretion fraction < 1

67. Which nephron segment contains the most diluted urine in central diabetes insipidus patient?

(a) Proximal convoluted tubules
(b) Distal convoluted tubules
(c) Collecting duct
(d) Loop of Henle

(Answer is C) Collecting duct

68. Which of the following is not a side effect of hydrochlorothiazide?

(a) Hypercholesterolemia
(b) Hyperuricemia
(c) Hypoglycemia
(d) Hypercalcemia

(Answer is C) Hypoglycemia

69. In which condition creatinine levels can not be 1200 mg/dl?

(a) An aspirate of pelvic urinoma
(b) In untreated end-stage renal failure disease
(c) A sample from a wound drain after pyeloplasty
(d) A sample from suprapubic catheter

(Answer is B) In untreated end-stage renal failure disease

70. What is false about "purple urine bag syndrome"?

(a) Occurs due to the interaction between the chemical components of the urine and polyvinyl chloride material in the urine bag
(b) It is commonly symptomless
(c) More common in female nursing home residents
(d) Commonly implicated bacteria are K. pneumoniae, P. mirabilis, E. coli

(Answer is A) Occurs due to the interaction between the chemical components of the urine and polyvinyl chloride material in the urine bag

71. What is false concerning the collecting system structures of a typical kidney?

(a) The renal pelvis could be intra or extra renal
(b) The renal pelvis divides into 2 or 3 major calyces
(c) Major calyces divide into 2 or 3 minor calyces
(d) Unlike lateral calyces, polar calyces are often paired

(Answer is D) Unlike lateral calyces, polar calyces are often paired

72. What could cause renal cortical necrosis in pregnancy?

(a) Amniotic fluid embolism
(b) Disseminated intravascular coagulopathy
(c) Intrauterine fetal demise
(d) All of the above

(Answer is D) All of the above

73. False about flank approach for renal surgery:

(a) Retroperitoneal structures better exposed
(b) May compromise pulmonary function and venous return
(c) Preferred in Kyphosis
(d) Table flexed between iliac crest and costal margin

(Answer is C) Preferred in Kyphosis

74. False about Dorsal lumbotomy approach:

(a) Typically reserved for elderly and bilateral nephrectomy
(b) No muscle is transected
(c) Disadvantage is poor exposure to hilum
(d) Increases work of breathing

(Answer is A) Typically reserved for elderly and bilateral nephrectomy

CHAPTER

9

Upper Urinary Tract Obstruction and Trauma

1. **Urinary enzymes elevated in patients with obstructed kidney is all *except:***
   (a) Leucine aminopeptidase
   (b) N-acetyl-α-D-glucosaminidase
   (c) Acid phosphatise
   (d) α-glutamyltransferase

(Answer is C) Urinary enzymes (derived from the proximal tubule) elevated in patients with obstructed kidneys such as:

- Alkaline phosphatase
- α-glutamyltransferase
- N-acetyl-α-D-glucosaminidase
- Leucine aminopeptidase

2. **All statements are true regarding UUO *except:***
   (a) Triphasic pattern is seen only in UUO
   (b) In first phase UUO, RBF increase is accompanied by a high PT
   (c) In a second phase pressure parameters remain elevated along with RBF
   (d) In third phase, decline in RBF, is paralleled by a decrease in PT

(Answer is C) With UUO, RBF increases during the first 1 to 2 hours and is accompanied by a high PT and collecting system pressure because of the obstruction. In a second phase lasting 3 to 4 hours, these pressure parameters remain elevated but RBF begins to decline. A third phase beginning about 5 hours after obstruction is characterized by a further decline in RBF, now paralleled by a decrease in PT and collecting system pressure.

3. **Which statement regarding BUO is not true?**
   (a) Triphasic pattern is seen in UUO and not in BUO
   (b) Initially there is a profound increase in RBF with BUO as compare to UUO
   (c) In BUO, later phase there is prolonged and profound decrease in RBF that is greater than that found with UUO
   (d) Postobstructive diuresis is much greater with BUO

(Answer is B) In contrast to the early robust renal vasodilation with UUO, there is a modest increase in RBF with BUO lasting approximately 90 minutes followed by a prolonged and profound decrease in RBF that is greater than that found with UUO.

4. **Which factor contributes to the profound diuresis and natriuresis in BUO?**
   (a) Aldosterone (b) Renin
   (c) Angiotensin (d) ANP

(Answer is D) ANP contributes to a profound diuresis and natriuresis.

5. **Which statement is not true for both UUO and BUO?**
   (a) Increase in urine flow
   (b) Increase in FE_{Na}
   (c) Increase in FE_K
   (d) Decrease acidification

(Answer is C) There is decrease of FE_K in UUO and increase in BUO.

6. **Aquaporin 2 is present at:**
   (a) Proximal tubule (b) LOH
   (c) Distal tubule (d) Collecting duct

(Answer is D) Aquaporin 2 (AQP2) with the apical membranes of the collecting duct cells.

7. **Normal urine concentrating ability requires a hypertonic medullary interstitial gradient because of active salt reabsorption from which part of nephron?**
   (a) Medullary collecting duct
   (b) Cortical collecting duct
   (c) Thick ascending LOH
   (d) Thin ascending LOH

(Answer is C) Normal urine concentrating ability requires a hypertonic medullary interstitial gradient because of active salt reabsorption from the thick ascending limb of Henle.

8. **Renal obstruction provokes a number of changes in the metabolic cascade *except:***
   (a) Shift from anaerobic respiration to oxidative metabolism
   (b) Reduction in ATP
   (c) Increase in ADP
   (d) Increase in the renal lactate-to-pyruvate ratio

(Answer is A) Renal obstruction provokes a number of changes in the metabolic cascade. There is a shift from oxidative metabolism to anaerobic respiration.

9. **Factors that have shown to play role in cellular level leading to fibrosis following urinary tract obstruction are all *except:***
   (a) TGF-β (b) Angiotensin II
   (c) TNF-α (d) IL-6

(Answer is D) A number of cytokines and growth factors have been shown to play roles in development of tubulointerstitial fibrosis, tubular atrophy and apoptosis, and interstitial inflammation, among which the most prominent include TGF-β, angiotensin II, nuclear factor eB (NFeB), and tumor necrosis factor α (TNF-α).

10. **Factors that have a positive influence on functional recovery include all *except:***
    (a) Smaller degree of obstruction
    (b) Greater compliance of the collecting system
    (c) Absence of pyelolymphatic backflow
    (d) Young age

(Answer is C) Factors that have a positive influence on functional recovery include a smaller degree of obstruction, greater compliance of the collecting system, and presence of pyelolymphatic backflow. Conversely, older age and decreased renal cortical thickness are predictors of diminished recovery of renal function.

11. **The RI is defined as:**
    (a) PSV minus EDV divided by the PSV
    (b) EDV minus PSV divided by the PSV
    (c) PSV minus EDV divided by the EDV
    (d) EDV minus PSV divided by the EDV

(Answer is A) The RI is defined as peak systolic velocity (PSV) minus the end-diastolic velocity (EDV) divided by the PSV.

12. **Obstruction is indicated at above what intrapelvic pressure?**
    (a) Greater than 7 (b) Greater than 15
    (c) Greater than 22 (d) Greater than 30

(Answer is C) A true intrapelvic pressure of less than 15 cm H_2O is considered normal, greater than 22 cm H_2O indicative of obstruction, and between 15 and 22 cm H_2O indeterminate.

13. **Sensitivity and specificity of Whitaker test is:**
    (a) 80% and 50% respectively
    (b) 50% and 80% respectively
    (c) 40% and 60% respectively
    (d) 60% and 40% respectively

(Answer is A) Sensitivity and specificity of whitaker test is 79% and 50% respectively.

14. Ureteral stenting is best effective for treating patients with:

(a) Diagnosis of cancer
(b) Metastatic disease requiring chemotherapy or radiation
(c) Renal insufficiency
(d) Intrinsic ureteral obstruction

(Answer is D) Ureteral stenting may not be as effective for treating patients with extrinsic ureteral obstruction. A diagnosis of cancer, metastatic disease requiring chemotherapy or radiation, and renal insufficiency were predictors of stent failure.

15. Which drug is not associated with RPF?

(a) Methyldopa (b) Hydralazine
(c) β blockers (d) ACE inhibitors

(Answer is D)

Drugs
Methysergide
Hydralazine
Reserpine
Haloperidol
LSD
Methyldopa
β blockers
Ergotamine alkaloids
Phenacetin
Amphetamines

16. Which statement regarding retroperitoneal fibrosis is not true?

(a) 3:1 male-to-female ratio
(b) Definitive etiology of retroperitoneal fibrosis is found in only 30% of cases
(c) An underlying malignancy is reported to be present in 8% to 10% of such cases
(d) Unilateral ureterolysis is recommended, in the setting of unilateral disease

(Answer is D) Bilateral ureterolysis is recommended, even in the setting of unilateral disease, as the disease typically progresses to involve the contralateral side.

17. On excretory urography, the bladder characteristically assumes a pear or gourd shape in:

(a) RPF
(b) Pelvic lipomatosis
(c) Tubo-ovarian abscess
(d) Pregnancy

(Answer is B) On excretory urography, the bladder characteristically assumes a pear or gourd shape, extrinsically compressed and elongated, and the bladder base is frequently elevated.

18. Which statement is not true regarding HDN of pregnancy?

(a) The left kidney becomes hydronephrotic more commonly than the right
(b) USG findings are hydroureteronephrosis extending to the pelvic brim
(c) MRU has been advocated as a noninvasive, nonradiating method of assessing those with hydronephrosis of pregnancy
(d) The majority of patients with symptomatic hydronephrosis of pregnancy can be managed with conservative measures

(Answer is A) The right kidney becomes hydronephrotic two to three times more commonly than the left in pregnancy. The typical ultrasonographic findings of this entity are hydroureteronephrosis extending to the pelvic brim.

19. Which statement is not true regarding endometriosis?

(a) Endometriosis of the urinary tract is predominantly found in the bladder
(b) Eighty percent of ureteral endometriosis is intrinsic and primarily involves the distal ureter

(c) The left side is more often affected
(d) Significant portion of patients with ureteral endometriosis do not have genitourinary symptoms

(Answer is B) Eighty percent of ureteral endometriosis is extrinsic and primarily involves the distal ureter.

20. Which statement regarding ovarian/testicular vein thrombophlebitis is not correct?

(a) Ovarian vein pathology causing ureteral obstruction occur more commonly on right side
(b) Majority of patients require ureterolysis and excision of thrombosed vein
(c) Thrombophlebitis of the left testicular vein causing extrinsic obstruction of the left ureter
(d) Ureterolysis and excision of the thrombosed testicular vein eradicate obstruction

(Answer is B) The majority of patients with ovarian vein thrombophlebitis respond to conservative measures, including antibiotic therapy.

21. Retrocaval ureter is due to:

(a) Failure of the supracardinal vein to develop into the suprarenal IVC
(b) Failure of the infracardinal vein to develop into the suprarenal IVC
(c) Failure of the supracardinal vein to develop into the infrarenal IVC
(d) Failure of the infracardinal vein to develop into the infrarenal IVC

(Answer is C) Failure of the supracardinal vein to develop into the infrarenal IVC leads to retrocaval ureter.

22. Incidence of crossing vessels in PUJ obstruction and in normal kidneys respectively is:

(a) 20% and 0 (b) 40% and 0
(c) 20% and 10% (d) 40% and 20%

(Answer is D) Significant crossing vessels have been noted in as many as 40% of cases of UPJ obstruction but as little as 20% of cases of normal kidneys.

23. Which scan is best to differentiate between UPJO and MCKD?

(a) 99^{m}Tc-DTPA (b) 99^{m}Tc-DMSA
(c) MAG-3 (d) Gallium scan

(Answer is A) Nuclear renography should be performed. Specifically, a technetium 99^{m}-labelled diethylene-triaminepentaacetic acid (99^{m}Tc-DTPA) scan allows differentiation of these two entities.

24. Who coined the term endopyelotomy?

(a) Ramsay (b) Badlani
(c) Lingeman (d) Perminger

(Answer is B) Endourologic management of UPJ obstruction was introduced by Ramsay and colleagues in 1984 as a "percutaneous pyelolysis" and then popularized in the United States by Badlani and coworkers, who coined the term *endopyelotomy.*

25. Contraindications to a percutaneous endopyelotomy includes all *except:*

(a) >2 cm of obstruction
(b) Active infection
(c) Uncorrected coagulopathy
(d) Presence of crossing vessel

(Answer is D) Contraindications to a percutaneous endopyelotomy are similar to the contraindications to any endourologic approach and include a long segment (>2 cm) of obstruction, active infection, or untreated coagulopathy. Whereas the impact of crossing vessels is controversial, the mere presence of crossing vessels is not a contraindication to an endopyelotomy.

26. During endopyelotomy incision should be made in which direction to avoid injury to crossing vessel?

(a) Anteriorly (b) Posteriorly
(c) Laterally (d) Medially

(Answer is C) Anatomic studies have shown the incision should generally be made laterally, because this is the location devoid of crossing vessels.

27. Aberrant or accessory lower pole vessels when found in association with the UPJ obstruction, which is the best pyeloplasty option?

(a) Dismembered pyeloplasty
(b) Foley YV plasty
(c) Culp-DeWeerd spiral flap
(d) Scardino-Prince vertical flap

(Answer is A) In the event that aberrant or accessory lower pole vessels are found in association with the UPJ obstruction, a dismembered pyeloplasty allows transposition of the UPJ in relation to these vessels.

28. Which pyeloplasty was originally designed for repair of PUJO with high insertion of ureter?

(a) Dismembered pyeloplasty
(b) Foley YV plasty
(c) Culp-DeWeerd spiral flap
(d) Scardino-Prince vertical flap

(Answer is B) The Foley YV plasty was originally designed for repair of a UPJ obstruction secondary to a high ureteral insertion.

29. UPJ obstruction with a relatively long segment of proximal ureteral narrowing or stricture. Best pyeloplasty is:

(a) Dismembered pyeloplasty
(b) Foley YV plasty
(c) Culp-DeWeerd spiral flap
(d) Scardino-Prince vertical flap

(Answer is C) The spiral flap may be of significant value when both UPJ obstruction and a relatively long segment of proximal ureteral narrowing or stricture occur in the same setting.

30. When a dependent UPJ is situated at the medial margin of a large, square ("boxshaped") extrarenal pelvis. Best pyeloplasty is:

(a) Dismembered pyeloplasty
(b) Foley YV plasty
(c) Culp-DeWeerd spiral flap
(d) Scardino-Prince vertical flap

(Answer is D) The Scardino-Prince vertical flap technique generally has limited clinical application, because it may be used appropriately only when a dependent UPJ is situated at the medial margin of a large, square ("box-shaped") extrarenal pelvis.

31. Ureterocalycostomy may be used as a primary reconstructive procedure in all *except:*

(a) Box shaped pelvis
(b) Failed pyeloplasty
(c) Horseshoe kidney
(d) Small intrarenal pelvis

(Answer is A) Ureterocalycostomy may be used as a primary reconstructive procedure whenever a UPJ obstruction or proximal ureteral stricture is associated with a relatively small intrarenal pelvis. When the UPJ is associated with rotational anomalies such as horseshoe kidney, ureterocalycostomy may be useful to provide completely dependent drainage.

Furthermore, ureterocalycostomy is a well-accepted salvage technique for the failed pyeloplasty.

32. Which statement is not true regarding retrocaval ureter?

(a) Procedural intervention is not indicated in all the patients
(b) This vascular anomaly is not always associated with ureteral obstruction
(c) Left side retrocaval ureter is not reported
(d) It occurs as a consequence of the persistence of the posterior cardinal veins

(Answer is C) Majority involve the right ureter, although left-sided circumcaval ureter has been reported in association with a duplicated IVC and in association with situs inversus. It occurs as a consequence of the persistence of the posterior cardinal veins during embryologic development. Procedural intervention is indicated in the presence of functionally significant obstruction leading to pain or renal function deterioration.

33. Minimum function required before starting endourologic therapy is:

(a) At any function, endourological therapy can be undertaken
(b) 10%
(c) 25%
(d) 50%

(Answer is C) It is critical to assess the renal unit for function before starting treatment, because endourologic therapies generally require 25% function of the ipsilateral moiety to have reasonable success rates.

34. How much of ureteral defect can be bridged with boari flap?

(a) 10-12 cm (b) 12-15 cm
(c) 15-18 cm (d) 8-10 cm

(Answer is B)

Technique	*Ureteral defect length (cm)*
Ureteroureterostomy	2–3
Ureteroneocystostomy	4–5
Psoas hitch	6–10
Boari flap	12–15
Renal descensus	5–8

35. In psoas hitch, which nerve is susceptible for injury while taking sutures?

(a) Genitofemoral nerve and obturator nerve
(b) Femoral nerve and obturator nerve
(c) Genitofemoral nerve and femoral nerve
(d) Genitofemoral nerve and sacral nerve

(Answer is C) Care should be taken to avoid injury to the genitofemoral nerve and the femoral nerve in the vicinity when placing the sutures.

36. Which statement is not true regarding psoas hitch?

(a) Small, contracted bladder with limited mobility is considered as a contraindication
(b) Additional mobility can be achieved by dividing the ipsilateral superior vesical artery
(c) The ipsilateral bladder dome is secured to the psoas minor tendon or the psoas major muscle using several absorbable sutures
(d) Ureteral defect extending proximal to the pelvic brim usually requires more than a psoas hitch alone

(Answer is B) Additional mobility can be achieved by dividing the contralateral superior vesical artery.

37. Which statement is not true regarding technique of boari flap?

(a) Base of the flap being at least 4 cm in width
(b) Tip of the flap being at least 3 cm in width
(c) The flap length should equal the estimated ureteral defect plus an addition of 3 to 4 cm if a nonrefluxing anastomosis is planned
(d) Ratio of flap length to base width should be 5:1

(Answer is D) The flap continues obliquely across the anterior bladder wall, with the base of the flap being at least 4 cm in width and the tip of the flap being atleast 3 cm in width. The flap length should equal the estimated ureteral defeet plus an addition of 3 to 4 cm if a nonrefluxing anastomosis is planned. Furthermore, the ratio of flap length to base width should not be greater than 3:1 to help minimize flap ischemia.

38. Relative contraindications to transureteroureterostomy is all *except:*

(a) History of nephrolithiasis
(b) Retroperitoneal fibrosis
(c) Chronic pyelonephritis
(d) Insufficient length of the donor ureter

(Answer is D) Absolute contraindication is insufficient

length of the donor ureter to reach the contralateral recipient ureter in a tension-free manner. Relative contraindications include history of nephrolithiasis, retroperitoneal fibrosis, urothelial malignancy, chronic pyelonephritis, and abdominopelvic radiation.

39. General contraindications to an ileal ureteral substitution are all *except:*

(a) Serum creatinine value of greater than 2 mg/dl
(b) IBD
(c) Bladder dysfunction or outlet obstruction
(d) High insertion of ureter

(Answer is D) General contraindications to an ileal ureteral substitution are baseline renal insufficiency with a serum creatinine value of greater than 2 mg/dl, bladder dysfunction or outlet obstruction, inflammatory bowel disease, or radiation enteritis.

40. Which statement is not true regarding retroperitoneal fibrosis?

(a) Lymphoma is the most common malignancy in RPF cases
(b) Retroperitoneal fibrotic mass generally centers around the distal aorta at L4-L5
(c) In approximately 30% of the cases, the disease is idiopathic
(d) Most common primary medical management has been corticosteroid therapy

(Answer is C) In approximately 70% of the cases, the disease is idiopathic.

41. Renal trauma with >1 cm parenchymal depth of renal cortex without collecting system rupture or urinary extravasation:

(a) Grade I (b) Grade II
(c) Grade III (d) Grade IV

(Answer is C) >1 cm parenchymal depth of renal cortex without collecting system rupture or urinary extravasation is classified under Grade III injury.

42. All *except* one group of patients will require CT to evaluate for renal trauma:

(a) All blunt trauma patients with gross hematuria
(b) All blunt trauma patients with microscopic hematuria
(c) All penetrating trauma patients with gross hematuria
(d) All penetrating trauma patients with microscopic hematuria

(Answer is B) All blunt trauma patients with gross hematuria and patients with microscopic hematuria and shock (systolic blood pressure <90 mm Hg any time during evaluation and resuscitation) should undergo renal imaging, usually CT with intravenous contrast.

43. Single shot IVU is done at what time after intravenous injection?

(a) 2 min (b) 5 min
(c) 10 min (d) 30 min

(Answer is C) The technique is key to gaining important information and minimizing the time involved: only a single film is taken 10 minutes after intravenous injection (IV push) of 2 ml/kg of contrast material.

44. Absolute indications for renal exploration in trauma is all *except:*

(a) Persistent renal bleeding
(b) Expanding perirenal hematoma
(c) Pulsatile perirenal hematoma
(d) Segmental arterial injury

(Answer is D) Absolute indications include evidence of persistent renal bleeding, expanding perirenal hematoma, and pulsatile perirenal hematoma. Relative indications include urinary extravasation, nonviable tissue, delayed diagnosis of arterial injury, segmental arterial injury, and incomplete staging.

45. More than 50% transaction in ureteral injury is graded as:

(a) Grade II (b) Grade III
(c) Grade IV (d) Grade V

(Answer is B)

III	Laceration	50% transection

46. Which surgery is most commonly associated with ureteral injury?

(a) Hysterectomy
(b) Colorectal surgery
(c) Transabdominal urethropexy
(d) Abdominal vascular surgery

(Answer is A) Hysterectomy was responsible for the majorit y (54%) of surgical ureteral injuries.

47. Options of reconstruction after ureteral injury in upper third of ureter:

(a) Ureteroureterostomy
(b) Transureteroureterostomy
(c) Ureterocalycostomy
(d) Illeal transposition

(Answer is D) Options of reconstruction after ureteral injury

Upper third:

- Ureteroureterostomy.
- Transureteroureterostomy.
- Ureterocalycostomy.

Middle third:

- Ureteroureterostomy.
- Transureteroureterostomy.
- Boari flap and reimplantation.

Lower third:

- Direct reimplantation.
- Psoas hitch.
- Blandy cystoplasty.

Complete:

- Ileal interposition.
- Autotransplantation.

48. What causes ureteral dilation during pregnancy is:

(a) Mechanical compression by the gravid uterus
(b) Physiological increase urine flow during pregnancy
(c) Elevated levels of progesterone
(d) Reflex inhibition of ureteral contractions

(Answer is A) Mechanical compression by the gravid uterus

49. What is false regarding gestational hydronephrosis?

(a) The incidence of dilation is lesser in nulliparous ladies
(b) Occurs in the second trimester
(c) Mostly, hydronephrosis disappears on its own in about 6 weeks after delivery
(d) Commoner in the right ureter

(Answer is A) The incidence of dilation is lesser in nulliparous ladies

50. What is true concerning hydronephrosis in pregnancy?

(a) Occurs because pregnancy increases the renal blood flow to up to 75% and approximately 50% increase in the GFR
(b) Typically, ureteral dilation does not occur below the pelvic brim
(c) Affects almost 13% of pregnancies by the 26th and 28th weeks
(d) Always asymptomatic

(Answer is B) Typically, ureteral dilation does not occur below the pelvic brim

51. As per the AAST kidney injury scale, to which grade does a parenchymal laceration extending through renal cortex, medulla and collecting system belong to?

(a) II (b) III
(c) IV (d) V

(Answer is C) IV

52. As per the AAST kidney injury scale, to which grade does a contusion injury causing hematuria with normal radiologic studies belong to?

(a) 0 (b) I
(c) II (d) III

(Answer is B) I

53. Indications for emergency exploration of renal trauma patients include all of the following, *except:*

(a) Hemodynamic instability
(b) Expanding hematomas
(c) The possibility of high-grade renal injury
(d) Stable patients with penetrating trauma

(Answer is D) Stable patients with penetrating trauma

54. What is false concerning renal trauma?

(a) The degree of hematuria corresponds well to the stage of injury
(b) Blunt traumas are commoner than sharp injuries
(c) Delayed contrast CT images, extravasated urine can be distinguished from blood
(d) Ultrasonography cannot identify vascular pedicle injuries or segmental infarcts

(Answer is A) The degree of hematuria corresponds well to the stage of injury

55. What statement is false concerning renal traumas caused by a major deceleration injury?

(a) Children are more prone to this mechanism of injury
(b) Could result from a motor vehicle accident or a fall from a height
(c) Might cause a tear of renal artery intima that results in vessel occlusion
(d) Such injuries, typically, result in severe subcapsular, nonexpanding hematoma without parenchymal laceration

(Answer is D) Such injuries, typically, result in severe subcapsular, nonexpanding hematoma without parenchymal laceration

56. What is false concerning renal trauma in pediatric patients?

(a) Anatomy, children are more prone to renal traumas
(b) Contrast to children, adults can maintain a normal blood pressure in spite of extensive blood loss
(c) Contrast CT is the best study for staging a solid organ injury
(d) Brisk flexion-extension motion might avulse the ureteropelvic junction

(Answer is B) Contrast to children, adults can maintain a normal blood pressure in spite of extensive blood loss

57. What is false regarding renal traumas?

(a) Renal parenchymal injury patients with urinary extravasation should be explored albeit they show stable hemodynamics
(b) Hemodynamically unstable patients with no response to resuscitation must undergo an immediate intervention
(c) After abdominal contrast CT for evaluating blunt abdominal trauma, delayed images should be taken if a renal injury was suspected
(d) Blunt injuries tend to track between the segmental vessels, while sharp injuries sever them

(Answer is A) Renal parenchymal injury patients with urinary extravasation should be explored albeit they show stable hemodynamics

58. Among all trauma cases, renal traumas constitute about:

(a) 0.2 – 1% (b) 1 – 5%
(c) 6 – 9% (d) 10 – 12%

(Answer is B) 1 – 5 %

59. What is false concerning blood loss in renal traumas?

(a) Hematuria that is out of proportion to the history of trauma might suggest a pre-existing pathology
(b) Urine dipstick is not reliable to evaluate hematuria as it has high false negatives
(c) Hemodynamically stable patients, serial hematocrit testing is part of the close monitoring
(d) All of the above

(Answer is B) Urine dipstick is not reliable to evaluate hematuria as it has high false negatives

60. What is false concerning renal imaging in trauma cases?

(a) Nuclear scintigraphy is recommended in 3 months post renal trauma for follow-up
(b) The diagnostic accuracy of MRI is not superior to CT for renal traumas
(c) Contrast enhanced ultrasonography (CEUS) with microbubbles helps diagnose injuries to the renal pelvis and/or ureter
(d) Plain KUB has a value in diagnosing renal trauma

(Answer is C) Contrast enhanced ultrasonography (CEUS) with microbubbles helps diagnose injuries to the renal pelvis and/or ureter

61. What is true regarding operating on acutely traumatized kidney and ureter?

(a) A renal vascular injury was suspected, surgical exploration must be performed through a midline abdominal incision
(b) Grade IV renal trauma, segmental artery occlusion, is an absolute indication for immediate surgical exploration
(c) Placing a vascular graft surrounding a traumatized ureter, overly, results in a vascular fistula
(d) Ureteral pelvic junction disruption is a relative indication for renal exploration through a flank incision

(Answer is A) A renal vascular injury was suspected, surgical exploration must be performed through a midline abdominal incision

62. Which management plan of complicated ureteral injuries is incorrect?

(a) When the ureter cannot be adequately repaired, it should be ligated with placement of nephrostomy tube
(b) When the uterus is removed, the uterine artery can be used to supply the devascularized lower ureter
(c) Complete ureteral transections should be repaired within 3 days of the injury, or delayed for secondary repair in 6 weeks
(d) Multiple ureteral injuries at different levels could result in page kidney

(Answer is D) Multiple ureteral injuries at different levels could result in page kidney

63. What is the ideal repair of a midureteral injury caused by a sharp object?

(a) Ureterocutaneus diversion
(b) Ureteroureterostomy
(c) Vesico-psoas hitch and/or Boari flap
(d) Transureteroureterostomy

(Answer is B) Ureteroureterostomy

64. What is most important on performing ureteroureterostomy?

(a) Repair should be under magnification
(b) Ensure leak-proof realignment
(c) Using DJ ureteral stent
(d) Applying the wound drain under negative pressure

(Answer is C) Using DJ ureteral stent

65. As per AAST ureteral trauma scale, to which grade does a < 2 cm complete transection with devascularisation belong to?

(a) II (b) III
(c) IV (d) V

(Answer is C) IV

66. The second most common cause of surgical ureteral injuries is:

(a) Obstetric and gynecologic operations
(b) Vascular operations
(c) Laparoscopic operations
(d) Colorectal operations

(Answer is D) Colorectal operations

67. How common are ureteral injuries during robot-assisted prostatectomies?

(a) Uncommon
(b) Not uncommon
(c) Common
(d) Exceedingly common

(Answer is A) Uncommon

68. In women, surgical injuries to the right ureter might present as any of the following, *except:*

(a) Anuria and renal failure
(b) Flank pain and vaginal discharge
(c) Fever and sepsis
(d) Fistula and urinoma

(Answer is A) Anuria and renal failure

69. Most surgical injuries to the ureters are:

(a) Detected on table
(b) Missed
(c) Diagnosed post operatively
(d) Avulsions

(Answer is C) Diagnosed post operatively

70. Which of the following is an absolute contraindication to transureteroureterostomy?

(a) Small-capacity bladder
(b) Short donor ureter
(c) Significant bladder outlet obstruction
(d) Urothelial tumor

(Answer is B) Short donor ureter

71. Which of the following is not a contraindication to ileal ureteral substitution?

(a) Short ureter
(b) Neurogenic bladder
(c) Bladder outlet obstruction
(d) Inflammatory disease

(Answer is A) Short ureter

72. What is the most sensitive radiographic study for diagnosing a ureteral injury?

(a) Antegrade ureterography
(b) Retrograde pyelography
(c) Contrast enhanced ultrasonography with microbubbles
(d) Intravenous urography

(Answer is B) Retrograde pyelography

73. Partial ureteral transections due to gunshot wounds should be:

(a) Repaired primarily
(b) Resected with 2 cm margin, and the edges re-approximated
(c) Stented
(d) Observed closely

(Answer is B) Resected with 2 cm margin, and the edges re-approximated

74. What is false concerning repairing lower ureteral injuries?

(a) Vesicopsoas hitch bridges an 8 – 12 cm defect
(b) Ureteroneocystostomy repairs defects up to 5 cm
(c) Boari flap provides an additional 12–15 cm of length
(d) The base of Boari flap should be $\geq$ 4 cm

(Answer is A) Vesicopsoas hitch bridges an 8 – 12 cm defect

75. **Following a blunt abdominal trauma to a 34 years woman, urethral catheterization drains gross hematuria. What could be the cause?**
    (a) Intravesical bladder rupture
    (b) Extravesical bladder rupture
    (c) Renal contusion
    (d) Any of the above

(Answer is D) Any of the above

76. **What is the primary lesion in an acute renal artery thrombosis following deceleration injury?**
    (a) Avulsion of the posterior segmental artery
    (b) Laceration of the anterior segmental artery
    (c) Tear in the arterial intima
    (d) Contusion of the renal pedicle

(Answer is C) Tear in the arterial intima

77. **What is the most important criterion of the gun shot that determines the magnitude of tissue damage?**
    (a) Entry and exit sites of the bullet
    (b) Velocity of the bullet
    (c) Length of the track inside the body
    (d) Firing range

(Answer is B) Velocity of the bullet

78. **During an emergency abdominal hysterectomy the lowest part of the left ureter is lacerated and bleeding. What would be next step?**
    (a) Place intraoperative ureteral stent
    (b) Segmental resection and end-to-end anastomosis
    (c) Ligate the ureter and insert post op. nephrostomy tube
    (d) Segmental resection and ureteral reimplantation

(Answer is A) Place intraoperative ureteral stent

79. **During transabdominal O'Connor's operation for vesicovaginal fistula repair, which omental arteries should be saved most?**
    (a) Gastroduodenal
    (b) Gastroepiploic
    (c) Inferior mesenteric
    (d) Pancreaticodeuodenal

(Answer is B) Gastroepiploic

80. **On day 5 post abdominal hysterectomy, the patient starts to have a watery vaginal discharge alongside the right flank pain and fever. IVU shows hydroureteronephrosis and lower ureteral leak of the dye. What should be next step?**
    (a) Inserting a nephrostomy tube
    (b) Simultaneous cystoscopy and vaginoscopy with fistula track fulguration
    (c) Cystoscopy a retrograde ureteral stenting
    (d) Exploration and primary repair

(Answer is A) Inserting a nephrostomy tube

81. **False about ureteric stricture:**
    (a) Goblet sign is seen classically in radiography in a case of transitional cell carcinoma
    (b) CT scan is necessary in a presumed case of idiopathic stricture
    (c) Endourologic therapy requires atleast 15% function of the ipsilateral moiety
    (d) Use of stenting is less successful in ureteric obstruction due to extrinsic compression

(Answer is C) Endourologic therapy requires atleast 15% function of the ipsilateral moiety

82. **True about endoureterotomy for ureteric stricture:**
    (a) Antegrade approach is preferred
    (b) Lower ureter stricture is incised in anteromedial direction
    (c) Upper ureteric stricture is incised medially
    (d) Incision is made upto muscle layer

(Answer is B) Lower ureter stricture is incised in anteromedial direction

83. All are true about ureteral injury *except:*

(a) Iatrogenic injury is the most common cause
(b) Most commonly affects distal 1/3 of ureter
(c) Urologic surgeries are the main cause
(d) High grade injuries with endoscopic surgery is rare

(Answer is C) Urologic surgeries are the main cause

84. All are true about diagnosis of ureteral injury *except:*

(a) Only 36% cases are recognized at the time of initial surgery
(b) Absence of hematuria usually rules out a clinically significant ureteral injury
(c) Gold standard investigation for diagnosis is cystography with retrograde urography
(d) Early diagnosis and management gives better prognosis

(Answer is B) Absence of hematuria usually rules out a clinically significant ureteral injury

85. All are true about management of ureteric injury *except:*

(a) Traumatic ureteral injuries should be repaired at the time of exploration in stable patients
(b) Absorbable sutures are used for repair
(c) Mucosa to mucosa repair is done
(d) A non-refluxing type of reimplantation is preferred in an acute setting

(Answer is D) A non-refluxing type of reimplantation is preferred in an acute setting

86. Complete transection with > 2 cm devascularisation of ureter is classified as which grade of ureter injury?

(a) 3 (b) 4
(c) 5 (d) 2

(Answer is C) 5

87. Most common cause of ureteric avulsion:

(a) Excess force applied to a basketed stone
(b) Forceful stenting
(c) Pneumatic lithotripsy
(d) Surgery in duplex ureter

(Answer is A) Excess force applied to a basketed stone

88. False about ureteral catheterization for elective abdominal surgeries:

(a) Do not decrease the risk of ureteral injury
(b) Helps in identification of ureteral injury
(c) Decreases the risk of acute kidney injury in the post operative setting
(d) May be required for acute diverticulitis requiring surgery

(Answer is C) Decreases the risk of acute kidney injury in the post operative setting

89. According to Waaldijk classification ureterovaginal fistula is type:

(a) II A (b) II B
(c) III (d) IV

(Answer is C) III

90. False about ureterovaginal fistula:

(a) Occurs more commonly after radical hysterectomy than a benign hysterectomy
(b) Usually a normal voiding pattern is present with constant urinary leakage
(c) Open repair most commonly involves ureteroneocystostomy
(d) Most common presenting symptom is incontinence 1-4 weeks after surgery

(Answer is A) Occurs more commonly after radical hysterectomy than a benign hysterectomy

CHAPTER

10 Renal Failure and Transplant

1. **Which of the following pair is not correct:**
   (a) RBC cast–AGN
   (b) WBC casts–AIN
   (c) Pigmented granular casts–ATN
   (d) Fatty casts–Urinary tract obstruction

(Answer is D) Urine Sediment in Acute Renal Failure

Sediment Findings	*Diagnosis*
Normal	Prerenal /obstruction
Red blood cell casts, red blood cells	AGN
Eosinophils, WBC and sterile urine	AIN
Pigmented granular casts	ATN

2. **Permanent renal failure in adults is commonly defined as an irreversible glomerular filtration rate of less than:**
   (a) 5 ml/min (b) 10 ml/min
   (c) 20 ml/min (d) 25 ml/min

(Answer is B) Permanent renal failure in adults is commonly defined as an irreversible glomerular filtration rate of less than 10 ml/min or a serum creatinine level of greater than 8 mg/dl (United Network for Organ Sharing [UNOS], 1994).

3. **In ESRD predominant form of renal replacement therapy for adults and children respectively is:**
   (a) In center hemodialysis for both
   (b) Renal transplant for both
   (c) In center hemodialysis and renal transplant respectively
   (d) Renal transplant and in center hemodialysis respectively

(Answer is C) In center hemodialysis is the predominant form of therapy for adults with ESRD. Transplantation, however, is the predominant mode of care for patients younger than 20 years.

4. **Unsuitable characteristics of patients for chronic peritoneal dialysis are all *except:***
   (a) Diabetes mellitus
   (b) Obesity
   (c) Hernia
   (d) Inflammatory bowel disease

(Answer is A) Unsuitable characteristics of patients for chronic peritoneal dialysis are considered to be obesity, hernias, poor hygiene, inflammatory bowel disease, and obliterated peritoneal space.

5. **Patients especially suited for peritoneal dialysis are all *except:***
   (a) Cardiac disease (b) Poor hygiene
   (c) Small stature (d) Desire for self care

(Answer is B) A desire for self-care, a long distance from a hemodialysis unit, difficulties with hemodialysis therapy, serious cardiac disease, diabetes mellitus, and small stature are characteristics of patients especially suited for peritoneal dialysis.

6. **First human renal allograft was performed by:**
   (a) Voronoy in 1933 (b) Carrel in 1912
   (c) Goodwin in 1963 (d) Collins in 1969

(Answer is A) In 1933, the first human renal allograft was performed by Voronoy in the Ukraine.

7. All *except* which patients should be counseled about the significant probability of disease recurrence and the risk of secondary graft failure?

(a) Focal segmental glomerulosclerosis
(b) Hemolytic-uremic syndrome
(c) Primary oxalosis
(d) Renal amyloidosis

(Answer is D) Patients with focal segmental glomerulosclerosis, hemolytic-uremic syndrome, and primary oxalosis should be counselled about the significant probability of disease recurrence and the risk of secondary graft failure.

8. All are indications for pretransplant nephrectomy *except:*

(a) Solid renal tumors
(b) Renal stones not cleared by minimally invasive techniques or lithotripsy
(c) Significant proteinuria
(d) Grade 3 hydronephrosis

(Answer is D) Indications for pretransplant nephrectomy

- Renal stones not cleared by minimally invasive techniques.
- Solid renal tumors.
- Larg PCKD.
- Persistent antiglomenulars basements membrane antibody.
- Significant proteinuria.
- Recurrent pyelonephritis.
- Grade 4 or 5 hydronephrosis.

9. Best renal imaging technique for living renal donor is:

(a) Doppler USG with X-ray KUB
(b) Intravenous Urogram + Arteriogram
(c) 30 Helical CT angiogram with and without intravenous contrast
(d) Magnetic Resonance Imaging + Intravenous Gadolinium

(Answer is C) Three-dimensional CT angiography without and with intravenous contrast material followed by plain radiography of the abdomen has been widely accepted because it satisfactorily excludes stone disease, demonstrates renal and vascular anatomy, and defines the urinary collecting system.

10. After living renal donor nephrectomy, endogenous creatinine clearance of donor approaches upto what preoperative levels?

(a) 60% to 70%
(b) 70% to 80%
(c) 80% to 90%
(d) 90% to 100%

(Answer is B) Endogenous creatinine clearance rapidly approaches 70% to 80% of the preoperative level, and this has been shown to be sustained for more than 10 years.

11. The advantages of LDN when compared with of ODN have been all *except:*

(a) Decreased analgesic requirement
(b) Decreased length of hospital stay
(c) Earlier return to work
(d) Better graft function

(Answer is D) The reported advantages of LDN when compared with historical cases of ODN have been decreased analgesic requirement, decreased length of hospital stay, and an earlier return to work. The disadvantages have been reported to be increased operating time, donor surgeon preference for the left kidney, an increased need for special equipment, a longer warm ischemia time, and delayed graft function.

12. During warm ischemic injury due to ATP depletion all *except* one change occurs in the cell:

(a) Decrease in K
(b) Increase in Mg
(c) Increase in Ca
(d) Lysosomal enzymes are activated

(Answer is B) When the sodium-potassium pump is

impaired, sodium chloride and water passively diffuse into the cells, resulting in cellular swelling and the "no-reflow" phenomenon after renal revascularization. Cellular potassium and magnesium are lost, calcium is gained, anaerobic glycolysis and acidosis occur, and lysosomal enzymes are activated. This results in cell death.

13. In renal transplant renal artery is usually anastomosed to:

(a) Side of internal iliac artery or end of external iliac artery
(b) End of internal iliac artery or side of external iliac artery
(c) Side of internal iliac artery or end of common iliac artery
(d) End of internal iliac artery or side of common iliac artery

(Answer is B) The renal artery is usually anastomosed to the end of the internal iliac artery or to the side of the external iliac artery.

14. In renal transplant end of renal vein is usually anastomosed to:

(a) Side of internal iliac vein
(b) Side of external iliac vein
(c) End of internal iliac vein
(d) End of external iliac vein

(Answer is B) The renal vein, with or without an extension, is usually anastomosed to the side of external iliac vein or to the junction of the external and common iliac veins.

15. In renal transplant urinary tract reconstruction is usually done by:

(a) Antireflux ureteroneocystostomy
(b) Reflux ureteroneocystostomy
(c) Ureteroureterostomy
(d) Ureteropyelostomy

(Answer is A) Urinary tract reconstruction is usually by antireflux ureteroneocystostomy.

16. MHC genes are encoded on:

(a) Long arm of chromosome 6
(b) Short arm of chromosome 6
(c) Long arm of chromosome 3
(d) Short arm of chromosome 3

(Answer is B) The MHC antigens are glycoproteins on the cell membrane. They are encoded by MHC genes on the short arm of chromosome 6

17. Which statement regarding transplant rejection is not true?

(a) Hyperacute rejection is a reversible process mediated by preformed circulating cytotoxic antibodies
(b) Hyperacute rejection is very rare when the microlymphocytotoxicity crossmatch between recipient serum and donor lymphocytes is negative
(c) Accelerated rejection is mediated by humoral and cellular components of the immune response
(d) Accelerated rejection occurs within days to weeks and often does not respond to antirejection therapy

(Answer is A) It is an irreversible process mediated by preformed circulating cytotoxic antibodies that develop after pregnancy, blood transfusions, or an earlier failed transplantation. It is very rare when the microlymphocytotoxicity crossmatch between recipient serum and donor lymphocytes is negative.

18. The Banff classification is accepted as the standard schema for diagnosing:

(a) Renal failure
(b) Transplant rejection
(c) Prostate cancer
(d) BPH

(Answer is B) The Banff classification is now accepted as the standard schema for diagnosing rejection.

19. Triple maintenance immunosuppression includes all *except:*

(a) Prednisone
(b) Tacrolimus
(c) Mycophenolate mofetil
(d) Basiliximab

(Answer is D) Triple maintenance immunosuppression with prednisone; cyclosporine or tacrolimus; and azathioprine or mycophenolate mofetil is common.

20. All are true regarding mode of action *except:*

(a) Mycophenolate mofetil–Inhibits purine synthesis
(b) Cyclosporine–Inhibits calcineurin and interleukin-2 production
(c) Sirolimus–Depletes T lymphocytes
(d) Basiliximab–Blocks interleukin-2 receptor

(Answer is C)

Drugs	*Mechanism of action*
Mycophenolate mofetil	Inhibits purine synthesis
Sirolimus progression	Inhibits cell cycle proliferation
Cyclosporine	Inhibits calcineurin and interleukin-2 production
Basiliximab	Blocks interleukin-2 receptor

21. Drugs that inhibit cytochrome P-450 enzyme system which result in increased blood or plasma levels of cyclosporine and tacrolimus includes all *except:*

(a) Diltiazem
(b) Erythromycin
(c) Ketoconazole
(d) Isoniazid

(Answer is D) Rifampin, isoniazid, phenytoin are the drugs which will decrease the blood levels of cyclosporine and tacrolimus.

22. Calcineurin inhibitor toxicity can be differentiated from acute rejection by all *except:*

(a) No fever
(b) No graft tenderness
(c) Normal urine output
(d) Rapid rise in serum creatinine

(Answer is D) Differentiation of calcineurin inhibitor toxicity from acute rejection.

Characteristic	*Tacrolimus or cyclosporine toxicity*	*Acute Rejection*
Fever	No	Yes
Urinary output	Usually maintained	Decreased
Graft tenderness	No	Yes
Graft size	Stable	Increased
Serum creatinine level rise	Slow	Rapid
Cyclosporine/ tacrolimus blood level	High	Normal or low
Graft biopsy	May be normal	Cellular infiltration, vasculitis, tubulitis

23. Impregnation should be delayed for how many years after transplantation?

(a) 1
(b) 2
(c) 3
(d) 4

(Answer is A) It is recommended that impregnation be delayed for at least 1 year after transplantation.

24. Kidney transplant recipients are more likely to develop all *except* following cancer:

(a) Kaposi's sarcoma
(b) Non-Hodgkin's lymphomas
(c) Non-melanoma skin cancers
(d) Hodgkin's lymphomas

(Answer is D) Kidney transplant recipients are more likely to develop cancer than age-matched subjects in the general population and patients wait-listed for deceased donor renal transplantation. This was especially true for Kaposi's sarcoma, non-Hodgkin's lymphomas, non-melanoma skin cancers and kidney cancer.

25. Which statement is not true regarding hepatorenal syndrome (HRS)?

(a) HRS represents a unique, severe form of prerenal azotemia
(b) Kidneys suffer from tubular hyalinization and cannot be considered for renal transplant
(c) Diagnosis is one of exclusion
(d) Diagnosis of HRS requires a lack of improvement in renal function after discontinuation of potential nephrotoxins and a trial of fluid repletion

(Answer is B) HRS is a prerenal disease, because the kidneys are normal histologically and have been successfully used in renal transplantation

26. To diagnose urine extravasation, ratio of drain creatinine to serum creatinine should be:

(a) 1:1 (b) 1:10
(c) 10:1 (d) 5:1

(Answer is C) Diagnosis of urinary extravasation requires analysis of fluid from the area near the reconstructed site. The drain creatinine is compared with the SCr. Ratios of 10:1 are virtually diagnostic for extravasation.

27. Urinalysis findings of sterile pyuria, white blood cell casts, and eosinophiluria is suggestive of:

(a) ATN
(b) AIN
(c) AGN
(d) Atheroembolic renal disease

(Answer is B) The diagnosis of ARF secondary to AIN may be suggested by the urinalysis findings of sterile pyuria, white blood cell casts, and eosinophiluria (using Hansel's stain).

28. Greatest risk of ischemic renal injury is to:

(a) S1 portion of proximal tubule
(b) S3 portion of proximal tubule
(c) Medullary thick ascending limb
(d) Medullary thick descending limb

(Answer is B) The S3 portion of the proximal tubule sustains the most severe injury. Other structures that sustain injury in this region include the medullary thick ascending limb (mTAL), which is metabolically active and rich in the energy requiring Na+/K+-ATPase.

29. Pigmented (muddy brown) granular casts and renal tubular epithelial cells, are seen in:

(a) AGN (b) ATN
(c) AIN (d) Prerenal

(Answer is B) The classic sediment of ATN includes pigmented (muddy brown) granular casts and renal tubular epithelial cells, which may be seen in nearly 80% of cases of oliguric ARF.

30. All *except* one are suggestive of prerenal/acute glomerulonephritis:

(a) Urinary [Na+] mEq /l <20
(b) Urine: plasma creatinine <30
(c) Renal failure index<1
(d) FENa<1

(Answer is B) Patterns of urinary indices in acute renal failure

	Prerenal/Acute Glomerulo-nephritis	*Acute Tubular Necrosis/ Obstruction*
Urinary [Na+] mEq/l	<20	>40
Urine: plasma creatinine	>30	<20
Renal failure index	<1	>1
FENa	<1	>1
Urinary osmolality	>500	<400

31. All are complications of acute renal failure *except:*

(a) Hypernatremia
(b) Hyperkalemia
(c) Hypermagnesemia
(d) Hypocalcemia

(Answer is A) Electrolyte imbalance includes hyponatremia, hypocalcemia, hyperkalemia and hypermagnesemia.

32. Best initial treatment for pigment nephropathy is:

(a) Mannitol (b) Dopamine
(c) ANP (d) Alkaline diuresis

(Answer is D) Early recognition of this pigment nephropathy is crucial, because a forced alkaline diuresis is indicated to minimize nephrotoxicity.

33. With hyperkalemia, the earliest change seen in ECG is:

(a) Broadening of the PR interval
(b) QRS broadening
(c) U wave
(d) Tall T waves

(Answer is D) With hyperkalemia, the earliest changes demonstrate peaked T waves with subsequent broadening of the PR interval and eventual QRS broadening, which may mature into a sine wave form.

34. Mortality rate for patients with ATN is:

(a) 25% (b) 50%
(c) 75% (d) 100%

(Answer is B) The mortality rate for patients with ATN is nearly 50%.

35. In hypetkalemia stabilizing the membrane of the cardiac conduction system may be accomplished with:

(a) Intravenous calcium
(b) Intravenous sodium bicarbonate
(c) Intravenous glucose and insulin
(d) Intravenous furosemide

(Answer is A) Stabilizing the membrane of the cardiac conduction system may be accomplished with intravenous calcium salts, which have an immediate effect and a rather short duration of action.

36. (K/DOQI) Advisory Board recommended that "chronic kidney disease" should be defined as sustained kidney damage of:

(a) > 3 months resulting in a GFR of less than 30 ml/min/1.73 m^2
(b) > 3 months resulting in a GFR of less than 60 ml/min/1.73 m^2
(c) > 6 months resulting in a GFR of less than 30 ml/min/1.73 m^2
(d) > 6 months resulting in a GFR of less than 60 ml/min /1.73 m^2

(Answer is B) Workgroup of the U.S. National Kidney Foundation, Kidney Disease Outcomes Quality Initiative (K/DOQI) Advisory Board recommended that "chronic kidney disease" should be defined as sustained kidney damage greater than 3 months resulting in a GFR of less than 60 ml/min/1.73 m^2.

37. GFR between 30 and 59 is graded as:

(a) CKD 1 (b) CKD 2
(c) CKD 3 (d) CKD 4

(Answer is C) Clinical action plan for chronic kidney disease by glomerular filtration rate levels.

Stage	*Description*	*GFR (ml/min/1.73 m^2)*
1.	Kidney damage with normal or increased GFR	=90
2.	Kidney damage decrease in GFR	60 to 89
3.	Moderate decrease in GFR	30 to 59
4.	Severe decrease in GFR	15 to 29
5.	Kidney failure	<15 (or dialysis)

38. According to NIH patients with CKD be referred to a nephrologist when the S Cr value has increased to what level in males?

(a) 1.0 (b) 1.5
(c) 2.0 (d) 2.5

(Answer is C) The National Institutes of Health (NIH) Consensus Conference of 1993 recommended that patients with CKD be referred to a nephrologist when the S Cr value has increased to 1.5 mg/dl in females and 2.0 mg/dl in males (National Institutes of Health,1994).

39. Proposed criteria for initiation of renal replacement therapy includes all *except:*

(a) Oliguria (urine output < 200 ml/12 hr)
(b) Hyperkalemia ([K+] > 6.5 mmol/l)
(c) Severe dysnatremia ([Na] > 160 or < 115 mmol/l)
(d) Severe acidemia (pH < 7.3)

(Answer is D) Proposed criteria for initiation of renal replacement therapy includes severe academia (pH < 7. 1).

40. Relentless progressive loss of renal function ensues even when the initial insult becomes inactive occurs when GFR is less than:

(a) 10% (b) 25%
(c) 50% (d) 75%

(Answer is C) At a set point (usually > 50% reduction in GFR), a relentless progressive loss of renal function ensues even when the initial insult becomes inactive.

41. The most common causes of CKD is:

(a) Hypertension
(b) DM
(c) Glomerulonephritis
(d) Interstitial nephritis/pyelonephritis

(Answer is B) The most common causes of CKD are diabetes and hypertension.

42. Causes of anemia in CRF:

(a) Decrease erythropoietin production
(b) Blood loss from hemodialysis
(c) Excessive destruction of RBC
(d) All of the above

(Answer is D)

Causes of anemia in CRF includes:

- Does not make enough erythropoietin.
- Blood loss from hemodialysis.
- Low levels of iron and folic acid.
- Excessive destruction of red blood cells.

43. Which agent should be avoided during living-related donor nephrectomy?

(a) Ice slush (b) Heparin
(c) Norepinephrine (d) Methylene blue

(Answer is C) Norepinephrine

44. Which of the following does NOT affect serum creatinine?

(a) Gender
(b) Age
(c) Obstructing stone at left lower ureter
(d) Rhabdomyolysis

(Answer is C) Obstructing stone at left lower ureter

45. What is the most significant complication of cyclosporine?

(a) Hepatic toxicity (b) Renal toxicity
(c) Neural toxicity (d) Cardiac toxicity

(Answer is B) Renal toxicity

46. MCC of renal transplant failure in children:

(a) Vascular thrombosis
(b) Chronic graft nephropathy
(c) Recurrent obstructive uropathy
(d) Post transplant lymphoproliferative disease

(Answer is B) Chronic graft nephropathy

47. False about hematuria after renal transplant is:

(a) More common with Lich Gregoir anastomosis
(b) Majority of AV fistula after renal biopsy resolves spontaneously
(c) BK virus nephropathy is an important cause for microscopic hematuria
(d) Hematuria during the immediate postoperative period is typically related to the ureterovesical anastomosis

(Answer is A) More common with Lich Gregoir anastomosis

48. False regarding urine leak after renal transplantation:

(a) Ureteral stent decreases ureteral stricture and urinary leak
(b) Most common early urologic complication after transplant
(c) Compromising the blood supply to the proximal ureter during organ procurement is the main risk factor for ureteral necrosis and urine leak
(d) Early exploration and reconstructive surgery should be offered to patients with a proximal large leak

(Answer is C) Compromising the blood supply to the proximal ureter during organ procurement is the main risk factor for ureteral necrosis and urine leak

49. All are true about post transplant lymphocele *except:*

(a) Peak incidence at 6 months
(b) It's a pseudocyst with hard fibrous capsule
(c) Majority are asymptomatic
(d) Open drainage should be considered in patients with wound complications and those with a small lymphocele adjacent to vital renal structures

(Answer is A) Peak incidence at 6 months

50. False about nephrolithiasis in transplant kidney:

(a) 1% incidence
(b) Most commonly uric acid stones
(c) Cyclosporine induces hyperuricemia
(d) Calcineurin inhibitors induces hyperoxaluria and hypocitraturia

(Answer is B) Most commonly uric acid stones

51. Wrong statement about post transplant malignancy:

(a) Most common renal tumor is clear cell type
(b) Increased incidence of renal tumor than general population
(c) Similar incidence of carcinoma prostate as in general population
(d) Increased risk of carcinoma bladder compared to general population

(Answer is A) Most common renal tumor is clear cell type

CHAPTER 11

Urinary Urolithiasis and Endourology

1. **Regarding demography of stone disease all are correct:**
   (a) Highest prevalence of stone disease in whites, followed by Hispanics, Asians and African-Americans
   (b) Higher prevalence of stone disease is in northeast
   (c) Highest incidence of stone disease in the summer months, July through September
   (d) Adult men more commonly affected than adult women

(Answer is B) Demography of stone disease

- Incidence has increased in all age groups and in both men and women.
- Peak incidence in men from 30 to 69 years.
- Adult men more commonly affected than adult women (struvite stones are more common in women).
- Highest prevalence of stone disease in whites, followed by Hispanics, Asians and African-Americans.
- Higher prevalence of stone disease is in southeast.
- Highest incidence of stone disease in the summer months, July through September.
- Heat exposure and dehydration constitute occupational risk factors for stone disease.
- Obesity and weight gain are risk factors.

2. **Which one of the following event does not occur in metastable states of saturation in urine?**
   (a) Spontaneous nucleation does not occur
   (b) Precipitation does not occur
   (c) Urine is not supersaturated
   (d) It is in this area that modulation of factors controlling stone formation can occur

(Answer is C) In metastable state, spontaneous nucleation or precipitation does not occur despite urine that is supersaturated.

3. **Which statement regarding Tamm-Horsfall protein is not true?**
   (a) Most abundant protein found in the urine
   (b) It is secreted by thick ascending LOH
   (c) Potent inhibitor of calcium oxalate monohydrate crystal aggregation
   (d) Potent inhibitor of calcium oxalate monohydrate crystal growth

(Answer is D) Tamm-Horsfall is the most abundant protein found in the urine and a potent inhibitor of calcium oxalate monohydrate crystal aggregation, but not growth.

4. **Citrate does not act as an inhibitor of stone formation by which action?**
   (a) It complexes with calcium, reducing the availability of ionic calcium
   (b) It directly inhibits the spontaneous precipitation of calcium oxalate
   (c) Reduces the rate of calcium oxalate crystal growth in vitro
   (d) Prevents heterogeneous nucleation of calcium oxalate by monosodium urate

(Answer is C) Citrate has limited inhibitory effect on calcium oxalate crystal growth, it has more potent activity in reducing calcium phosphate growth.

Magnesium reduces the rate of calcium oxalate crystal growth in vitro.

5. **Which statement regarding matrix stone is not true?**
   (a) Crysta lline component of renal stone is termed as matrix
   (b) Accounts for about 2.5% of the weight of the stone
   (c) The exact composition of matrix is difficult to ascertain as only 25% of it is soluble
   (d) Substance A is immunologically unique and present in the matrix component of all stone formers

(Answer is A) Renal calculi consist of both crystalline and noncrystalline components. The non-crystalline component is termed matrix.

6. **What portion of dietary calcium is absorbed and in which portion of intestine?**
   (a) 20% to 30% of dietary calcium is absorbed, with most being absorbed in small intestine
   (b) 30% to 40% of dietary calcium is absorbed, with most being absorbed in small intestine
   (c) 20% to 30% of dietary calcium is absorbed, with most being absorbed in colon
   (d) 30% to 40% of dietary calcium is absorbed, with most being absorbed in colon

(Answer is B) Thirty to 40 percent of dietary calcium is absorbed from the intestine, with most being absorbed in the small intestine and only approximately 10% absorbed in the colon.

7. **Which statement regarding calcium metabolism is not correct?**
   (a) Calcium is absorbed in the ionic state
   (b) Calcium phosphate formation is dependent on pH
   (c) Calcium oxalate complex formation is pH dependent
   (d) Transcellular calcium absorption is mediated by calcitriol

(Answer is C) Calcium oxalate complex formation displays less pH dependence and complex formation is less reversible.

8. **Which statement regarding calcium metabolism is not correct?**
   (a) 1,25(OH) 203, is the most potent stimulator of intestinal calcium absorption
   (b) 25-hydroxy vitamin D3, is hydroxylated in the proximal renal tubule to 1,25(OH)2D3
   (c) PTH enhances renal calciurn reabsorption and reduces renal tubular reabsorption of phosphate
   (d) PTH directly enhances intestinal calcium absorption

(Answer is D) The active form of vitamin D, 1,25(OH)2D3, is the most potent stimulator of intestinal calcium absorption. 25- hydroxy-vitamin D3, is hydroxylated in the proximal renal tubule to 1,25(OH)2D3. PTH has no direct effect on intestinal calcium absorption.

9. **Which statement regarding oxalate metabolism is not correct?**
   (a) Hyperoxaluric stone formers absorb more oxalate in response to an oral oxalate load than stone formers with normal oxalate excretion
   (b) In patients with small bowel disease or intestinal resection and an intact colon, oxalate absorption is markedly increased
   (c) Oxalate-degrading bacteria, notably oxalobacter formigenes, utilize oxalate as an energy source and consequently reduce intestinal oxalate absorption
   (d) Up to 20% of urinary oxalate is derived from endogenous production in the liver and 80% or more is derived from dietary sources

(Answer is D) Upto 80% of urinary oxalate is derived from endogenous production in the liver (40% from ascorbic acid, 40% from glycine) and 20% or more is derived from dietary sources.

10. Which one is not the feature of absorptive hypercalciuria?

(a) Increase in PTH
(b) Transient increase in serum calcium
(c) Increase in urine calcium
(d) Normal fasting urinary calcium

(Answer is A) The added systemic load of calcium due to intestinal calcium hyperabsorption results in a transient increase in serum calcium, which suppresses serum PTH and results in increased renal filtration of calcium, ultimately leading to hypercalciuria. Because the increase in intestinal absorption of calcium is matched by enhanced renal calcium excretion, serum calcium level remains normal.

11. Absorptive hypercalciuria 1 is differentiated from absorptive hypercalciuria 2 on what basis?

(a) PTH (b) Serum calcium
(c) Urine calcium (d) Calcitriol

(Answer is C) AH is classified as type I when urinary calcium remains high despite a low calcium diet and type II when urinary calcium normalizes with a restricted calcium intake.

12. Characteristic of renal hypercalciuria is:

(a) High fasting urinary calcium levels with normal serum calcium
(b) Low fasting urinary calcium levels with normal serum calcium
(c) Normal fasting urinary calcium levels with high serum calcium
(d) Normal fasting urinary calcium levels with low serum calcium

(Answer is A) High fasting urinary calcium levels (> 0.11 mg/dl glomerular filtration) with a normal serum calcium value are characteristic of renal hypercalciuria.

13. Primary hyperparathyroidism is the cause of nephrolithiasis in:

(a) 1% (b) 2%
(c) 5% (d) 10%

(Answer is C) Primary hyperparathyroidism is the cause of nephrolithiasis in about 5% of cases.

14. Most common cause of hypercalcemia in an outpatient setting:

(a) Tuberculosis
(b) Primary hyperparathyroidism
(c) Malignancy
(d) Vitamin D toxicity

(Answer is B) Primary hyperparathyroidism is the most common cause of hypercalcemia in an outpatient setting, malignancy is the main cause of hypercalcemia in hospitalized patients.

15. Most common malignancy-associated hypercalcemia is:

(a) Lung and breast
(b) Renal cell carcinoma
(c) Head and neck malignancies
(d) Lymphoma and myeloma

(Answer is A) Lung and breast cancers account for about 60% of malignancy-associated hypercalcemia, whereas renal cell (10% to 15%), head and neck (10%), and hematologic cancers such as lymphoma and myeloma (10%) account for the rest.

16. Which statement regarding hyperuricosuria is not correct?

(a) The most common cause of hyperuricosuria is increased dietary purine intake
(b) Hyperuricosuria is defined by urinary uric acid exceeding 600 mg/day
(c) At pH less than 5.5, sodium urate formation promotes uric acid stone formation through heterologous nucleation
(d) Uric acid may reduce the effectiveness of naturally occurring inhibitors of crystallization

(Answer is C) At pH less than 5.5, the undissociated form of uric acid predominates, leading to uric acid and/or calcium oxalate stone formation. At pH greater than 5.5, sodium urate formation promotes calcium oxalate stone formation through heterologous nucleation.

17. Hypocitraturia exists as an isolated abnormality in how many patients of calcium stone formers?

(a) 5% (b) 10%
(c) 15% (d) 20%

(Answer is B) Hypocitraturia is an important and correctable abnormality associated with nephrolithiasis that exists as an isolated abnormality in upto 10% of calcium stone formers.

18. Which statement regarding type I RTA is not correct?

(a) It is the most common form of RTA
(b) RTA most frequently associated with stone formation
(c) Findings include hypokalemic, hyperchloremic, non-anion gap metabolic acidosis
(d) RTA occurs as a result of impairment of reabsorption of bicarbonate

(Answer is D) RTA occurs as a result of impairment of net excretion of acid into the urine (type I) or of reabsorption of bicarbonate (type II).

19. The most common type of stone associated with distal RTA is:

(a) Calcium phosphate
(b) Calcium oxalate monohydrate
(c) Calcium oxalate dihydrate
(d) Uric acid

(Answer is A) The most common type of stone associated with distal RTA is calcium phosphate as a result of hypercalciuria, hypocitraturia, and increased urinary pH.

20. In distal RTA most common cause of stone formation is:

(a) Hyperoxaluria (b) Hypercalciuria
(c) Hypocitraturia (d) Decrease urine pH

(Answer is C) Profound hypocitraturia, perhaps the most important factor in stone formation, is due to impaired citrate excretion as a result of metabolic acidosis.

21. Which statement regarding type 4 RTA is not correct?

(a) Seen in diabetic nephropathy
(b) Hypokalemia
(c) Hyperchloremia
(d) Metabolic acidosis

(Answer is B) Reduction in glomerular filtration results in hyperkalemic, hyperchloremic metabolic acidosis due to loss of HCO-3 in the urine and decreased excretion of ammonium.

22. Most important pathogenetic factor for uric acid stone formation is:

(a) Low urine pH (b) Low urine volume
(c) Hyperuricosuria (d) Hypercalciuria

(Answer is A) The three main determinants of uric acid stone formation are low pH, low urine volume, and hyperuricosuria. The most important pathogenetic factor is low urine pH, because most patients with uric acid stones have normal uric acid excretion but invariably demonstrate persistent low urine pH.

23. Low urine pH in patients with uric acid stones with DM is due to:

(a) Impaired ammoniagenesis
(b) Impaired urine bicarbonate excretion
(c) Ketoacidosis
(d) Lactic acidosis

(Answer is A) Impaired ammonium production or excretion as a result of insulin resistance could leave hydrogen ions unbuffered in the urine, thereby leading to reduction in urine pH.

24. Which statement regarding cystine stones is not correct?

(a) Cystinuria is an AD disorder
(b) It is characterized by a defect in both intestinal and renal tubular transport of dibasic amino acids
(c) Under normal conditions amino acids are freely filtered and completely reabsorbed in the proximal tubules
(d) There is no specific inhibitor of cystine crystallization in the urine

(Answer is A) Cystinuria is an autosomal recessive disorder characterized by a defect in intestinal and renal tubular transport of dibasic amino acids.

25. Most common organism associated with infection stones:

(a) E. coli
(b) Pseudomonas
(c) Proteus
(d) Staphylococcus

(Answer is C) Proteus mirabilis the most common organism associated with infection stones.

26. Which stone occurs more commonly in females?

(a) Uric acid
(b) Calcium oxalate monohydrate
(c) Calcium phosphate
(d) Struvite

(Answer is D) Struvite stones occur more often in women than men by a ratio of 2:1.

27. Which statement regarding matrix stones are not correct?

(a) Radiolucent
(b) Contains 65% of protein
(c) Best treated with ESWL
(d) Associated with urea splitting organism

(Answer is C) Matrix stones are typically radiolucent. The matrix component of calcium-based stones comprises only 2.5% of the dry weight of the stone, whereas pure matrix stones may contain upward of 65% protein. SWL is not an effective treatment modality for patients with these stones.

28. Which statement regarding diuretics and formation of stone is not correct?

(a) Thiazides cause intracellular acidosis and subsequent hypocitraturia
(b) Loop diuretics inhibit sodium and calcium resorption in the thick ascending LOH, which in addition to a diuretic effect results in hypercalciuria
(c) In LBW infants receiving furosemide therapy, stones are consistently composed of uric acid
(d) Acetazolamide block resorption of sodium bicarbonate in the PT, leading to urinary alkalinization

(Answer is C) In LBW infants receiving furosemide therapy, stones are consistently composed of calcium oxalate.

29. Which statement regarding anatomical obstruction and formation of stone is correct?

(a) The incidence of renal calculi in patients with UPJ obstruction is nearly 20%
(b) Correction of the UPJ obstruction did not prevent recurrent stones in most patients
(c) Horseshoe kidneys have an associated rate of renal calculi of 20%
(d) Caliceal diverticula are associated with stones in up to 20% of patients

(Answer is D) Caliceal diverticula are associated with stones in up to 40% of patients

30. Which statement regarding stones in pregnancy is not correct?

(a) The majority of symptomatic stones occur in the first trimester of pregnancy
(b) Most stones pass spontaneously and complications are rare
(c) USG constitutes the first-line imaging modality when renal colic is suspected
(d) Physiologic hydronephrosis occurs in up to 90% of pregnant women and persists up to 4 to 6 weeks postpartum

(Answer is A) The majority of symptomatic stones occur in the second and third trimester of pregnancy.

31. Risk of recurrence for first stone formers within the subsequent 10 years is:

(a) 10% (b) 30%
(c) 50% (d) 75%

(Answer is C) First-time stone formers have often been estimated to have a 50% risk of recurrence within the subsequent 10 years.

32. Indications for a metabolic stone evaluation includes all *except:*

(a) Recurrent stone formers
(b) Osteoporosis
(c) Personal history of gout
(d) Stones composed of calcium oxalate

(Answer is D) Indications for a metabolic stone evaluation

- Recurrent stone formers.
- Strong family history of stones.
- Intestinal disease (particularly chronic diarrhea).
- Pathologic skeletal fractures.
- Osteoporosis.
- History of urinary tract infection with calculi.
- Personal history of gout.
- Solitary kidney.
- Anatomic abnormalities.
- Renal insufficiency.
- Stones composed of cystine, uric acid, or struvite.

33. Which one is not the correct pair?

(a) Calcium oxalate monohydrate–Hourglass
(b) Calcium oxalate dihydrate–Envelope
(c) Brushite–Needle shaped
(d) Uric acid–Hexagonal

(Answer is D)

Calcium oxalate monohydrate	Hourglass
Calcium oxalate dihydrate	Envelope, tetrahedral
Calcium phosphate–apatite	Amorphous
Brushite	Needle shaped
Magnesium ammonium phosphate (struvite)	Rectangular, coffin-lid
Cystine	Hexagonal
Uric acid	Amorphous shards, plates

34. Which one is not a radiolucent stone?

(a) Uric acid (b) Cystine
(c) Xanthine (d) Triamterene

(Answer is B) Radiolucent stones: Uric acid, xanthine, triamterene.

35. Which statement is not true regarding enteric hyperoxaluria?

(a) Low urine pH (b) Hypocitraturia
(c) Low urine volumes (d) Hypercalciuria

(Answer is D) The main hallmark is, hyperoxaluria with values that can be quite high (i.e., >50 mg/day). Urine calcium excretion is often low because of the saponification of oral calcium with poorly absorbed fats in the intestinal tract.

36. Incidence of renal stone in patients with distal RTA is:

(a) 20% (b) 50%
(c) 70% (d) 90%

(Answer is C) Upto 70% of adults with distal renal tubular acidosis have kidney stones.

37. Causes of acquired renal tubular acidosis are all *except:*

(a) ATN
(b) Renal transplantation
(c) Sarcoidosis
(d) Thyrotoxicosis

(Answer is D) Causes of acquired renal tubular acidosis

Recurrent pyelonephritis
Acute tubular necrosis
Renal transplantation
Analgesic nephropathy
Sarcoidosis
Idiopathic hypercalciuria
Primary hyperparathyroidism

38. Which one is not the correct pair?

(a) Calcium oxalate monohydrate–Weddellite
(b) Calcium hydrogen phosphate dehydrate–Brushite
(c) Tricalcium phosphate–Whitlockite
(d) Magnesium ammonium phosphate–Struvite

(Answer is A)

Calcium oxalate monohydrate	Whewellite
Calcium oxalate dihydrate	Weddellite
Calcium hydrogen phosphate dihydrate	Brushite
Tricalcium phosphate	Whitlockite
Carbonite-apatite	Carbonite-apatite
Magnesium ammonium phosphate	Struvite
Cystine	None
Uric acid	None

39. Which drink does not decrease the incidence of stone formation?

(a) Tea (b) Beer
(c) Wine (d) Apple juice

(Answer is D) For both men and women, there was a decrease in the risk of nephrolithiasis for those who consumed increased volumes of water, caffeinated or decaffeinated coffee, tea, beer and wine. Conversely, daily servings of apple or grape fruit juice increased the risk of stone events.

40. Which statement regarding formation of stone is not correct?

(a) Obesity is an independent risk factor for nephrolithiasis, particularly for women
(b) Obese patients have a higher propensity for struvite stones
(c) High-protein diets may increase the risk of stone formation
(d) Low-carbohydrate diets may increase the risk of stone formation

(Answer is B) Obese patients have a higher propensity for uric acid calculi.

41. Which one of the following is not the recommendation for prevention of stone disease?

(a) Low calcium diet
(b) Low sodium diet
(c) Low oxalate diet
(d) Vitamin C intake to a maximum daily dose of less than 2 g

(Answer is A) Older recommendations to significantly restrict calcium intake probably led to an increase in available intestinal oxalate.

42. The major goal in the management of gouty diathesis is to maintain the urine pH:

(a) Between 4.5 and 5.0
(b) Between 5.5 and 6.0
(c) Between 6.5 and 7.0
(d) Between 7.5 and 8.0

(Answer is C) The major goal in the management of gouty diathesis is to increase the urine pH above 5.5, preferably between 6.5 and 7.0.

43. Best medication for cystinuria includes:

(a) D-penicillamine
(b) α-mercaptopropionylglycine
(c) Captopril
(d) Allopurinol

(Answer is B) α-mercaptopropionylglycine is better tolerated than D-penicillamine and therefore enjoys clinical superiority.

44. Urease inhibitor used for struvite stone is:

(a) D-penicillamine
(b) α-mercaptopropionylglycine
(c) Captopril
(d) Acetohydroxamic acid

(Answer is D) Acetohydroxamic acid, a urease inhibitor, may reduce the urine saturation of struvite and therefore retard stone formation.

45. Major side effect of acetohydroxamic acid is:

(a) GI intolerance
(b) DVT
(c) Peripheral neuropathy
(d) Renal stones

(Answer is B) Significant percentage of patients receiving chronic acetohydroxamic acid therapy have experienced minor side effects, and 15% developed deep venous thrombosis.

46. Stone undetectable on CT is:

(a) Cystine (b) Triamterene
(c) Indinavir (d) Xanthine

(Answer is C) Difficulties may arise during diagnosis as indinavir stones may not be visible on plain film radiography and may even be undetectable on stone protocol CT.

47. Bladder stones in infected and non-infected urine respectively is mostly composed of:

(a) Uric acid and struvite
(b) Struvite and uric acid
(c) Calcium oxalate and struvite
(d) Struvite and calcium oxalate

(Answer is B) Bladder stones are usually composed of uric acid (in non-infected urine) or struvite (in infected urine).

48. Limited intravenous pyelography in pregnancy includes:

(a) Only scout film
(b) Scout film and 30 minutes film
(c) Scout film, 30 and 60 minutes film
(d) Scout film, 30 and 60 minutes and post void film

(Answer is B) Limited intravenous pyelography may be performed that consists of one scout image followed by one plate taken approximately 30 minutes after the injection of contrast material.

49. Which match is not correct?

(a) Multiple radial nephrotomies by Wickham
(b) Inferior pyelonephrolithotomy by Zucker-kandl
(c) Extended pyelolithotomy by Gil-Vernet
(d) Anatrophic nephrolithotomy by Brodel

(Answer is D) Smith and Boyce described anatrophic nephrolithotomy

50. Father of endourology is:

(a) Arthur Smith (b) Gil Yernet
(c) Badlani (d) Johannson

(Answer is A) Arthur Smith defined the term endourology as closed controlled manipulation within the genitourinary tract.

51. Stones can be satisfactorily treated by ESWL in:

(a) 70% - 75% (b) 75% - 80%
(c) 80% - 85% (d) 85% - 90%

(Answer is C) Most (about 80% to 85%) patients harboring "simple" renal calculi can be treated satisfactorily with SWL.

52. Single most important factor in determining the appropriate treatment modality for a patient with renal calculi is:

(a) Size (b) Anatomy
(c) Location (d) Composition

(Answer is A) Stone burden (size and number) is perhaps the single most important factor in determining the appropriate treatment modality for a patient with renal calculi.

53. Best predictor of post-PNL urosepsis is:

(a) Blood culture
(b) Mid stream urine culture
(c) Bladder urine culture
(d) Renal pelvic urine culture

(Answer is D) The best predictor of post-PNL urosepsis is stone culture or renal pelvic urine culture results, rather than bladder urine culture results.

54. Patients who have evidence suggestive of struvite or in whom infection is suspected should receive a minimum of how many days of antibiotics before surgery?

(a) 2 days (b) 5 days
(c) 2 weeks (d) 5 weeks

(Answer is C) Patients who have radiographic or clinical features suggestive of struvite or in whom infection is suspected should receive a minimum of 2 weeks of broad-spectrum antibiotics before surgery to reduce the risk of sepsis.

55. Asymptomatic calyceal stone more than what size will need intervention?

(a) Any size (b) 2 mm
(c) 5mm (d) 10 mm

(Answer is C) The necessity of treating patients with small (<5 mm), nonobstructive, asymptomatic stones in a prophylactic fashion remains undetermined. For larger stones absence of intervention, are likely to increase in size, causing symptoms of pain or infection. Cumulative 5-year probability of a symptomatic event is 48.5%; half of these events required active intervention.

56. Most staghorn stones are composed of:

(a) Uric acid
(b) Calcium oxalate monohydrate
(c) Struvite
(d) Cystine

(Answer is C) Most staghorn stones are composed of struvite, and factors that predispose to urinary tract infection and retained urine increase the likelihood of struvite stone formation.

57. The mean overall stone-free rates of SWL for the treatment of patients with solitary stones for stones 10 mm or less, 11 to 20 mm, and larger than 20 mm, respectively is:

(a) 90%, 80% and 70%
(b) 90%, 65% and 40%
(c) 80%, 65% and 55%
(d) 80%, 50% and 30%

(Answer is C) The mean overall stone-free rates of SWL for the treatment of patients with solitary stones stratified by size are 79.9% (range, 63% to 90%), 64.1% (range, 50% to 82.7%), and 53.7% (range, 33.3% to 81.4%) for stones 10 mm or less, 11 to 20 mm, and larger than 20 mm, respectively.

58. Stone most resistant to SWL is:

(a) Cystine
(b) Calcium oxalate monohydrate
(c) Struvite
(d) Calcium oxalate dihydrate

(Answer is A) Cystine and brushite calculi are the most resistant to SWL, followed by calcium oxalate monohydrate; following, in descending order of resistance to fragmentation, are struvite, calcium oxalate dihydrate, and uric acid stones.

59. Stone most resistant to SWL is:

(a) Uric acid
(b) Calcium oxalate monohydrate
(c) Struvite
(d) Calcium oxalate dihydrate

(Answer is B) Adjusted for size, cystine and brushite calculi are the most resistant to SWL, followed by calcium oxalate monohydrate; following, in descending order of resistance to fragmentation, are struvite, calcium oxalate dihydrate, and uric acid stones.

60. Increase risk for residual, "insignificant" fragments leading to stone regrowth after ESWL is particularly important with:

(a) Uric acid
(b) Calcium oxalate monohydrate

(c) Struvite
(d) Calcium oxalate dihydrate

(Answer is C) The use of SWL monotherapy in treating struvite stones may be particularly problematic because residual , "insignificant" fragments can prevent the sterilization of urine, increasing the risk of stone regrowth.

61. Which statement regarding calyceal diverticula is not correct?

(a) Congenital
(b) Secretory
(c) Urothelium lined
(d) Present in < 1% of patients

(Answer is B) Calyceal diverticula are congenitally derived, nonsecretory, urothelium-lined eventrations of the renal collecting system that are filled with urine. Calyceal diverticula are uncommon, having been reported as incidental findings in 0.2% to 0.6% of individuals undergoing renal imaging.

62. Calyceal diverticulum is best treated:

(a) Direct percutaneous approach for stone extraction
(b) Direct percutaneous approach for stone extraction with dilation of diverticular neck
(c) Direct percutaneous approach for stone extraction with dilation and incision of diverticular neck
(d) Direct percutaneous approach for stone extraction with dilation and incision of diverticular neck and fulgration of diverticular epithelium

(Answer is D) A direct percutaneous approach to the calyceal diverticulum is preferable because it allows use of a rigid nephroscope for stone extraction, dilation and incision of the diverticular neck, and fulguration of the diverticular epithelium.

63. In HSK, SWL can achieve satisfactory results with a stone burden smaller than:

(a) 0.5 cm (b) 1.0 cm
(c) 1.5 cm (d) 2.0 cm

(Answer is C) In HSK, SWL can achieve satisfactory results in the properly selected patient with a stone burden smaller than 1.5 cm and non-obstructed urine drainage.

64. Which statement regarding horseshoe kidney is not true?

(a) The results of PNL for patients with calculi in a horseshoe kidney are generally superior to those achieved with SWL
(b) Optimal point of entry for these kidneys is through a posterior calyx
(c) Vessels tend to enter the kidney posteriorly
(d) In most cases, the lower pole calyces are anterior and inaccessible percutaneously

(Answer is C) Vessels tend to enter the kidney anteriorly. An upper pole collecting system puncture is often appealing as the entire kidney is usually subcostal.

65. Successful outcome for lower pole calculi by ESWL includes:

(a) Stones less than 15 mm
(b) Infundibulopelvic angle of 90 degrees or lesser
(c) Infundibular length of less than 3 cm
(d) Infundibular width of more than 5 mm

(Answer is B) The combination of an infundibulopelvic angle of 90 degrees or greater, an infundibular length of less than 3 cm, and an infundibular width of more than 5 mm was associated with a successful outcome for lower pole calculi of 15 mm or less.

66. Fifteen mm renal pelvic stone in a patient with coagulopathy should be managed with:

(a) ESWL
(b) PNL
(c) Expectant management
(d) Flexible ureteroscopy

(Answer is D) Although SWL or PNL treatment of patients with uncorrected coagulopathy can result in life-threatening hemorrhage, such patients can be safely treated once the bleeding diathesis has been corrected. However, if the patient's coagulopathy is the result of a pharmacologic therapy that cannot be safely discontinued, ureteroscopy with holmium:YAG laser Iithotripsy is the preferable approach.

67. Clinically insignificant residual fragments were initially defined as:

(a) 2 mm (b) 4 mm
(c) 6 mm (d) 7 mm

(Answer is B) Clinically insignificant residual fragments were initially defined as residual fragments 4 mm or smaller in diameter associated with sterile urine in an otherwise asymptomatic patient.

68. Radiologic evaluation of asymptomatic patients after SWL includes:

(a) Abdominal radiography
(b) Abdominal radiography and ultrasonography
(c) Ultrasonography
(d) Non contrast CT

(Answer is B) Routine radiologic evaluation of asymptomatic patients after SWL could be limited to abdominal radiography and ultrasonography.

69. "Gold standard" for assessment of residual stones after PNL includes:

(a) Abdominal radiography and ultrasonography
(b) Noncontrast CT
(c) Flexible nephroscopy
(d) Flexible ureteroscopy

(Answer is C) Flexible nephroscopy may be considered the "gold standard" for assessment of residual stones after PNL.

70. Primary method for evaluation of patients after PNL includes:

(a) Abdominal radiography and ultrasonography
(b) Noncontrast CT
(c) Flexible nephroscopy
(d) Flexible ureteroscopy

(Answer is B) Given its wide availability and high sensitivity, non-contrast-enhanced CT is likely to become the primary method for evaluation of patients after PNL.

71. Regarding ureteral stone which is the most significant factor affecting the likelihood of stone passage?

(a) Location
(b) Size
(c) Composition
(d) Degree of obstruction

(Answer is B) Regarding ureteral stone the width of the stone is the most significant measurement affecting the likelihood of stone passage.

72. Rates of spontaneous passage for stones smaller than 4 mm, 4 to 6 mm, and larger than 6 mm respectively is:

(a) 90%, 80% and 40%
(b) 90%, 65% and 30%
(c) 80%, 60% and 20%
(d) 80%, 50% and 30%

(Answer is C) Those with stones smaller than 4 mm, 4 to 6 mm, and larger than 6 mm experienced rates of spontaneous passage of 80%, 59% and 21%, respectively.

73. Rate of spontaneous passage for distal, middle and proximal ureter stones respectively is:

(a) 80%, 60% and 40%
(b) 80%, 65% and 30%
(c) 70%, 60% and 30%

(d) 70%, 45% and 20%

(Answer is D) The rate of spontaneous passage is highly dependent on stone location; passage rates from the proximal, middle and distal ureter were 22%, 46% and 71%, respectively.

74. Conservative management should be considered for ureteric stone less than:

(a) 2mm (b) 5mm
(c) 7mm (d) 10mm

(Answer is B) For patients with stones of 5 mm or less in ureter, conservative management should be considered.

75. Stent placement before ESWL is useful because of all the following reasons *except:*

(a) Facilitated passage
(b) Improvement in stone fragmentation
(c) Mandatory in pati ents who have a solitary obstructed kidney
(d) In the treatment of difficult-to-visualize stones

(Answer is B) Initial experience with SWL suggested that placement of a ureteral stent before treatment facilitated stone fragmentation and passage. However, the AUA meta-analysis demonstrated no improvement in stone fragmentation for these patients, so this practice was discouraged.

76. Primary approach for stones smaller than 1 cm in the proximal ureter:

(a) ESWL
(b) PNL
(c) Flexible ureteroscopy
(d) Lap ureterolithotomy

(Answer is A) Because of its greater efficacy and lower morbidity, the panel suggested that SWL, either *in situ* or after push back, should be the primary approach for stones smaller than 1 cm in the proximal ureter.

77. Best approach for impacted stone of 2.5 cm in the proximal ureter:

(a) ESWL
(b) PNL
(c) Flexible ureteroscopy
(d) Lap ureterolithotomy

(Answer is D) Stones that could not be accessed ureteroscopically or did not fragment with other treatment modalities as well as large (> 1.5 cm) proximal ureteral stones as indications for the uretreolithotomy.

78. An impacted stone may be defined as a stone that remains at the same site in the ureter for more than:

(a) 1 month (b) 2 months
(c) 3 months (d) 4 months

(Answer is B) An impacted stone may be defined as a stone that cannot be bypassed by a wire or catheter or a stone that remains at the same site in the ureter for more than 2 months.

79. Which statement regarding renal stones in pregnancy is not true?

(a) Incidence of symptomatic urinary calculi has been calculated to be more in pregnant women
(b) Upper tract dilation is seen in up to 90% of pregnant women by the third trimester
(c) The right ureter tends to be more dilated than the left
(d) Humoral as well as mechanical factors have been implicated in the etiology of hydronephrosis

(Answer is A) Incidence of symptomatic urinary calculi has been calculated to be the same for pregnant women as for non-pregnant women of childbearing age.

80. All *except* one are the physiological changes in pregnancy:

(a) The increase in renal plasma flow and glomerular filtration
(b) Normal ranges of serum creatinine and blood urea nitrogen are approximately 25% lower for the pregnant patient
(c) Increases the filtered loads of sodium, calcium and uric acid, causing a state of hypercalciuria and hyperuricosuria
(d) Increase in the excretion of urinary citrate and decrease in urinary excretion of magnesium

(Answer is D) Potentially lithogenic physiologic changes are offset by an increase in the excretion of urinary inhibitors, such as citrate and magnesium, as well as an increase in urine output.

81. Preferred approach for renal diversion in pregnant patient with 6 mm upper ureteric stone at 12th week and 32nd week, who has failed conservative management respectively is:

(a) Placement of JJ stent and nephrostomy tube
(b) Placement of nephrostomy tube and JJ stent
(c) Flexible ureteroscopy and JJ stent
(d) JJ stent and flexible ureteroscopy

(Answer is B) Ureteral stent placements should be considered in later stages of pregnancy (after 22 weeks) and placing a nephrostomy tube in early pregnancy.

82. Which treatment modality is safe in pregnancy?

(a) ESWL
(b) Electrohydraulic lithotripters
(c) Ballistic lithotripters
(d) Ultrasonic lithotripters

(Answer is C) If lithotripsy is required, both the holmium: YAG laser and the pneumatic lithotrite devices are safe. Ultrasonic lithotripters should be avoided as the high-pitched audible sound may induce hearing injury in the fetus.

83. Highest incidence of ureteral perforation occurs with which lithotripter?

(a) EHL (b) Holmium
(c) Ultrasonic (d) Ballistic

(Answer is A) The incidence of ureteral perforation varies among the different intracorporeal lithotrites; the highest incidence of ureteral perforation occurs with EHL.

84. Laser is an acronym for:

(a) Light amplification by simulated emission of radiation
(b) Light amplification by stimulated emission of radiation
(c) Light anticipation by simulated emission of radiation
(d) Light anticipation by stimulated emission of radiation

(Answer is B) Laser is an acronym for light amplification by stimulated emission of radiation.

85. The coumarin wavelength (504 nm) is absorbed by all stone materials *except:*

(a) Uric acid
(b) Struvite
(c) Cystine
(d) Calcium oxalate monohydrate

(Answer is C) The coumarin wavelength (504 nm) was chosen because it is absorbed by all stone materials except cystine but not by surrounding tissues.

86. Which laser has ability to fragment all stones regardless of composition?

(a) EHL (b) Ballistic
(c) Ultrasonic (d) Holmium

(Answer is D) The ability of the holmium laser to fragment all stones regardless of composition is a clear advantage over the coumarin pulsed-dye laser. Successful fragmentation of ureteral stones of all compositions has been reported in 91% to 100% of cases, with a mean stone-free rate of 95%.

87. Which one of the safest, most effective and most versatile intracorporeal lithotripters?

(a) EHL (b) Holmium
(c) Ultrasonic (d) Ballistic

(Answer is B) Holmium laser is one of the safest, most effective, and most versatile intracorporeal lithotripters.

88. Which should not be done while performing holmium lithotripsy?

(a) Start at low settings and increase only as necessary
(b) Work from the inside of the stone outward
(c) Keep the fiber tip at least 2 mm from the urothelium
(d) One person should control the fiber and another the foot pedal

(Answer is D)

- Do not have one person controlling the fiber and another the foot pedal.
- Do not discharge the laser fiber inside the working channel or on guide wires and baskets.
- Do not pass the fiber tip through the back wall of stones. ·
- Do not get impatient–holmium:YAG laser lithotripsy is not necessarily fast.

89. Preferred initial setting of holmium laser for ureteric stone is:

(a) 1J with pulse rate of 6 Hz
(b) 6J with pulse rate of 10 Hz
(c) 0.6J with pulse rate of 6 Hz
(d) 0.6J with pulse rate of 10 Hz

(Answer is C) It is recommended that treatment be commenced with low-pulse energy (e.g., 0.6J) with a pulse rate of 6 Hz and that pulse frequency be increased (in preference to increasing pulse energy) as needed to speed fragmentation.

90. Which intracorporeal lithotripters has highest rate of stone retropulsion?

(a) EHL (b) Holmium
(c) Ultrasonic (d) Pnuematic

(Answer is D) Ballistic lithotripsy is associated with a relatively high rate of stone retropulsion.

91. Which lithotripsy has the advantage of combination of stone fragmentation and simultaneous fragment removal?

(a) EHL (b) Holmium
(c) Ultrasonic (d) Ballistic

(Answer is C) The major advantage of ultrasonic lithotripsy is the efficient combination of stone fragmentation and simultaneous fragment removal.

92. Regarding electrohydraulic shockwave lithotripter which statement is not true?

(a) Cylindrical expanding shockwave is generated
(b) Effective in breaking kidney stones
(c) Substantial pressure fluctuations from shock to shock
(d) Relatively short electrode life

(Answer is A) In the electrohydraulic shockwave lithotripter, a spherically expanding shockwave is generated by an underwater spark discharge.

93. Regarding electromagnetic shockwave lithotripter which statement is not true?

(a) More controllable and reproducible generator
(b) Introduction of energy into the patient's body over a small skin area
(c) Small focal point can be achieved with high-energy densities
(d) Increased rate of subcapsular hematoma formation

(Answer is B) Advantages include the introduction of energy into the patient's body over a large skin area, which may cause less pain. In addition, a small focal point can be achieved with high-energy densities, which may increase its effectiveness in breaking stones.

94. Regarding piezoelectric shockwave lithotripter which statement is not true?

(a) Poor focusing accuracy
(b) Long service life
(c) Produces plane shockwaves with directly converging shock fronts
(d) Insufficient power it delivers, which hampers its ability to effectively break renal stones

(Answer is A) The advantages of this generator include the focusing accuracy, a long service life, and the possibility of an anesthetic-free treatment because of the relatively low energy density at the skin entry point of the shockwave.

95. EMLA cream, a eutectic mixture of:

(a) Lignocaine and alfentanil
(b) Lidocaine and prilocaine
(c) Midazolam and lignocaine
(d) Midazolam and propofol

(Answer is B) EMLA cream, a eutectic mixture of lidocaine and prilocaine, has been shown significantly to reduce anesthesia requirements during SWL.

96. Shock wave ratio of the positive to negative peak pressures is:

(a) 2 (b) 3
(c) 4 (d) 5

(Answer is D) Typical shock wave ratio of the positive to negative peak pressures is approximately 5.

97. The first mechanism by which a stone might break is through?

(a) Cavitation (b) Squeezing
(c) Shear stress (d) Spall fracture

(Answer is D) The first mechanism by which a stone might break is through spall fracture. Second is squeezing and splitting. Third is shear stress. Fourth is superfocusing. Fifth is cavitation .

98. Risk Factors for shockwave lithotripsy are all *except:*

(a) Diabetes mellitus
(b) Preexisting hypertension
(c) Coagulopathies
(d) Thyrotoxicosis

(Answer is D) *Acute renal side effects:* Risk factors for shockwave lithotripsy are hypertension, DM, coronary heart disease, thrombocytopenia.

99. Absolute contraindication to PNL is:

(a) Pelvic kidney
(b) 4 cm renal stone
(c) Morbidly obese
(d) Uncorrected coagulopathy

(Answer is D) Absolute contraindication to PNL, such as uncorrected coagulopathy, as well as those with an active, untreated urinary tract infection.

100. All urologic endoscopic procedures are regarded as:

(a) Clean
(b) Clean contaminated
(c) Contaminated
(d) Dirty

(Answer is B) All urologic endoscopic procedures are regarded as clean contaminated.

101. In PNL the most common secondarily infecting organism is:

(a) Staph. epidermidis (b) Staph. aureus
(c) Streptococcus (d) Pseudomonas

(Answer is A) Cephalosporins are the most appropriate antibiotic for prophylaxis before surgical procedures in noninfected patients as the most common secondarily infecting organism is S. epidermidis.

102. A supracostal puncture is usually necessary in all *except:*

(a) Associated ureteropelvic junction stricture requiring endopyelotomy
(b) Multiple upper pole infundibula and calyces containing stone material

(c) Associated ureteral stone
(d) Horseshoe kidneys

(Answer is B) A supracostal puncture is usually necessary when the predominant distribution of stone material is in the upper of stone material is in the upper calyces, when there is an associated ureteropelvic junction stricture requiring endopyelotomy, in cases of multiple lower pole infundibula and calyces containing stone material or an associated ureteral stone, in staghorn calculi with substantial upper pole stone burden, and in horseshoe kidneys.

103. Factors increasing the risk of colon injury include all *except:*

(a) Posterior calyceal puncture
(b) Previous extensive renal surgery
(c) Horseshoe kidney
(d) Kyphoscoliosis

(Answer is A) Factors increasing the risk of colon injury include anterior calyceal puncture, previous extensive renal surgery, horseshoe kidney, and kyphoscoliosis; retrorenal colon is more commonly found on the left.

104. Which statement regarding closed system in PNL is not true?

(a) Low flow and high pressure system
(b) Lead to low fluid absorption
(c) Nephroscope serving as its own sheath
(d) Nephrostomy track is smaller

(Answer is B) Closed , high-pressure system with the nephroscope serving as its own sheath. The advantages of the closed system are that the nephrostomy track is smaller, hydrodistention of the collecting system occurs, and bleeding may be reduced. However, a closed system is a low-flow, high-pressure (16 to 33 cm H_2O) system that can lead to significant fluid absorption.

105. Most significant complication of PNL is:

(a) Bleeding
(b) Infection
(c) Chest compilication
(d) Incomplete stone removal

(Answer is A) Hemorrhage is the most significant complication of PNL, with transfusion rates reported to be from less than 1% to 10%.

106. In PNL if bleeding persists despite the placement of a nephrostomy tube, next step is:

(a) Kaye nephrostomy tamponade balloon catheter should be placed
(b) Clamp the tube
(c) Surgical exploration
(d) Angiography

(Answer is B) If bleeding persists despite the placement of a nephrostomy tube, clamping the tube for a time may facilitate the tamponade of any bleeding points. If these measures do not control the hemorrhage, a Kaye nephrostomy tamponade balloon catheter should be placed.

107. Which statement regarding steinstrasse is not true?

(a) This complication has been reported in 2% to 10% of SWL cases
(b) Directly correlates with increasing stone burden
(c) More than 70% of steinstrasse occurs in the distal ureter
(d) The placement of a ureteral stent before SWL will eliminate risk of steinstrasse

(Answer is D) The placement of a ureteral stent before SWL therapy may decrease although not eliminate the risk of steinstrasse.

108. Best management for steinstrasse is:

(a) ESWL (b) PCN
(c) PCNL (d) URS

(Answer is D) In summary, steinstrasse is a well-known complication of SWL, with most cases resolving spontaneously. When intervention is required, percutaneous nephrostomy alone has a success rate of more than 70%. Ureteroscopic intervention is definitive and predictable with an immediate success rate approaching 100%.

109. Indications for flexible ureteroscopy included all *except:*

(a) Single renal stone of 1.2 cm
(b) Two renal stones smaller than 5 mm
(c) Renal stones associated with intrarenal stenosis
(d) Patients with a need for complete stone removal (e.g., pilots)

(Answer is A) Indications for ureteroscopy included patients whose SWL treatment failed (single stone smaller than 1 cm or up to five stones smaller than 5 mm.

110. The advantages of the semirigid ureteroscope include all *except:*

(a) Large working channel
(b) Faster irrigation flow
(c) Large field of view
(d) Less trauma to ureter

(Answer is D) The advantages of the semirigid ureteroscope include a large working channel, faster irrigation flow, and a larger field of view because of the larger number of fiberoptic bundles compared with the corresponding flexible instruments. Disadvantages: May be more traumatic to the urethra/ureter, limited access within the ureter.

111. Which statement is not true regarding hydrophilic-tipped guide wires?

(a) Require sterile water or saline flushes through the holding jacket before use
(b) Decreased coefficient of friction
(c) Becomes slippery to facilitate manipulation past tight obstructions
(d) Stenting over a hydrophilic wire is easy

(Answer is D) The main disadvantage of the hydrophilic wire is also its slipperiness, which allows it to slide easily out of the ureter. Stenting over a hydrophilic wire is difficult.

112. Regarding ureteroscopy access (UAS) sheath which statement is not true?

(a) Shorter operating room times and greater cost savings
(b) UASs may cause ureteral ischemia and necrosis
(c) Stone-free rate was higher in patients using UAS
(d) UASs can limit endoscope damage

(Answer is B) Shorter operating room times and greater cost savings have been demonstrated when UASs are utilized in conjunction with ureteroscopy. Previous concerns that UASs may cause ureteral ischemia and necrosis resulting in a ureteral stricture have been unfounded, as the stricture incidence has been demonstrated to be the same as that with ureteroscopy alone (~1.4%).

113. Which statement regarding holmium: YAG laser is not true?

(a) The method of stone fragmentation is photoacoustic
(b) Wavelength is 2100 nm
(c) Penetration is 0.5 to 1 mm in liquid medium
(d) Effective in fragmenting all stone composition

(Answer is A) The method of stone fragmentation using the holmium:YAG laser differs from the photoacoustic method utilized by other lasers. Energy from the holmium:YAG laser produces a photothermal effect resulting in vaporization of the stone.

114. Indications for ureteral stent placement following ureteroscopy are all *except:*

(a) Ureteral perforation intraoperatively
(b) Ureteral dilation greater than 6 Fr

(c) Failure to advance the ureteroscope due to a narrow ureter
(d) Large stone burden with many fragments remaining to pass

(Answer is B) Indications for ureteral stent placement following ureteroscopy:

- Ureteral perforation intraoperatively.
- Ureteral dilation greater than 10 Fr (either coaxial or balloon dilator).
- Significant ureteral edema due to stone (e.g., impacted stone).
- Failure to advance the ureteroscope due to a narrow ureter or ureteral orifice and in preparation for a subsequent ureteroscopy after 7 days.
- Infected urinary system with an obstructing system.
- Large stone burden with many fragments remaining to pass.
- Solitary kidney.

115. Most common polymer used in today's ureteral stents:

(a) Silicone
(b) Poly-L-lactic and glycolic acids
(c) Polyurethane
(d) Polyethylene

(Answer is C) Polyurethane, the most common polymer used in today's stents.

116. Indications for ureteroscopy rather than shockwave lithotripsy in stone ureteral disease are all *except:*

(a) Morbidly obese·
(b) Uncorrectable bleeding diathesis
(c) Multiple proximal ureteral stones
(d) Stones <1 cm

(Answer is D) Indications for ureteroscopy rather than shockwave lithotripsy in stone ureteral disease is:

- Known hard stone (calcium oxalate monohydrate, cystine, brushite).
- Morbidly obese (>300 lb or above the focusing limit of the lithotriptor).
- Uncorrectable bleeding diathesis (or in a patient in whom it is unsafe to discontinue anticoagulation).
- Multiple proximal ureteral stones.
- Stones > 1cm (decreased rate of success with SWL when stone is > 1 cm).
- Radiolucent stones.
- Patient's preference.
- Social reasons (i.e., for patients who must be completely stone free, such as pilots, bus drivers).

117. Incidence of ureteral stricture after ureteral perforation is:

(a) 3.5% (b) 6%
(c) 10% (d) 15%

(Answer is B) The reported ureteral stricture rate of approximately 3.5% increases to 5.9% if a ureteral perforation occurs.

118. Regarding Brödel type configuration which is true?

(a) Anterior calyx is long and medially directed, whereas the posterior calyx is shorter and more laterally directed
(b) Anterior calyx is short and medially directed, whereas the posterior calyx is longer and more laterally directed
(c) Anterior calyx is short and laterally directed, whereas the posterior calyx is longer and more medially directed
(d) Anterior calyx is long and laterally directed, whereas the posterior calyx is shorter and more medially directed

(Answer is B) In the Brödel type configuration, the anterior calyx is short and medially directed (forming a 70-degree angle to the frontal plane of the kidney), whereas the posterior calyx is longer and more laterally directed (positioned only 20 degrees from the frontal plane of the kidney).

119. Consistent finding regarding drainage pattern of pelvicalyceal system is:

(a) Superior calyceal group is drained by one midline infundibulum
(b) Middle calyceal group was drained by one midline infundibulum
(c) Inferior calyceal group was drained by one midline infundibulum
(d) Anterior calyceal group was drained by one midline infundibulum

(Answer is A) The only consistently noted findings were that the superior calyceal group was drained by only one midline infundibulum in 99% of the endocasts and that the midzone was drained by paired calyces arranged in two rows (anterior and posterior) in 96% of cases.

120. Most commonly injured vessel in endourologic procedures is:

(a) Anterior segmental artery
(b) Posterior segmental artery
(c) Lateral segmental artery
(d) Medial segmental artery

(Answer is B) The posterior segmental artery is the most commonly injured vessel in endourologic procedures.

121. The maximum yearly whole-body exposure recommended by the National Council on Radiation Protection is:

(a) 05 rem (b) 10 rem
(c) 15 rem (d) 20 rem

(Answer is A) The maximum yearly whole-body exposure recommended by the National Council on Radiation Protection is 5000 mrem, or 5 rem.

122. Boundaries of lumbar notch are all *except:*

(a) Superiorly by latissimus dorsi muscle
(b) Medially by sacrospinalis
(c) Laterally by transversus abdominis
(d) Laterally by internal oblique

(Answer is D) The lumbar notch, bounded superiorly by the latissimus dorsi muscle and the 12th rib, medially by the sacrospinalis and the quadratus lumborum muscles, and laterally by the transversus abdominis and the external oblique muscles, has been shown to be a useful anatomic window for successful blind percutaneous calyceal access.

123. For correct direction of needle advancement and for depth of needle insertion, C-arm should be in what position respectively?

(a) 30 degree and 0 degree
(b) 0 degree and 30 degree
(c) 45 degree and 0 degree
(d) 0 degree and 45 degree

(Answer is A) Correct direction of needle advancement by rotating the C-arm 30 degrees toward the surgeon and observing for the bull's-eye effect. The depth of needle penetration is monitored by rotating the C-arm back to the vertical position.

124. Increased risk of bleeding occurs in all situations *except:*

(a) Patients on anticoagulant therapy
(b) Multiple punctures
(c) Puncture into kidney with abnormal anatomy
(d) Excessive lateral puncture

(Answer is D) In particular, excessively medial punctures, multiple punctures, and punctures into kidneys with abnormal anatomy are associated with an increased risk of bleeding.

125. Which statement regarding perculex is not correct?

(a) Poor coil retention

(b) Good biocompatibility
(c) Relatively low coefficient of friction
(d) Excellent tensile strength

(Answer is A) Percuflex offers the best ratio of internal to external diameter, excellent tensile strength and coil retention, a relatively low coefficient of friction, and good biocompatibility.

126. Which is not correctly matched regarding nephrostomy tube drainage?

(a) Uncomplicated percutaneous renal surgery–tubeless
(b) Complicated percutaneous renal surgery-Councill tip catheter
(c) Post-endopyelotomy care–14Fr/7Fr
(d) Long term drainage–Malecot catheter

(Answer is D)

Choosing appropriate nephrostomy tube drainage

Clinical indication	*Suggested nephrostomy tube and tract management*
Acute obstruction, simple temporary drainage	Pigtail, cope loop catheter
Uncomplicated percutaneous renal surgery	Tubeless + cautery or hemostatic sealants, Malecot catheter, Balloon catheter
Complicated percutaneous renal surgery	Council tip catheter, kaye tamponade catheter
Minor mucosal damage or post-endopyelotomy care	Malecot re-entry tube, Smith endopyelotomy stent (14 Fr/7 Fr)
Long-term drainage, administration of topical chemotherapy, pyelopyelostomy	Circle loop nephrostomy tube

127. Robotic PAKY has proved to be a safe and efficacious method for management for:

(a) ESWL (b) PCNL
(c) Pyeloplasty (d) TURP

(Answer is B) Robotic PAKY has proved to be a safe and efficacious method of obtaining access before percutaneous nephrolithotomy.

128. Risk factors for SWL are all *except*:

(a) Obesity
(b) Thrombocytosis
(c) Pre-existing hypertension
(d) Diabetes mellitus

(Answer is B) Risk factors for SWL

- Age.
- Obesity.
- Coagulopathies.
- Thrombocytopenia.
- Diabetes mellitus.
- Coronary heart disease.
- Preexisting hypertension.

129. Which of the following is not a cause of hypocitraturia?

(a) High protein diet
(b) Hypokalaemia
(c) Proximal renal tubular acidosis
(d) Idiopathic

(Answer is C) Proximal renal tubular acidosis

130. To which region does pain, from the left mid ureter, refer to?

(a) The loin region
(b) The inguinal region
(c) The umbilical region
(d) The penis or clitoris

(Answer is B) The inguinal region

131. Which type of renal stone crystals is known as "coffin lid"?

(a) Oxalate (b) Struvite
(c) Urate (d) Cystine

(Answer is B) Struvite

132. How can hyperuricosuria cause calcium oxalate calculi?

(a) By increasing oxalate absorption

(b) By heterogeneous nucleation
(c) By inducing hyperoxaluria
(d) By reducing urate crystals saturation

(Answer is B) By heterogeneous nucleation

133. Which type of urinary casts are solidified Tamm-Horsfall mucoproteins secreted from the tubular epithelial cells of individual nephrons?

(a) Granular
(b) Hyaline
(c) Waxy
(d) Pigment

(Answer is B) Hyaline

134. What causes "pink diaper syndrome" is (are)?

(a) Staphylococcus epidermidis in the urine
(b) Dried urate crystals on the diaper
(c) Adenovirus 11 in the urine
(d) Candidiasis in the urine

(Answer is B) Dried urate crystals on the diaper

135. What is false about indinavir sulfate stones?

(a) Intratubular crystal formation might occur
(b) CT cannot reliably confirm the presence of indinavir calculi
(c) Stone formation is demonstrated in 80% of patients taking the medication
(d) Is a protease inhibitor with poor solubility and significant urinary excretion

(Answer is C) Stone formation is demonstrated in 80% of patients taking the medication

136. What stone is inherited as an autosomal recessive trait?

(a) Xanthine
(b) Ammonium urate
(c) Cystine
(d) Calcium oxalate dihydrate

(Answer is C) Cystine

137. As per the "fixed particle theory" of stone formation:

(a) The initial step is papillary plaque formation
(b) Crystals formation occurs inside the nephron
(c) Tubular precipitates form harmless crystalluria
(d) The attraction of organic compounds and activation crystallization is regulated by osteopontin

(Answer is A) The initial step is papillary plaque formation

138. What risk factor(s) promote(s) stone formation?

(a) Dehydration
(b) Metabolic disorders
(c) Congenital anomalies
(d) All of the above

(Answer is A) Dehydration

139. What are the expected findings on urinalysis in patients with acute renal colic?

(a) Blood cells more than pus cells
(b) Pus cells if infection was superadded
(c) Crystals might appear
(d) All of the above

(Answer is A) Blood cells more than pus cells

140. Worldwide, the most common type of urinary stones is:

(a) Calcium monohydrate
(b) Calcium oxalate
(c) Ammonium urate
(d) None of the above

(Answer is B) Calcium oxalate

141. What is false concerning primary bladder stones?

(a) Commoner in females than in males
(b) Pediatrics, are of calcium oxalate and/or ammonium urate composition
(c) Caused by bladder outlet obstruction

(d) Might result in bladder cancer

(Answer is A) Commoner in females than in males

142. What is false concerning staghorn calculus?

(a) Commonly unilateral
(b) Commonly due to repeated infections
(c) Urate stones are the second most common cause of staghorn calculi
(d) ESWL monotherapy with ureteral stenting is the ideal treatment

(Answer is D) ESWL monotherapy with ureteral stenting is the ideal treatment

143. What is false concerning cystine stones?

(a) Result from an inherited defect of renal tubular reabsorption of cysteine
(b) Characteristically, urate and cysteine stone are radiolucent
(c) Cysteine is a dibasic amino acid
(d) Plain X-ray, cysteine stones exhibit "ground-glass" appearance

(Answer is B) Characteristically, urate and cysteine stone are radiolucent

144. What is false concerning cystine stones?

(a) Have diagnostic hexagonal crystals
(b) Don't respond to ESWL therapy
(c) Are highly soluble in water
(d) Inherited in an autosomal recessive fashion

(Answer is C) Are highly soluble in water

145. What is false concerning struvite stones?

(a) The most common to form staghorn giant calculi
(b) Formed by urease producing bacteria
(c) Antibiotics have a role in the treatment
(d) Form at the two extremes of urinary pH range

(Answer is D) Form at the two extremes of urinary pH range

146. Which of the following bacteria split urea?

(a) Klebsiella pneumonia
(b) Morganella morganii
(c) Proteus mirabilis
(d) All of the above

(Answer is D) All of the above

147. Patients having what kind of stones should refrain from eating purines?

(a) Cysteine (b) Urate
(c) Calcium (d) None of the above

(Answer is D) None of the above

148. What congenital anomaly is unlikely to result in stone formation?

(a) Left ureterocele
(b) Bifid right renal pelvis
(c) Neurogenic bladder
(d) Bilateral UPJ stenosis

(Answer is B) Bifid right renal pelvis

149. In what kind of renal stones do antibiotics help most?

(a) Indinavir
(b) Magnesium ammonium phosphate
(c) Xanthine
(d) Matrix

(Answer is B) Magnesium ammonium phosphate

150. What medications do not cause renal stones?

(a) Ciprofloxacin (b) Indinavir
(c) Thiazides (d) Triamterene

(Answer is C) Thiazides

151. What stones are radiopaque on plain X-ray film?

(a) 2,8 dihydroxyadenine stones
(b) Sulfa medications-induced stones
(c) Calcium oxalate stones
(d) Matrix stones

(Answer is C) Calcium oxalate stones

152. What is the proper sequence of the following stones when ordered from most radiopaque to most radiolucent as they appear on plain X-ray film?

(a) Ca. oxalate, Ca. phosphate, Na.urate, cystine
(b) Ca. phosphate, Ca. oxalate, cystine, Na. urate
(c) Ca. oxalate, Ca. phosphate, cystine, Na. urate
(d) Ca. phosphate, Ca. oxalate, Na. urate, cystine

(Answer is B) Ca. phosphate, Ca. oxalate, cystine, Na. urate

153. What does not appear as a filling defect in the renal pelvis on IVU?

(a) Fungal ball
(b) Radiolucent stone
(c) Urothelial growth
(d) Upper end of DJ ureteral stent

(Answer is D) Upper end of DJ ureteral stent

154. What is true concerning uric acid stones?

(a) They are metabolic stones that form at high urinary pH
(b) They score 800 – 1000 HU on CT
(c) Only 25% of affected patients have gout disease
(d) Affected patients must stop eating animal protein

(Answer is C) Only 25% of affected patients have gout disease

155. What condition might not cause uric acid stones?

(a) Tumor lysis syndrome
(b) Hypoparathyroidism
(c) Myeloproliferative disorder
(d) Lesch-Nyhan syndrome

(Answer is B) Hypoparathyroidism

156. What is the composition of brushite stones?

(a) Calcium phosphate
(b) Calcium oxalate monohydrate
(c) Sodium urate
(d) 2,8 dihydroxyadenine

(Answer is A) Calcium phosphate

157. When should renal stone patients be evaluated for metabolic diseases?

(a) When stones are multiple and/or recurrent
(b) When stones form in childhood
(c) Cases where nephrocalcinosis and urolithiasis are present
(d) All of the above

(Answer is D) All of the above

158. What is (are) the indication(s) of hospitalization of ureteral stone patients?

(a) Steinstrasse
(b) A stone in ureterocele
(c) Fever, leucocytosis, pain
(d) Brushite stones

(Answer is C) Fever, leucocytosis, pain

159. A 24-hour urine collection of a recurrent Ca. oxalate stone former patient having Crohn's disease might reveal:

(a) High citrate, high oxalate
(b) Low citrate, low oxalate
(c) High citrate, low oxalate
(d) Low citrate, high oxalate

(Answer is D) Low citrate, high oxalate

160. How is primary oxaluria treated?

(a) Terminal ilium resection
(b) Liver transplantation
(c) Kidney transplantation
(d) Regular hemodialysis

(Answer is C) Kidney transplantation

161. What type of stones do laxative abusers might develop?

(a) Ammonium urate
(b) Sodium urate
(c) Calcium oxalate
(d) Calcium phosphate

(Answer is A) Ammonium urate

162. What does nephrocalcin do?

(a) Dissolves cystine stones
(b) Enhances nephrocalcinosis process over old scared areas
(c) Inhibits Ca. oxalate aggregation and crystallization
(d) Plays a secondary role in metastatic calcification process

(Answer is C) Inhibits Ca. oxalate aggregation and crystallization

163. What bowel surgery could result in enteric hyperoxaluria?

(a) Right hemicolectomy
(b) Small bowel resection
(c) Roux-en-Y gastric bypass
(d) B and C

(Answer is D) B and C

164. How does oral Mg. citrate inhibit Ca. oxalate stone formation?

(a) Lowering urinary saturation of Ca. oxalate
(b) Preventing heterogeneous nucleation of Ca. oxalate
(c) Inhibiting spontaneous precipitation and agglomeration of Ca. oxalate
(d) All of the above

(Answer is D) All of the above

165. When urine reaches a high tendency to form stones, the situation is called:

(a) Lithogenic anion to cation ratio
(b) Randall cut off
(c) Saturation index
(d) Solubility product

(Answer is C) Saturation index

166. What type of stones is soft, resilient, composed of mucoproteins of urine and serum?

(a) Matrix
(b) Indinavir
(c) Brushite
(d) 2,8 dihydroxyadenine

(Answer is A) Matrix

167. What is the principal defect in renal hypercalciuria?

(a) Impaired renal tubular calcium reabsorption
(b) Excessive glomerular leak of calcium
(c) Deficiency of the enzyme xanthine oxidase
(d) Hypercalcemia

(Answer is A) Impaired renal tubular calcium reabsorption

168. Why do patients with cystic fibrosis form stones?

(a) Because urine and body secretions are highly concentrated
(b) Due to renal leak hypercalciuria
(c) A result of distal renal tubular acidosis type I
(d) Because of reduced or absent of oxalobacter formigenes colonization

(Answer is D) Because of reduced or absent of oxalobacter formigenes colonization

169. The process where nucleation and further precipitations occur by different components to form urinary stones, is called:

(a) Classical nucleation theory
(b) Heterogeneous nucleation

(c) Suspension solution
(d) Concentric lamination

(Answer is B) Heterogeneous nucleation

170. Where do Randall plaques originate from?

(a) Transitional epithelium lining minor calyces
(b) Transitional epithelium lining major calyces
(c) Basement membrane of the loops of Henle
(d) Papillary tips of polar pyramids

(Answer is C) Basement membrane of the loops of Henle

171. What does the treatment of hyperuricemia with urate stones include?

(a) Oral potassium sodium hydrogen citrate granules
(b) Increase hydration
(c) Allopurinol
(d) All of the above

(Answer is D) All of the above

172. What is the sure diagnostic finding of Ca. oxalate stones?

(a) Chemical analysis of a recovered stone
(b) Hypercalcemia
(c) CT finding
(d) High breakability on ESWL

(Answer is A) Chemical analysis of a recovered stone

173. On treating uric acid stones, excessive alkalinization with potassium citrate could result in all of the following, *except:*

(a) Formation of triple-phosphate stones
(b) Infection with proteus species
(c) Increase production of endogenous uric acid
(d) Increase level of uric acid in the blood

(Answer is C) Increase production of endogenous uric acid

174. What medication(s) could be helpful in the management of cystinuria?

(a) α-Mercaptopropionylglycine
(b) d-Penicillamine
(c) A and B
(d) None of the above

(Answer is C) A and B

175. What medication could help in managing carbonate apatite stones?

(a) α-mercaptopropionylglycine
(b) Acetohydroxamic acid
(c) Carbonic anhydrase inhibitors
(d) Xanthine oxidase inhibitors

(Answer is B) Acetohydroxamic acid

176. What is false concerning recurrent stone formation?

(a) Best treated by total parathyroidectomy
(b) First-time stone formers are at a 50% risk for recurrence
(c) Males have higher recurrence rate than females
(d) Stone formers produce stones of the same type every time

(Answer is A) Best treated by total parathyroidectomy

177. What is the most important parameter that determines the treatment modality of a kidney stone?

(a) Stone chemical composition
(b) Stone burden
(c) First stone vs. Recurrent
(d) Stone density

(Answer is B) Stone burden

178. What kind of stones is most amenable to ESWL?

(a) Cystine
(b) Brushite

(c) Ca. oxalate monohydrate
(d) Ca. oxalate dihydrate

(Answer is D) Ca. oxalate dihydrate

179. What parameter impairs the kidney stone-free rate, after ESWL?

(a) Short skin-to-stone distance (SSD)
(b) End-stage renal failure
(c) A stone in the upper calyx
(d) The presence of a 30 cm, 4.7 Fr ureteral stent in situ

(Answer is B) End-stage renal failure

180. Which of the following factors, positively, affect lower calyceal stone clearance after ESWL?

(a) Short and wide infundibulum
(b) Large lower-pole infundibulo-pelvic angle
(c) The adjunct usage of PCNL
(d) All of the above

(Answer is D) All of the above

181. Which statement is false concerning renal stones related to hyperparathyroidism (HPT)?

(a) Renal stones are found in 20% of patients with primary HPT
(b) "Acidic arrest" promotes crystallisation of calcium phosphate stones related to HPT
(c) HPT, vitamin D excess, and malignancy could lead to hypercalcemia and hypercalciuria
(d) Only surgery can cure primary HPT

(Answer is B) "Acidic arrest" promotes crystallisation of calcium phosphate stones related to HPT

182. What parameter is not considered in the "stone burden" concept?

(a) The surface area of the stones
(b) The volume of the stones
(c) The density of the stones
(d) The number of the stones

(Answer is C) The density of the stones

183. What metabolic disturbances could result from renal tubular acidosis type I?

(a) Hypercalciuria and hypocitraturia
(b) Hypercalciuria and hypercitraturia
(c) Hypocalciuria and hypocitraturia
(d) Hypocalciuria and hypercitraturia

(Answer is A) Hypercalciuria and hypocitraturia

184. What could high dietary protein result in?

(a) Increase urinary calcium, oxalate and uric acid excretion
(b) Decrease urinary calcium; but increase oxalate, and uric acid excretion
(c) Increased urinary calcium and uric acid; but decrease oxalate excretion
(d) Decreased urinary calcium, oxalate, and uric acid excretion

(Answer is A) Increase urinary calcium, oxalate and uric acid excretion

185. What could high level of sulfate in 24-hour urine collection mean?

(a) Dissolving homogenous nucleation
(b) High tendency to form cystine sulfate stones
(c) Indicates the amount of dietary protein
(d) Post ESWL therapy

(Answer is C) Indicates the amount of dietary protein

186. What is the fatality risk if a triple-phosphate staghorn stone left untreated?

(a) 0 – 10%
(b) 10 – 20%
(c) 20 – 30%
(d) 30 – 40%

(Answer is C) 20 – 30%

187. What is the treatment of choice for a 15 mm stone in the lower calyx with a narrow infundibulum?

(a) ESWL
(b) PCNL
(c) Radial nephrolithotomy

(d) Pyelolithotomy with ureteral stenting

(Answer is B) PCNL

188. What is the treatment of choice for a 15 mm stone in a mid calyceal diverticulum?

(a) ESWL
(b) PCNL with fulguration of the diverticulum
(c) Ureteroscopy with fulguration of the diverticulum
(d) Pyelolithotomy with diverticulectomy

(Answer is B) PCNL with fulguration of the diverticulum

189. What type of stones is most effectively treated with PCNL?

(a) Ca. oxalate monohydrate
(b) Cystine
(c) Matrix
(d) Ca. oxalate dihydrate

(Answer is C) Matrix

190. For how long a completely obstructed ureter could be respited with no expected permanent damage to renal functions?

(a) 2 days (b) 2 weeks
(c) 2 months (d) 4 – 6 hours

(Answer is B) 2 weeks

191. Expectant therapy for ureteral stones is indicated when:

(a) Stone size of $\leq$ 4 mm
(b) Stone burden of $\geq$ 22 mm
(c) There is a distal partial obstruction
(d) The patient has end-stage renal failure

(Answer is A) Stone size of $\leq$ 4 mm

192. What is the preferred drug for medical expulsive therapy for lower ureteral stones?

(a) Furosemide (b) Tamsulosin
(c) Nifedipine (d) Diclofenac

(Answer is B) Tamsulosin

193. Which of the following is a relative contra-indication to ESWL?

(a) Renal insufficiency
(b) Active urinary tract infection
(c) Uncorrected bleeding disorder
(d) Third trimester pregnancy

(Answer is A) Renal insufficiency

194. What is (are) true concerning ESWL?

(a) A stone is fragmented when the force of the shockwaves overcomes the tensile strength of the stone
(b) Fragmentation occurs as a result of compressive and tensile forces, erosion, shearing, spalling and cavitation
(c) The generation of compressive and tensile forces and cavitation are thought to be the most important
(d) All of the above

(Answer is D) All of the above

195. What type of shockwaves is generated by spark-gap technology?

(a) Piezoelectric (b) Electrohydraulic
(c) Electromagnetic (d) Microexplosive

(Answer is B) Electrohydraulic

196. Ureteral stones of $\geq$ 7 mm:

(a) Should be treated with more analgesics
(b) Must undergo metabolic worked out
(c) Are unlikely to pass out spontaneously
(d) Chemolysis should be tried first

(Answer is C) Are unlikely to pass out spontaneously

197. Invasive intervention in stone patients is not indicated in the following condition:

(a) Stone size
(b) Unrelieved obstruction
(c) Infection and septicemia

(d) Recurrent stone formation

(Answer is D) Recurrent stone formation

198. What is (are) the indication(s) of ureteral stenting before ESWL?

(a) Stones in a solitary kidney
(b) Ureteral stones causing bilateral obstructions
(c) A kidney stone of $\geq$ 2.5 cm in size
(d) All of the above

(Answer is D) All of the above

199. What statement is false concerning the use of desmopressin (DDAVP) in renal colic patients?

(a) Causes reduction in the mean intra-ureteral pressure
(b) Reduces the pain of acute renal colic
(c) Has a direct relaxing effect on the renal pelvis and ureteral musculature
(d) Is indicated when stones are $\leq$ 4 mm in diameter

(Answer is D) Is indicated when stones are $\leq$ 4 mm in diameter

200. What is false concerning the use of antibiotics in stone patients?

(a) They are mandatory when urine shows $\geq$ 10 WBCs/hpf in symptomatic patients
(b) They aim at treating pyonephrosis and urosepsis
(c) They should cover Escherichia coli and Staphylococcus, Enterobacter, Proteus and Klebsiella species
(d) All of the above

(Answer is D) All of the above

201. What is true concerning the use of intravenous fluids in renal colic cases?

(a) Patients should be given large amounts of fluids to hasten stones passage
(b) Fluids are given to keep the patient well hydrated
(c) The recommended regimen is 2 l of Ringer's lactate over 2 hours
(d) Fluids are contraindicated if desmopressin (DDAVP) was given

(Answer is B) Fluids are given to keep the patient well hydrated

202. What is the immediate management of ureteral avulsion on retrieving an upper ureteral stone by a basket?

(a) Placement of a percutaneous nephrostomy drain
(b) Surgical exploration and primary repair
(c) Conservative management
(d) Endoscopic retrograde ureteral stenting

(Answer is A) Placement of a percutaneous nephrostomy drain

203. What is the incidence risk of ureteral strictures following ureteroscopy?

(a) 3 – 6%
(b) 12 – 15%
(c) 0.4 – 0.8%
(d) 0.09 – 0.14%

(Answer is A) 3 – 6%

204. What kind of stones is more likely to recur with infections if not removed completely?

(a) Urate
(b) Triple phosphate
(c) Oxalate monohydrate
(d) Matrix

(Answer is B) Triple phosphate

205. What is the least serious complications of PCNL?

(a) Uncontrollable bleeding
(b) Incomplete removal of stones
(c) Pneumothorax
(d) Colonic perforation

(Answer is B) Incomplete removal of stones

206. Which event is unlikely to occur after placing a DJ ureteral stent?

(a) Can be forgotten in place
(b) Vesico-renal reflux
(c) Calyceal perforation
(d) Detrusor irritability and/or hematuria

(Answer is C) Calyceal perforation

207. What is false regarding DJ ureteral stents?

(a) Can be introduced from the bladder or kidney or any part of the ureter's course
(b) The standard adult size is 32 cm long, 4 mm calibre
(c) Might result in encrustations and ureteral obstruction
(d) Might result in ureteral dilation

(Answer is B) The standard adult size is 32 cm long, 4 mm calibre

208. What is (are) the indication(s) of using DJ ureteral catheters?

(a) Stent the ureter after ureteral surgery
(b) Facilitate stone passage
(c) After a tough ureteroscopy procedure
(d) All of the above

(Answer is D) All of the above

209. What is true regarding DJ ureteral stents?

(a) Can be placed through perc. nephrostomy
(b) Might slip out, especially in females
(c) Usually radiopaque
(d) All of the above

(Answer is D) All of the above

210. During pyelolithotomy for removing a staghorn urate stone; how to ensure a complete removal of calyceal branches?

(a) Performing intra-operative ultrasonography
(b) Performing radial nephrotomies
(c) Performing adjunct PCLN
(d) Taking a scout KUB film

(Answer is A) Performing intra-operative ultrasonography

211. Which patient is at lowest risk for the development of perinephric hematoma after ESWL?

(a) Hypertensive patient
(b) Patient on aspirin withheld 5 days prior to ESWL
(c) A stone in a scared poorly functioning kidney
(d) ESWL every other day

(Answer is C) A stone in a scared poorly functioning kidney

212. ESWL in pediatric patients is characterized by all of the following, *except:*

(a) Often need sedation or anesthesia
(b) Vesico-ureteral reflux must be excluded
(c) Pediatrics have a higher clearance rate of stones when compared to adults
(d) Safety measures must be taken to avoid lung contusions

(Answer is B) Vesico-ureteral reflux must be excluded

213. What is the least likely condition to form bladder stones?

(a) Spinal cord injury
(b) Senile enlargement of prostate
(c) Augmented bladder
(d) Neurogenic hyper-reflexive bladder

(Answer is D) Neurogenic hyper-reflexive bladder

214. What is false concerning prostatic stones?

(a) Composed of calcium phosphate and calcium carbonate
(b) The vast majority are asymptomatic

(c) Most of the calculi are found in the transitional zone
(d) They don't affect PSA levels

(Answer is C) Most of the calculi are found in the transitional zone

215. What is true regarding prostatic stones?

(a) They are multiple and small in size
(b) Usually, they are voided spontaneously
(c) They, rarely, form large stones within the peripheral zone
(d) Contrast CT is the conventional method for diagnosis

(Answer is A) They are multiple and small in size

216. Which method of the following stone analysis techniques is based on the interaction of polarized light with the stone crystals?

(a) Wet chemical analysis
(b) Thermogravimetry
(c) Scanning electron microscopy
(d) None of the above

(Answer is D) None of the above

217. Which of the following dietary advice is recommended for Ca. oxalate stone formers?

(a) Limit beef, chicken, pork, eggs, fish, shellfish and other animal proteins
(b) Limit beans, nuts, chocolate, coffee, dark green vegetables and soda
(c) Limit canned, packaged, and fast foods
(d) Limit milk, cheese, and other dairy products

(Answer is B) Limit beans, nuts, chocolate, coffee, dark green vegetables and soda

218. What is false concerning urethral stones?

(a) Stones at posterior urethra could be pushed back to the bladder
(b) Stones at anterior urethra have to undergo a trial of "milking out", using copious intraurethral xylocaine gel
(c) Often respond to a two-week course of tamsulosin
(d) Respond to Holmium laser treatment

(Answer is C) Often respond to a two-week course of tamsulosin

219. What is true regarding a stone in a urethral diverticulum?

(a) Symptomless
(b) Should undergo a trial of milking out
(c) Diverticulectomy and stone extraction is the treatment of choice
(d) ESWL is the preferred treatment option

(Answer is C) Diverticulectomy and stone extraction is the treatment of choice

220. What is false concerning preputial stones?

(a) Form due to inspissated smegma
(b) Form due to stasis of urinary salts
(c) Cause inguinal lymphadenopathy
(d) Often associated with phimosis in uncircumcised males

(Answer is C) Cause inguinal lymphadenopathy

221. What type of urinary diversion carries the highest risk of stone formation?

(a) Kock pouch
(b) Neobladder-to-urethra diversion
(c) Florida pouch
(d) Indiana pouch

(Answer is A) Kock pouch

222. What is false concerning primary bladder stones?

(a) Commonly occur in patients with senile prostatic enlargement
(b) Common in children exposed to low-protein, low-phosphate diet

(c) Rarely recur after treatment
(d) Respond to ESWL

(Answer is A) Commonly occur in patients with senile prostatic enlargement

223. What is false concerning patient's preparation for PCNL?

(a) Active UTI is an absolute contraindication
(b) Fluoroquinolone is the first choice for antimicrobial prophylaxis
(c) Withholding aspirin for only 10 days is enough
(d) Despite sterile urine, stone fragmentation might release hidden bacterial endotoxins and viable bacteria

(Answer is B) Fluoroquinolone is the first choice for antimicrobial prophylaxis

224. How can the effectiveness of ESWL treatment session be enhanced?

(a) Ensuring optimal coupling of the patient to the lithotripter
(b) Running the treatment at a slower rate (60 shocks/min)
(c) Running the treatment with general anesthesia
(d) All of the above

(Answer is D) All of the above

225. What could the discomfort experienced during ESWL session be related to?

(a) The energy density of the shock waves as they pass through the skin
(b) The size of the focal point
(c) A and B
(d) None of the above

(Answer is C) A and B

226. What is the unfavorable stone characteristic for a rigid URS treatment?

(a) Size of 5 mm
(b) Location at the lower calyx
(c) Density of 400 HU
(d) Being recurrent

(Answer is B) Location at the lower calyx

227. What is the favorable stone characteristic for ESWL treatment?

(a) 1000 - 1300 HU density
(b) 5 - 10 mm diameter
(c) Lower calyx location
(d) Mid ureteral location

(Answer is B) 5 - 10 mm diameter

228. What is the most favorable stone characteristic for PCNL treatment?

(a) ≥ 2 cm diameter
(b) Upper calyx location
(c) Na. urate composition
(d) 600 - 800 HU density

(Answer is A) ≥ 2 cm diameter

229. What is the most favorable stone characteristics for laparoscopic and robotic approaches for the treatment of a kidney stone?

(a) A stone in the lower calyx with a wide mouth of infundibulum and obtuse lower calyx to ureter angle
(b) A stone in an anterior group calyceal diverticulum with thin overlying renal parenchyma
(c) 5 mm calcium-containing stone in an intrarenal pelvis and wide UPJ
(d) 6 years post anatrophic nephrolithotomy, recurrent mid calyceal stone

(Answer is B) A stone in an anterior group calyceal diverticulum with thin overlying renal parenchyma

230. What is the first-line treatment of kidney stones of a burden greater than 2 cm?

(a) ESWL (b) URS

(c) PCNL (d) None of the above

(Answer is C) PCNL

231. What is false regarding hypomagnesuric calcium nephrolithiasis?

(a) Is characterized by low urinary magnesium and citrate
(b) Magnesium increases renal tubular citrate resorption
(c) Diarrheal is a remarkable side effect of magnesium therapy
(d) Potassium-magnesium preparations might restore urinary magnesium and citrate levels

(Answer is B) Magnesium increases renal tubular citrate resorption

232. What is the most common composition of ureteral stones?

(a) Ca. phosphate (b) Ca. oxalate
(c) Na. urate (d) Struvite

(Answer is B) Ca. oxalate

233. What sequence of ureteral parts represents the most to least favorable stone response to ESWL treatment?

(a) Upper, lower, mid
(b) Lower, upper, mid
(c) Mid, upper, lower
(d) Mid, lower, upper

(Answer is A) Upper, lower, mid

234. What is false concerning obesity and urinary stone formation?

(a) Obese patients have a higher tendency for uric acid stone formation
(b) High-protein, low-carbohydrate diet might increase the risk of stone formation and bone loss
(c) Metabolic syndrome is associated with high urinary pH
(d) Roux-en-Y-gastric bypass surgery may increase the risk for stone formation

(Answer is C) Metabolic syndrome is associated with high urinary pH

235. What is true concerning primary hyperparathyroidism and stone formation?

(a) Orthophosphates may have a role in the treatment
(b) Hyperparathyroidectomy and levothyroxine replacement is the optimum treatment
(c) Management includes calcium chelating agent and repeat 24 hours urine collection in 3 months
(d) Surgical excision of the adenoma(s) is the treatment of choice

(Answer is D) Surgical excision of the adenoma(s) is the treatment of choice

236. What is a remarkable disadvantage of ultrasonic imaging for ESWL?

(a) Localization of stones in the ureter is difficult or impossible
(b) Inability to visualize stones breaking down in real time
(c) Patient's position on ESWL table is uncomfortable
(d) Inability to visualize radiolucent stones

(Answer is A) Localization of stones in the ureter is difficult or impossible

237. What is the most common organism that might complicate PCNL?

(a) Proteus mirabilis
(b) E. coli
(c) Pseudomonas aeruginosa
(d) Staphylococcus epidermidis

(Answer is D) Staphylococcus epidermidis

238. What is the preferred entry point into the collecting system for PCNL for a 2.4 cm renal pelvis stone?

(a) Anterior lower pole calyx
(b) Posterior lower pole calyx
(c) Anterior upper pole calyx
(d) Posterior upper pole calyx

(Answer is B) Posterior lower pole calyx

239. What could carry the least risk of colon injury during PCNL?

(a) Subcostal puncture performed during full expiration
(b) Previous open nephrolithotomy
(c) Access lateral to the posterior axillary line
(d) Horseshoe kidney

(Answer is B) Previous open nephrolithotomy

240. What situation carries lower risk for lung injury during supracostal upper pole access for PCNL?

(a) Placing the patient in anti-trendelenburg position
(b) Making the puncture under local anesthesia
(c) Injection CO_2 gas to create a safety space under the diaphragm before puncturing
(d) Making the puncture during full expiration

(Answer is D) Making the puncture during full expiration

241. What is the preferred irrigation fluid during PCNL?

(a) Physiological saline 0.9%
(b) Glycine 1.5%
(c) Balanced salt solution
(d) Distilled water

(Answer is A) Physiological saline 0.9%

242. What is false concerning PCNL in horseshoe kidneys?

(a) The preferred access into the collecting system is through a posterior calyx
(b) The posterior calyceal group is typically more medial than in the normal kidney
(c) Most cases the lower pole calyces are posterior
(d) Is desirable to make an upper pole collecting system puncture

(Answer is C) Most cases the lower pole calyces are posterior

243. What is the treatment of choice for a moderately symptomatic right ureteral stone in a pregnant woman?

(a) Conservative management with hydration and analgesics
(b) ESWL
(c) Cystoscopy and DJ ureteral stent insertion
(d) Perc. nephrostomy

(Answer is A) Conservative management with hydration and analgesics

244. Which of the following states is not induced by pregnancy?

(a) Enteric hyperoxaluria
(b) Absorptive hypercalciuria
(c) Hypercitraturia
(d) High urinary output

(Answer is A) Enteric hyperoxaluria

245. False about electrohydraulic lithotripsy:

(a) Can't be used with flexible ureteroscopy
(b) Rapidly expanding plasma shock wave is created
(c) Chemical composition of stone affects efficacy of fragmentation
(d) Uric acid stone requires more time to fragment

(Answer is A) Can't be used with flexible ureteroscopy

246. False about pneumatic lithotripsy:

(a) Main disadvantage is stone migration
(b) Increasing probe size increases efficacy of fragmentation

(c) Less efficacious in very soft stones
(d) Most damage to ureter compared to other lithotripters

(Answer is D) Most damage to ureter compared to other lithotripters

247. Gold standard imaging for urolithiasis:

(a) Non contrast CT
(b) Ultrasonography
(c) MRI
(d) Intravenous urogram

(Answer is A) Non contrast CT

248. Microscopy showing needle shaped crystals correspond to stones of the type:

(a) Calcium oxalate dihydrate
(b) Brushite
(c) Magnesium ammonium phosphate
(d) Calcium phosphate

(Answer is B) Brushite

249. Calcium phosphate stone differs from calcium oxalate stone in all *except:*

(a) Affects more women than men
(b) Presents at younger age
(c) Most common type associated with renal tubular acidosis
(d) Associated with acidic urine pH

(Answer is D) Associated with acidic urine pH

250. False about Brushite stones:

(a) Extremely hard stones
(b) Strongly associated with metabolic abnormalities
(c) Needle shaped crystals
(d) Associated with hyperoxaluria

(Answer is D) Associated with hyperoxaluria

251. Citrate acts as inhibitor of calcium stone formation by following mechanisms *except:*

(a) Complexes with calcium and reduces urinary concentration of calcium
(b) Prevents spontaneous nucleation of calcium oxalate
(c) Inhibits the effects of Tamm-Horsfall glycoprotein
(d) Inhibits agglomeration and sedimentation of calcium oxalate crystals

(Answer is C) Inhibits the effects of Tamm-Horsfall glycoprotein

252. All are conditions associated with hypercitraturia *except:*

(a) Elevated PTH
(b) Elevated estrogen
(c) Elevated Mg
(d) Low vitamin D levels

(Answer is D) Low vitamin D levels

253. Idiopathic uric acid nephrolithiasis is characterized by:

(a) Increased fractional excretion of urate
(b) High urinary uric acid levels
(c) Acidic urine
(d) Hypercalciuria

(Answer is C) Acidic urine

254. All increase the risk of uric acid stone formation *except:*

(a) Obesity
(b) Metabolic syndrome
(c) Diabetes mellitus
(d) Hyperthyroidism

(Answer is D) Hyperthyroidism

255. False about Allopurinol:

(a) A common cause for Stevens-Johnson syndrome
(b) Dose reduction is needed in decreased renal function

(c) First line therapy in patient with uric acid stones
(d) Common side effect is skin rash and muscle pain

(**Answer is C)** First line therapy in patient with uric acid stones

256. Thiol drug of choice for cystinuria is:

(a) D pencillamine
(b) Captopril
(c) Tiopronin
(d) Potassium citrate

(**Answer is C)** Tiopronin

257. Acetohydroxamic acid is useful in:

(a) Brushite calculi
(b) Xanthine stone
(c) Infection stone
(d) Cystine stone

(**Answer is C)** Infection stone

258. Antibiotic from which urinary calculi may be formed is:

(a) Trimethoprim-sulfamethoxazole
(b) Ciprofloxacin
(c) Azithromycin
(d) Nitrofurantoin

(**Answer is A, B, C)** Trimethoprim-sulfamethoxazole, Ciprofloxacin, Azithromycin

259. Preferred treatment approach for most matrix stones is:

(a) PCNL
(b) ESWL
(c) Medical management
(d) Open stone removal

(**Answer is A)** PCNL

260. False about calyceal diverticulum:

(a) Urothelium lined non secretory cystic dilatation of intrarenal collecting system
(b) More common in lower pole calyces
(c) Stone formation occurs in 10-50% cases
(d) PCNL is the first line treatment modality

(**Answer is B)** More common in lower pole calyces

261. Factors impending lower pole stone clearance in ESWL are all *except:*

(a) Infundibular length > 3 cms
(b) Infundibular width < 5 mm
(c) Infundibulopelvic angle < 70 degrees
(d) Single infundibulum

(**Answer is D)** Single infundibulum

262. The chief determinant of stone passage in the ureter is:

(a) Diameter of stone in transverse axis
(b) Diameter of stone in longitudinal axis
(c) Composition of stone
(d) Hydrostatic pressure

(**Answer is A)** Diameter of stone in transverse axis

263. For patients on antiplatelet therapy the treatment modality of choice for upper ureteric calculi is:

(a) PCNL
(b) ESWL
(c) URS with laser lithotripsy
(d) URS with pneumatic lithotripsy

(**Answer is C)** URS with laser lithotripsy

264. Primary types of shock wave generators (ESWL) are all *except:*

(a) Electrohydraulic (b) Electromagnetic
(c) Piezoelectric (d) LASER

(**Answer is D)** LASER

265. All are ways to improve ESWL outcomes *except:*

(a) General anesthesia
(b) Ureteral stent
(c) Use of alpha blocker for expulsion

(d) Diuresis

(Answer is B) Ureteral stent

266. About complications of PCNL all are true *except:*

(a) Hemorrhage risk increases with increasing stone burden and procedure duration
(b) Sepsis occurs in one in four patients
(c) Pneumothorax and pleural effusion is more for supracostal puncture
(d) Bleeding is usually arterial

(Answer is D) Bleeding is usually arterial

267. Treatment of extraperitoneal colonic injury after PCNL is:

(a) Observation and IV antibiotics
(b) Immediate exploration
(c) Ileostomy
(d) Ureteral stenting and placement of nephrostomy tube as colostomy tube

(Answer is D) Ureteral stenting and placement of nephrostomy tube as colostomy tube

CHAPTER 12

Neoplasm of Upper Urinary Tract

1. **Features suggestive of malignancy on intravenous pyelography include all *except:***
   (a) Calcification within mass
   (b) Decreased tissue density
   (c) Irregularity of the margin
   (d) Distortion of collecting system

(Answer is B) Features suggestive of malignancy on intravenous pyelography include:

- Calcification within the mass.
- Increased tissue density.
- Irregularity of the margin.
- Distortion of the collecting system.

2. **Single most important test to delineate the nature renal mass is:**
   (a) IVU (b) USG
   (c) CECT (d) MRI

(Answer is C) A dedicated (thin-slice) renal CT scan remains the single most important radiographic test for delineating the nature of a renal mass.

3. **Renal mass should enhance how much to prove RCC?**
   (a) 10 HU (b) 15 HU
   (c) 20 HU (d) 25 HU

(Answer is B) In general, any renal mass that enhances with intravenous administration of contrast material on CT scanning by more than 15 Hounsfield units (HU) should be considered a renal cell carcinoma (RCC) until proved otherwise.

4. **How much negative attenuation is required to diagnose AML?**
   (a) –10 HU (b) –15 HU
   (c) –20 HU (d) –25 HU

(Answer is C) Solid masses that also have substantial areas of negative CT attenuation numbers (below –20 HU) indicative of fat are diagnostic of AMLs.

5. **Diagnosis of a pseudotumor can be confirmed by:**
   (a) CECT (b) MRI
   (c) DMSA scan (d) DTPA scan

(Answer is C) The diagnosis of a pseudotumor can be confirmed by isotope renography with technetium-labelled dimercaptosuccinic acid.

6. **FNAB is indicated when there is clinical suspicion of all *except:***
   (a) Renal abscess
   (b) Metastatic malignancy
   (c) Lymphoma
   (d) Oncocytoma

(Answer is D) The primary indications for needle aspiration or biopsy of a renal mass are when a renal abscess or infected cyst is suspected and when RCC must be differentiated from metastatic malignant disease or renal lymphoma.

7. **The radiographic features including an irregular margin, thickened septa, and thick irregular calcification is classified as:**
   (a) Bosniak category I
   (b) Bosniak category II
   (c) Bosniak category III
   (d) Bosniak category IV

(Answer is C) The radiographic features include an irregular margin, thickened septa, and thick irregular calcification.

8. **Which one of the following is not the Bosniak category II cyst?**
   (a) Septated cyst
   (b) Infected cyst
   (c) Hyperdense cyst
   (d) Hemorrhagic cyst

(Answer is D) Benign multiloculated, hemorrhagic, or densely calcified cysts are Bosniak category III.

9. **Small, solid, CT-enhancing renal masses with features suggestive of RCC prove to be benign after surgical excision in how many patients?**
   (a) Nil (b) 0% to 10%
   (c) 10% to 20% (d) 20% to 30%

(Answer is C) Approximately 10% to 20% of small, solid, CT-enhancing renal masses with features suggestive of RCC prove to be benign after surgical excision.

10. **The risk of malignancy for category II renal cysts is:**
    (a) Nil (b) 0% to 5%
    (c) 5% to 10% (d) 10% to 15%

(Answer is B) The risk of malignancy for category II renal cysts is 0% to 5%, and these lesions should be observed with periodic renal imaging.

11. **Which statement regarding simple renal cyst is not true?**
    (a) Most common benign renal lesions
    (b) Represent more than 70% of all asymptomatic renal masses
    (c) More common in men
    (d) Prevalence decreases with age

(Answer is D) Prevalence increases with age, and renal cysts can be found in more than 50% of patients older than 50 years.

12. **Which statement is not true regarding renal cortical adenoma?**
    (a) More common in patients with VHL disease and ARCD associated with ESRD
    (b) It is a small, well-circumscribed lesion characterized by uniform basophilic or eosinophilic cells with monotonous nuclear and cellular characteristics
    (c) Exhibit trisomy of chromosomes 7 and 17
    (d) Most adenomas are detectable radiographically because of large size

(Answer is D) The overwhelming majority of renal adenomas remain asymptomatic, and most are undetectable radiographically because of size less than 1 cm.

13. **Which statement is not true regarding oncocytoma?**
    (a) A central scar is commonly found
    (b) Has prominent necrosis or hypervascularity
    (c) Packed with numerous large mitochondria, which contributes to their distinctive staining characteristics
    (d) On microscopic examination, uniform round or polygonal eosinophilic cells predominate

(Answer is B) Prominent necrosis or hypervascularity is lacking.

14. **55-year-old-man has a 4 cm central renal mass, biopsy of which reveals oncocytoma:**
    (a) Observation with follow-up with CT annually
    (b) Observation with follow-up with CXR yearly CT two yearly
    (c) Partial nephrectomy
    (d) Radical nephrectomy

(Answer is C) A nephron-sparing approach is clearly desirable if oncocytoma is suspected and if tumor size and location are amenable.

15. **Which statement is true regarding AML?**
    (a) It is a malignant neoplasm of adipose tissue, smooth muscle, thick walled vessels

(b) Fat is must on CT for diagnosis of AML
(c) Angiography shows "spoke wheel" and "lucent rim" pattern
(d) Surgery is required when symptomatic and >4 cm

(Answer is D) Spoke wheel pattern of feeding arteries observed on angiography can suggest the diagnosis of oncocytoma. In 14% of AMLs, fat cannot be identified with CT, presumably related to a reduced proportion of mature adipose tissue, and a definite diagnosis cannot be made AML is benign lesion.

16. All are true about AML associated with TS *except:*

(a) Approximately 20% to 30% of AMLs are found in patients with TS
(b) 50% of patients with TS develop AMLs
(c) Mean age at presentation is fifth and sixth decade
(d) Female-to-male predominance of 2:1 has been observed

(Answer is C) 70% to 80% of patients with AML who do not have TS, a more pronounced female predominance is found, and most patients present later in life, during the fifth or sixth decade.

17. HMB-45 is characteristic for:

(a) AML
(b) Oncocytoma
(c) RCC
(d) Metanephric adenoma

(Answer is A) Positive immunoreactivity for HMB-45, a monoclonal antibody raised against a melanoma-associated antigen, is characteristic for AML.

18. Retroperitoneal hemorrhage from which disease is, also known as Wunderlich's syndrome?

(a) AML
(b) Oncocytoma
(c) RCC
(d) Metanephric adenoma

(Answer is A) Massive retroperitoneal hemorrhage from AML, also known as Wunderlich's syndrome.

19. Sixty-year-female with 5 cm AML on CT has developed massive life threatening retroperitoneal hemorrhage, which will be the best treatment option?

(a) Total nephrectomy
(b) Partial nephrectomy
(c) Embolisation
(d) Observation

(Answer is A) Most patients with acute or potentially life-threatening hemorrhage require total nephrectomy if it is explored.

20. Forty-year-female with 5 cm bilateral AML on CT, which will be the best treatment option?

(a) Total nephrectomy
(b) Partial nephrectomy
(c) Embolisation
(d) Observation

(Answer is C) If a patient has TS, bilateral disease, preexisting renal insufficiency, or other medical or urologic disease that could affect renal function in the future, selective embolization should be considered. In such circumstances, selective embolization can temporize and in many cases prove definitive.

21. Which statement is not true regarding cystic nephroma in adult?

(a) Female predominance is observed in adults
(b) Most common presentation is abdominal mass
(c) Class III-IV in Bosniak's classification scheme
(d) Most cystic nephromas in adults have traditionally been managed with radical nephrectomy because of the concern for malignancy

(Answer is B) Children tend to present with an asymptomatic abdominal mass detected on routine physical examination, whereas symptomatic presentation with abdominal pain, hematuria, urinary tract infection, or hypertension is more common in adults.

22. Which statement is not true for reninoma?

(a) Derived from the juxtaglomerular cell
(b) Most are small (<3 cm), solitary
(c) Clinical presentation includes hypertension and hypokalemia
(d) Treatment is mainly medical (anti-hypertensive drugs)

(Answer is D) Almost all patients may be cured with surgical excision, which typically leads to normalization of blood pressure and resolution of other related symptoms.

23. Which is the most lethal tumor?

(a) RCC
(b) Carcinoma urinary bladder
(c) Carcinoma prostate
(d) Carcinoma testis

(Answer is A) More than 40% of patients with RCC have died of their cancer, in contrast with the 20% mortality rates associated with prostate and bladder carcinomas.

24. Which statement regarding RCC is not correct?

(a) RCC accounts for 2% to 3% of all adult malignant neoplasms
(b) Incidental detection of RCC is increasing
(c) Typical presentation in the sixth and seventh decades of life
(d) RCC is as common as Wilms' tumor during the first decade of life

(Answer is D) Although Wilms' tumor is much more common in younger children, RCC is as common as Wilms' tumor during the second decade of life.

25. Familial renal cell carcinoma syndrome includes all *except:*

(a) VHL
(b) Tuberous sclerosis
(c) Birt-Hogg-Dube
(d) Familial leiomyomatosis

(Answer is B) Familial renal cell carcinoma syndromes does not include TS.

26. About VHL disease which statement is not correct?

(a) It is hereditary tumor syndrome predisposing to RCCand pheochromocytoma
(b) It is not associated with sporadic RCC
(c) RCC develops in 50% of patients with VHL and has low age of onset with increase bilateral and multifocal involvement
(d) Both alleles of the VHL gene must be mutated for development of the disease

(Answer is B) VHL gene, which is located at chromosome 3p25-26, has now been completely sequenced, and its role as a tumor suppressor gene for both the sporadic and the familial forms of clear cell RCC has been confirmed.

27. Most common cause of mortality in patients with von Hippel-Lindau disease is:

(a) RCC
(b) Pheochromocytoma
(c) Islet cell tumor
(d) Hemangioblastoma

(Answer is A) RCC has now become the most common cause of mortality in patients with von Hippel-Lindau disease.

28. Regarding type 2 papillary RCC all are true *except:*

(a) Commonly develop cutaneous and uterine leiomyomas
(b) They are often multiple and bilateral
(c) More likely to be aggressive
(d) Collecting duct RCC, has also been observed in this syndrome

(Answer is B) Renal tumors in this syndrome are unusual for familial RCC in that they are often solitary and unilateral.

29. Renal tumors in Birt-Hogg-Dube syndrome includes all *except:*

(a) Cutaneous fibrofolliculomas
(b) Chromophobe RCC
(c) Oncocytomas
(d) Angiomyolipomas

(Answer is D) The renal tumors typically include chromophobe RCC, oncocytomas, and hybrid or transitional tumors that exhibit features of both of these entities.

30. RCC express which tumor associated antigen?

(a) RAGE (b) PAGE
(c) MAGE (d) CAGE

(Answer is A) RCC has been shown to express a variety of tumor-associated antigens, including PRAME, RAGE-I, MUC-1, gp47, and CA-9, which contribute to its immunogenicity.

31. Of the tumor-associated antigens for RCC, which has demonstrated the most specificity?

(a) HIF-1 (b) CA-9
(c) PRAME (d) gp47

(Answer is B) Of the tumor-associated antigens for RCC, CA-9 (also known as MN-9) has demonstrated the most specificity.

32. Response rates of immunotherapy for RCC is:

(a) 0 to 10% (b) 10% to 20%
(c) 20% to 30% (d) 30% to 40%

(Answer is B) Response rates of immunotherapy for RCC have been disappointing, typically ranging from 15% to 20% despite a variety of creative treatment strategies, suggesting immune tolerance.

33. The primary angiogenesis inducer in clear cell RCC is:

(a) VEGF (b) PDGF
(c) FGF (d) TGF

(Answer is A) The primary angiogenesis inducer in clear cell RCC appears to be VEGF, which is suppressed by the wild-type VHL protein under normal conditions and is dramatically upregulated during tumor development.

34. Which variant of RCC can be infiltrative?

(a) Chromophilic RCC
(b) Chromophobic RCC
(c) Collecting duct RCC
(d) Medullary RCC

(Answer is C) RCCs are not grossly infiltrative, with the notable exception of collecting duct RCC and some sarcomatoid variants.

35. Fuhrman's classification system in renal cell carcinoma is based on all *except:*

(a) Cell size (b) Nucleus size
(c) Presence of nucleoli (d) Nuclear outline

(Answer is A) Fuhrman's classification system for nuclear grade in renal cell carcinoma

Grade	*Nuclear size*	*Nuclear Outline*	*Nucleoli*
1	10 mm	Round, uniform	Absent or inconspicuous
2	15 mm	Irregular	Small (visible at 400 × magnification)
3	20 mm	Irregular	Prominent
4	>20 mm	Bizarre, often multilobed	Prominent, heavy chromatin clumps present

36. Which statement regarding conventional RCC is not correct?

(a) Conventional RCC is more likely to exhibit venous tumor extension than is any other subtype of RCC
(b) Conventional RCC have a worse prognosis compared with chromophilic or chromophobic RCC
(c) Most responders in immunotherapy protocols have non-conventional RCC
(d) Chromosome 3 alterations and VHL mutations are common in conventional RCC

(Answer is C) Most responders in immunotherapy protocols have had conventional RCC, and these protocols are now being reserved primarily for this population.

37. Which statement regarding chromophilic RCC is not correct?

(a) Include trisomy of chromosomes 7 and 17 and loss of the Y chromosome

(b) Unique feature of chromophilic RCC is its tendency toward multicentricity

(c) More likely to be hypovascular, perhaps owing to the lack of VHL mutations

(d) More aggressive type 1 variant, has eosinophilic cells and abundant granular cytoplasm

(Answer is D) Two subtypes of chromophilic RCC: type 1, consisting of basophilic cells with scant cytoplasm; and the potentially more aggressive type 2 variant, with eosinophilic cells and abundant granular cytoplasm.

38. Which variant of RCC is more common in patients with ESRD and ARCD?

(a) Chromophilic RCC

(b) Chromophobic RCC

(c) Collecting duct RCC

(d) Medullary RCC

(Answer is A) Chromophilic is more commonly found in certain populations, such as patients with end-stage renal failure and acquired renal cystic disease.

39. Affinity for the Ulex europaeus lectin and expression of high-molecular-weight keratins (34βE12) supports:

(a) Chromophilic RCC

(b) Chromophobic RCC

(c) Collecting duct RCC

(d) Medullary RCC

(Answer is C) Affinity for the Ulex europaeus lectin and expression of high-molecular-weight keratins (34βE12) support a collecting duct origin.

40. Which is not true regarding histological variant of RCC?

(a) Conventional variety of RCC represents garden variety of RCC and YHL mutations are common

(b) Chromophilic RCC typically exhibit a relatively transparent cytoplasm with a fine reticular pattern that has been described as a "plant cell" appearance

(c) Chromophobe RCC is defined by perinuclear halo and microvessels

(d) Renal medullary carcinoma is almost exclusively associated with sickle cell trait

(Answer is B) Chromophobe cell carcinoma, exhibit a relatively transparent cytoplasm with a fine reticular pattern that has been described as a "plant cell" appearance.

41. Paraneoplastic syndromes are found in how many patients with RCC?

(a) 10% (b) 20%

(c) 30% (d) 40%

(Answer is B) Paraneoplastic syndromes are found in 20% of patients with RCC.

42. Paraneoplastic syndrome of RCC in which medical therapy has proved beneficial?

(a) Hypercalcemia (b) Hyperglycemia

(c) Stauffer syndrome (d) Hypertension

(Answer is A) In hypercalcemia medical management predominates and includes vigorous hydration followed by diuresis with furosemide and the selective use of bisphosphonates, corticosteroids, or calcitonin.

43. Regarding Stauffer syndrome which statement is not correct?

(a) Metastatic hepatic dysfunction

(b) Biopsy, when it is indicated, often demonstrates non-specific hepatitis associated with a prominent lymphocytic infiltrate

(c) Hepatic function normalizes after nephrectomy in 60% to 70% of cases
(d) Persistence of hepatic dysfunction is almost always indicative of the presence of viable tumor and thus represents a poor prognostic finding

(Answer is A) Non-metastatic hepatic dysfunction, or Stauffer's syndrome.

44. Target population of screening includes all *except:*

(a) End stage renal failure
(b) VHL
(c) ADPKD
(d) Tuberous sclerosis

(Answer is C) Routine screening is not justified in ADPKD.

45. According to TNM staging in RCC, stage division of T1a and T1b is on what size?

(a) 2 cm (b) 2.5 cm
(c) 4 cm (d) 5 cm

(Answer is C)

T1a: Tumor = 4.0 cm and confined to the kidney.

T1b: Tumor > 4.0 cm and = 7.0 cm and confined to the kidney.

T2: Tumor > 7.0 cm and confined to the kidney.

46. Involvement of adrenals is classified into which stage?

(a) T 3b (b) T 3a
(c) T 3c (d) T 4

(Answer is D) Extension to adrenal gland–T4.

47. Premier study for evaluation and staging of IVC thrombus is:

(a) MRI
(b) IV cavography
(c) Transesophageal echo
(d) Doppler USG

(Answer is A) MRI is well established as the premier study for the evaluation and staging of inferior vena caval tumor thrombus, although recent data suggest that multiplanar CT may be equivalent.

48. For evaluation of patients with RCC and IVC thrombus in whom MRI is contraindicated, next best test is:

(a) MRI
(b) IV cavography
(c) Transesophageal echo
(d) Doppler USG

(Answer is B) Venacavography is now best reserved for patients with equivocal MRI findings and for patients who cannot tolerate MRI or have other contraindications to MRI.

49. Which statement regarding prognostication of RCC is not correct?

(a) High CA-9 expression has correlated with improved survival in this population
(b) Decreased proliferative index assessed by Ki-67 has correlated with improved survival
(c) Downregulation of E-cadherin has correlated with good outcomes
(d) Increased expression of proteases, such as plasmin and the matrix metalloproteinases, has correlated with reduced survival in RCC

(Answer is C) Downregulation of E-cadherin and cadherin-6, which mediate adhesion between cancer cells, is well documented in RCC and has correlated with poor outcomes.

50. UCLA Integrated Staging System for patients with renal cell carcinoma includes all the following prognostic factors *except:*

(a) Size
(b) Shape
(c) Grade
(d) ECOG performance status

(Answer is A) UCLA Integrated Staging System for patients with renal cell carcinoma does not include size.

51. The prototypical concept of radical nephrectomy encompasses all *except:*

(a) Early ligation of the renal artery and vein
(b) Removal of the kidney inside Gerota's fascia
(c) Excision of the ipsilateral adrenal gland
(d) Complete regional lymphadenectomy from the crus of the diaphragm to the aortic bifurcation

(Answer is B) The prototypical concept of radical nephrectomy encompasses the basic principles of early ligation of the renal artery and vein, removal of the kidney outside Gerota's fascia, excision of the ipsilateral adrenal gland, and performance of a complete regional lymphadenectomy from the crus of the diaphragm to the aortic bifurcation.

52. Which statement regarding RCC is not correct?

(a) Cystic degeneration is found in 10% to 20% of RCCs
(b) Calcification can be stippled or plaquelike and is found in 10% to 20% of RCCs
(c) Frank invasion and perforation of the collecting system or renal capsule are found in approximately 20% of cases
(d) 10% to 20%% of localized RCCs manifest perinephric fat involvement

(Answer is D) Performance of a perifascial nephrectomy is of undoubted importance in preventing postoperative local tumor recurrence because approximately 25% of localized RCCs manifest perinephric fat involvement.

53. 60-year-old male, was diagnosed as a case of RCC. He has tumor mass of 8 cm but confined to kidney and with no other venous or lymphatic involvement. Radical nephrectomy is performed for patient. Follow-up will be:

(a) No follow-up required
(b) Yearly clinical examination and no imaging studies
(c) Yearly clinical examination and CXR and abdominal CT every 2 years
(d) 6 monthly clinical examination and CXR with yearly abdominal CT

(Answer is C) Patient belongs to stage T2N0M0.

Pathologic tumor stage	*History, examination and blood tests*	*Chest radiograph*	*Abdominal CT scan*
T1 N0 M0[*]	Yearly	–	–
T2 N0 M0[*]	Yearly	Yearly	Every 2 years
T3 N0 M0	Every 6 months for 3 years, then yearly	Every 6 months for 3 years, then yearly	At 1 year, then every 2 years

54. Which statement is true regarding nephron sparing surgery for RCC?

(a) There are no significant biologic differences between centrally and peripherally located small, solitary, unilateral RCCs
(b) Local tumor recurrence rate is 20% in operated kidney
(c) Three-dimensional USG can accurately depict the renal parenchymal and vascular anatomy
(d) Increase risk of mesangioproliferative glomerulosclerosis in remnant kidney

(Answer is A) The major disadvantage of nephron-sparing surgery is the risk of postoperative local recurrence in the kidney that was operated on, which has occurred in up to 10% of patients. Patients with more than 50% reduction in overall renal mass were found to be at increased risk for development of proteinuria, focal segmental glomerulosclerosis. Three-dimensional volume-rendered CT (or MRI) is now established as a noninvasive imaging modality that can accurately depict the renal parenchymal and vascular anatomy.

55. After partial nephrectomy minimum functioning renal remnant required of one normal kidney to avoid end-stage renal failure:

(a) 10%
(b) 20%

(c) 30% (d) 40%

(Answer is B) A functioning renal remnant of at least 20% of one normal kidney is necessary to avoid end-stage renal failure.

56. 30-year-old male, was diagnosed as a case of RCC. He has tumor mass of 5 cm but confined to kidney and with no other venous or lymphatic involvement. Radical nephrectomy is performed for patient. Follow-up imagimg will be:

(a) No follow-up imaging required
(b) 6 monthly CXR and CT abdomen
(c) Yearly CXR and CT abdomen
(d) 2 yearly CXR and CT abdomen

(Answer is A) Patient belongs to T1N0M0 post-operative surveillance after partial nephrectomy for localized renal cell carcinoma.

Pathologic tumor stage	*History, examination and bood tests*	*Chest radiograph*	*Abdominal CT scan*
T1 N0 M0[*]	Yearly	–	–
T2 N0 M0[*]	Yearly	Yearly	Every 2 years
T3 N0 M0	Every 6 months for 3 years, then yearly	Every 6 months for 3 years, then yearly	Every 6 months for 3 years, then every 2 years

57. In patients with a solitary remnant kidney to screen for hyperfiltration nephropathy which test should be performed?

(a) Renal biopsy
(b) Serum creatinine
(c) 24-hour urinary protein measurement
(d) BUN levels

(Answer is C) Because proteinuria is the initial manifestation of this phenomenon, a 24-hour urinary protein measurement should be obtained yearly in patients with a solitary remnant kidney to screen for hyperfiltration nephropathy.

58. In patients with RCC and von Hippel-Lindau disease excision of lesion should be considered above what size?

(a) Any size (b) >I cm
(c) >2 cm (d) >3 cm

(Answer is D) Partial nephrectomy can provide effective initial treatment of patients with RCC and von Hippel-Lindau disease but should be withheld until tumor size reaches or eclipses 3.0 cm.

59. Target lethal temperature which should be achieved while cryosurgery in RCC is:

(a) 0°C (b) –10°C
(c) –20°C (d) –176°C

(Answer is C) Target lethal temperature of –20°C was achieved at a distance of 3. 1 mm inside the leading edge of the ice ball as visualized by real-time ultrasonography.

60. Involvement of the IVC with RCC occurs in:

(a) 0 to 5% (b) 5% to 10%
(c) 10% to 15% (d) 15% to 20%

(Answer is B) Overall, involvement of the IVC with RCC occurs in 4% to 10% of patients.

61. Stage III level of IVC thrombus is:

(a) Tumor thrombus till renal ostium
(b) Infrahepatic tumor thrombus
(c) Intrahepatic tumor thrombus
(d) Suprahepatic tumor thrombus

(Answer is C) Staging of the level of IVC thrombus is as follows: I. adjacent to the ostium of renal vein; II. extending up to the lower aspect of the liver; III. involving the intrahepatic portion of the IVC but below the diaphragm; and IV. extending above the diaphragm.

62. Correct order of sequential clamping required for level 2 thrombus is:

(a) Initially caudal IVC, then contralateral renal vein, and then cephalad IVC

(b) Initially cephalad IVC, then contralateral renal vein, and then caudal IVC
(c) Initially caudal IVC, then cephalad IVC and then contralateral renal vein
(d) Initially cephalad IVC, then caudal IVC, and then contralateral renal vein

(Answer is A) Level II thrombi require sequential clamping of the caudal IVC, contralateral renal vein, and cephalad IVC along with mobilization of the relevant segment of the IVC and occlusion of lumbar veins.

63. Which therapy has the best success rate for RCC?

(a) Interferon alfa
(b) Interferon alfa + CRA
(c) Interferon alfa + vinblastine
(d) Interferon alfa + IL-2 + 5-FU

(Answer is D) Overall survival increases with 31% with Interferon alfa + IL-2 + 5-FU.

64. Fifty-five years healthy male is diagnosed with 7 cm RCC and a 2 cm lung metastasis, best treatment option will be:

(a) Observation
(b) Cytoreductive nephrectomy with later pulmonary lobectomy with later
(c) Cytoreductive nephrectomy with simultaneous pulmonary lobectomy
(d) Cytoreductive nephrectomy with simultaneous pulmonary lobectomy followed by interferon therapy

(Answer is D) Data support the concept of cytoreductive nephrectomy before systemic therapy with a cytokine such as interferon. Metastectomy either before or after administration of systemic therapy should be considered in patients with solitary or limited pulmonary metastasis.

65. Poor prognostic factors in patients with metastatic renal cancer includes all *except:*

(a) Erythrocyte segmentation rate more than 30
(b) Time from diagnosis of metastatic disease less than 12 months
(c) Lactate dehydrogenase level more than 1.5 times the upper limit of normal
(d) Corrected calcium concentration above 10.0 mg/dl

(Answer is A) Prognostic factors in patients with metastatic renal cancer: Karnofsky performance status below 80%; time from diagnosis of metastatic disease less than 12 months; hemoglobin level below the lower limit of normal; lactate dehydrogenase level more than 1.5 times the upper limit of normal; corrected calcium concentration above 10.0 mg/dl.

66. Which drug is a IgG1 monoclonal antibody recognizing and binding all VEGF isoforms?

(a) Sorafenib (b) Sunitinib
(c) Bevacizumab (d) Erlotinib

(Answer is C) Bevacizumab is an IgG1 monoclonal antibody recognizing and binding all VEGF isoforms.

67. Which statement regarding renal sarcoma is true?

(a) Renal sarcoma represents 10% renal tumours in adults
(b) Renal sarcoma are less lethal than sarcoma of prostate, bladder or testis
(c) Follows hypervascular pattern on angiography
(d) Sarcoma tend to grow to large size in the absence of lymphadenopathy

(Answer is D) Sarcomas represent 1% to 2% of all malignant renal tumors in adults, with a peak incidence in the fifth decade of life. Renal sarcoma is less common but more lethal than sarcoma of any other genitourinary site. Sarcoma follows hypovascular pattern on angiography.

68. Most common histologic subtype of renal sarcoma is:

(a) Liposarcoma
(b) Leiomyosarcoma
(c) Rhabdomyosarcoma
(d) Osteosarcoma

(Answer is B) Leiomyosarcoma is the most common histologic subtype of renal sarcoma, accounting for 50% to 60% of such tumors.

69. All are true regarding renal lymphoma *except:*

(a) More common with non Hodgkin's lymphoma than Hodgkin's lymphoma
(b) Hematogenous dissemination of lymphoma to kidney is most common
(c) CT is radiographic modality of choice for diagnosis and follow-up
(d) Radical nephrectomy remains treatment of choice

(Answer is D) Extirpative surgery should be avoided if renal lymphoma and leukemia are suspected because the treatment of these processes is generally systemic chemotherapy with or without radiation therapy.

70. How much does upper urinary tract urothelial tumors involving the renal pelvis or ureter account for renal tumors?

(a) 0% to 3% (b) 3% to 5%
(c) 5% to 7% (d) 7% to 10%

(Answer is C) Upper urinary tract urothelial tumors involving the renal pelvis or ureter are relatively uncommon, accounting for about 5% to 7% of all renal tumors and about 5% of all urothelial tumors.

71. Which one of the following is not included in the etiology of upper urinary tract urothelial tumors?

(a) Smoking
(b) Thorotrast
(c) Chronic inflammation
(d) Aniline dyes

(Answer is B) Thorotrast is involved in renal malignancies and not upper tract urothelial tumors.

72. Which hereditary disorder is associated with upper urinary tract urothelial tumors?

(a) VHL
(b) Bitt-Hogg-Dube
(c) Tuberous sclerosis
(d) Lynch syndrome II

(Answer is D) Lynch syndrome II, for example, is characterized by the early development of colonic tumors (without polyposis) and extracolonic neoplasms, including upper tract urothelial tumors.

73. Most common site of upper tract urothelial tumor is:

(a) Upper ureter (b) Middle ureter
(c) Lower ureter (d) Renal pelvis

(Answer is D) Tumors of the renal pelvis are slightly more common than ureteral tumors. Ureteral tumors occur more commonly in the lower than in the upper ureter. Overall, about 70% of ureteral tumors occur in the distal ureter, 25% in the midureter, and 5% in the proximal ureter.

74. Most common determinant of outcome in upper urinary tract tumors is:

(a) Grade (b) Stage
(c) Size (d) Site

(Answer is B) Stage is currently the most important predictor of survival in patients with upper tract urothelial tumors.

75. Most common predictor of invasiveness in upper urinary tract tumors is:

(a) Grade (b) Stage
(c) Size (d) Site

(Answer is A) Tumors of high grade are more likely to invade into the underlying connective tissue, muscle and surrounding tissues.

76. Most common finding on imaging studies in upper urinary tract tumors is:

(a) Filling defect (b) Non visualization
(c) Hydronephrosis (d) Mass lesion

(Answer is A) A filling defect is the most common finding on imaging studies.

77. In transitional cell cancers density range from:

(a) 70 to –10 HU (b) 10 to 10 HU
(c) 10 to 70 HU (d) 70 to 90 HU

(Answer is C) Transitional cell cancers have an average density of 46 Hounsfield units (HU) and a range of 10 to 70 HU.

78. Most common type of renal pelvic tumors are:

(a) Papillary, non invasive
(b) Papillary, invasive
(c) Sessile, non invasive
(d) Sessile, invasive

(Answer is B) Approximately 85% of renal pelvic tumors are papillary and the remainder sessile. 50% to 60% of renal pelvic tumors are invasive into either the lamina propria or muscle.

79. Which is the most common site and histological variant of ureteral tumors?

(a) Upper ureter, low grade, low stage
(b) Upper ureter, high grade, high stage
(c) Lower ureter, low grade, low stage
(d) Lower ureter, high grade, high stage

(Answer is C) 55% to 75% of ureteral tumors are low grade and low stage.

80. What is the incidence of upper tract tumor after bladder tumor?

(a) 0 to 2% (b) 2 to 4%
(c) 4 to 8% (d) 8 to 16%

(Answer is B) The incidence of upper tract tumor after bladder tumor is 2% to 4% with a mean time to occurrence of 70 months.

81. Sixty-year-old man with a solitary kidney develops a 4 cm tumor in renal pelvis. It is grade II invasive and is organ confined. Best chance of cure for this patient will be:

(a) Pyelotomy, tumor ablation and partial nephrectomy
(b) Radical nephroureterectomy and dialysis
(c) Pylectomy alone
(d) External beam radiation and chemotherapy

(Answer is B) Radical nephroureterectomy and dialysis still offer the best chance of cure and survival in patients with a large, invasive, high-grade, organ-confined renal pelvis tumor (T2, N0, M0) in a solitary kidney.

82. A 48-year-old male has grade II ureteral tumor in mid ureter in volving 3 cm of ureter. Disease is organ confined and non-invasive. Ideal treatment will be:

(a) Radical nephroureterectomy
(b) Segmental ureterectomy and regional lymphadenectomy
(c) Segmental ureterectomy without regional lymphadenectomy
(d) Subtotal ureterectomy

(Answer is B) Segmental ureterectomy and ureteroureterostomy are indicated for noninvasive grade 1 and grade 2 tumors of the proximal ureter or midureter that are too large for complete endoscopic ablation.

83. A 63-year-old female has a grade III stage T2 tumor of proximal ureter. She underwent a radical nephroureterectomy and regional lymphadenectomy. Management regarding ureter removal will be:

(a) Ligation as far as exposure will allow
(b) Ligation of ureter with 2 cm margin
(c) Ligation of abdominal ureter (Till iliac vessels)
(d) Ligation of whole ureter with a bladder cuff

(Answer is D) Radical nephroureterectomy with excision of a bladder cuff is recommended for large, high-grade, invasive tumors of the renal pelvis and proximal ureter.

84. HIV patient on indinavir for 8 years started developing hematuria. IVU shows renal pelvic filling defect. Urine is suspicious of malignant cells. Lesion has soft tissue density on CT scan. Next step will be:

(a) Nephroureterectomy
(b) Abdominal MRI
(c) Percutaneous nephroscopy and pyeloscopy
(d) Discontinuation of indinavir, hydration and reimaging

(Answer is D) Indinavir can lead to urolithiasis.

85. About combining regional lymphadenectomy with radical nephroureterectomy which of the following statement is true?

(a) Significantly increased operative time
(b) Significantly increased morbidity
(c) Important for prognosis
(d) Is of great significance and should be performed

(Answer is C) The usefulness of regional lymphadenectomy in this disease has not been firmly established. Although it is recommended by many investigators, little therapeutic value has been established, and nearly every patient with positive nodal metastases has developed early systemic metastases.

86. Percutaneous antegrade approach in upper urinary tract tumors is associated with all *except:*

(a) Larger instruments can be introduced and deeper biopsies can be taken
(b) Can assess lower pole calyx and urinary tract of patients with urinary diversion
(c) Increase morbidity as compare to ureteroscopic approach
(d) Decrease possibility of tumor seedling

(Answer is D) The main disadvantages are the increased morbidity compared with ureteroscopy and the potential for tumor seeding outside the urinary tract.

87. Fifty-four-year-old male presenting with hematuria has an isolated positive urine cytology, otherwise he has normal IVP, RGP and negative cystoscopy and negative biopsy from bladder and urethra. Ideal management for this patient will be:

(a) Radical nephroureterectomy
(b) Ureteropyeloscopy
(c) Observation
(d) Instillation of chemotherapic agents

(Answer is B) Ureteropyeloscopy is indicated in such cases because the yield for direct visualization of small lesions is superior to that of retrograde pyelography.

88. Pluck technique is performed for:

(a) Renal tumor
(b) Upper tract urothelial tumor
(c) Bladder tumor
(d) Urethral tumor

(Answer is B) TUR of ureteric orifice is, also referred to as the pluck technique, should be reserved for proximal, low-grade tumors.

89. Which statement regarding upper tract urothelial tumor is not correct?

(a) Systemic chemotherapy regimens offered for treatment are the same as those used for transitional cell carcinoma of the bladder
(b) Complete responses are rare and the duration of response is limited
(c) Upper tract urothelial cancer is chemo-resistant
(d) Overall survival of approximately 12 to 24 months

(Answer is C) Upper tract urothelial cancer, like bladder cancer, is chemosensitive.

90. After what period of warm ischemia, there is generally significant, immediate functional loss, and late recovery of renal function is either incomplete or absent?

(a) 10 minutes (b) 20 minutes
(c) 30 minutes (d) 40 minutes

(Answer is C) For periods of warm ischemia beyond 30 minutes, there is generally significant, immediate functional loss, and late recovery of renal function is either incomplete or absent.

91. Incidence of renal ischemia was less in all the following situation *except:*

(a) Solitary kidney is more resistant to ischemic damage
(b) Temporary arterial occlusion is the presence of an extensive collateral vascular supply
(c) When the renal artery alone is occluded
(d) Intermittent clamping of the renal artery with short periods of recirculation is less damaging than continuous arterial occlusion

(Answer is D) Intermittent clamping of the renal artery with short periods of recirculation is also more damaging than continuous arterial occlusion, possibly because of the release and trapping of damaging vasoconstrictor agents within the kidney.

92. Mannitol is most effective when it is given:

(a) 10 minutes before arterial occlusion
(b) 30 minutes before arterial occlusion
(c) 10 minutes after arterial occlusion
(d) 30 minutes after arterial occlusion

(Answer is A) Mannitol is most effective when it is given 5 to 15 minutes before arterial occlusion.

93. The optimum temperature for hypothermic in situ renal preservation is:

(a) 0°C (b) 5°C
(c) 15°C (d) 25°C

(Answer is C) The optimum temperature for hypothermic in situ renal preservation is 15°C.

94. Surface cooling of the kidney with ice slush allows how much time of safe ischemia without permanent renal injury?

(a) 1 hour (b) 2 hours
(c) 3 hours (d) 4 hours

(Answer is C) Both animal and human studies have shown that this level of hypothermia provides complete renal protection from arterial occlusion of up to 3 hours. Surface cooling of the kidney with ice slush allows up to 3 hours of safe ischemia without permanent renal injury.

95. The major advantage of dorsal lumbotomy are all *except:*

(a) This approach is preferred for removal of a small kidney, for bilateral nephrectomy in patients with ESRD
(b) This approach is more rapid, provides strong wound closure with less postoperative pain
(c) No muscles are transected, and access to the kidney is obtained by simply incising the posterior fascial layers
(d) Good access to the kidney and renal vessels

(Answer is D) The major disadvantage of dorsal lumbotomy is its limited access to the kidney and renal vessels, which can pose a problem if there are intraoperative complications such as migration of a calculus or injury to major renal vessels with bleeding.

96. The thoracoabdominal approach is desirable for performing radical nephrectomy in patients with:

(a) RCC with extensive lymphadenopathy
(b) RCC with large central hilar tumor
(c) Right side large upper pole RCC
(d) Left side large upper pole RCC

(Answer is C) The thoracoabdominal approach is desirable for performing radical nephrectomy in patients with large tumors involving the upper portion of the kidney. It is particularly advantageous on the right side.

97. **An extraperitoneal flank approach is usually preferable in all *except:***
   (a) Kidney is chronically infected
   (b) When the patient is obese
   (c) When multiple prior abdominal operations have been performed
   (d) Cases of traumatic renal injury

(Answer is D) A transperitoneal approach is preferable in patients who cannot tolerate the flank position, in patients with end-stage renal disease undergoing bilateral nephrectomy for polycystic kidney disease, and in cases of traumatic renal injury in which early access to the pedicle is necessary.

98. **Hypothermic circulatory arrest can be safely maintained for how much time without incurring a cerebral ischemic event?**
   (a) 10 min (b) 20 min
   (c) 30 min (d) 40 min

(Answer is D) Hypothermic circulatory arrest can be safely maintained for at least 40 minutes without incurring a cerebral ischemic event.

99. **Venovenous bypass in the form of a caval-atrial shunt is a useful technique for:**
   (a) Infradiaphragmatic vena caval tumor thrombi
   (b) Non-adherent supradiaphragmatic vena caval tumor thrombi not extending into right atrium
   (c) Adherent supradiaphragmatic vena caval tumor thrombi not extending into right atrium
   (d) Supradiaphragmatic vena caval tumor thrombi just extending into right atrium

(Answer is B) In patients with nonadherent supradiaphragmatic vena caval tumor thrombi that do not extend into the right atrium, venovenous bypass in the form of a caval-atrial shunt is a useful technique.

100. **The major disadvantage of partial nephrectomy for RCC is the risk of:**
   (a) Post operative bleeding
   (b) Post operative tumor recurrence in renal remnant
   (c) Post operative distant renal metastasis
   (d) Post operative tumor recurrence in lymph nodes

(Answer is B) The major disadvantage of partial nephrectomy for RCC is the risk of postoperative local tumor recurrence in the kidney that was operated on, which has been observed in 4% to 6% of patients. These local recurrences are most likely a manifestation of undetected microscopic multifocal RCC in the renal remnant.

101. **In performing a transverse resection of the upper part of the kidney, care must be taken to avoid injury to the:**
   (a) Posterior segmental renal arterial branch
   (b) Anterior segmental renal arterial branch
   (c) Apical segmental renal arterial branch
   (d) Basal segmental renal arterial branch

(Answer is A) In performing a transverse resection of the upper part of the kidney, care must be taken to avoid injury to the posterior segmental renal arterial branch.

102. **Two most common complication after partial nephrectomy is:**
   (a) Hemorrhage and urinary fistula formation
   (b) Ureteral obstruction and hemorrhage
   (c) Renal insufficiency and urinary tract fistula
   (d) Infection and renal insufficiency

(Answer is A) Two most common complication after partial nephrectomy is hemorrhage and urinary fistula formation.

103. **Renal artery aneurysms may require repair in all *except:***
   (a) Significant hypertension
   (b) More than 2 cm, non calcified

(c) Women of reproductive age
(d) More than 2 cm, calcified

(Answer is D) Renal artery aneurysms may require repair if they result in significant hypertension or for prevention of rupture when they are larger than 2 cm and noncalcified. This is a particular concern in women of reproductive age because of the predisposition for rupture during pregnancy.

104. Progressive obstruction resulting in ischemic renal atrophy is least common with:

(a) Medial fibroplasia
(b) Perimedial fibroplasia
(c) Intimal fibroplasia
(d) True fibromuscular hyperplasia

(Answer is A) Medical management of medial fibroplasia is the initial approach because loss of renal function from progressive obstruction is uncommon, and intervention is reserved for those patients with difficult-to-control hypertension. Renal artery disease due to intimal or perimedial fibroplasia is often associated with progressive obstruction, which can result in ischemic renal atrophy.

105. Primary indication of endovascular stenting is:

(a) Ostial atherosclerosis
(b) Nonostial atherosclerosis
(c) Perimedial fibroplasia
(d) True fibromuscular hyperplasia

(Answer is A) The results with endovascular stenting for ostial lesions are better than those with PTA; however, surgical revascularization remains the definitive long-term therapy for these patients.

106. Revascularisation is indicated in which situation with best results?

(a) Unilateral RAS with 50% stenosis with creatinine of 5.0 mg/dl
(b) Unilateral RAS with 80% stenosis with creatinine of 5.0 mg/dl
(c) Unilateral RAS with 80% stenosis with creatinine of 3.0 mg/dl
(d) Bilateral RAS with 80% stenosis with creatinine of 3.0 mg/dl

(Answer is D) Those at highest risk of renal failure are patients with high-grade stenosis (>75%) involving the entire renal mass (bilateral disease or disease in a solitary kidney). Intervention is indicated in such patients for purpose of preserving renal function. However, surgical revascularization is generally not worthwhile for patients with advanced azotemia (serum creatinine concentration of more than 4 m g/dl) because of significant underlying renal parenchymal disease.

107. For aortorenal bypass which remains the preferred method in patients with a nondiseased abdominal aorta:

(a) Hypogastric artery (b) Saphenous vein
(c) Gonadal vein (d) PTFE

(Answer is B) Although a variety of surgical revascularization techniques are available for treatment of patients with renal artery disease, aortorenal bypass with a free graft of autogenous saphenous vein or hypogastric artery remains the preferred method in patients with a nondiseased abdominal aorta. Although an arterial autograft is theoretically advantageous, use of the hypogastric artery as a bypass graft is limited by its short length and frequent involvement with atherosclerosis.

108. Which is the single piece hand assisted laparoscopic device?

(a) Gelport (b) Lapdisc
(c) Omniport (d) All of the above

(Answer is B) Lapdisc is single piece device while omniport and gelport are 2 piece and 3 piece device respectively.

109. Factors that may make a patient unsuitable for percutaneous biopsy are all *except:*

(a) Morbid obesity
(b) Multiple bilateral cyst
(c) Solitary functioning kidney
(d) Uncontrolled hypertension

(Answer is D) Factors that may make a patient unsuitable for percutaneous biopsy include morbid obesity, multiple bilateral cysts, a body habitus that makes localization impossible, and a solitary functioning kidney.

110. In nephroptosis indication of surgery is:

(a) Descent of the symptomatic kidney by one vertebral body with diminished blood flow
(b) Descent of the symptomatic kidney by one vertebral body with or without diminished blood flow
(c) Descent of the symptomatic kidney by two vertebral body and obstruction or diminished flow
(d) Descent of the symptomatic kidney by two vertebral body with or without diminished flow

(Answer is C) Descent of the symptomatic kidney by two vertebral bodies and obstruction or diminished flow to the symptomatic side should be documented before surgical repair.

111. Indication of laparoscopic ureterolithotomy are all *except:*

(a) Failed ESWL of large upper ureteric stone
(b) Failed ureteroscopy for large upper ureteric stone
(c) Pelvic ectopic kidney with large renal stone
(d) UVJO with large lower ureteric stone

(Answer is D) Individuals to be considered for laparoscopic approach include those who have failed ESWL or percutaneous or ureteroscopic procedures, patients with unusual anatomy such as the pelvic kidney, and patients with stones resistant to fragmentation, such as those of cystine composition. In addition, patients with ureteropelvic junction obstruction and renal stones undergoing laparoscopic reconstruction can have stones removed during the same procedure using a flexible cystoscope

112. Indication for laparoscopic treatment of renal stone in calyceal diverticula are all *except:*

(a) Large peripheral diverticula with renal stone
(b) Diverticula located near the renal hilum
(c) Diverticula in posterior location
(d) Diverticula in anterior location

(Answer is C) Large peripheral diverticula, those located medially near the renal hilum and those in an anterior location, may be treated using laparoscopic techniques.

113. Prevention of port site seeding during laparoscopy for malignancy includes all *except:*

(a) Maximize direct tumor handling
(b) Place all tissues within an impermeable laparoscopic sac before morcellation or tissue extraction
(c) Re-drape port sites at time of tissue removal
(d) Ensure wide en-bloc dissection of tumor and surrounding tissues

(Answer is A) Minimize direct tumor handling to prevent iatrogenic spread.

114. Indication of laparoscopic nephrectomy includes all *except:*

(a) Patients with tumor thrombus extending into adrenals
(b) Patients with tumor thrombus extending into the renal vein
(c) Patients with a RCC with prior history of ipsilateral renal surgery and perinephric inflammation
(d) Patients with tumor thrombus extending into the subdiaphragmatic IVC

(Answer is D) Laparoscopic radical nephrectomy is indicated in patients with Tl to T3a renal tumors. Some patients with tumor thrombus extending into the renal vein can also be treated with laparoscopic radical nephrectomy. Patients with a prior history of ipsilateral renal surgery, perinephric inflammation, or extensive intra-abdominal surgery are still candidates for laparoscopic surgery.

115. Advantage of retroperitoneal approach over transperitoneal approach are all *except:*

(a) Patients with a history of multiple abdominal surgical procedures or peritonitis
(b) Patients with abnormalities on the posterior surface of the kidney (exophytic cyst or mass)
(c) More direct access to the renal vessels for early control
(d) More working space can make trocar placement, instrument movement, and organ manipulation easy

(Answer is D) The small working space can make trocar placement, instrument movement and organ manipulation difficult.

116. Conversion from laparoscopic to open, occurs most often during procedure performed for:

(a) Stones (b) Malignancy
(c) Infection (d) Obstruction

(Answer is C) The majority of patients converted to open surgery had infectious causes of renal abnormality as the leading indication for kidney removal.

117. Most common cause of conversion from laparoscopic to open surgery in renal surgery is:

(a) Bleeding
(b) Adhesions
(c) Inability to identify ureter
(d) Inability to approach renal hilum

(Answer is A) Bleeding was the most common cause of open conversion, followed by the surgeon's inability to visualize the renal hilum for dissection.

118. Ablation of renal tumor is documented by:

(a) Negative biopsy
(b) Progressive shrinking on USG
(c) Loss of enhancement on follow-up CT or MRI
(d) Loss of enhancement on follow-up CT or MRI and also progressive shrinking after therapy

(Answer is D) Complete loss of contrast enhancement on follow-up CT or MRI scans has been considered a sign of complete tissue destruction. The lesion should also show progressive shrinking after therapy as proof of remission.

119. In cryoablation complete destruction of renal parenchyma occurs below which temperature?

(a) –10°C (b) –20°C
(c) –30°C (d) –40°C

(Answer is B) Complete destruction of normal renal parenchyma occurs at temperatures below –19.4°C.

120. Minimum temperature required for complete ablation of tumor in RFA is:

(a) 30°C (b) 50°C
(c) 70°C (d) 90°C

(Answer is C) Temperatures over 70°C throughout the entire target zone are needed for complete ablation.

121. Energy ablation techniques provides reliable results in:

(a) Hilar tumor less than 3 cm
(b) Peripheral tumor less than 3 cm
(c) Multifocal small tumors
(d) Recurrent small tumors

(Answer is B) Reliable results are obtained with peripheral tumors less than 3 cm in diameter.

122. The most common neoplasms that metastasize to kidneys come from:

(a) Breasts (b) Thyroids
(c) Lungs (d) Liver

(Answer is C) Lungs

123. The etiology of renal cysts includes all of the following, *except:*

(a) Autosomal dominant polycystic kidney disease (ADPKD)
(b) Developmental cystic renal disease
(c) Inherited cystic renal disease
(d) Systemic disease with associated renal cysts

(Answer is A) Autosomal dominant polycystic kidney disease (ADPKD)

124. Inherited renal cystic disease(s) include(s) the following:

(a) Glomerulocystic kidney disease (GCKD)
(b) Juvenile nephronophthisis (JNPHP)
(c) Medullary cystic kidney disease
(d) All of the above

(Answer is D) All of the above

125. What is (are) true regarding the etiology of medullary cystic kidney disease (MCKD)?

(a) Mutations in the $MCKD_1$ (chromosome 1q21) gene
(b) Mutations in the $MCKD_2$ (chromosome 16q12) gene
(c) Inherited in an autosomal dominant fashion
(d) All of the above

(Answer is D) All of the above

126. What is the proper terminology of a renal cyst with the following characteristics: well-marginated, anechoic, with thin visible back wall, positive posterior acoustic enhancement, no septations, and no calcifications?

(a) Hyperattenuating renal cyst
(b) Solitary renal cyst
(c) Uncomplicated renal cyst
(d) Focal renal cyst

(Answer is C) Uncomplicated renal cyst

127. What is the likelihood that Bosniak type III renal cysts accompany malignant masses?

(a) Never (b) Unlikely
(c) Likely (d) Always

(Answer is C) Likely

128. What type of Bosniak renal cysts accompanies tumor masses in 5% of cases?

(a) I (b) II
(c) III (d) IV

(Answer is B) II

129. Regarding simple renal cysts, fluid attenuation on non-contrast CT series is:

(a) < -10 HU (b) < -20 HU
(c) < 10 HU (d) < 20 HU

(Answer is D) < 20 HU

130. What is false concerning end-stage renal disease (ESRD)?

(a) ARPKD accounts for 5% of ESRD in children
(b) More than one-half of patients with ARPKD require kidney transplant before age 20 years
(c) ADPKD is a common cause of ESRD
(d) Uncommonly, juvenile nephronophthisis causes ESRD in children

(Answer is D) Uncommonly, juvenile nephronophthisis causes ESRD in children

131. What is false concerning renal malignancy?

(a) RCC occurs in < 5% of patients with tuberous sclerosis
(b) Glomerulocystic kidney disease, renal tumors are typically solitary, large with central necrosis
(c) Von Hippel-Lindau syndrome, renal tumors are frequently bilateral and multicentric

(d) Acquired cystic disease, tumors are commonly bilateral, and metastatic in 15% of cases

(Answer is B) Glomerulocystic kidney disease, renal tumors are typically solitary, large with central necrosis

132. What is true regarding cancer incidence in renal cystic diseases?

(a) > 90% in Bosniak type IV renal cysts
(b) Patients receiving renal transplants for polycystic kidney disease is 48% higher than that expected in the general population
(c) All of the above
(d) Simple renal cysts might turn malignant in < 4% of cases

(Answer is C) All of the above

133. What is false concerning ADPKD patients?

(a) Hepatic cysts are the most common extra-renal manifestation
(b) Might experience cyst hemorrhage, renal infection, or nephrolithiasis
(c) Typically, complain of flank pain or intermittent hematuria in the early twenties
(d) Hypertension and CRF commonly occur in the fifth decade of life

(Answer is C) Typically, complain of flank pain or intermittent hematuria in the early twenties

134. What is true regarding ADPKD patients?

(a) Progress to ESRD in the sixth decade of life
(b) Hypertension is seen in 80% of patients with ADPKD aged 20-34 years
(c) Aortic valve stenosis in 25%
(d) Manifestations are more significant in patients with the PKD_2 genotype

(Answer is A) Progress to ESRD in the sixth decade of life

135. Antenatal sonography is the diagnostic tool for the following condition:

(a) Glomerulocystic kidney disease
(b) Developmental cystic renal disease
(c) Juvenile nephronophthisis
(d) Medullary cystic kidney disease

(Answer is B) Developmental cystic renal disease

136. The likelihood of malignancy in category IIF (indeterminate) renal cysts is:

(a) 20% (b) 30%
(c) 40% (d) 50%

(Answer is A) 20%

137. What is the treatment of a 3 cm renal mass suggestive of RCC adjacent to a huge renal cyst?

(a) Cyst aspiration and sclerosis
(b) Partial nephrectomy
(c) Endoscopic marsupialization and fulguration of the cyst
(d) Administration of TKIs

(Answer is B) Partial nephrectomy

138. Which of the following conditions carries the best prognosis?

(a) Acquired cystic renal disease
(b) Juvenile nephronophthisis
(c) Medullary sponge kidney
(d) Bilateral multicystic dysplastic kidney

(Answer is C) Medullary sponge kidney

139. Which of the following conditions carries the worst prognosis?

(a) Acquired cystic renal disease
(b) Juvenile nephronophthisis
(c) Medullary sponge kidney
(d) Bilateral multicystic dysplastic kidney

(Answer is D) Bilateral multicystic dysplastic kidney

140. What cannot be a manifestation of a renal tumor?

(a) Right hydrocele (b) Left varicocele
(c) Painless hematuria (d) Hypertension

(Answer is A) Right hydrocele

141. Which of the following is not a risk factor for RCC?

(a) Type II DM, especially in males
(b) Hypertension
(c) Obesity, especially in females
(d) Cigarette smoking

(Answer is A) Type II DM, especially in males

142. After radical nephrectomy, what is the 5-year survival rate for stage I RCC?

(a) 80% (b) 85%
(c) 90% (d) 95%

(Answer is D) 95%

143. Which of the following factors is associated with increased survival in patients with metastatic kidney tumors?

(a) Physically active patients with good performance status
(b) Extirpation of the primary tumor
(c) Long disease-free interval between initial nephrectomy and the emergence of secondaries
(d) All of the above

(Answer is D) All of the above

144. In renal mass(es), the main indication to take a renal biopsy is the suspicion of:

(a) Papillary RCC
(b) Renal metastases
(c) Renal oncocytoma
(d) Renal xanthogranuloma

(Answer is B) Renal metastases

145. On ultrasonography, what are the percentages of incidentally discovered renal masses that will later be malignant on further workup?

(a) 70 - 85% (b) 55 - 70%
(c) 40 - 55% (d) 25 - 40%

(Answer is A) 70 - 85%

146. What type of renal adenomas is a precursor to papillary RCC?

(a) Adenoma with clear cell
(b) Papillary adenoma
(c) Metanephric adenoma
(d) None of the above

(Answer is B) Papillary adenoma

147. What is false concerning renal angiomyolipoma (AML)?

(a) Most lesions $\leq$ 4 cm are asymptomatic
(b) Renal masses with fat content is pathognomonic for AML
(c) Renal biopsy from AML carries a high risk of hemorrhage
(d) May coexist with malignant lesions, such as sarcomas and RCCs

(Answer is B) Renal masses with fat content is pathognomonic for AML

148. What is true regarding renal angiomyolipoma (AML)?

(a) Most classic AMLs eventually undergo malignant transformation to sarcomatoid and epithelioid AML
(b) The preferred treatment is nephrouretere-ctomy followed by active surveillance
(c) Angiographic embolization and/or nephron-sparing surgery is advised for symptomatic AMLs greater than 4 cm
(d) Extra-renal sites include the pancreas, salivary glands and thyroids

(Answer is C) Angiographic embolization and / or nephron-sparing surgery is advised for symptomatic AMLs greater than 4 cm

149. What is false concerning renal oncocytoma?

(a) The central scar on CT or MRI, and the spoke-wheel pattern of vessels on angiograms are not specific to oncocytoma

(b) Calcification, necrosis and hemorrhage are rare in oncocytomas
(c) Is thought to arise from the basement membrane of proximal convoluted tubules
(d) Treatment is partial nephrectomy or tumor excision

(Answer is C) Is thought to arise from the basement membrane of proximal convoluted tubules

150. The diagnosis of renal adenoma is commonly made:

(a) Autopsy
(b) Staining positive for human melanoma black (HMB)-45
(c) Fine-needle aspiration cytology
(d) Exclusion

(Answer is A) Autopsy

151. What is false regarding multiloculated cystic nephromas?

(a) They follow a benign clinical course
(b) They have a bimodal age distribution
(c) They are more common in men than in women
(d) None of the above

(Answer is C) They are more common in men than in women

152. What is false concerning metanephric adenoma?

(a) Radiographically, it is indistinguishable from RCC
(b) Has a female predominance
(c) Has a benign clinical course
(d) Has a peak incidence in the third decade of life

(Answer is D) Has a peak incidence in the third decade of life

153. On histological examination of a resected renal tumor, the presence of multiple mitochondria observed on electron microscopy is diagnostic for:

(a) Renal oncocytoma
(b) Multiloculated cystic nephromas
(c) Metanephric adenoma
(d) Adenoma with clear cell

(Answer is A) Renal oncocytoma

154. On histological examination of a resected renal tumor, positive staining for human melanoma black (HMB)-45 is a distinctive and diagnostic feature for:

(a) Multiloculated cystic nephromas
(b) Angiomyolipoma
(c) Metanephric adenoma
(d) Adenoma with clear cell

(Answer is B) Angiomyolipoma

155. What is (are) the risk factor(s) for developing simple renal cysts?

(a) Male gender (b) Hypertension
(c) Renal insufficiency (d) All of the above

(Answer is D) All of the above

156. What is the likelihood that simple renal cysts increase in size and number over time?

(a) Never (b) Unlikely
(c) Likely (d) Always

(Answer is D) Always

157. CT shows a renal mass with calcifications associated with fat. What could the lesion be?

(a) RCC (b) AML
(c) Teratoma (d) Any of the above

(Answer is A) RCC

158. After radical nephrectomy for organ-confined RCC, what is (are) the recommended surveillance radiologic examination(s)?

(a) Chest X-ray and abdominal ultrasonography every 3 months for the first year, and then annually for 3 years
(b) Annual chest X-ray for 3 years

(c) Abdominal and chest CT every 6 months for the first year, and then annually for 3 years
(d) Radiological examination required

(Answer is B) Annual chest X-ray for 3 years

159. What is the most powerful single predictor of oncologic outcomes in RCC cases?

(a) Margin status and grade
(b) Tumor size
(c) Tumor stage
(d) The time interval between the tumor emergence and excision

(Answer is C) Tumor stage

160. Which of the following renal tumors carries the best prognosis?

(a) Fibrosarcoma
(b) Leiomyosarcoma
(c) Carcinoid
(d) Adult Wilms' tumor

(Answer is C) Carcinoid

161. Which RCC subtype is most likely to benefit from targeted molecular therapy?

(a) Clear cell
(b) Chromophobe
(c) Papillary
(d) Renal medullary

(Answer is A) Clear cell

162. What does determine the renal function status after partial nephrectomy of a single kidney?

(a) The quality of the kidney and renal function prior to surgery
(b) The quantity of vascularized parenchymal mass preserved after excision of the tumor
(c) Warm ischemia time
(d) All of the above

(Answer is D) All of the above

163. What is the most common histologic subtype of renal sarcomas?

(a) Rhabdomyosarcoma
(b) Nephrosarcoma
(c) Leiomyosarcoma
(d) Neurosarcoma

(Answer is C) Leiomyosarcoma

164. What is false concerning "targeted molecular therapy"?

(a) A personalized medical therapy devised to meet each person's individual needs for cancer's specifications
(b) Treats cancer by interrupting unique molecular abnormalities that drive cancer growth
(c) Some cancer types have different molecular targets
(d) None of the above

(Answer is D) None of the above

165. What is not an indication for simple nephrectomy?

(a) Symptomatic chronic renal infection with poor function
(b) Some cases of renovascular hypertension
(c) Symptomatic calculus disease with poor renal function
(d) Prior to kidney transplant

(Answer is D) Prior to kidney transplant

166. What is an indication for radical nephrectomy?

(a) A 6 cm, polar tumor
(b) Bilateral RCC
(c) Locally advanced RCC
(d) Unilateral RCC with a functioning opposite kidney, but at risk for future impairment

(Answer is C) Locally advanced RCC

167. What is the relapse rate for completely resected RCC after radical nephrectomy?

(a) 1- 10%
(b) 10 - 20%
(c) 20 - 30%
(d) 30 - 40%

(Answer is C) 20 - 30%

168. What is false concerning imaging studies for preoperative evaluation of RCC case?

(a) Case of bone pain or elevated serum calcium and/or alkaline phosphatase levels, an isotopic bone scan is required
(b) Renal arteriography accurately localizes central scaring and tumor necrosis
(c) Transesophageal echocardiography helps assess vena caval and right atrial tumor thrombi
(d) CT can detect renal vein involvement in 82-95% of cases and vena caval involvement in 95-100% of cases

(Answer is B) Renal arteriography accurately localizes central scaring and tumor necrosis

169. In RCC, ipsilateral adrenal metastasis occurs in:

(a) 0.3 - 2% (b) 2 - 10%
(c) 11 - 18% (d) 19 - 26%

(Answer is B) 2 - 10%

170. What is false regarding radical nephrectomy operation?

(a) Nodal involvement doesn't influence prognosis
(b) Renal artery should be ligated before the vein to avoid kidney ballooning
(c) Cardiopulmonary bypass with deep hypothermic circulatory arrest is performed in patients with supra-diaphragmatic tumor thrombi
(d) Renal vein thrombi can be resected after incising the vein between 2 vascular clamps

(Answer is A) Nodal involvement doesn't influence prognosis

171. Manifestations of paraneoplastic syndrome associated with RCC include all of the following, *except:*

(a) Anemia and erythrocytosis
(b) Hepatic dysfunction and elevated human chorionic gonadotropin levels
(c) Hypocalcemia
(d) Hypertension

(Answer is C) Hypocalcemia

172. Metastatic tumors to the kidney are common from all of the following organs, *except:*

(a) Lungs (b) Thyroid
(c) Breasts (d) Melanoma

(Answer is B) Thyroid

173. The second most common RCC subtype is:

(a) Collecting duct (b) Clear cell
(c) Papillary (d) Chromophobe

(Answer is C) Papillary

174. What is false concerning renal cancers?

(a) Papillary subtype of RCC has a tendency to multifocality
(b) Chromosome 13 alterations are common in the development of clear cell renal carcinoma
(c) A solid mass on CT that enhances more than 15 HU is suggestive of RCC
(d) Bilateral involvement in RCC either synchronously or metachronously occurs in 2% to 4% of patients

(Answer is B) Chromosome 13 alterations are common in the development of clear cell renal carcinoma

175. According to Fuhrman's classification system for nuclear grading in RCC, nuclear size of 20 µg with irregular outline and prominent nucleoli is grade:

(a) 1 (b) 2
(c) 3 (d) 4

(Answer is C) 3

176. Fuhrman's grading system for renal cell carcinoma relies on:

(a) Nuclear size, outline and nucleoli
(b) Cohesiveness and the degree of cellular atypia
(c) Chromatin structure and content of the interphase nucleus
(d) Multinucleation and mitosis

(Answer is A) Nuclear size, outline and nucleoli

177. In RCC cases where IVC involvement with tumor thrombi are suspected, venacavography:

(a) The first and most reliable radiologic examination to study IVC thrombi
(b) Reserved for patients with equivocal MRI or CT findings
(c) Obsolete and has fallen out of use
(d) Carries a risk of IVC terrible bleeding that outweighs the diagnostic merits

(Answer is B) Reserved for patients with equivocal MRI or CT findings

178. Routine metastatic evaluation in RCC cases should include all of the following, *except:*

(a) Abdominal CT
(b) Chest X-ray
(c) Renal function test
(d) Liver function test

(Answer is B) Chest X-ray

179. In a localized RCC, local recurrence after tumor ablation therapy is managed by any of the following options, *except:*

(a) Repeat ablation
(b) Active surveillance
(c) Salvage surgery
(d) Radical nephrectomy

(Answer is D) Radical nephrectomy

180. Regarding ureteral cancers, what is the most common part of tumor development?

(a) Upper ureter (b) Middle ureter
(c) Lower ureter (d) Comparable

(Answer is C) Lower ureter

181. Which of the following is a risk factor for developing upper urinary tract tumors?

(a) Obesity
(b) Consuming artificial sweeteners
(c) Asbestosis
(d) Analgesic abuse

(Answer is D) Analgesic abuse

182. What is the most common manifestation of upper tract urothelial carcinomas?

(a) Obstructive uropathy
(b) Painless hematuria
(c) Pain radiating to the groin
(d) Locally advanced tumor

(Answer is B) Painless hematuria

183. Evaluation of painless hematuria includes all of the following, *except:*

(a) Urine cytology
(b) CT urography
(c) Cystoscopy
(d) Renal function tests

(Answer is D) Renal function tests

184. Concerning upper tract urothelial tumors, what is the single most important predictor of outcome?

(a) Tumor stage
(b) Tumor grade
(c) Lymphovascular invasion
(d) Lymph node spread

(Answer is A) Tumor stage

185. In what percentages of patients do bilateral upper tract tumors occur either synchronously or metachronously?

(a) 0.6 - 2% (b) 2 - 6%
(c) 6 - 10% (d) 12 - 16%

(Answer is B) 2 - 6%

186. What is the likelihood that inverted papillomas of the upper urinary tract accompany tumors?

(a) Never (b) Unlikely
(c) Likely (d) Always

(Answer is B) Unlikely

187. CARMENA trial is for:

(a) VEGF inhibitors
(b) Cytoreductive nephrectomy
(c) Immunotherapy
(d) Tyrosine kinase inhibitors

(Answer is B) Cytoreductive nephrectomy

188. False about metastatic RCC:

(a) One third of RCC cases diagnosed have synchronous metastases
(b) Metastatic RCC has survival around 50% at 10 years
(c) Nephrectomy as the sole therapeutic intervention in the context of metastatic disease is unlikely to alter outcome
(d) There are no prospective, randomized studies demonstrating a favorable outcome with metastasectomy.

(Answer is B) Metastatic RCC has survival around 50% at 10 years

189. Not a component of IMDC risk grouping of metastatic RCC:

(a) Karnofsky Performance score <80
(b) Neutrophilia
(c) Anemia
(d) Elevated LDH

(Answer is D) Elevated LDH

190. False about Sunitinib:

(a) Oral VEGFR kinase inhibitor
(b) Oral tyrosine Kinase inhibitor
(c) Hypertension is an important side effect
(d) Hyperthyroidism is an important side effect

(Answer is D) Hyperthyroidism is an important side effect

191. False about complications of laparoscopic renal surgery:

(a) Vascular injuries are the most common complication
(b) Unrecognised bowel injury has mortality of 3%
(c) Most common cause of unrecognized bowel injury is the use of thermal energy
(d) Less risk of rhabdomyolysis compared to open surgery

(Answer is D) Less risk of rhabdomyolysis compared to open surgery

192. Adrenalectomy is indicated along with radical nephrectomy in all *except:*

(a) >7 cm tumor
(b) Extrarenal tumor extension
(c) Tumor thrombus
(d) Lymphadenopathy

(Answer is A) >7 cm tumor

193. Risk of malignancy in Bosniak 2F cyst:

(a) 3-10% (b) 10-20%
(c) 1-2% (d) 30%

(Answer is A) 3-10%

194. Risk of malignancy in Bosniak 3 cyst:

(a) 30% (b) 10%
(c) 50% (d) 70%

(Answer is C) 50%

195. False regarding vascular injury during radical nephrectomy:

(a) IMA ligation usually won't lead to catastrophic complications
(b) SMA ligation is a catastrophic event
(c) IMV ligation is a catastrophic event

(d) Laparostomy is usually required if SMV injury

(Answer is C) IMV ligation is a catastrophic event

196. All are contraindications for partial nephrectomy *except:*

(a) T4 disease
(b) Regional lymphadenopathy
(c) < 35% of global renal mass retained
(d) Cold ischemia time >45 minutes

(Answer is C) < 35% of global renal mass retained

197. All are measures to reduce post operative renal failure after partial nephrectomy *except:*

(a) Pack kidney with ice slush for 15 minutes
(b) Vascular clamping instead of parenchymal clamping
(c) Warm ischemia time < 20 minutes
(d) Cold ischemia time <35 minutes

(Answer is B) Vascular clamping instead of parenchymal clamping

198. Clavien dingo grade for intervention under GA is:

(a) II
(b) III A
(c) III B
(d) IV

(Answer is C) III B

199. All are true about upper tract urothelial carcinoma *except:*

(a) Concurrent bladder tumor is seen in 17%
(b) Ureter is involved twice more than pelvis
(c) Higher incidence in people from Balkan countries
(d) Recurrence in bladder occurs in 22-47% cases

(Answer is B) Ureter is involved twice more than pelvis

200. False about renal lymphoma:

(a) 90% cases are primary lymphoma
(b) Extirpative surgery should be avoided
(c) Typically managed with chemotherapy
(d) Renal involvement is more with non Hodgkin lymphoma

(Answer is A) 90% cases are primary lymphoma

201. False about imaging in renal lymphoma:

(a) CT scan is the imaging modality of choice
(b) Typically hypervascular
(c) Most commonly presents as multiple renal masses
(d) Diffuse renal infiltration is a common pattern

(Answer is B) Typically hypervascular

202. False about metastatic tumors of the kidney:

(a) They are the 2nd most common malignant neoplasms of the kidney
(b) Most common solid organ tumor to metastasize to kidney is carcinoma lung
(c) Most are multifocal
(d) CT typically shows isodense masses with moderate enhancement

(Answer is A) They are the 2nd most common malignant neoplasms of the kidney

203. False about clinical trials in adjuvant treatment of RCC:

(a) ASSURE trial– Sunitinib vs Sorafenib
(b) S-TRAC trial– Sunitinib vs Pazopanib
(c) EVEREST trial– Everolimus for RCC
(d) ATLAS trial– Axitinib for RCC

(Answer is B) S-TRAC trial– Sunitinib vs Pazopanib

204. False about local recurrence of RCC after nephrectomy:

(a) Occurs in 2-4% of patients after radical nephrectomy
(b) Occurs in 1.4-10% patients after partial nephrectomy

(c) Majority have systemic disease also
(d) Majority of patients with positive margins after partial nephrectomy are managed with completion nephrectomy

(Answer is D) Majority of patients with positive margins after partial nephrectomy are managed with completion nephrectomy

205. False about RCC with venous thrombi:

(a) 4-10% cases of RCC has venous system involvement
(b) 45-70% cases of IVC thrombus can be cured with nephrectomy and thrombectomy
(c) Venous thrombus should be suspected in RCC associated with proteinuria
(d) Level II thrombus involves hepatic veins

(Answer is D) Level II thrombus involves hepatic veins

206. False about management of RCC with IVC thrombus:

(a) Preservation of atleast 50% lumen of IVC is needed
(b) Patients with completely occluded IVC may not need reconstruction after IVC resection
(c) Bland thrombus may be left in situ
(d) For level II thrombus liver mobilization is often needed

(Answer is D) For level II thrombus liver mobilization is often needed

207. False about renal mass biopsy for RCC:

(a) Relatively safe procedure
(b) Tumor seeding of the track is the main reported complication
(c) Positive biopsy has 96% specificity
(d) Histological subtype evaluation is dependable

(Answer is B) Tumor seeding of the track is the main reported complication

208. __% of clinical T1 renal mass is potentially aggressive RCC:

(a) 60% (b) 20%
(c) 30% (d) 40%

(Answer is B) 20%

CHAPTER

13

The Adrenals

1. **Zonation is complete by:**

(a) 6 months (b) 12 months
(c) 18 months (d) 24 months

(Answer is C) Zonation is complete by–18 months, but adult configuration is not reached until the age of 10 to 12 years.

2. **Which statement regarding adrenal gland is not correct?**

(a) The adrenal glands are paired retroperitoneal organs that lie within perinephric fat at the anterosuperior and medial aspects of the kidneys
(b) They measure up to 5 cm in length by 3 cm in width and are 1 cm thick
(c) Weight increases with age
(d) Adrenal is susceptible to hemorrhage at the time of birth

(Answer is C) Weight at birth is large (5 to 10 g) because of the fetal adrenal cortex.

3. **Adrenal hemorrhage at the time of birth is best diagnosed by:**

(a) USG (b) CT
(c) MRI (d) MIBG

(Answer is C) Adrenal is susceptible to hemorrhage at the time of birth, a condition now readily diagnosed by magnetic resonance imaging.

4. **Which statement regarding adrenal gland is not correct?**

(a) The adrenal cortex develops from mesoderm
(b) Mature adrenal cortex constitutes 90% of the gland
(c) Zonation is complete by 18 months
(d) The zona glomerulosa is less prominent in humans than in other species and is the site of glucocorticoids production

(Answer is D) The zona glomerulosa is less prominent in humans than in other species and is the site of aldosterone production.

5. **Primary physiologic control of aldosterone secretion is:**

(a) Renin (b) Angiotensin II
(c) Potassium (d) Sodium

(Answer is B) Primary physiologic control of aldosterone secretion is angiotensin II.

6. **Angiotensinogen is activated by all *except:***

(a) Decrease perfusion pressure
(b) Decrease sodium intake
(c) Prostaglandins
(d) Increase cellular cAMP

(Answer is D) Angiotensinogen is activated by decrease in cAMP.

7. **Most common source of ectopic ACTH:**

(a) Carcinoma liver
(b) Carcinoma lung
(c) Thymoma
(d) Carcinoma pancreas

(Answer is B) Most common source of ectopic ACTH is carcinoma lung.

8. **Most common cause of Cushing's syndrome is:**
   (a) Exogenous steroids
   (b) Ectopic corticotropin syndrome
   (c) Adrenal adenoma
   (d) Adrenal carcinoma

(Answer is A) Exogenous source of Cushing's syndrome should always be excluded first because therapeutic steroids are the most common cause.

9. **Cause of pseudo-Cushing's syndrome is:**
   (a) Depression
   (b) Diabetes mellitus
   (c) Hypertension
   (d) Congestive heart failure

(Answer is A) In pseudo-Cushing's syndrome, abnormally regulated cortical secretion, albeit mild, may exist in as many as 80% of patients with major depression and can occur commonly in patients with chronic alcoholism.

10. **Most direct and reliable index of cortisol secretion is:**
    (a) Low dose dexamethasone suppression test
    (b) High dose dexamethasone suppression test
    (c) Adrenal MRI
    (d) 24-hour excretion of cortisol in the urine

(Answer is D) The determination of 24-hour excretion of cortisol in the urine is the most direct and reliable index of cortisol secretion.

11. **Low dose suppression tests are now reserved primarily for patients with:**
    (a) Adrenal adenoma
    (b) Adrenal carcinoma
    (c) Pheochromocytoma
    (d) Pseudo-Cushing's syndrome

(Answer is D) Low-dose suppression tests are now reserved primarily for patients with equivocal 24-hour urinary cortisol excretion and are especially useful for identifying patients with pseudo-Cushing's syndrome.

12. **Ideal way to determine whether a patient has ACTH-dependent or ACTH-independent hypercortisolism is:**
    (a) 24-hour excretion of cortisol
    (b) Low dose dexamethasone test
    (c) Measurement of both plasma ACTH
    (d) Concurrent measurement of both plasma ACTH and cortisol

(Answer is D) Ideal way to determine whether a patient has ACTH-dependent or ACTH-independent hyper-cortisolism is the concurrent measurement of both plasma ACTH and cortisol.

13. **Ideal time to measure ACTH and cortisol is:**
    (a) Midnight and 2 AM
    (b) 6 AM to 8 AM
    (c) 12 noon to 2 PM
    (d) 6 PM to 8 PM

(Answer is A) Ideal time to measure ACTH and cortisol is between midnight and 2 AM.

14. **Most direct way to demonstrate pituitary hypersecretion of ACTH is:**
    (a) Urinary cortisol levels
    (b) Serum ACTH levels
    (c) Adrenal vein sampling of ACTH
    (d) Petrous vein sampling of ACTH

(Answer is D) Most direct way to demonstrate pituitary hypersecretion of ACTH is to measure its level in the petrosal venous sinus and compare the level with the peripheral level.

15. **Adrenal carcinomas are often indistinguishable from adenomas *except* for the:**
    (a) Size
    (b) Site
    (c) Number
    (d) Heterogenecity on CT

(Answer is A) Adrenal carcinomas are often indistinguishable from adenomas except for the larger size (> 6 cm). Large benign adenomas (5 cm or larger) often show calcification, heterogenicity, and cystic characteristics on CT and have regions of high signal intensity on T2-weighted MRI.

16. Which statement is not true regarding Nelson syndrome?

(a) May arise many years after bilateral adrenalectomy
(b) 10% to 20% of patients subsequently developed chromophobe adenomas
(c) After adrenalectomy patients must be followed up with determination of ACTH levels and evaluation of the sella turcica
(d) May be prevented by pituitary ablation

(Answer is D) The development of Nelson's syndrome may be prevented by prophylactic pituitary radiotherapy.

17. Exploration of adrenal mass should be performed when the lesion is beyond what size on CT or MRI?

(a) Any size exploration is must
(b) 2 cm
(c) 5 cm
(d) 6 cm

(Answer is C) CT scanning may underestimate the size of an adrenal lesion, and we suggest that exploration be performed when the lesion is larger than 5 cm on CT or MRI.

18. Incidentally detected all adrenal masses should be removed *except:*

(a) Functional
(b) More than 5 cm and solid component present
(c) Less than 5 cm with low signal T2 on MRI
(d) Less than 5 cm, cystic but increasing in size on CT follow-up

(Answer is C) All functional tumors, more than 5 cm with solid component and tumors with high signal T2 on MRI should be removed.

19. All are true regarding myelolipoma *except:*

(a) Nonfunctioning benign lesion
(b) Generally smaller than 5 cm, unilateral, asymptomatic
(c) Excludes the need for extensive metabolic evaluation or surgical exploration
(d) Calcified and hormonally active

(Answer is D) Lesions are rarely calcified or hormonally active. Hormone levels should be obtained, however, because coexisting functional cortical adenoma and myelolipoma have been reported.

20. Weiss criterion is used for:

(a) Pheochromocytoma
(b) Adrenocortical carcinoma
(c) Adrenal adenoma
(d) Adrenal metastasis

(Answer is B) Adrenocortical carcinoma: Weiss criteria.

21. Adrenal is site of metastasis most commonly from:

(a) Contralateral adrenal
(b) Kidney
(c) Urinary bladder
(d) Liver

(Answer is B) Adrenal has been found to be a site of metastasis in more than 50% of patients with melanomas and carcinomas ofthe breast and lung; in 40% of patients with renal cell carcinomas; and in patients with, in order of frequency, carcinomas of the contralateral adrenal, bladder, colon, esophagus, gallbladder, liver, pancreas, prostate, stomach and uterus.

22. Most common variety of adrenal cyst is:

(a) Endothelial or lymphangiomatous cysts
(b) Adrenal pseudocysts
(c) Parasitic cysts

(d) True epithelial cysts

(Answer is A) Endothelial or lymphangiomatous cysts account for nearly 45% of these lesions and are usually small, measuring 0.1 to 1.5 cm in diameter.

23. Treatment of asymptomatic simple adrenal cyst is:

(a) Sclerotherapy
(b) Laparoscopic cyst deroofing
(c) Laparoscopic removal of cyst
(d) Observation

(Answer is D) Most cystic adrenal lesions are found incidentally and can be observed; symptomatic cysts can be percutaneously drained or laparoscopically decorticated.

24. The classic triad of adrenal insufficiency includes:

(a) Hyponatremia, hypokalemia and azotemia
(b) Hypernatremia, hypokalemia and hypotension
(c) Hypernatremia, hyperkalemia and hypotension
(d) Hyponatremia, hyperkalemia and azotemia

(Answer is D) The classic triad of adrenal insufficiency includes hyponatremia, hyperkalemia and azotemia was present in only 50% to 60% of cases.

25. Patients who are most likely to respond favorably to adrenalectomy are:

(a) Limited effect on aldosterone production by maneuvers that affect angiotensin II level
(b) Increased levels of aldosterone biosynthetic precursors
(c) Decreased levels of "hybrid" steroids
(d) Lateralization of aldosterone secretion to one adrenal gland

(Answer is C) Patients who are most likely to respond favorably to surgery are those in whom aldosterone production is highly autonomous from renin-angiotensin. Elevated levels of "hybrid" steroids (e.g., urinary cortisol C-18-methyloxygenated metabolites [18-hydroxycortisol and 18-oxocortisol]) is one of them.

26. Which statement regarding hyperaldosteronism is not correct?

(a) In primary aldosteronism, an adrenal neoplasm or bilateral hyperplasia is the initiating event
(b) Secondary aldosteronism is most commonly seen in edematous disorders
(c) Primary hyperaldosteronism is identified by hypertension and high urine and plasma aldosterone levels
(d) Secondary hyperaldosteronism has low plasma renin activity

(Answer is D) Secondary aldosteronism is most commonly seen in edematous disorders (e.g., cirrhosis, renal failure), in which the elevated renin levels are a physiologic adjustment to a contracted blood volume.

27. Medical therapy in primary aldosteronism caused by idiopathic hyperaldosteronism is:

(a) Spironolactone
(b) Phenoxybenzamine
(c) Propranolol
(d) Captopril

(Answer is A) The cornerstone of medical therapy in PAL caused by idiopathic hyperaldosteronism is a mineralocorticoid receptor antagonist (i.e., spironolactone, eplerenone).

28. In pheochromocytoma percentage of patients with normal blood pressure is:

(a) 1% (b) 5%
(c) 10% (d) 15%

(Answer is C) About 10% of pheochromocytomas are found in normotensive patients.

29. Hereditary forms of pheochromocytoma includes all *except:*

(a) MEN I (b) MEN II
(c) MEN III (d) NF I

(Answer is A) Pheochromocytomas occur in MEA II, a triad including pheochromocytoma, MCT, and parathyroid adenomas. Pheochromocytoma may also be a part of MEN III.

30. "Light bulb" image on T2-weighted study is characteristic finding of:

(a) Pheochromocytoma
(b) Adrenocortical carcinoma
(c) Adrenal adenoma
(d) Adrenal metastasis

(Answer is A) In pheochromocytoma MRI appears to be as accurate as CT in identifying lesions while having a characteristically bright, "light bulb" image on T2-weighted study.

31. Regarding pre-operative management of pheochromocytoma which statement is not true?

(a) Only β-adrenergic blockers
(b) Only α-adrenergic blockers
(c) α-adrenergic blockers added on β-adrenergic blockers
(d) β-adrenergic blockers added on α-adrenergic blockers

(Answer is D) β-Adrenergic blockers, such as propranolol, have been added to α blockers to prepare patients for anesthesia and surgery. The β blockers protect against arrhythmias and permit reduction in the amount of α-adrenergic blockers necessary to control blood pressure.

32. Which one of the following is not the absolute contraindication for laparoscopic adrenalectomy?

(a) Adrenal vein tumor thrombus
(b) Invasive adrenocortical tumor
(c) Adrenal tumor with thrombus extending into IVC
(d) 8 cm adrenal tumor

(Answer is D) Known adrenal vein or vena caval involvement is an absolute contraindication to laparoscopic surgery. Tumor size is a relative contraindication to laparoscopic surgery.

33. Which statement regarding adrenal gland is not true?

(a) The left adrenal gland tends to lie more cephalad than the right adrenal gland
(b) The left adrenal gland is often more elongated than the right adrenal gland
(c) The left adrenal gland will lie in a more superomedial position to the kidney
(d) The right adrenal vein drains into the vena cava directly on the right

(Answer is A) The right adrenal gland tends to lie more cephalad than the left adrenal gland.

34. Patients undergoing surgery for large adrenal masses is to be counseled about the possibility of concurrent:

(a) Splenectomy for left side adrenal masses
(b) Hepatectomy for right side adrenal masses
(c) Nephrectomy
(d) Pleural effusion

(Answer is C) It is imperative for all patients undergoing surgery for large adrenal masses to be counseled about the possibility of concurrent en bloc nephrectomy.

35. Indications for partial adrenalectomy are all *except:*

(a) Solitary adrenal gland
(b) Von Hippel-Lindau syndrome
(c) Multiple endocrine neoplasia type IIA
(d) Multiple endocrine neoplasia type IIIA

(Answer is D) The main indications for partial adrenalectomy are solitary adrenal gland, bilateral disease, and patients with familial syndromes. Pheochromocytoma has been treated with partial adrenalectomy, especially in patients with von Hippel-Lindau syndrome, familial pheochromocytoma, or multiple endocrine neoplasia type IIA.

36. Which statement is not true regarding pheochromocytoma?

(a) 10% familial
(b) 10% pediatric
(c) 10% malignant
(d) 10% of all incidentalomas pheochromocytomas

(Answer is C) Pheochromocytoma

- 10% are found in normotensive patients.
- 10% familial.
- 10% pediatric.
- 5% of all incidentalomas are pheochromocytomas.
- 25% of all pheochromocytomas are found incidentally.
- 10% to 20% are malignant.

37. Triad of pheochromocytoma includes all *except:*

(a) Headache (b) Hypertension
(c) Perspiration (d) Tachycardia

(Answer is B) Classic hallmark of pheochromocytoma-triad of headache, episodic sudden perspiration, and tachycardia.

38. What is the nerve supply of the adrenal gland?

(a) Sympathetic to the medulla
(b) Parasympathetic to the medulla
(c) Sympathetic to the cortex
(d) Parasympathetic to the cortex

(Answer is A) Sympathetic to the medulla

39. Which of the following is not related to von Hippel-Lindau disease?

(a) Retinal hemangioblastoma
(b) Ureteral atresia
(c) Pheochromocytomas
(d) Multiple cysts in the pancreas and kidneys

(Answer is B) Ureteral atresia

40. Which of the following is false regarding zona glomeruloza?

(a) The most superficial layer of the adrenal cortex
(b) Responses to increased potassium levels, renin or decreased renal blood flow
(c) It causes pheochromocytoma
(d) Secretes aldosterone

(Answer is C) It causes pheochromocytoma

41. Which of the following is false regarding Addison's disease?

(a) Autoimmune disease in 70% of the cases
(b) Diagnosed by the rapid ACTH stimulationtest
(c) Characterized by low serum sodium and high potassium
(d) May coexist with hyperthyroidism and diabetes mellitus

(Answer is D) May coexist with hyperthyroidism and diabetes mellitus

CHAPTER 14

Urine Transport Storage and Emptying

1. **Latent pacemaker cells are present in:**
   (a) Upper ureter
   (b) Middle ureter
   (c) Lower ureter
   (d) All regions of ureter

(Answer is D) Latent pacemaker cells are present in all regions of the ureter.

2. **Nutritive functions of the cell is performed by:**
   (a) Mitochondria
   (b) Endoplasmic reticulum
   (c) Nucleus
   (d) Golgi bodies

(Answer is A) Mitochondria in the cytoplasm perform many of the nutritive functions of the cell.

3. **Which organelle is responsible for Ca^{2+} storage sites?**
   (a) Mitochondria
   (b) Endoplasmic reticulum
   (c) Nucleus
   (d) Golgi bodies

(Answer is B) Endoplasmic reticulum and sarcoplasmic reticulum dispersed in the cytoplasm serve as Ca^{2+} storage sites.

4. **Which one of the following substance is responsible for recanalization process of ureter?**
   (a) Aldosterone (b) Angiotensin II
   (c) Acetylcholine (d) Epinephrine

(Answer is B) At a point during development, the ureteral lumen is obliterated, and then it recanalizes. It appears that angiotensin acting through the angiotensin II receptor is involved in the recanalization process.

5. **The RMP of ureteral cell is determined by which ion?**
   (a) Na (b) K
   (c) Cl (d) H

(Answer is B) The RMP of the ureteral cell is approximately –33 to –70 mV and is determined primarily by the distribution of K^+ ions across the cell membrane and the relatively selective permeability of the resting cell membrane to K^+.

6. **Plateau phase of ureteral cell is related to:**
   (a) Efflux of Ca and influx of Na
   (b) Efflux of Na and influx of Ca
   (c) Efflux of Ca and Na
   (d) Influx of Ca and Na

(Answer is D) The plateau appears to be related to a persisting inward Ca^{2+} current and to an influx of Na^+.

7. **Conduction velocity in the ureter is:**
   (a) 0 to 4 cm /sec (b) 2 to 6 cm/sec
   (c) 4 to 8 cm/sec (a) 6 to 10 cm/sec

(Answer is B) Conduction velocity in the ureter is 2 to 6 cm/sec.

8. **Primary pacemaker cell in human are present:**
   (a) Near pelvicalyceal border
   (b) Pelvicalyceal border to UPJ
   (c) Near UPJ
   (d) From UPJ to UVJ

(Answer is A) Species with a multicalyceal system, such as the pig, sheep, and human, the "pacemaker cells" are located near the pelvicalyceal border.

9. How many ureteral contractions occur in a minute?

(a) 0 to 4 (b) 2 to 6
(c) 4 to 8 (d) 6 to 10

(Answer is B) Baseline, or resting, ureteral pressure is approximately 0 to 5 cm H_2O, and superimposed ureteral contractions ranging from 20 to 80 cm H_2O occur two to six times per minute.

10. Substances required for the conversion of ATP to cAMP:

(a) GTP and Ca^{2+} (b) GTP and Mg^{2+}
(c) GMP and Ca^{2+} (d) GMP and Mg^{2}

(Answer is B) In the presence of magnesium (Mg^{2+}) and a guanine nucleotide (GTP), adenylyl cyclase catalyzes the conversion within the cell of ATP to cAMP.

11. All agent increase intracellular cAMP levels *except:*

(a) Isoproterenol (b) Norepinephrine
(c) Papaverine (d) Theophylline

(Answer is B) Agents that either increase adenylyl cyclase activity, such as the β-adrenergic agonist isoproterenol, or decrease phosphodiesterase activity, that is, phosphodiesterase inhibitors such as theophylline and papaverine, increase intracellular cAMP levels and cause smooth muscle relaxation.

12. NO is formed from:

(a) Arginine and NADPH
(b) Arginine and NADP
(c) Citrulline and NADP
(d) Citrulline and NADPH

(Answer is A) Nitric oxide synthase (NOS) converts L-arginine to NO and L-citrulline in a reaction that requires reduced nicotinamide adenine dinucleotide phosphate (NADPH).

13. Which nitric oxide synthase (NOS) is NADPH dependent but Ca^{2+} independent?

(a) n NOS (b) i NOS
(c) e NOS (d) d NOS

(Answer is B) An inducible NOS isoform (i NOS) is NADPH dependent but Ca^{2+} independent.

14. The ureter has been shown to decompensate at which intravesical pressure approaches at?

(a) 20 cm H_2O (b) 40 cm H_2O
(c) 60 cm H_2O (d) 80 cm H_2O

(Answer is B) The ureter has been shown to decompensate when intravesical pressure approaches 40 cm H_2O.

15. Which one of the following has inhibitory effect on ureter?

(a) Bethanechol (b) Physostigmine
(c) Norepinephrine (d) Isoproterenol

(Answer is D) Isoproterenol, a β-adrenergic agonist, depresses contractility.

16. Which one of the following has inhibitory effect on ureter and UVJ?

(a) HI receptor agonist
(b) H2 receptor agonist
(c) Angiotensin
(d) Morphine

(Answer is B) Histamine's excitatory effect on the ureter and UVJ appears to be mediated by H1 receptors as it is inhibited by the H1 receptor antagonists. The H2 receptor mediates inhibitory effects of histamine.

17. Laplace eqation is:

(a) Pressure=Tension × wall thickness/Radius
(b) Tension=Pressure × wall thickness/Radius
(c) Pressurec=Tension × Radius/wall thickness
(d) Tension=Pressure × Radius/wall thickness

(Answer is A) The Laplace equation expresses the relation between the variables that affect intraluminal pressure=Pressure=Tension × wall thickness *I* Radius.

18. Onuf nucleus is present at:

(a) Lateral border of ventral horn
(b) Medal border of ventral horn
(c) Lateral border of dorsal horn
(d) Lateral border of ventral horn

(Answer is A) The external urethral sphincter motoneurons are located along the lateral border of the ventral horn, commonly referred to as Onuf's nucleus.

19. The prototypic cholinergic agonist is ACh, which serves as the neurotransmitter at all *except:*

(a) Preganglionic parasympathetic
(b) Preganglionic sympathetic
(c) Postganglionic parasympathetic
(d) Postganglionic sympathetic

(Answer is D) The prototypic cholinergic agonist is ACh, which serves as the neurotransmitter at (1) neuromuscular junctions of somatic motor nerves (nicotinic sites), (2) preganglionic parasympathetic and sympathetic neuroeffector junctions (nicotinic sites), and (3) postganglionic parasympathetic neuroeffector sites (muscarinic sites).

20. Which is the correct equation?

(a) Pdet = Pves - Pabd
(b) Pves= Pdet - Pabd
(c) Pabd = Pves - Pdet
(d) Pdet = Pabd - Pves

(Answer is A) Intravesical pressure reflects the combined factors of abdominal (Pabd) and detrusor (Pdet) pressures. Therefore, Pdet = Pves - Pabd.

21. In poorly compliant bladder, there is increase in:

(a) Collagen type I (b) Collagen type II
(c) Collagen type III (d) Collagen type IV

(Answer is C) Poorly compliant bladders is secondary to an alteration in the connective tissue content of the bladder wall, especially increased collagen type III.

22. Regarding umbrella cells that form the primary urine-plasma barrier are unique in all *except:*

(a) Ability to increase and to decrease considerably their surface area
(b) They may multinucleate
(c) Asymmetrical unit membrane, with the inner leaflet consisting of protein plaques and lipid and with a lipid outer leaflet
(d) Extremely high gradient between the plasma and the urine in terms of water concentration, urea concentration, potassium concentration, osmolality and pH

(Answer is C) The large umbrella cells that form the primary urine-plasma barrier are unique in several ways, they have an unusual apical surface membrane, which is described as an asymmetrical unit membrane, with the outer leaflet consisting of protein plaques and lipid and with a lipid inner leaflet.

23. In the male, the rhabdosphincter consists of:

(a) 35% fast-twitch and 65% slow-twitch fibers
(b) 65% fast-twitch and 35% slow-twitch fibers
(c) 45% fast-twitch and 55% slow-twitch fibers
(d) 55% fast-twitch and 45% slow-twitch fibers

(Answer is A) In the male, the rhabdosphincter consists of 35% fast-twitch and 65% slow-twitch fibers.

24. Initial event in expulsion phase of micturition is:

(a) Contraction of bladder
(b) Increase in bladder pressure
(c) Relaxation of urethral sphincter
(d) Relaxation of bladder neck

(Answer is C) The expulsion phase consists of an initial relaxation of the urethral sphincter followed in a few seconds by a contraction of the bladder, an increase in bladder pressure, and the flow of urine.

25. Excitatory transmitter in the CNS pathway facilitating micturition is:

(a) Serotonin (b) GABA
(c) Glutamate (d) Norepinephrine

(Answer is C) Pharmacologic experiments revealed that glutamic acid is the excitatory transmitter in these pathways.

26. Which muscarinic receptor predominate in human bladder?

(a) M1 (b) M2
(c) M3 (d) M4

(Answer is B) Although ligand receptor binding studies revealed that M2 receptors predominate, M3 receptors mediate cholinergic contractions.

27. Relaxation induced by adrenergic stimulation of the human detrusor is mediated mainly through:

(a) β1 (b) β2
(c) β3 (d) β5

(Answer is C) The relaxation induced by adrenergic stimulation of the human detrusor is mediated mainly through β3 adrenoceptor activation.

28. In human bladder mucosa, most potent to contract detrusor is:

(a) PGF2α (b) PGE
(c) PGI2 (d) TXA2

(Answer is A) Specimens of human bladder mucosa contain prostaglandin (PG)12, PGE2, PGE2α, and thromboxane A. In decreasing order of potency, PGF2α, PGE and PGE2 contract human detrusor.

29. Normal micturition is associated with:

(a) Myelinated Aδ afferents
(b) Unmyelinated Aδ afferents
(c) Myelinated Aδ and C afferents
(d) Unmyelinated Aδ and C afferents

(Answer is A) Normal micturition is associated with a spinobulbospinal reflex mediated by lightly myelinated Aδ afferents.

30. The most important afferents for initiating and maintaining normal micturition are those in the:

(a) Pelvic nerve (b) Pudendal nerve
(c) Cavernosal nerve (d) Hypogastric nerve

(Answer is A) The most important afferents for initiating and maintaining normal micturition are those in the pelvic nerve, relaying to the sacral spinal cord.

31. Which one of the following event does not occur during bladder filling?

(a) Passive phenomenon dependent on the elastic and viscoelastic properties of the bladder wall
(b) Increase in parasympathetic excitatory input
(c) Sympathetic reflex also contributes to storage by increasing outlet resistance by increasing tension on the smooth sphincter
(d) Increase in striated sphincter activity, on a reflex basis

(Answer is B) Lack of parasympathetic excitatory input occurs during bladder filling.

32. Which one of the following event does not occur during bladder emptying?

(a) Excitation of the spinal somatic and sympathetic reflexes
(b) Activation of the vesical parasympathetic pathways
(c) Cessation of the somatic and sympathetic spinal reflexes
(d) Nitric oxide, released by parasympathetic stimulation

(Answer is A) Inhibition of the spinal somatic and sympathetic reflexes occurs during bladder emptying.

33. The continence point in women is at:

(a) Proximal urethra

(b) Mid urethra
(c) Distal urethra
(d) Equal in all parts

(Answer is B) The continence point in women (highest point of pressure transmission) is at the midurethra.

34. Therapy to facilitate urine storage/bladder filling are all *except:*

(a) Calcium antagonists
(b) Potassium channel openers
(c) Prostaglandin inhibitors
(d) β-adrenergic antagonists

(Answer is D) Drugs that facilitate bladder filling are:

- Calcium antagonists.
- Potassium channel openers.
- Prostaglandin inhibitors.
- β-Adrenergic agonists.

35. Lower urinary tract dysfunction in a classic T10 level paraplegic patient after spinal shock has passed would include all *except:*

(a) Overactive neurogenic detrusor function
(b) Normal sensation
(c) Low capacity
(d) Normal compliance

(Answer is B) Lower urinary tract dysfunction in a classic T10 level paraplegic patient after spinal shock has passed would be classified in the ICS system as follows:

Storage phase–Overactive neurogenic detrusor function, absent sensation, low capacity, normal compliance, normal urethral closure function.

Voiding phase–Overactive obstructive urethral function, overactive detrusor function.

36. Detrusor hyperreflexia is now known as:

(a) Idiopathic detrusor overactivity
(b) Detrusor instability
(c) Neurogenic detrusor overactivity
(d) A contractile bladder

(Answer is C) If the condition is caused by neurologic disease, the term neurogenic detrusor overactivity (previously, detrusor hyperreflexia) is used; if not, the term idiopathic detrusor overactivity (previously, detrusor instability) is applied.

37. Sensory neurogenic bladder results from all *except:*

(a) Diabetes mellitus (b) Tabes dorsalis
(c) Pernicious anemia (d) Herpes zoster

(Answer is D) A sensory neurogenic bladder results from disease that selectively interrupts the sensory fibers between the bladder and the spinal cord or the afferent tracts to the brain. Diabetes mellitus, tabes dorsalis, and pernicious anemia are most commonly responsible.

38. The term urodynamics was first defined by:

(a) D K Rose (b) David M Davis
(c) Drake (d) Nitti

(Answer is B) The term urodynamics was first defined by David M Davis in 1953 to denote the study of the storage and emptying phases of the urinary bladder.

39. Indications and selection of patients for conduction of urodynamics includes all *except:*

(a) Children with daytime urgency and urge incontinence
(b) Children with persistent diurnal enuresis
(c) Children with spinal dysraphism
(d) Children with persistent nocturnal enuresis

(Answer is D) Indications and selection of patients for conduction of urodynamics:

- Children with daytime urgency and urge incontinence.
- Children with persistent diurnal enuresis.
- Children with spinal dysraphism.

40. Physiologic filling rate for cystometry is:

(a) Body weight (in kg)/4

(b) Body weight (in kg)/2
(c) Body height (in cm)/4
(d) Body height (in cm)/2

(Answer is A) Physiologic filling rate for cystometry: Rate = body weight (in kg)/4, expressed as ml/min.

41. Uroflowmetry in women all are correct *except:*

(a) In the normal woman Qmax can be greater than 30 ml/sec
(b) The flow curve is bell shaped as in men
(c) Flow time is shorter
(d) Maximum flow in women decreases with age

(Answer is D) In the normal woman Qmax can be greater than 30 ml/sec, the flow curve is bell shaped as in men, and the flow time is shorter. Maximum flow in women does not seem to be dependent upon age.

42. During the course of cystometry, information is gained regarding all the following bladder characteristics *except:*

(a) Capacity
(b) Residual urine
(c) Involuntary contraction
(d) Compliance

(Answer is B) During the course of cystometry, information is gained regarding four bladder characteristics; capacity, sensation, compliance, and the occurrence of involuntary contractions.

43. Functional bladder capacity is defined as:

(a) Bladder volume at the end of the filling CMG
(b) Bladder volume voided as determined by a voiding diary
(c) Bladder volume of the bladder after filling under general anesthesia
(d) Bladder volume of the bladder after filling under spinal anesthesia

(Answer is B) The functional bladder capacity is the largest volume voided as determined by a voiding diary.

44. MUCP is defined as:

(a) Maximum difference between the urethral pressure and the intravesical pressure
(b) Maximum difference between the intravesical pressure and the urethral pressure
(c) Maximum difference between the detrusor pressure and the intravesical pressure
(d) Maximum difference between the intravesical pressure and the detrusor pressure

(Answer is A) Maximum urethral closure pressure (MUCP): The maximum difference between the urethral pressure and the intravesical pressure.

45. Which statement regarding bladder compliance is not true?

(a) It is calculated by dividing the detrusor pressure change (dPdet) by the change in volume (dV)
(b) It is generally calculated between two points: the Pdet with the bladder empty at the start of filling and the Pdet at either the maximal cystometric capacity
(c) During the filling and storage phase of the CMG, increasing intravesical volumes should occur with little or no change in intravesical pressure
(d) Normal bladder compliance should be less than 12.5 ml/cm H_2O

(Answer is A) Bladder compliance is the relationship between change in volume and change in pressure. It is calculated by dividing the volume change (dV) by the change in detrusor pressure (dPdet) and expressed in ml/cm H_2O.

46. Patients with urge incontinence who do not have detrusor overactivity on a CMG is:

(a) 10% (b) 20%
(c) 30% (d) 40%

(Answer is D) The mere absence of documented overactivity on a CMG does not rule out its existence. Up to 40% of patients with urge incontinence do not have detrusor overactivity on a CMG.

47. Test used to differentiate "upper" from "lower" motor neuron lesions is:

(a) Bethanechol
(b) Ice water test
(c) Pressure flow study
(d) Video urodynamics

(Answer is B) The ice water test was first described by Bors and Blinn as a way to differentiate "upper" from "lower" motor neuron lesions.

48. What detrusor opening pressure may indicate outflow obstruction?

(a) 60 cm H_2O (b) 80 cm H_2O
(c) 100 cm H_2O (d) 120 cm H_2O

(Answer is B) The detrusor opening pressure is the detrusor pressure recorded at the onset of measured flow. It tends to be elevated in patients with infravesical obstruction, and pressures greater than 80 cm H_2O may indicate outflow obstruction.

49. What detrusor pressure at maximal flow implies the presence of outlet obstruction?

(a) 60 cm H_2O (b) 80 cm H_2O
(c) 100 cm H_2O (d) 120 cm H_2O

(Answer is C) The detrusor pressure at maximal flow is the magnitude of the detrusor contraction at the time when the flow rate is at its maximum. If this pressure is greater than 100 cm H_2O, it implies the presence of outlet obstruction even if the flow rate is normal.

50. Which statement is not true regarding pressure flow study (PFS)?

(a) Ideal to differentiate between patients with low flow because of obstruction and those with poor bladder contractility
(b) PFSs alone cannot identify the location of the obstruction
(c) The absence of residual urine exclude infravesical obstruction or bladder dysfunction
(d) The normal male generally voids with a Pdet of 40 to 60 cm H_2O, and women typically void with lower pressures

(Answer is C) The absence of residual urine does not exclude infravesical obstruction or bladder dysfunction.

51. AG number is:

(a) PdetQmax – 2 Qmax
(b) PdetQmax – 4 Qmax
(c) PdetQmax × 2 Qmax
(d) PdetQmax × 4 Qmax

(Answer is A) AG number = PdetQmax – 2 Qmax. A value greater than 40 defines obstruction; a value less than 20, no obstruction. A range of 20 to 40 is designated as equivocal.

52. Bladder contractility index is defined as:

(a) PdetQmax + 2 Qmax
(b) PdetQmax + 3 Qmax
(c) PdetQmax + 4 Qmax
(d) PdetQmax + 5 Qmax

(Answer is D) Using this formula for the BCI (i.e., BCI = PdetQmax + 5 Qmax), it is possible to define ranges of bladder contractility: BCI greater than 150 is strong, BCI less than 100 is weak, and BCI of 100 to 150 is normal contractility.

53. Which statement is not true regarding sphincter activity?

(a) Just before the onset of voiding, sphincter activity increases and remains so for the duration of micturition
(b) Failure of the sphincter to relax during micturition, when it occurs in patients with neurologic disease, it is termed DESD
(c) DESD typically occurs in patients with suprasacral spinal cord injury
(d) Failure of sphincter to relax in the absence of neurologic disease, the term pelvic floor hyperactivity is used

(Answer is A) Just before the onset of voiding, sphincter activity ceases and remains so for the duration of micturition.

54. DLPP greater than what level are higher risk for upper tract deterioration?

(a) 20 cm H_2O (b) 40 cm H_2O
(c) 60 cm H_2O (d) 80 cm H_2O

(Answer is B) Those with a DLPP greater than 40 cm H_2O were at significantly higher risk for upper tract deterioration (hydronephrosis, reflux) than those with DLPPs less than 40 cm H_2O.

55. At what level of VLPP suggest urethral hypermobility and minimal ISD?

(a) Greater than 70 cm
(b) Greater than 90 cm
(c) Greater than 100 cm
(d) Greater than 120 cm

(Answer is B) A VLPP less than 60 cm H_2O indicates the presence of significant ISD; a VLPP of 60 to 90 cm H_2O is equivocal, suggesting a combination of urethral hypermobility and some component of ISD; and pressures greater than 90 cm H_2O suggest urethral hypermobility and minimal ISD.

56. Voiding pattern in parkinson disease is:

(a) Detrusor–Overactivity, compliance-Normal, Smooth and striated sphincter-synergy
(b) Detrusor–Underactivity, compliance-Normal, Smooth and striated sphincter-synergy
(c) Detrusor–Overactivity, compliance-decreased, Smooth and striated sphincter -synergy
(d) Detrusor–Overactivity, compliance-Normal, Smooth and striated sphincter-dyssynergy

(Answer is A)

Parkinson's disease	Overactive detrusor, Normal compliance, smooth and striated sphincter synergy

57. Voiding pattern in autonomic hyperreflexia is:

(a) Detrusor–Overactivity, compliance-Normal, Smooth and striated sphincter-synergy
(b) Detrusor–Underactivity, compliance-Normal, Smooth and striated sphincter-synergy
(c) Detrusor–Overactivity, compliance-decreased, Smooth and striated sphincter-synergy
(d) Detrusor–Overactivity, compliance-Normal, Smooth and striated sphincter-dyssynergy

(Answer is D)

Autonomic hyperreflexia	Detrusor Overactivity, Normal compliance smooth and striated sphincter-dyssynergy

58. Patients with complete lesions of the spinal cord between spinal cord level T6 and S2, after they recover from spinal shock, generally exhibit:

(a) Detrusor–Overactivity, Smooth and striated sphincter-synergy
(b) Detrusor–Underactivity, Smooth sphincter-dyssynergy and striated sphincter-synergy
(c) Detrusor–Overactivity, Smooth and striated sphincter-dyssynergy
(d) Detrusor–Overactivity, Smooth sphincter synergy and striated sphincter-dyssynergy

(Answer is D) Patients with complete lesions of the spinal cord between spinal cord level T6 and S2, after they recover from spinal shock, generally exhibit involuntary bladder contractions without sensation, smooth sphincter synergy, but striated sphincter dyssynergia. Those with lesions above spinal cord level T6 may experience, in addition, smooth sphincter dyssynergia and autonomic hyperreflexia.

59. The most common long-term expression of lower urinary tract dysfunction after CVA is:

(a) Phasic detrusor overactivity
(b) Terminal detrusor overactivity

(c) Smooth sphincter overactivity
(d) Smooth sphincter underactivity

(Answer is A) The most common long-term expression of lower urinary tract dysfunction after CVA is phasic detrusor overactivity. Smooth sphincter activity is generally unaffected (synergic) by CVA. Pseudodyssynergia may indeed occur.

60. Most frequently involved area with associated micturition dysfunction are:

(a) Superior aspects of the frontal lobe
(b) Inferior aspects of the frontal lobe
(c) Superior aspects of the temporal lobe
(d) Inferior aspects of the temporal lobe

(Answer is A) The areas that are most frequently involved with associated micturition dysfunction are the superior aspects of the frontal lobe.

61. Spinal shock includes all *except:*

(a) Suppression of autonomic activity as well as somatic activity
(b) Bladder is acontractile and areflexic
(c) Radiologically, the bladder has evidence of trabeculation
(d) The bladder neck is generally closed and competent

(Answer is C) Radiologically, the bladder has a smooth contour with no evidence of trabeculation. The bladder neck is generally closed and competent.

62. Pseudodyssynergia and bradykinesia occurs in:

(a) CVA
(b) Cerebral palsy
(c) Normal pressure hydrocephalus
(d) Parkinson disease

(Answer is D) In parkinsonism pseudodyssynergia may occur, as well as a delay in striated sphincter relaxation (bradykinesia) at the onset of voluntary micturition.

63. The characteristic pattern that results when a patient has a complete lesion above the sacral spinal cord is all *except:*

(a) Detrusor overactivity
(b) Smooth sphincter synergia
(c) Striated sphincter dyssynergia
(d) Absent sensation above the level of the lesion

(Answer is D) Generally, complete spinal cord lesions above the sacral spinal cord, but below the area of the sympathetic outflow, result in detrusor overactivity, absent sensation below the level of the lesion, smooth sphincter synergia, and striated sphincter dyssynergia.

64. Dysfunctions that occur with interruption of the peripheral reflex arc are all *except:*

(a) Detrusor areflexia
(b) Normal compliance
(c) Smooth sphincter area may be relatively incompetent
(d) Striated sphincter area may exhibit fixed residual tone not amenable to voluntary relaxation

(Answer is B) The dysfunctions that occur with interruption of the peripheral reflex arc may be very similar to those of distal spinal cord or nerve root injury. Detrusor areflexia often develops, low compliance may result, the smooth sphincter area may be relatively incompetent, and the striated sphincter area may exhibit fixed residual tone not amenable to voluntary relaxation.

65. Which is not true about autonomic hyper-reflexia?

(a) Autonomic hyperreflexia is a syndrome of exaggerated sympathetic activity in response to stimuli above the level of the lesion
(b) The symptoms are pounding headache, hypertension, and flushing of the face and body above the level of the lesion
(c) Any endoscopic procedure in susceptible

patients should be done under spinal anesthesia

(d) Sublingual nifedipine had been reported to be capable of alleviating this syndrome when given during cystoscopy

(Answer is A) Autonomic hyperreflexia is a syndrome of exaggerated sympathetic activity in response to stimuli below the level of the lesion.

66. The "typical" myelodysplastic patient shows:

(a) Areflexic bladder with open bladder neck
(b) Hypercontractile bladder with open bladder neck
(c) Areflexic bladder with closed bladder neck
(d) Hypercontractile bladder with open bladder neck

(Answer is A) The "typical " myelodysplastic patient shows an areflexic bladder with an open bladder neck.

67. Which is not true about tethered cord syndrome?

(a) TCS is defined as a stretch-induced functional disorder of the spinal cord with its caudal part anchored by inelastic structures
(b) There is no typical dysfunction in TCS
(c) If present dysfunction may appear till teenage
(d) Urgency (67%) and urge incontinence (50%) are the most common findings

(Answer is C) If present dysfunction may not be present until the teenage years.

68. "Classic" diabetic cystopathy may not include:

(a) Impaired bladder sensation
(b) Decreased cystometric capacity
(c) Decreased bladder contractility
(d) Impaired uroflow

(Answer is B) The typically described classic urodynamic findings include impaired bladder sensation, increased cystometric capacity, decreased bladder contractility, impaired uroflow, and, later, increased residual urine volume.

69. Which is not true about DESD?

(a) DESD, unless specified otherwise, refers to dyssynergia of the striated sphincter
(b) In type I, there are sporadic contractions of the striated sphincter throughout the detrusor contraction
(c) Without proper treatment, over 50% of men with DESD will develop significant complications
(d) Oral medical therapy directed toward the striated sphincter has not provided wide success

(Answer is B) In type 2, there are sporadic contractions of the striated sphincter throughout the detrusor contraction.

70. Hinman syndrome is also termed as all *except:*

(a) Neurogenic bladder
(b) Occult voiding dysfunction
(c) Occult neuropathic bladder
(d) Learned voiding dysfunction

(Answer is A) Non-neurogenic neurogenic bladder, occult voiding dysfunction, occult neuropathic bladder, learned voiding dysfunction.

71. The Fowler syndrome all are true *except:*

(a) Syndrome of urinary retention in young women in the absence of overt neurologic disease
(b) A bladder capacity of over 1 liter with no sensation of urgency is necessary for the diagnosis
(c) Efforts to treat this condition by neuro-modulation have been unsuccessful
(d) The urodynamic problem is detrusor acontractility

(Answer is C) Efforts to treat this condition by hormonal manipulation, pharmacologic therapy, or injections of botulinum toxin have been unsuccessful. This condition is highly responsive to neuromodulation (success rate approaching 70%) even in women who have been in retention for many months or years.

72. Which one of the following is not the symptom?

(a) Stress incontinence
(b) Urge incontinence
(c) Mixed incontinence
(d) Overflow incontinence

(Answer is D) Overflow incontinence is not a symptom or condition but rather a term used to describe leakage of urine associated with urinary retention.

73. The micturition reflex is organized in the:

(a) Midbrain (b) Pons
(c) Medulla (d) Cerebellum

(Answer is B) The micturition reflex is normally under voluntary control and is organized in the rostral brainstem (the pontine micturition center).

74. During micturition the first recorded event is:

(a) Rise in abdominal pressure
(b) Complete electrical silence of the sphincter electromyogram
(c) Rise in detrusor pressure
(d) Fall in urethral pressure as the bladder and proximal urethra

(Answer is B) The first recorded event is sudden and complete relaxation of the striated sphincteric muscles, characterized by complete electrical silence of the sphincter electromyogram.

75. Midurethral complex is formed by:

(a) Arcus tendineus fascia pelvis
(b) Endopelvic fascia (abdominal side) and the pubocervical fascia (vaginal side)
(c) Pubocervical fascia and pubourethral ligaments
(d) Pubourethral ligament and pubourethralis muscle

(Answer is D) Anterior support of the urethra is provided by the pubourethral ligaments, attaching the midurethra to the inferior aspect of the pubic bone. These work in conjunction with the pubourethralis muscle of the levator ani complex, which forms a sling around the proximal urethra and prevents rotational descent. Together, the two structures form the midurethral complex.

76. Which statement regarding proximal urethral sphincter (PUS) is not correct?

(a) The PUS consists of the bladder neck and prostate
(b) PUS is innervated by autonomic parasympathetic fibers from the pelvic nerve
(c) PUS portion of the continence mechanism is removed during prostatectomy, leaving only the DUS to prevent urinary leakage
(d) The male PUS complex is composed of the prostatomembranous urethra, cylindrical rhabdosphincter

(Answer is D) The male DUS compfex is composed of the prostatomembranous urethra, cylindrical rhabdosphincter (external sphincter muscle) surrounding the prostatomembranous urethra, and extrinsic paraurethral musculature and connective tissue structures of the pelvis.

77. In which type of OAB the patient is aware of involuntary detrusor contraction and can voluntarily contract the sphincter and momentarily prevent incontinence, but the patient is unable to abort the detrusor contraction and when the sphincter fatigues, incontinence ensues?

(a) Type 1 (b) Type 2
(c) Type 3 (d) Type 4

(Answer is C) Type 3, there are involuntary detrusor contractions, the patient is aware of them and can voluntarily contract the sphincter and momentarily prevent incontinence, but the patient is unable to abort the detrusor contraction and when the sphincter fatigues, incontinence ensues.

78. Causes of low bladder compliance includes all *except:*

(a) Tuberculous cystitis
(b) Cerebral palsy
(c) Radical hysterectomy
(d) Chronic indwelling catheter

(Answer is B) Causes of low bladder compliance:

- Neurogenic.
- Myelodysplasia.
- Shy-Drager syndrome.
- Suprasacral spinal cord injury/lesion.
- Radical hysterectomy.
- Abdominoperineal resection.
- Non-neurogenic (Increased Collagen).
- Tuberculous cystitis.
- Radiation cystitis.
- Chronic indwelling catheter.
- Bladder outlet obstruction.

79. Which statement regarding bulbocavernosus reflex is not true?

(a) It can be checked by suddenly squeezing the glans penis or clitoris
(b) Reflex may be initiated by suddenly pulling the balloon of the Foley catheter against the bladder neck
(c) The absence of this reflex in men is almost always associated with a neurologic lesion
(d) The absence of this reflex in women is almost always associated with a neurologic lesion

(Answer is D) The absence of this reflex in men is almost always associated with a neurologic lesion, but the reflex is not detectable in up to 30% of otherwise normal women.

80. Precise diagnosis of urinary incontinence is made by:

(a) CMG study
(b) Pad test
(c) Q tip test
(d) Direct observation by examiner

(Answer is D) Sine qua non for a precise diagnosis is that the urinary in continence is actually witnessed by the examiner.

81. Hypermobility is defined as a resting or straining angle greater than:

(a) 30 degrees (b) 60 degrees
(c) 90 degrees (d) 20 degrees

(Answer is A) Hypermobility is defined as a resting or straining angle greater than 30 degrees from the horizontal.

82. According to AHCPR guidelines, how much of PVR signlfies adequate bladder emptying and inadequate emptying respectively?

(a) 0 ml and 100 ml (b) 20 ml and 120 ml
(c) 50 ml and 150 ml (d) 50 ml and 200 ml

(Answer is D) The Agency for Health Care Policy and Research (AHCPR) guidelines state that, in general, a PVR less than 50 ml is adequate bladder emptying and a PVR more than 200 ml is inadequate emptying.

83. Which statement regarding ALPP is not correct?

(a) It is a measure of sphincter strength (its ability to resist changes in abdominal pressure)
(b) Defined as the intravesical pressure at which urine leakage occurs because of increased abdominal pressure in the absence of a detrusor contraction
(c) Higher the ALPP, the weaker the sphincter
(d) There is no normal ALPP

(Answer is C) Conceptually, the lower the ALPP, the weaker the sphincter. There is no normal ALPP.

84. Which statement regarding DLPP is not correct?

(a) Defined as the lowest detrusor pressure at which urine leakage occurs because of increased abdominal pressure in the absence of a detrusor contraction

(b) The higher the DLPP, the higher the urethral resistance

(c) The higher the DLPP, the more likely is upper tract damage as intravesical pressure is transferred to the kidneys

(d) From a clinical perspective DLPP is most useful in patients with lower motor neuron disease affecting the bladder and in non-neurogenic patients with low bladder compliance

(Answer is A) Detrusor leak point pressure (DLPP), which is a measure of detrusor pressure in patients with decreased bladder compliance. It is defined as the lowest detrusor pressure at which urine leakage occurs in the absence of either a detrusor contraction or increased abdominal pressure.

85. Functional urethral length and MUCP in continent women is:

(a) 2 cm and 20 to 40 cm of H_2O
(b) 3 cm and 20 to 40 cm of H_2O
(c) 2 cm and 40 to 60 cm of H_2O
(d) 3 cm and 40 to 60 cm of H_2O

(Answer is D) In most continent women, the functional urethral length is approximately 3 cm and the MUCP is 40 to 60 cm H_2O.

86. Most precise diagnostic tool for evaluating disturbances of micturition:

(a) Pressure flow study
(b) Cystometrogram
(c) Uroflowmetry
(d) Videourodynamics

(Answer is D) VUDS is the most precise diagnostic tool for evaluating disturbances of micturition.

87. Receptor believed to be the most important for detrusor contraction:

(a) M1 (b) M2
(c) M3 (d) M5

(Answer is C) In human as well as in animal detrusor, the M3 receptors are believed to be the most important for contraction.

88. Antimuscarinic with grade A recommendation for OAB are all *except:*

(a) Darifenacin (b) Oxybutynin
(c) Trospium (d) Propantheline

(Answer is D)

Antimuscarinic drug	*Grade of recommendation[*]*
Darifenacin	A
Oxybutynin[†]	A
Propiverine[†]	A
Tolterodine	A
Trospium	A
Solifenacin	A
Propantheline	B
Hyoscyamine	C

89. Which statement regarding use of botolinum toxin in OAB is true?

(a) BTX-B is the most commonly used botox for OAB

(b) 1 million units of BTX injected at 20 to 30 different sites

(c) A favorable response to BTX-A occurs in about 30 days

(d) A favorable response should last for 2 to 3 years

(Answer is C) A favorable response to BTX-A occurs in about 7 days, although it can take up to 30 days to see a maximal response. A favorable response should last for 6 to 9 months.

90. Which statement regarding sacral nerve stimulation (SNS) is not correct?

(a) SNS has established itself as a second-line treatment for incontinence secondary to the overactive detrusor

(b) Based on the induction of somatic afferent inhibition of sensory processing in the spinal cord

(c) Technically, the treatment is done in two steps. Stage I is a "screening test"

(d) In Stage II permanent neurostimulator is implanted next to the dorsal root of L3

(Answer is D) Stage I is a "screening test" in which a stimulation lead (temporary or permanent) is placed next to the dorsal root of S3 and stimulated for a period of days (temporary) to weeks (permanent). If the patient has a positive response (usually defined as greater than 50% improvement in symptoms), the patient may go on to stage 2, in which a permanent neurostimulator or "pacemaker" is implanted in the soft tissue of the buttock after connection to the S3 lead.

91. Which symptom is not included in OAB?

(a) Frequency (b) Urgency

(c) Nocturia (d) Dysuria

(Answer is D) The overactive bladder (OAB) is defined as urgency, with or without urge incontinence, usually with frequency and nocturia.

92. Which statement is not true regarding OAB?

(a) Urgency is usually described as being felt lower down than the sensations of bladder filling

(b) In men urge is felt in the perineum/base of penis and in women in the vagina/urethra

(c) In OAB sensation builds to discomfort and then to pain and is felt suprapubically

(d) Urgency tends to come on quickly and resolve quickly

(Answer is C) It is in PBS that sensation build to discomfort and then to pain and is felt suprapubically even if the patient also has perineal (urethral/vaginal/penile) discomfort/pain and not in OAB.

93. Which symptom is rare in PBS?

(a) Incontinence (b) Voluntary leakage

(c) Pain (d) Urgency

(Answer is A) Incontinence in PBS is rare, but voluntary (deliberate) leakage can occur because of great pain, whereas in OAB incontinence follows urgency and is involuntary, and much more common, with a prevalence of 30% to 50% in OAB sufferers.

94. Which statement is not true regarding terminal detrusor overactivity?

(a) Terminal detrusor overactivity is defined as a single involuntary detrusor contraction occurring at cystometric capacity

(b) It cannot be suppressed, and causes incontinence, which often results in complete bladder emptying

(c) It is most characteristically seen in the elderly person with "precipitant voiding"

(d) Such patients have a negative ice water test

(Answer is D) Terminal detrusor overactivity is defined as a single involuntary detrusor contraction occurring at cystometric capacity, which cannot be suppressed, and causes incontinence, which often results in complete bladder emptying (voiding). Such patients have a positive ice water test.

95. All are true regarding tertiary anticholinergic compounds *except:*

(a) Higher lipophilicity

(b) More molecular charge

(c) They are generally well absorbed from the gastrointestinal tract

(d) Theoretically be able to pass into the central nervous system

(Answer is B) Tertiary compounds generally have higher lipophilicity and less molecular charge than quaternary agents.

96. Which statement is not true regarding tolterodine?

(a) Tolterodine is a tertiary amine, rapidly absorbed and extensively metabolized by the cytochrome P-450 system

(b) The plasma half-life of both tolterodine and its metabolite is 24 hours

(c) Tolterodine has no selectivity for muscarinic receptor subtypes
(d) It has functional selectivity for the bladder over the salivary glands

(Answer is B) The plasma half-life of both tolterodine and its metabolite is only 2 to 3 hours.

97. All *except* one are the trials done for overactive bladder:

(a) ACET (b) OPERA
(c) OBJECT (d) IMAGE

(Answer is D) Comparative RCTs, such as the OBJECT (Overactive Bladder: Judging Effective Control and Treatment) and the OPERA (Overactive Bladder: Performance of Extended Release Agents) studies, have further supported effectiveness of anticholinergics. In the ACET (Antimuscarinic Clinical Effectiveness Trial) study, patients with OAB were randomized to 8 weeks of open-label treatment with either 2 mg or 4 mg of once-daily tolterodine ER and in the other trial to 5 mg or 10 mg of oxybutynin ER.

98. Which statement is not true regarding darifenacin?

(a) It is a tertiary amine
(b) Extensively metabolized in the liver by the cytochrome P-450 isoforms
(c) The most common adverse events were mild to moderate dry mouth and constipation
(d) Relatively selective muscarinic M2 receptor antagonist

(Answer is D) Darifenacin is a tertiary amine. Darifenacin is a relatively selective muscarinic M3 receptor antagonist.

99. Which drug may be active during the filling phase of the bladder, abolishing DO with no effect on normal bladder contraction?

(a) Tolterodine (b) Trospium
(c) Cromakalim (d) Nimodipine

(Answer is C) Potassium channel openers drugs may be active during the filling phase of the bladder, abolishing DO with no effect on normal bladder contraction.

100. Among following which one is quaternary ammonium compound?

(a) Trospium (b) Tolterodine
(c) Darifenacin (d) Solfenacin

(Answer is A) Trospium chloride is a quaternary ammonium compound.

101. Which one is not the pharmacological effect of oxybutynin?

(a) Antimuscarinic
(b) Direct muscle relaxant
(c) Local anesthetic
(d) Ca^{2+} channels blocker

(Answer is D) Oxybutynin has several pharmacologic effects, some of which seem difficult to relate to its effectiveness in the treatment of DO. It has both an antimuscarinic and a direct muscle relaxant effect and, in addition, local anesthetic actions.

102. All *except* one is the major pharmacologic actions of tricyclic antidepressants:

(a) They have central and peripheral antimuscarinic effects
(b) Block the active transport system in the presynaptic nerve ending that is responsible for the reuptake of the released amine neurotransmitters norepinephrine and serotonin
(c) Antihistaminic properties
(d) Local anaesthetic properties

(Answer is D) Tricyclic antidepressants possess varying degrees of at least three major pharmacologic actions: (1) they have central and peripheral antimuscarinic effects at some but not all sites; (2) they block the active transport system in the presynaptic nerve ending that is responsible for the reuptake of the released amine neurotransmitters norepinephrine and serotonin; and (3) they are sedatives, an action that occurs presumably on a central basis but is perhaps related to antihistaminic properties.

103. Regarding response rate of BTX-A which statement is true?

(a) Occur in week and last for 3 to 6 months
(b) Occur in month and last for 3 to 6 months
(c) Occur in 1 week and last for 6 to 9 months
(d) Occur in 1 month and last for 6 to 9 months

(Answer is C) A good response· rate of BTX-A appears to occur within 1 week and to last from 6 to 9 months before reinjection is necessary.

104. Which statement regarding resiniferatoxin is not true?

(a) RTX is an analog of capsaicin
(b) The rationale for intravesical instillations ofvanilloids is based on the involvement of C fibers
(c) RTX is approximately 1000 times more potent for excitation than capsaicin
(d) C fibers are not implicated in the normal voiding reflex

(Answer is C) Resiniferatoxin (RTX) is an analog of capsaicin, approximately 1000 times more potent for desensitization than capsaicin but only a few hundred times more potent for excitation.

105. Which drug has level A recommendation for stress incontinence?

(a) Duloxetine (b) Imipramine
(c) Methoxamine (d) Midodrine

(Answer is A)

	Level of evidence	*Forde of recommendation*
Duloxetine	1	A
Imipramine	3	D
Methoxamine	2	D
Midodrine	2	C

106. Which statement regarding duloxetine is not true?

(a) Duloxetine hydrochloride, a combifled norepinephrine and acetylcholine reuptake inhibitor
(b) The sphincteric effects were reversed by α1-adrenergic and 5-HT2 serotonergic antagonism
(c) Nausea the most common reason for discontinuation
(d) Duloxetine 40 mg twice daily improved incontinence and quality of life

(Answer is A) Duloxetine hydrochloride, a combined norepinephrine and serotonin reuptake inhibitor.

107. Which statement regarding desmopressin is not true?

(a) Bioavailability is low (less than 1% compared with 2% to 10% after intranasal administration
(b) Synthetic vasopressin analog has a pronounced antidiuretic effect with vasopressor actions
(c) Positive effects of desmopressín on nocturia in adults also have been documented
(d) There is a risk of water retention and hyponatremia

(Answer is B) Synthetic vasopressin analog has a pronounced antidiuretic effect but practically lacking vasopressor actions.

108. To facilitate bladder emptying which group constitute the most reasonable group for a trial of bethanechol:

(a) Incomplete lower motoneuron lesions
(b) Complete lower motoneuron lesions
(c) Incomplete upper motoneuron lesions
(d) Complete upper motoneuron lesions

(Answer is A) Patients with incomplete lower motoneuron lesions constitute the most reasonable group for a trial of bethanechol.

109. Prostaglandins and thromboxane A_2 is present in human bladder in which of the following quantitative order?

(a) $PGE_1 > PGE_2 > PGF_{2\alpha} >$ thromboxane A_2
(b) $PGE_1 > PGE_1 > PGF_{2\alpha} >$ thromboxane A_2
(c) $PGE_1 > PGE_2 >$ thromboxane $A_2 > PGF_{2\alpha}$
(d) $PGE_2 > PGF_1 >$ thromboxane $A_2 > PGF_{2\alpha}$

(Answer is B) Prostaglandins and thromboxane A_2 is shown to be present in human bladder in the following quantitative order: $PGE_2 > PGE_1 > PGF_{2\alpha}$ > thromboxane A_2.

110. Which statement regarding receptors is not correct?

(a) The smooth muscle of the bladder base and proximal urethra contains predominantly α adrenoceptors
(b) The bladder body contains both varieties of adrenergic receptors, with β3 subtype being more common
(c) The human lower urinary tract contains more α_1 than α_2 adrenoceptors
(d) Prostatic smooth muscle contraction and human lower urinary tract smooth muscle contraction are mediated largely, if not exclusively, by α1 adrenoceptors.

(Answer is C) The human lower urinary tract contains more α_2 than α_1 adrenoceptors, but prostatic smooth muscle contraction and human lower urinary tract smooth muscle contraction are mediated largely, if not exclusively, by α1 adrenoceptors.

111. Which statement is not correct?

(a) Phenoxybenzamine has blocking properties at both α_1 and α_2 adrenoceptor sites
(b) Terazosin and doxazosin are two highly selective postsynaptic α_1 adrenoceptor antagonists
(c) Dantrolene (Dantrium) exerts its effects by a direct peripheral action on skeletal muscle
(d) The $GABA_B$ receptor is activated by baclofen

(Answer is D) The $GABA_B$ receptor is activated by baclofen

112. Which statement regarding pessary is not correct?

(a) Pessaries used for prolapse only should be fitted with an empty bladder for patient comfort
(b) Pessaries intended for use in SUI should be fitted with the bladder at a comfortable fullness
(c) If OAB or other LUTS resolve with the pessary, the patient may elect to use the device either temporarily until a convenient time for surgery
(d) If symptoms do not resolve after appropriate support with a pessary the patient can be considered for successful repair of the anatomic defect

(Answer is D) If symptoms do not resolve after appropriate support with a pessary the patient should be counseled that they are more likely to persist even after successful repair of the anatomic defect.

113. Botox-A injections are currently FDA approved for:

(a) Urgency incontinence
(b) Urge frequency syndrome
(c) Idiopathic urinary retention
(d) None of the above

(Answer is D) Neuromodulation is FDA approved for urgency incontinence, urge frequency syndrome, and idiopathic urinary retention. Botox-A injections are not currently FDA approved for any application in the urinary tract.

114. For women with SUI which statement is not true?

(a) PFMT and vaginal cones have similar effect
(b) PFMT is inferior to electrical stimulation
(c) PFMT is less effective than surgery
(d) PFMT and adrenergic agonists have similar effect

(Answer is B) For women with SUI:

- PFMT and vaginal cones have similar effect.
- PFMT is superior to electrical stimulation.
- PFMT is less effective than surgery.
- PFMT and adrenergic agonists have similar effect.

115. For women with incontinence which statement is not correct?

(a) For women with all types of incontinence-PFMT and bladder training have similar effect

(b) For women with SUI with UUI-PFMT and a adrenergic agonists have similar effect

(c) For women with detrusor overactivity with or without SUI-PFMT is superior to oxybutynin

(d) For women with SUI without UUI-PFMT is superior to α adrenergic agonists

(Answer is D) For women with SUI with or without UUI-PFMT and adrenergic agonists have similar effect.

116. For optimal bladder emptying to be achieved, sacral anterior root stimulation with posterior rhizotomies is required for:

(a) Sl, S2 and S3 (b) S2, S3 and S4

(c) S3, S4 and S5 (d) L5, S1 and S2

(Answer is B) Data showed that for optimal bladder emptying to be achieved, sacral anterior root stimulation with posterior rhizotomies of S2, S3 and S4 would be required.

117. Which motor or sensory response is not correct in relation to S2?

(a) Plantar flexion of the entire foot with lateral rotation

(b) Clamp movement of the anal sphincter

(c) Sensations in the leg and buttock

(d) Bellows reflex

(Answer is D)

Sacral Nerve	*Motor and Sensory Response*
S2	Motor: Plantar flexion of the entire foot with lateral rotation and clamp movement of the anal sphincter Sensory: Sensations in the leg and buttock
S3	Motor: Dorsiflexion of the great toe and a bellows reflex (anal wink) Sensory: Paresthesias or sensation of pulling in the rectum, scrotum or vagina
S4	Motor: Bellows reflex only.

118. For erectile stimulation electrode are placed at:

(a) Primarily by S3 and to a smaller extent by S2 or S4

(b) Primarily by S2 and to a smaller extent by S3 or S4

(c) All three roots equally

(d) Chiefly by S2 with a small contribution from S3

(Answer is D) The detrusor is usually innervated primarily by S3 and to a smaller extent by S2 or S4. Rectal stimulation is by means of all three roots equally. Erectile stimulation is chiefly by S2 with a small contribution from S3 and none from S4.

119. Which statement is not true regarding retropubic suspension procedure?

(a) A retropubic approach for the correction of anatomic SUI is indicated for a patient undergoing a laparotomy for concomitant abdominal surgery that cannot be performed vaginally

(b) When SUI exists solely due to intrinsic sphincter deficiency, a retropubic suspension procedure has good results

(c) With short-term follow-up, vaginal and open retropubic suspension procedures have similar success rates in the treatment of stress incontinence

(d) With longer follow-up, patients who have retropubic procedures fare better

(Answer is B) When SUI exists solely due to intrinsic sphincter deficiency, a retropubic suspension procedure is not indicated.

120. Which is not correctly paired?

(a) MMK procedure–chromic catgut
(b) Burch procedure–polydioxanone
(c) VOS procedure–polyglycolic acid
(d) Paravaginal repair–silicon-coated Dacron

(Answer is B) Absorbable sutures were used in the original descriptions of the MMK procedure (chromic catgut), Burch procedure (chromic catgut), and VOS procedure (polyglycolic acid or polydioxanone), whereas the original paravaginal repair used nonabsorbable sutures (silicon-coated Dacron).

121. Which is considered to be standard open retropubic colposuspension procedure?

(a) Burch
(b) MMK
(c) Paravaginal repair
(d) Vaginal obturator shelf repair

(Answer is A) Trials comparing the Burch colposuspension and the MMK procedure, Burch technique results in higher cure rates. Thus, it should be regarded as the standard open retropubic colposuspension procedure.

122. Which is the most effective procedure for incontinence?

(a) Retropubic suspension
(b) Needle suspension
(c) Anterior colporrhaphies
(d) Posterior colporrhaphies

(Answer is A) Retropubic suspensions to be more effective than either needle suspensions or anterior colporrhaphies.

123. Which type of incontinence predominates in young and older women respectively?

(a) Stress and urge incontinence
(b) Stress incontinence in both age groups
(c) Urge and stress incontinence
(d) Urge incontinence in both age groups

(Answer is A) Stress incontinence predominates in young and middle aged women, whereas mixed and urge incontinence predominate in older women.

124. Which is not the risk factor for pelvic organ prolapse?

(a) Menopause (b) Pregnancy
(c) Obesity (d) Constipation

(Answer is A) Menopause has not been found to be a risk factor for pelvic organ prolapse.

125. Which muscle can be palpated during physical examination of the pelvis on the lateral side walls of vagina?

(a) Iliococcygeus (b) Pubococcygeus
(c) Ischiococcygeus (d) Coccygeus

(Answer is B) The pubococcygeus can be palpated during physical examination of the pelvis as a bulky muscular ridge on both right and left lateral side walls of the vagina, superior to the hymen.

126. Levator plate, the shelf on which the pelvic organs rest is formed by the fusion of:

(a) Iliococcygeus and the posterior fibers of the pubococcygeus muscles
(b) Iliococcygeus and the anterior fibers of the pubococcygeus muscles
(c) Ischiococcygeus and the posterior fibers of the pubococcygeus muscles
(d) Ischiococcygeus and the anterior fibers of the pubococcygeus muscles

(Answer is A) This median raphe between the anus and the coccyx is called the levator plate, the shelf on which the pelvic organs rest. It is formed by the fusion of the iliococcygeus and the posterior fibers of the pubococcygeus muscles.

127. Which one of the following is not the prolapse of middle compartment?

(a) Central cystocele
(b) Lateral cystocele
(c) Enterocele
(d) Rectocele

(Answer is D) Rectocele is prolapse of posterior vaginal wall.

128. After hysterectomy, the vaginal cuff will have dimples at the 3 and 9 O'clock areas, at the locations of:

(a) Iliococygeus
(b) Arcus tendineus fasciae pelvis
(c) Cardinal uterosacral ligament attachments
(d) Levator ani

(Answer is C) After hysterectomy, the vaginal cuff will have dimples at the 3 and 9 O'clock areas, at the l ocations of the cardinal uterosacral ligament attachments.

129. When most distal portion of the prolapse protrudes more than 1 cm below the hymen but protrudes no farther than 2 cm less than the total vaginal length is staged as:

(a) Stage I (b) Stage II
(c) Stage III (d) Stage IV

(Answer is C)

Stage III–The most distal portion of the prolapse protruoes more than 1 cm below the hymen but protrudes no farther than 2 cm less than the total vaginal length (i.e., not all of the vagina has prolapsed).

130. In POPQ system which is considered as reference point?

(a) Introitus (b) Symphysis pubis
(c) Midplane of vagina (d) Hymenal ring

(Answer is D) The pelvic organ prolapse quantification (POPQ) system uses the hymenal ring as the principal reference point.

131. Transvaginal suspensions to be a good option for all *except:*

(a) Those with urethral hypermobility
(b) Those with smaller volume incontinence
(c) Those with intrinsic urethral sphincter deficiency
(d) Those who are willing to accept worse long-term benefit in favor·of lower immediate morbidity

(Answer is C) Transvaginal suspensions is a good option for the appropriate women with stress incontinence, those with smaller volume incontinence, those with less intrinsic urethral sphincter deficiency, and those who are willing to accept worse long-term benefit in favor of lower immediate morbidity.

132. Surgical obliteration of cul-de-sac to treat or prevent enterocele is termed as:

(a) Colpocleisis (b) Colporrhaphy
(c) Culdoplasty (d) Colpopexy

(Answer is C) Culdoplasty-surgical obliteration of cul-de-sac to treat or prevent enterocele.

133. Principal risks of sacrospinous ligament fixation for vaginal apical repairs are all *except:*

(a) Postoperative anterior prolapse
(b) Injury to pudendal and inferior gluteal arteries
(c) Injury to pudendal and sciatic nerves
(d) Rectal and ureteral injury

(Answer is D)

Procedure	*Major risks*	*Major benefits*
Sacrospinous ligament	• Postoperative anterior prolapse • Injury to pudendal and inferior gluteal arteries and pudendal and sciatic nerves • Ligament may be atrophied in elderly • More difficult to teach and learn	• No ureteral injury; rectal injury rare

134. Use of autologous rectus fascia for sling has all the following disadvantage *except:*

(a) Increase urethral erosion
(b) Increase operative time
(c) Increase in postoperative pain
(d) Surapubic tissue seroma

(Answer is A) One advantage of this material is complete biocompatibility without tissue rejection. Urethral erosion of autologous rectus fascial slings is extremely rare. Disadvantages include increased operative time, relative increase in postoperative pain and suprapubic tissue seromas.

135. Autologous fascial sling is indicated in all *except:*

(a) Urethra that will be subjected to lifelong intermittent catheterization
(b) Proximal urethral incompetence
(c) Low-compliance bladder
(d) Patients with a low-pressure urethra

(Answer is C) A low-compliance bladder of any cause should be identified and treated before treatment of putative urethral dysfunction is undertaken.

136. All the following causes low compliant bladder *except:*

(a) Pelvic irradiation
(b) Pelvic trauma
(c) Pelvic extirpative study
(d) Chronic Foley catheter treatment

(Answer is B) Low-compliance bladder occurs after pelvic irradiation for malignant disease, in neurogenic conditions, after chronic Foley catheter treatment, and after bladder decentralization syndromes, for example, those occasionally associated with radical pelvic extirpative surgery.

137. Degree of urethral dysfunction leading to stress incontinence is measured by:

(a) DLPP
(b) VLPP
(c) Pressure flow study
(d) MCUP

(Answer is B) Measurement of the abdominal pressure required to produce leakage from an incompetent urethra (variously called the Valsalva, abdominal, or cough leak point pressure) has been used to characterize the degree of urethral dysfunction leading to stress incontinence.

138. Pubovaginal sling placement is done at:

(a) Bladder neck and proximal urethra
(b) Midurethra
(c) Distal urethra
(d) Can be placed at any level

(Answer is A) The sling should be located at the level of the bladder neck and proximal urethra, and both ends of the sling should be in the retropubic space.

139. All are properties of type 1 mesh *except:*

(a) Synthetic polypropylene monofilament mesh
(b) Pore size under 150 mm
(c) Material prevents optimal migration of host inflammatory components
(d) Optimal for inciting fibrous tissue in growth

(Answer is C) A synthetic polypropylene monofilament mesh with pore size under 150 mm. Also, this material allows optimal migration of host inflammatory components (leukocytes and macrophages) into the mesh for purposes of infectious surveillance and host wound healing (imbibition and inosculation).

140. During TVT which degree lens is used to exclude subtle tangential injury?

(a) 0 degree (b) 30 degree
(c) 70 degree (d) 120 degree

(Answer is C) Cystoscopy is performed to exclude needle penetration of the lower urinary tract. The use of a 70 degree lens is essential, as is complete distention of the bladder with irrigant to exclude subtle tangential injury.

141. Which statement is not true regarding TOT tape?

(a) Tape penetrate the adductor longus muscle
(b) In 70% of studied cases, the implanted material did traverse the adductor magnus, adductor brevis, and gracilis muscles during its path into the pelvis
(c) At the level of the obturator foramen, the tape was noted to traverse both the obturator externus and internus muscles as well as the obturator membrane
(d) The tape remained outside the pelvic space and did not penetrate the levator ani muscular group

(Answer is A) Tape never penetrate the adductor longus muscle, thus being a safe distance from neurovascular structures.

142. The ideal patient for the use of injectables has been:

(a) ISD
(b) Overactive bladder
(c) Poorly compliant bladder
(d) Poor anatomical support

(Answer is A) The ideal patient for the use of injectables has been described as one with poor urethral function (ISD), normal bladder capacity and compliance, and good anatomic support.

143. To be effective, injectable material must be injected at:

(a) Superior to external sphincter
(b) At external sphincter
(c) Inferior to external sphincter
(d) Bladder neck

(Answer is A) To be effective, injectable material must be injected in the urethra superior to the external sphincter.

144. At present the most widely used injectable agent is:

(a) GAX-collagen (b) PTFE
(c) Slicone polymers (d) Durasphere

(Answer is A) GAX-collagen does have the potential for eliciting an allergic reaction and, although it is more compatible than PTFE in biologic systems, it is considerably more expensive and requires more treatment sessions to attain continence. At present the most widely used injectable agent is GAX-collagen.

145. In injectable technique compare to transurethral approach which is not true regarding periurethral approach?

(a) Decreases bleeding complications
(b) Much longer learning curve
(c) Increase rate of urinary retention
(d) Volume of material injected was lower

(Answer is D) Each approach has similar success rates, but the rate of urinary retention and the volume of material injected was higher in the periurethral group.

146. Management in postprostatectomy urethra if material extravasation occurs in all quadrants during injection is:

(a) Reinjection can be done at the same time
(b) Reinjection can be done after 2 weeks
(c) Reinjection can be done after 4 weeks
(d) Reinjection should never be considered again

(Answer is C) In postprostatectomy urethra if material extravasation occurs in all quadrants during injection, the procedure should be terminated and rescheduled after 4 weeks.

147. Incidence of bladder rupture after therapeutic bladder overdistension is:

(a) 0 to 5% (b) 5% to 10%
(c) 10% to 15% (d) 15% to 20%

(Answer is B) Potential complications of bladder overdistention include bladder rupture (5% to 10%), hematuria and retention.

148. Procedures involving construction of a neourethra from the posterior surface of the bladder wall and trigone is:

(a) Young-Dees principle
(b) Tanagho procedure
(c) Pippe sale procedure
(d) Leadbetter politano procedure

(Answer is A) Procedures using the Young-Dees principle involve construction of a neourethra from the posterior surface of the bladder wall and trigone. In the male, the prostatic urethra affords additional substance for closure and increase in outlet resistance.

149. Which is not true regarding suprapubic urethral catheter?

(a) Does not obviate urethral leakage with detrusor contractions
(b) Does not provide better drainage
(c) Less leakage in patients with sphincteric incontinence
(d) Difficult to change this type of catheter without physician assistance

(Answer is C) Use of a suprapubic catheter does not, obviate urethral leakage with detrusor contractions, nor does it provide better drainage or less leakage in patients with sphincteric incontinence.

150. Which statement regarding external compression or Valsalva maneuver is not correct?

(a) Most effective in patients with decreased bladder tone who can generate an intravesical pressure greater than 50 cm H_2O
(b) Such "voiding'' is unphysiologic and is resisted by the same forces that normally resist stress incontinence
(c) Adaptive changes (funneling) of the bladder outlet occur
(d) Vesicoureteral reflux is a relative contra-indication to external compression or Val-salva maneuver

(Answer is C) Adaptive changes (funneling) of the bladder outlet generally do not occur with external compression maneuvers of any kind.

151. The most effective method of initiating a reflex contraction "trigger voiding" is:

(a) By pulling the skin or hair of the pubis, scrotum
(b) By squeezing the clitoris
(c) By digital rectal stimulation
(d) Rhythmic suprapubic manual pressure

(Answer is D) "Trigger voiding" is sometimes induced by pulling the skin or hair of the pubis, scrotum, or thigh; by squeezing the clitoris; or by digital rectal stimulation. According to the classic reference, the most effective method of initiating a reflex contraction is rhythmic suprapubic manual pressure.

152. For the management of DESD sphincterotomy is done at:

(a) 6 O'clock
(b) 5 and 7 O'clock
(c) 12 O'clock
(d) 3 and 9 O'clock

(Answer is C) The 12 O'clock sphincterotomy, remains the procedure of choice for a number of reasons. The anatomy of the striated sphincter is such that its main bulk is anteromedial. The blood supply is primarily lateral, and thus there is little chance of significant hemorrhage with a 12 O'clock incision.

153. Most reliable urodynamic parameter to predict the risk of upper tract complications after sphincterotomy:

(a) DLPP   (b) VLPP

(c) PVR (d) Qmax

(Answer is A) Detrusor leak point pressure as the most reliable urodynamic parameter to predict the risk of upper tract complications after sphincterotomy.

154. All *except* one decline with age in women:

(a) Urethral length
(b) Maximum closure pressure
(c) Striated muscle cells
(d) Bladder capacity

(Answer is D) Bladder capacity does not change with age, bladder sensation, contractility, and the ability to postpone voiding decline in both sexes, whereas urethral length and maximum closure pressure, as well as striated muscle cells in the rhabdosphincter, probably decline with age in women.

155. Most common form of lower urinary tract dysfunction in the elderly is:

(a) Detrusor underactivity
(b) Poor compliance
(c) Detrusor overactivity with preserved contraction
(d) Detrusor overactivity with impaired contraction

(Answer is D) Detrusor overactivity is the most common type of lower urinary tract dysfunction in incontinent elderly of either sex. Detrusor overactivity in the elderly exists as two physiologic subsets: one in which contractile function is preserved and one in which it is impaired.The latter condition is termed detrusor hyperactivity with impaired contractility (DHIC) and is likely the most common form of detrusor overactivity in the elderly.

156. All are principles of indwelling catheter care *except:*

(a) Empty the bag every 8 hours
(b) Do not routinely irrigate the catheter
(c) Avoid frequent cleaning of the urethral meatus
(d) Adding disinfectants to the catheter bag is effective

(Answer is D) Adding disinfectants to the catheter bag is ineffective.

157. In the developing world, VVF most commonly results from:

(a) Gynecologic, urologic, or other pelvic surgery
(b) Malignant disease
(c) Pelvic irradiation
(d) Obstetric trauma

(Answer is D) In the developing world, where routine perinatal obstetric care may be limited, VVF most commonly results from prolonged obstructed labor due to cephalopelvic disproportion, with resulting pressure necrosis to the anterior vaginal wall bladder, bladder neck, and proximal urethra from the baby.

158. Most common type of acquired fistula of the urinary tract:

(a) Vesicovaginal fistulas
(b) Ureterovaginal fistulas
(c) Colovesical fistula
(d) Vesicoureterine fistula

(Answer is A) Vesicovaginal fistulas represent, by far, the most common type of acquired fistula of the urinary tract.

159. Incidence of postsurgical VVFs associated with ureteral injury or ureterovaginal fistula is:

(a) 2% (b) 12%
(c) 22% (d) 32%

(Answer is B) Upto 12% of postsurgical VVFs have an associated ureteral injury or ureterovaginal fistula.

160. The median interval from completion of radiation therapy to presentation of VVF is:

(a) Immediately after radiation therapy
(b) 3 to 6 months
(c) 6 to 12 months

(d) 6 to 12 years

(Answer is C) The median interval from completion of radiation therapy to presentation of VVF is 8.7 months.

161. Radiation induced VVF should be repaired after:

(a) Immediately after radiation therapy
(b) 3 to 6 weeks
(c) 3 to 6 months
(d) 6 to 12 months

(Answer is D) 6 to 12 months, have been advocated for radiation-induced fistulas which are often associated with a severe obliterative endarteritis and reduced tissue vascularity.

162. Uncomplicated postgynecologic urinary tract fistulas may be repaired:

(a) As soon as they are identified
(b) 3 to 6 weeks
(c) 3 to 6 months
(d) 6 to 12 months

(Answer is A) Uncomplicated postgynecologic urinary tract fistulas may be repaired as soon as they are identified and confirmed, thereby minimizing the patient's discomfort and anguish.

163. The relative advantages of a transvaginal approach compared with an abdominal approach are all *except:*

(a) Shorter operative times
(b) Briefer hospital stay
(c) Less blood loss
(d) Lesser risk for vaginal shortening

(Answer is D) The principal disadvantages of the transvaginal approach include the relative lack of familiarity of the vaginal cuff anatomy to many urologists; the potential for vaginal shortening, especially with the Latzko approach; and the difficulty in exposing high or retracted fistulas near the vaginal cuff, especially in deep, narrow vaginas or those without any apical prolapse.

164. Which one of the following is not the transvaginal approach?

(a) Raz (b) Latzko
(c) Webster (d) O'Conor

(Answer is D) As classically described by O'Conor and colleagues, the bladder is approached extraperitoneally; however, in some cases, the peritoneum is entered.

165. Which statement is not true regarding martius flap?

(a) Blood supply is provided inferiorly with posterior labial vessels
(b) Blood supply is provided superiorly by external pudendal artery
(c) Blood supply is provided laterally by obturator artery
(d) Inferior blood supply is sacrificed during mobilization of the flap

(Answer is D) The blood supply to the flap is provided inferiorly by the posterior labial vessels (off the internal pudendal artery), superiorly by the external pudendal artery, and laterally by the obturator artery. The lateral blood supply is sacrificed during mobilization of the flap.

166. Which statement regarding ureterovaginal fistula is not correct?

(a) Most ureterovaginal fistulas occur during procedures for malignant as opposed to benign indications
(b) If ureteral patency is demonstrated, a trial of an indwelling ureteral stent may result in resolution of the fistula
(c) The most common presenting symptom is the onset of constant urinary incontinence 1 to 4 weeks after surgery
(d) Patients will continue to report normal voiding habits as bladder filling

(Answer is A) Most ureterovaginal fistulas occur during procedures for benign as opposed to malignant indications.

167. Youssef's syndrome describes the presenting symptom complex of all *except:*

(a) Menouria
(b) Cyclic hematuria with associated apparent menorrhagia
(c) Infertility
(d) Urinary continence in a patient who has undergone prior low-segment cesarean section

(Answer is B) Youssef's syndrome describes the presenting symptom complex of vesicouterine fistula: menouria, cyclic hematuria with associated apparent amenorrhea, infertility, and urinary continence in a patient who has undergone prior low-segment cesarean section.

168. Which statement is not true regarding urethrovaginal fistula?

(a) Distal urethrovaginal fistulas are often asymptomatic, whereas proximal fistulas may present with intermittent or constant urine leakage
(b) Urethrovaginal fistulas due to surgical trauma may be difficult to visualize on cystoscopy
(c) Diagnosis of a urethrovaginal fistula is best made with retrograde urethrography
(d) Repair of urethrovaginal fistula can be challenging and often involves an interpositional tissue flap because of the relative lack of surrounding connective tissue in the mid and distal urethra

(Answer is C) Diagnosis of a urethrovaginal fistula is best made with voiding cystourethrography.

169. Most common cause of colovesical fistula is:

(a) Colorectal carcinoma
(b) Diverticulitis
(c) Crohn's disease
(d) External penetrating trauma

(Answer is B) Vesicoenteric fistulas commonly occur in the setting of bowel disease, such as diverticulitis, colorectal carcinoma, and Crohn's disease. Less common causes include irradiation, infection, and trauma (external penetrating trauma as well as iatrogenic surgical trauma). Diverticulitis is the most common cause of colovesical fistula in most series, accounting for approximately 70% of cases.

170. Findings on CT that are suggestive of colovesical fistula consists of all *except:*

(a) Bladder wall thickening adjacent to a loop of thickened colon
(b) Air in the bladder
(c) Presence of colonic diverticula
(d) Clear fluid in bowel adjacent to bladder

(Answer is D) The triad of findings on CT that are suggestive of colovesical fistula consists of (1) bladder wall thickening adjacent to a loop of thickened colon, (2) air in the bladder (in the absence of previous lower urinary tract manipulation), and (3) presence of colonic diverticula.

171. Gouverneur's syndrome is best described as all *except:*

(a) Classic presentation of vesicoureterine fistula
(b) Suprapubic pain
(c) Frequency and dysuria
(d) Tenesmus

(Answer is A) The classic presentation of vesicoenteric fistula is described as Gouverneur's syndrome and consists of suprapubic pain, urinary frequency, dysuria and tenesmus.

172. The Bourne test, can be a useful adjunctive study in the evaluation of:

(a) Ureterovaginal fistula
(b) Vesicoureterine fistula
(c) Colovesical fistula
(d) Urovascular fistula

(Answer is C) The Bourne test, however, can be a useful adjunctive study in the evaluation of colovesical fistula. As described, the Bourne test is performed after a nondiagnostic barium enema study. The first voided urine after the barium enema is immediately centrifuged and then examined radiographically. Radiodense particles in the urine are considered a positive test result and evidence for a vesicoenteric fistula.

173. Among following most common cause of ureteroarterial fistula is:

(a) Ureteral stenting
(b) Radiation therapy
(c) Prior vascular surgery
(d) Vascular pathology

(Answer is A)

Ureteral stenting	65%
Radiation therapy	46%
Prior vascular surgery	19%
Vascular pathology	19%

174. Which statement regarding congenital diverticula is not true?

(a) Usually present during childhood
(b) Usually solitary and almost exclusively in boys
(c) Located lateral and posterior to the ureteral orifice
(d) Found in significantly trabeculated bladder

(Answer is D) Congenital diverticula usually present during childhood , with a peak incidence in those younger than 10 years. These are usually solitary, occur almost exclusively in boys, and are located lateral and posterior to the ureteral orifice. Typically, congenital bladder diverticula are found in smooth-walled bladders and are not associated with significant trabeculation on cystoscopic examination.

175. The most common histologic type of malignant neoplasia seen within bladder diverticula is:

(a) Squamous cell carcinoma
(b) Transitional cell carcinoma
(c) Adenocarcinoma
(d) Carcinosarcoma

(Answer is B) The most common histologic type of malignant neoplasia seen within bladder diverticula is transitional cell carcinoma in approximately 70% to 80% of cases, followed by squamous cell carcinoma in 20% to 25% of cases.

176. The ostium of the urethral diverticulum is most often located:

(a) Posterolaterally at the level of the mid-urethra
(b) Anterolaterally at the level of the midurethra
(c) Posterolaterally at the level of the proximal urethra
(d) Anterolaterally at the level of the proximal urethra

(Answer is A) The ostium of the urethral diverticulum is most often located posterolaterally at the level of the midurethra but can be difficult to identify in some patients.

177. The most common malignant pathologic process in urethral diverticula is:

(a) Adenocarcinoma
(b) Transitional cell carcinoma
(c) Squamous cell carcinoma
(d) Malignant melanoma

(Answer is A) The most common malignant pathologic process in urethral diverticula is adenocarcinoma, followed by transitional cell and squamous cell carcinomas.

178. AUS cuff in children and women is placed at:

(a) Bladder neck (b) Proximal urethra
(c) Mid urethra (d) Distal urethra

(Answer is A) As is the case with women, the AUS cuff in children is placed at the bladder neck and is typically 6 to 8 cm in circumference.

179. In men with post-prostatectomy incontinence, classic route of implantation of AUS is:

(a) Bladder neck
(b) Membranous urethra
(c) Bulbar urethra
(d) Pendulous urethra

(Answer is C) In men with post-prostatectomy incontinence, the bulbous urethra is the classic route of implantation through a perineal incision.

180. Which is not correct pair?

(a) MMK procedure–(chromic catgut)
(b) Burch procedure–(chromic catgut)
(c) VOS procedure–(chromic catgut)
(d) Paravaginal repair–(silicon-coated Dacron)

(Answer is C) Sutures used in:

- MMK procedure–(chromic catgut).
- Burch procedure–(chromic catgut).
- VOS procedure–(polyglycolic acid or polydioxanone).
- Paravaginal repair–(silicon-coated Dacron).

181. Which statement explains the first event in the micturition reflex?

(a) Opening of internal bladder sphincter
(b) Fall in urethral pressure
(c) Rise in intravesical pressure
(d) Cessation of sphincter EMG activity

(Answer is D) Cessation of sphincter EMG activity

182. Which statement regarding post-obstructive diuresis (POD) is false?

(a) Urine production exceeding 200 ml/hr for 2 consecutive hours or producing greater than 3L of urine in 24 hours is diagnostic of POD
(b) Pathologic POD can be exacerbated by excessive fluid replacement
(c) The replacement fluid choice is Ringer's lactate
(d) Fluid resuscitation depends on the degree of dehydration

(Answer is C) The replacement fluid choice is Ringer's lactate

183. Which of the following conditions could result in white urine?

(a) Chyluria (b) Bacteriuria
(c) Phosphaturia (d) All of the above

(Answer is D) All of the above

184. Which statement concerning urine pH is false?

(a) Influenced by food and medications
(b) Renal stones form at the extremes of pH range
(c) Reliable only when measured by 24 hours urine collection
(d) Ranges from 4 – 7

(Answer is C) Reliable only when measured by 24 hours urine collection

185. All of the following medications may alleviate symptoms of urge incontinence, *except:*

(a) Duloxetine (b) Mirabegron
(c) Fesoterodine (d) Estrogen

(Answer is A) Duloxetine

186. Procedures that treat urge urinary incontinence include all of the following, *except:*

(a) Sacral nerve modulation
(b) Injection of neurotoxins
(c) Bladder neck lifting
(d) Bladder augmentation

(Answer is C) Bladder neck lifting

187. What type of urinary incontinence is characterized by involuntary leakage typically while exertion, sneezing or coughing; accompanied by urgency?

(a) Functional (b) Urge
(c) Stress (d) Mixed

(Answer is D) Mixed

188. What is false concerning stress incontinence pathophysiology?

(a) Physiologically, during sneezing, the intra-abdominal pressure increases over the bladder and the abdominal part of the urethra; ending in no leakage
(b) While leaking bladder pressure exceeds the urethral resistance
(c) During episodes of stress incontinence, leakage ceases when bladder pressure falls below urethral pressure
(d) The major cause of stress incontinence is intrinsic sphincter deficiency

(Answer is D) The major cause of stress incontinence is intrinsic sphincter deficiency

189. Repeated vaginal deliveries could result in stress incontinence due to:

(a) Connective tissue injuries
(b) Pelvic and/or pudendal nerves denervation
(c) Levator ani muscle tears
(d) Any of the above

(Answer is D) Any of the above

190. Which of the following is false concerning total urinary incontinence?

(a) Any significant breech in the storage capabilities of the bladder or urethra could end in total incontinence
(b) Urinary fistula and ectopic ureters are common examples
(c) Commonly results from mechanical or neurological injuries to both internal and external urinary sphincters
(d) Continuous leakage of urine, not uncommonly, presents with skin infections, frustrations and impaired life quality

(Answer is C) Commonly results from mechanical or neurological injuries to both internal and external urinary sphincters

191. What is the most common cause of intrinsic sphincter deficiency in men?

(a) Radical prostatectomy or TURP
(b) Pelvic trauma or neurologic dysfunction
(c) Idiopathic or as an aging process
(d) Pelvic fractures following high-impact deceleration injuries

(Answer is A) Radical prostatectomy or TURP

192. How common is urinary incontinence among elderly in long-term care facilities?

(a) Uncommon
(b) Not uncommon
(c) Common
(d) Exceedingly common

(Answer is C) Common

193. What is false concerning overflow incontinence?

(a) Symptoms are similar to those of mixed urinary incontinence
(b) May present with hydroureteronephrosis and renal failure
(c) Typical examples are bladder outlet obstruction and automatic bladder
(d) Urine leaks out when the intravesical pressure exceeds the resting urethral closure pressure

(Answer is C) Typical examples are bladder outlet obstruction and automatic bladder

194. Fluoroscopy and video urodynamic are valuable tools in the evaluation of:

(a) Ureterovesical and vesicovaginal fistula
(b) Complex stress incontinence cases
(c) Neurogenic non-neurogenic dysfunctional voiding in children
(d) Is the preferred method to diagnose detrusor-sphincter dyssynergia

(Answer is B) Complex stress incontinence cases

195. A 25 years man on treatment for chronic prostatitis, complains of post-micturition dribbling. What is the likelihood that diagnostic cystoscopy yields additional significant findings?

(a) Never (b) Unlikely
(c) Likely (d) Always

(Answer is B) Unlikely

196. What is false concerning neuromodulation?

(a) Has been used to treat fecal incontinence
(b) The primary innervation of the bladder is S_3
(c) To function, it requires effective communications between sacral outflow and the pontine micturition centre
(d) It suppresses neurons that cause inhibition at spinal the level

(Answer is D) It suppresses neurons that cause inhibition at spinal the level

197. Direct electrical stimulation to the bladder results in:

(a) Pain in the abdomen, pelvis, perineum and legs
(b) Defecation, erection and ejaculation
(c) Parasympathetic stimulation results in emptying of the bladder
(d) All of the above

(Answer is D) All of the above

198. Bladder hyperactivity accompanies genuine stress urinary incontinence in:

(a) 10% of cases (b) 20% of cases
(c) 30% of cases (d) 40% of cases

(Answer is C) 30% of cases

199. A 34 years multipara having stress urinary incontinence. What does not align with the diagnosis of intrinsic sphincter deficiency is:

(a) The advice to undergo retropubic colposuspension
(b) Leak point pressure < 60 cm H_2O
(c) Maximum urethral closure pressure < 20 cm H_2O
(d) The advice to take duloxetine 20 mg bid

(Answer is A) The advice to undergo retropubic colposuspension

200. In women, transobturator tape procedure is particularly helpful in treating urinary incontinence that results of:

(a) Urethral hypermobility
(b) Intrinsic sphincter deficiency
(c) Detrusor overactivity
(d) Genital prolapse

(Answer is A) Urethral hypermobility

201. Which urodynamic equation is true?

(a) The maximal urethral closure pressure is the maximum urethral pressure minus intravesical pressure
(b) The detrusor pressure is the intravesical pressure minus intra-abdominal pressure
(c) In children, bladder capacity in cm^3 is determined by adding the value 2 to the patient's age, and then multiplying the sum by 30
(d) All of the above

(Answer is D) All of the above

202. What is the likelihood that a woman with stress urinary incontinence status post sling excision gets incontinence again?

(a) Never (b) Unlikely
(c) Likely (d) Always

(Answer is C) Likely

203. In women with stress urinary incontinence, injectable agents are particularly helpful in treating cases that result of:

(a) Urethral hypermobility
(b) Intrinsic sphincter deficiency
(c) Detrusor over activity
(d) Genital prolapse

(Answer is B) Intrinsic sphincter deficiency

204. What is false concerning injecting bulking agents to treat stress incontinence due to IS:

(a) The material should be biocompatible and adhesive to host tissue

(b) Transurethral route of injection is far superior to paraurethral route

(c) The agent is allowed to cause little inflammatory reaction

(d) Microcrystalline particle's size should be > 100 μm to prevent migration

(Answer is B) Transurethral route of injection is far superior to paraurethral route

205. What is false concerning botulinum toxin A injections to treat detrusor over activity?

(a) It blocks neuromuscular transmission by inhibiting the release of acetylcholine

(b) The recommended dose of on a botulinum-toxin A is 200 U per treatment

(c) If symptoms recur, injection is indicated but no sooner than 2 weeks

(d) Injections should be to a depth of about 2 nun, distributed all around the bladder excluding the trigone

(Answer is C) If symptoms recur, injection is indicated but no sooner than 2 weeks

CHAPTER 15

Bladder, Lower Genitourinary Calculi and Trauma

1. **Most common nonepithelial benign tumor of the bladder:**
   (a) Leiomyoma
   (b) Leukoplakia
   (c) Papilloma
   (d) Nephrogenic adenoma

(Answer is A) Leiomyoma is the most common nonepithelial benign tumor of the bladder.

2. **Which of the following statement regarding bladder tumor is not correct?**
   (a) More common in males
   (b) Bladder cancer has almost never been reported as an incidental finding at autopsy
   (c) Mortality increases with age
   (d) Survival rate is better in females

(Answer is D) Males have higher 5-year survival rates than women.

3. **Which statement regarding bladder tumor in younger patients is not true?**
   (a) Younger patients appear to have a more favorable prognosis
   (b) Younger patients present more frequently with superficial, low-grade tumors
   (c) Risk for disease progression is the same, grade-for-grade, in younger patients as in older ones
   (d) Molecular and genetic aberrations in younger patients share close correlation with histologic grade and clinical behavior

(Answer is D) Molecular and genetic aberrations in bladder tumors in this population do not share the fairly close correlation with histologic grade and clinical behavior.

4. **Which statement regarding TP53 is not true?**
   (a) The TP53 gene is the most frequently altered gene in human cancers
   (b) Bladder cancers with TP53 abnormalities appear to have more aggressive behaviors
   (c) Wild-type TP53 induces the expression of a potent inhibitor of angiogenesis, TSP-1 whereas mutant TP53 does not
   (d) Impaired TP53 function, contributes to a more aggressive phenotype and may enhance resistance to some chemotherapeutic agents

(Answer is D) Impaired TP53 function, although contributing to a more aggressive phenotype, may paradoxically enhance sensitivity to some chemotherapeutic agents.

5. **Which statement regarding genetics of bladder tumor is not correct?**
   (a) 9q losses is associated with development of low grade superficial tumor
   (b) High grade cancers are associated with p53 and chromosome 17 deletions
   (c) Precise molecular analysis has been far from complete for chromosome 13 because most often entire chromosome is missing
   (d) Abnormal expression of RB occur primarily in aggressive TCCs

(Answer is C) Precise molecular analyses have been far more difficult for chromosome 9 than for 13q (RB) or 17p (TP53), because most often an entire chromosome is "missing".

6. **Gene most closely associated with bladder cancer is:**

(a) TP 53 (b) RAS
(c) ERBB2 (d) RB

(Answer is B) The one most closely associated with bladder cancer is RAS, a membrane-bound, mitogenic, signal transduction molecule.

7. **Not true regarding smoking and urinary bladder carcinoma is:**

(a) Higher number of p53 mutation occurs in smokers
(b) Risk correlates with number of cigarettes and duration of smoking
(c) Reduction of risk down to baseline occurs 10 years after cessation of smoking
(d) Cigarette smokers have up to a fourfold higher incidence of bladder cancer than do people who have never smoked

(Answer is C) The reduction of this risk down to baseline (age adjusted) takes nearly 20 years after cessation, a period far longer than that for the reduction of risk of cardiovascular disease and lung cancer after smoking has stopped.

8. **Predisposing factors for squamous cell carcinoma are all *except:***

(a) Chronic indwelling catheter
(b) Calculi
(c) S. haematobium
(d) Analgesic abuse

(Answer is D) Consumption of large quantities (5 to 15 kg over a 10-year period) of analgesic combinations containing phenacetin (which has a chemical structure similar to that of aniline dyes) is associated with an increased risk for TCC of the renal pelvis and bladder.

9. **Which statement regarding risk factors for bladder cancer is not true?**

(a) Between 2% and 10% of paraplegics with long-term indwelling catheters develop bladder cancer
(b) Women treated with radiation for carcinoma of the uterine cervix or ovary have a two-fold to four-fold increased risk
(c) Patients treated with cyclophosphamide have up to a twenty-fold increased risk
(d) Renal transplant recipient has increased risk

(Answer is C) Patients treated with cyclophosphamide have up to a nine-fold increased risk.

10. **Which disease is believed to be a response of the normal urothelium to noxious stimuli and is considered a premalignant lesion that may progress to SCC?**

(a) Nephrogenic adenoma
(b) Vesical leukoplakia
(c) Pseudosarcoma
(d) Inverted papilloma

(Answer is B) Vesical leukoplakia is believed to be a response of the normal urothelium to noxious stimuli and is generally considered a premalignant lesion that may progress to SCC in up to 20% of patients.

11. **Islands of benign-appearing urothelium situated in the lamina propria termed as:**

(a) Urothelial metaplasia
(b) Von Brunn's nest
(c) Cystitis cystica
(d) Cystitis glandularis

(Answer is B) Von Brunn's nests are islands of benign-appearing urothelium situated in the lamina propria.

12. **Carcinoma *in situ* all are true *except:***

(a) Endoscopically invisible
(b) Poorly differentiated TCC confined to urothelium
(c) May be asymptomatic
(d) Urine cytopathology is positive in only 60%-80% of cases

(Answer is D) Urine cytopathology is positive in 80% to 90% of patients with carcinoma *in situ.*

13. Which of the following is graded as low grade urothelial carcinoma by WHO and ISUP classification?

(a) Grade 0 (b) Grade 1
(c) Grade 2 (d) Grade 3

(Answer is C) WHO and ISUP classification

Grade 1	–	PUNLMP
Grade 2	–	Low Grade
Grade 3	–	High Grade

14. All are true regarding S. hematobium causing squamous cell carcinoma *except:*

(a) Patient is 10-20 years younger than TCC
(b) Cancers are exophytic, nodular, fungating lesions that are wholly well differentiated
(c) Liver is the most common site of metastasis
(d) Low incidence of lymph node and distant metastasis

(Answer is C) With bilharzial SCCs, bone is the most common site of distant metastases.

15. Which is not true regarding urachal carcinoma?

(a) Extremely rare tumor that arises outside bladder
(b) It is usually adenocarcinoma
(c) They have very poor prognosis
(d) Partial cystectomy has excellent results

(Answer is D) Histologically, these tumors exhibit wider and deeper infiltration of the bladder wall than expected, compromising the results of partial cystectomy.

16. Expression of which molecule decreases chances of malignancy?

(a) E-cadherin
(b) Matrix metalloproteinase
(c) Urokinase
(d) Tissue-plasminogen activator

(Answer is A) Reduced expressions of E-cadherin and a, b and/or g catenins have been found in invasive tumors and have been associated with decreased survival of bladder cancer patients.

17. Which is the most common pattern of local spread in bladder tumor?

(a) En block (b) Tentacle
(c) Lateral (d) Circumferential

(Answer is A) The most common is en bloc spread, which occurs in about 60% of tumors and is characterized by cancer cells invading in a broad front directly beneath the primary mucosal lesion.

18. Most common group of lymph node involved in bladder cancer is:

(a) Paravesical (b) Obturator
(c) External illiac (d) Internal illiac

(Answer is B) Paravesical nodes are involved in 16%, the obturator nodes in 74%, the external iliac nodes in 65%, and the presacral nodes in roughly 25%. Juxtaregional common iliac lymph nodes are involved in about 20% of patients.

19. Which statement regarding the natural history of bladder cancer is not correct?

(a) Forty to 45 percent of newly diagnosed bladder cancers are high-grade lesions
(b) Almost 25% of patients with newly diagnosed bladder cancer have muscle-invasive disease
(c) Almost 10% of patients with muscle-invasive bladder cancer already have occult distant metastases
(d) Ten to 20 percent of patients with superficial papillary tumors subsequently develop invasive or metastatic cancer

(Answer is C) Almost 50% of patients with muscle-invasive bladder cancer already have occult distant metastases.

20. Which statement regarding the grading of bladder cancer is not correct?

(a) Patients with high-grade superficial tumors have high likelihoods of recurrence and far higher chances of developing invasive and metastatic disease than do those with low-grade superficial tumors
(b) Some patients with low-grade tumors eventually develop higher-grade recurrences
(c) Completely resected high-grade cancers frequently recur as low-grade ones
(d) It is not common to have low-grade and high-grade lesions simultaneously in the same patient's bladder

(Answer is D) It is not uncommon to have low-grade and high-grade lesions simultaneously in the same patient's bladder.

21. Primary genetic abnormality in low grade bladder cancer is associated with:

(a) Long arm of chromosome 9
(b) Short arm of chromosome 9
(c) Long arm of chromosome 13
(d) Short arm of chromosome 13

(Answer is A) High-grade cancer with abnormalities in TP53 and possibly P21, P27, RB and P16 contributing to aggressive behavior and low-grade cancer with deletions of yet unidentified genes on the long arm of chromosome 9 being the primary genetic abnormality.

22. Which statement regarding fibronectin is not correct?

(a) It appears primarily in the basement membrane and submucosa and is absent from the luminal surface of urothelial cells
(b) Soluble fibronectin can inhibit BCG's adherence to the vesical wall
(c) Urinary fibronectin excretion are much higher in deeply invading malignancies
(d) Patients receiving BCG therapy who had higher urinary fibronectin levels before TUR had higher likelihood of being tumor free than did those with low fibronectin excretion

(Answer is D) Patients receiving BCG therapy who had lower urinary fibronectin levels before the initiation of treatment (but after TUR) had a much higher likelihood of being tumor free at 1 year than did those with elevated fibronectin excretion.

23. Marker of apoptosis:

(a) Survivin
(b) Ki67
(c) E cadherin
(d) Capsaces

(Answer is A) Survivin, an inhibitor for apoptosis, is upregulated in many cancers, including urothelial cancer. Detection of survivin in urine has had promising results as a diagnostic marker.

24. True regarding hematuria of carcinoma of urinary bladder is:

(a) Associated with painful voiding
(b) Nearly all patients with cystoscopically detectable bladder cancer have microhematuria
(c) It occurs continuously
(d) Second most common presentation is painless hematuria

(Answer is B) In reality, nearly all patients with cystoscopically detectable bladder cancer have at least microhematuria if enough urine samples are tested.

25. Which statement regarding urine cytology is not correct?

(a) The limitations of microscopic cytology are due to the cytologically normal appearance of cells from well-differentiated tumors
(b) Poorly-differentiated cancer cells are more cohesive, and are not readily shed into urine
(c) Even in patients with high-grade tumors, urinary cytology may be falsely negative in 20%
(d) False-positive cytology may occur in 1% to 12% of patients

(Answer is B) The limitations of microscopic cytology are due to the cytologically normal appearance of cells from well-differentiated tumors and because well-differentiated cancer cells are more cohesive, they are not readily shed into the urine.

26. Which technique has highest sensitivity in distinguishing muscle-invasive from superficial bladder cancer?

(a) Transurethral USG (b) CECT KUB
(c) MRI (d) PET

(Answer is A) Transurethral ultrasonic assessment using 5.5 MHz probes with 60-degree, 90-degree, and 120-degree transducers before and at the end of TUR was helpful in further distinguishing infiltration of superficial versus deep muscle and extravesical spread. One hundred percent sensitivity and more than 98% specificity in distinguishing muscle-invasive from superficial bladder cancers.

27. Which is not true regarding resection of bladder tumor?

(a) Resect first bulk of tumor, then deep portion then underlying bladder muscle
(b) Tumor near ureteric orifice should be resected without regard of ureteric orifice
(c) Tumor on lateral wall induces obturator nerve stimulation
(d) Tumor arising in bladder diverticula should be resected

(Answer is D) Tumors arising in bladder diverticula often should be sampled rather than resected.

28. Boundaries of staging lymphadenectomy is all *except:*

(a) Superiorly-Iliac bifurcation
(b) Inferiorly-Femoral canals
(c) Medially-Bladder pedicles
(d) Laterally-Obturator nerve

(Answer is D) The standard staging lymphadenectomy for bladder cancer includes removal of the nodes from slightly above the iliac bifurcations to the femoral canals and from the genitofemoral nerves to the bladder pedicles.

29. Recommended metastatic evaluation for invasive bladder cancer includes all *except:*

(a) IVU
(b) Abdomen and pelvic CT
(c) Chest CT
(d) LFT

(Answer is C) Recommended metastatic evaluation for patients with invasive bladder cancer includes a chest radiograph, abdominal-pelvic CT, bone scan and liver function tests.

30. In bladder cancer macroscopic extension of perivesical fat is staged as:

(a) T2a (b) T2b
(c) T3a (d) T3b

(Answer is D) T3b Macroscopic extension into perivesical fat.

31. Sixty-year-old man presenting as painless hematuria was diagnosed as a case of urinary bladder malignancy. CT suggested only microscopic involvement of perivesical fat. It also showed two lymph nodes each of 1.5 cm Bone scan and CXR did not suggest any metastasis. TNM staging for this patient will be:

(a) T2a N 2 MO (b) T3a N1MO
(c) T2a N1MO (d) T3a N2MO

(Answer is D)

T3a Microscopic extension into perivesical fat.

N1 Single positive node ≤2 cm in diameter, below common iliacs.

N2 Single positive node 2-5 cm in diameter or multiple positive nodes.

32. Which is the most common malignant mesenchymal tumor that arises in the bladder of adults?

(a) Leimyosarcoma (b) Liposarcoma
(c) Rhabdomyosarcoma (d) Angiosarcoma

(Answer is A) Leiomyosarcoma is the most common malignant mesenchymal tumor that arises in the bladder of adults.

33. Which statement regarding bladder pheochromocytomas is not correct?

(a) Bladder pheochromocytomas account for less than 1% of all bladder tumors and less than 1% of all pheochromocytomas
(b) TUR is generally contraindicated
(c) About 10% of pheochromocytomas are malignant
(d) Hematuria develops in 85% to 100% of patients

(Answer is D) Hematuria develops in only about half of patients.

34. The term superficial bladder cancer is applied till what stage?

(a) T cis (b) Ta
(c) T1 (d) T2a

(Answer is C) Traditionally known as superficial bladder cancer, malignant urothelial tumors that have not invaded the detrusor are more appropriately termed non-muscle-invasive tumors.

35. Which statement regarding bladder tumor is not correct?

(a) Approximately 70% of bladder tumors are non-muscle invasive at presentation
(b) Low-grade Ta lesions recur at a rate of 50% to 70% and progress in approximately 5% of cases
(c) High-grade T1 lesions recur in more than 80% of cases and progress in 50% of patients within 3 years
(d) Between 20% and 40% of patients with CIS will develop muscle invasion if untreated, especially if associated with papillary tumors

(Answer is D) Between 40% and 83% of patients with CIS will develop muscle invasion if untreated, especially if associated with papillary tumors.

36. Most important risk factor for progression is:

(a) Stage (b) Grade
(c) Multiplicity (d) Size

(Answer is B) Most important risk factor for progression is grade, not stage.

37. Role of repeat TURBT are all *except:*

(a) Residual tumor is identified at the site of the initial resection at least 40% of the time
(b) Repeat TUR can demonstrate worse prognostic findings in up to 25% of specimens
(c) The efficacy of BCG in preventing progression appears to be higher in patients with high-grade papillary tumors and CIS if a restaging TURBT was performed before instillation of BCG
(d) Consensus is that all patients with pTa and pT1 tumors merit repeat resection

(Answer is D) Consensus is that patients with pT1 and only high-grade Ta tumors merit repeat resection.

38. Which statement regarding perioperative intravesical therapy to prevent tumor implantation is not true?

(a) MMC appears to be the most effective adjuvant intravesical chemotherapeutic agent perioperatively
(b) A single dose administered within 6 hours lessens recurrence rates
(c) Dose administered after 24 hours later does not lessens recurrence rates
(d) Maintenance therapy reduces the risk further

(Answer is D) Maintenance therapy does not reduce the risk further.

39. All can decrease incidence of obturator reflex in TURBT *except:*

(a) TURIS minimize the risk of the obturator reflex
(b) Use of regional anesthesia prevents obturator reflex

(c) Direct injection of 20 to 30 ml of local anesthetic into the obturator nerve
(d) Laser therapy

(Answer is B) Use of general anesthesia with muscle-paralyzing agents prevents obturator reflex.

40. Which one of the following laser is not used in treatment of bladder carcinoma?

(a) Nd:YAG (b) Holmium:YAG
(c) KTP (d) CO_2

(Answer is D) The carbon dioxide laser is completely absorbed by fluid so is not appropriate for use in the treatment of bladder cancer.

41. Which one is true regarding laser treatment of bladder carcinoma?

(a) Increase bleeding
(b) Increase elicitation of obturator reflex
(c) Increase recurrence at site of treatment
(d) Increase perforation of hollow, viscus organ

(Answer is D) The most significant complication of laser therapy is forward scatter of laser energy to adjacent structures, resulting in perforation of a hollow, viscous organ such as overlying bowel.

42. Which statement regarding BCG therapy for bladder cancer is not true?

(a) BCG is an attenuated mycobacterium developed as a vaccine for tuberculosis
(b) The original regimen described by Morales included as intravesical dose
(c) The vaccine is reconstituted with 50 ml of saline and should be administered through a urethral catheter under gravity drainage soon thereafter
(d) After instillation, the patient should retain the solution for 2 hours

(Answer is B) The original regimen described by Morales and colleagues included a percutaneous dose.

43. 68 years old healthy man was diagnosed as a case of urinary bladder malignancy with stage T1. He underwent two courses of BCG. On follow up, he was found to have high grade T1 lesion at the site of treatment. Best management will be:

(a) Repeat BCG with interferon
(b) Immediate cystectomy
(c) External beam radiation therapy
(d) Nd:YAG laser therapy

(Answer is B) Additional courses of BCG to treat refractory patients after a second 6-week course are accompanied by a significant risk of tumor progression in 20% to 50% of patients. For persistent high-grade papillary disease after two courses of intravesical therapy, cystectomy is the standard of care and should not be considered "early".

44. Not true regarding BCG administration in carcinoma urinary bladder patient is:

(a) In CIS the initial tumor-free response rate is as high as 80%
(b) BCG reduces the risk of progression by 25%
(c) BCG can effectively treat residual papillary lesions with up to 60% response rate
(d) The average additional response to a second induction course is 10-15% in those patients treated for prophylaxis

(Answer is D) The average additional response to a second induction course is 25% in those patients treated for prophylaxis.

45. Treatment of serious complication related to BCG is all *except:*

(a) Isoniazid, 300 mg/day
(b) Rifampin, 600 mg/day
(c) Ethambutol, 15 mg/kg/day
(d) Pyrazinamide, 25 mg/kg/day

(Answer is D) BCG is almost uniformly resistant to pyrazinamide, so this drug has no role.

46. Absolute contraindication to BCG therapy includes all *except:*

(a) Immunosuppressed and immunocompromised patients
(b) Traumatic catheterization
(c) Total incontinence
(d) Urinary tract infection

(Answer is D) Urinary tract infection is a relative contraindication to BCG therapy.

47. Which drug is not used peri-operatively?

(a) Epirubicin (b) Thiotapa
(c) Interferon (d) Gemcitabine

(Answer is C) Interferon and BCG is not for peri-operative use.

48. Which drug has been approved by the FDA for treatment of BCG refractory CIS in patients who cannot tolerate cystectomy?

(a) Epirubicin (b) Valrubicin
(c) Interferon (d) Gemcitabine

(Answer is B) Valrubicin is a semisynthetic analog of doxorubicin that has been approved by the FDA for treatment of BCG refractory CIS in patients who cannot tolerate cystectomy.

49. Recurrence or persistence of disease of lesser degree, stage, or grade after an initial course, which then resolves with further BCG is termed as:

(a) BCG failure (b) BCG refractory
(c) BCG resistant (d) BCG relapse

(Answer is C) Persistent disease after BCG therapy can be categorized as BCG-refractory (non-improving or worsening disease despite BCG), BCG-resistant (recurrence or persistence of lesser degree, stage, or grade after an initial course, which then resolves with further BCG), or BCG-relapsing (recurrence after initial resolution with BCG).

50. Which marker will detect chromosomal changes before the development of phenotypic expression of malignancy, so leads to an "anticipatory positive" reading?

(a) BTA TRAK
(b) Immunocyte
(c) UroVision
(d) NMP22 BladderChek Test

(Answer is C) UroVision was the only marker whose specificity approaches that of cytology. It will, however; detect chromosomal changes before the development of phenotypic expression of malignancy, so leads to an "anticipatory positive" reading in some patients.

51. Recommendation for cystoscopic surveillance in high grade superficial bladder malignancy is:

(a) Monthly for first 3 months, three monthly for next 6 months and then six monthly
(b) Three monthly for first 6 months, six monthly for next 1 year and then annually
(c) Three monthly for first 1 year, six monthly for next 1 year and then annually
(d) Three monthly for first 2 years, six monthly for next 2 years and then annually

(Answer is D) High grade–Every 3 months for 2 years then semiannual for 2 years and then annually for lifetime.

52. Which statement regarding bladder malignancy is not true?

(a) For patients in whom an invasive lesion is suspected, axial staging should be accomplished before biopsy
(b) Presence of a palpable mass after TUR correlates significantly with stage T3 cancer and prognosis after treatment
(c) With PET scan success in identifying malignant lymphadenopathy has been lesser than that in staging primary bladder lesions

(d) Preoperative bone scan is not necessary for patients with clinically organ confined, muscle-invasive bladder carcinoma

(Answer is C) Success in identifying malignant lymphadenopathy has been greater than that in staging primary bladder lesions because concentration of the fluorodeoxyglucose tracer in urine obscures detail adjacent to the bladder lumen.

53. Which statement regarding pelvic lymphadenectomy is not true?

(a) Pelvic lymphadenectomy provides insight into the local extent of disease
(b) In extended pelvic lymphadenectomy percentage of patients with node-positive disease increases
(c) An extended lymph node dissection should include the distal para-aortic and paracaval lymph nodes as well as the presacral nodes
(d) Among patients with lymph node-positive disease, the total number of lymph nodes removed at the time of surgery has been shown to be of prognostic value

(Answer is B) An extended pelvic lymph node dissection may yield a greater number of positive and total number of lymph nodes compared with standard pelvic lymph node dissection. However, the percentage of patients with node-positive disease who are identified is similar between these two groups.

54. Regarding follow up after radical cystectomy which statement is not true?

(a) Annual screening with physical examination, serum chemistries, and chest radiograph for patients with pT1 disease
(b) Semiannual screening with physical examination, serum chemistries, and chest radiograph for patients with pT2 disease
(c) Quaterly screening with physical examination, serum chemistries, and chest radiograph for patients with pT3 disease
(d) Annual CT for pT2 a nd semiannual CT for pT3 is recommended

(Answer is D) Annual screening with physical examination, serum chemistries, and chest radiograph for patients with pT1 disease; semiannual evaluation for patients with pT2 disease; and quarterly evaluation for patients with pT3 disease. For the last group, semiannual CT scan was also recommended.

55. Which statement regarding adjunct to surgical therapy in radical cystectomy is not true?

(a) Data suggest that for patients with T3 disease, local control may be improved by preoperative radiotherapy
(b) Neoadjuvant cisplatin-based combination chemotherapy may offer a modest improvement in overall survival of 5% among patients with T3
(c) Difference in survival was identified when perioperative chemotherapy was used as compared to postoperative groups
(d) Adjuvant chemotherapy trials for bladder cancer suggested a 9% improvement in survival at 3 years for patients who received chemotherapy compared with controls

(Answer is C) No difference in survival was identified between the perioperative and postoperative groups.

56. Bladder preservation protocol can be applied in:

(a) Carcinoma *in situ*
(b) Mild HDN
(c) 4 cm tumor but completely resected with TUR
(d) Small multifocal tumor

(Answer is C) Structural and histologic features that argue against the use of bladder preservation are the presence of hydronephrosis; carcinoma *in situ,* which responds poorly to multimodality therapy; and a tumor that cannot be completely resected transurethrally.

57. Which statement is not true regarding systemic chemotherapy in management of urinary bladder malignancy?

(a) Metastatic bladder cancer is routinely treated with systemic chemotherapy
(b) Multi agent chemotherapy has greater activity than single agent
(c) Multi agent chemotherapy has greater toxicity than single agent
(d) Most common employed agent is bleomycin, etoposide and cisplatin (BEP)

(Answer is D) The combination of GC and MVAC is the most common regimen used.

58. Which statement is not true regarding systemic chemotherapy in management of urinary bladder malignancy?

(a) The combination of GC provided a survival advantage similar to that of MVAC
(b) The most significant toxic effects associated with GC combination chemotherapy are nausea, vomiting and mucositis
(c) Standard of care for patients with metastatic disease has shifted from MVAC to GC
(d) Toxoids are microtubule disassembly inhibitors

(Answer is B) The most significant toxic effects associated with GC combination chemotherapy are thrombocytopenia and neutropenia, which can occur in up to 50% of patients.

59. Which statement regarding TURBT is not correct?

(a) Water can be used as the bladder irrigant during the procedure
(b) If a lengthy resection is anticipated, glycine, sorbitol, or mannitol is used as irrigant
(c) If the bladder lesion is small, it may be amenable to cold-cup biopsy and fulguration
(d) Finer diameter loops project a more concentrated current and therefore produces better hemostasis

(Answer is D) Finer diameter loops project a more concentrated current and therefore cut more easily; the larger diameter loops produce better hemostasis.

60. Which statement regarding perforation during TURBT is not correct?

(a) Obturator nerve stimulation during resection of superior lateral tumor can increase the likelihood of perforation
(b) Small perforations are of no clinical significance and can be managed with catheter drainage
(c) Large extraperitoneal perforations often resolve with catheter drainage alone Intraperitoneal perforations may also do well with catheter drainage

(Answer is A) Obturator nerve stimulation during resection of an inferior lateral tumor can increase the likelihood of perforation.

61. TUR alone may be a reasonable option in all *except*:

(a) Small, solitary, stage T2 transitional cell carcinoma
(b) Well differentiated, sessile, stage T2 transitional cell carcinoma
(c) T3a lesions smaller than 2 cm in diameter at the tumor base
(d) Moderately differentiated T2 tumor

(Answer is B) There is probably a small subset of patients with stage T2 transitional cell carcinoma who may be candidates for resection therapy alone. These are likely to be patients with small, solitary, papillary, moderately differentiated, stage T2 or minimal stage T3a lesions smaller than 2 cm in diameter at the tumor base. Most important, the lesion must be completely resectable transurethrally.

62. For patients with single or multiple superficial Ta or T1 tumors, immediate intravesical mitomycin C has demonstrated reduction in tumor recurrences by:

(a) 10% (b) 25%
(c) 50% (d) 75%

(Answer is C) For patients with single or multiple superficial Ta or T1 tumors, immediate or early postoperative intravesical instillation of chemotherapy, such as mitomycin C (40 mg in 40 ml of normal saline for 1 hour), has demonstrated more than 50% reduction in tumor recurrences.

63. All are true regarding transverse incision *except:*

(a) More cosmetic
(b) Heal more securely
(c) Decrease inguinal hernia risk
(d) Difficult to perform in comparison with vertical incision

(Answer is C) Transverse incisions are more cosmetic and have been considered to heal more securely, but there may be an increased inguinal hernia risk with extended incisions. Vertical incisions may be midline or paramedian. Vertical midline incisions are easier to perform and can be extended superiorly.

64. About urethrectomy which is true?

(a) Surgery is done in exaggerated lithotomy position
(b) Urethrectomy should follow radical cystectomy by 2-3 weeks
(c) It is necessary to split glans to remove transitional cell epithelium till meatus
(d) Post operative drain is usually not required

(Answer is A) Surgery is done in exaggerated lithotomy position by raising the leg braces until the hips are flexed 60 degrees. As transitional epithelium does not typically extend to meatus, it is not necessary to perform dissetion. Urethrectomy is best done at time of radical cystectomy. A drain is placed in the bad of urethra.

65. Anterior exentration in females for urinary bladder malignancy includes all *except:*

(a) Cystectomy with uretherectomy
(b) Distal colectomy
(c) Bilateral pelvic lymphadenectomy
(d) Hysterectomy

(Answer is B) The anterior approach has advantages in that it allows simultaneous pelvic lymphadenectomy, cystectomy, urethrectomy, hysterectomy, salpingo-oophorectomy, and partial vaginectomy if clinically indicated for extensive carcinomatous involvement.

66. In females orthotopic neobladder has excellent continence rates with preservation of the distal urethra by:

(a) Removing only proximal 1 cm of urethra and ligating the pubourethral ligaments
(b) Removing proximal 2 cm of urethra and ligating pubourethral ligaments
(c) Removing proximal 1 cm of urethra and preserving the pubourethral ligaments
(d) Removing proximal 2 cm of urethra and preserving the pubourethral ligaments

(Answer is C) Orthotopic neobladder has excellent continence rates with preservation of the distal urethra, taking only the proximal 1 cm of urethra and preserving the pubourethral ligaments.

67. Indication of simple cystectomy includes all *except:*

(a) Radiation cystitis
(b) Cyclophosphamide cystitis
(c) Pyocystitis
(d) Tumor in bladder divetlicula

(Answer is D) Various benign conditions may warrant simple cystectomy, including pyocystis, neurogenic bladder, severe urinary incontinence, severe urethral trauma, large vesical fistula, cyclophosphamide cystitis, and radiation cystitis after treatment of other pelvic malignant neoplasms.

68. Which of the following is not a contraindication to partial cystectomy?

(a) Tumor located at trigone or bladder neck

(b) Multifocal tumors

(c) Tumor located at dome or posteriolateral wall of bladder

(d) Tumor requiring ureteric implantation

(Answer is C) An ideal patient for partial cystectomy is one who has a normally functioning bladder with good capacity, a first-time tumor recurrence with a solitary tumor, and a tumor location in an area that allows a 1 to 2 cm margin of resection, such as at the dome.

69. Which statement regarding boari flap is not correct?

(a) An anterolateral bladder flap based on the ipsilateral vesical pedicle is developed

(b) Flap somewhat longer and wider than anticipated should be developed

(c) Flap length-to-breadth ratio of 5:1 ensures good vascularity of its apex

(d) It is necessary to fix the bladder dome to the ipsilateral psoas muscle with absorbable 2-0 suture

(Answer is C) An anterolateral bladder flap based on the ipsilateral vesical pedicle is developed. A flap somewhat longer and wider than anticipated should be developed to ensure a tension-free anastomosis; flap length-to-breadth ratio of 3:1 ensures good vasculariy of its apex.

70. For laparoscopic bladder diverticulectomy:

(a) Bladder should be deflated and diverticular sac should be inflated with council catheter

(b) Bladder should be inflated and diverticular sac should be deflated with council catheter

(c) Both bladder and diverticula should be deflated

(d) Both bladder and diverticula should be inflated

(Answer is A) With the bladder deflated and the diverticulum sac distended by the council catheter, the peritoneum overlying the diverticulum is incised directly.

71. Regarding laparoscopic VVF repair which statement is not true?

(a) Adequate bladder drainage

(b) Wide excision of fibrous and scar tissue from the fistula edge

(c) Individual tension-free suture repair of the freshened fistula edges in the vagina and the bladder

(d) Interposition of a peritoneal or omental flap

(Answer is B) Circumferential excision of fibrous and scar tissue from the fistula edge is all that is necessary. Only the fibrotic VVF track and edges are excised; wide excision is unnecessary.

72. Which statement regarding partial cystectomy is not true?

(a) Less than 10% of patients in large series with bladder cancer are candidates for partial cystectomy

(b) In open partial cystectomy series, 5-year survival rates range from 50% to 70% in properly selected patients

(c) Contraindications to partial cystectomy include tumor involving the bladder neck

(d) Ongoing surveillance is not important once bladder margins are free from tumor

(Answer is D) Ongoing surveillance with cystoscopy and cytology is important because the local recurrence rate is high (40% to 78%).

73. All *except* one group of patients will require thorough evaluation for prostate and seminal vesicle-sparing laparoscopic radical cystectomy:

(a) Abnormal DRE findings

(b) PSA more than 3

(c) High percentage of free prostate-specific antigen (>12%)

(d) Hypoechoic nodule on transrectal ultrasonography

(Answer is C) Patients with abnormal findings on digital rectal examination, prostate-specific antigen concentration above 3 ng/ml, low percentage of free prostate-specific antigen (<12%), or hypoechoic nodule on transrectal ultrasonography must undergo thorough evaluation to exclude concomitant prostate cancer.

74. When stomach is used for bowel augmentation all are true *except:*

(a) The blood supply for stomach is based on either the left or right gastroepiploic artery
(b) It should not include a significant portion of the antrum
(c) Should never extend to the pylorus
(d) Lesser curve of the stomach is included

(Answer is D) When a wedge of fundus is employed, it should not include a significant portion of the antrum and should never extend to the pylorus or all the way to the lesser curve of the stomach.

75. Small bowel that may lie within the confines of the pelvis and as such may be exposed to pelvic irradiation and pelvic disease is:

(a) First 2 inches of the terminal ileum
(b) Last 2 inches of the terminal ileum
(c) 2 feet of small bowel beginning approximately 6 feet from the ligament of Treitz
(d) 5 feet of small bowel beginning approximately 6 feet from the iliocecal junction

(Answer is B) There are two portions of the small bowel that may lie within the confines of the pelvis and as such may be exposed to pelvic irradiation and pelvic disease: the last 2 inches of the terminal ileum, which is often fixed in the pelvis by ligamentous attachments; and 5 feet of small bowel beginning approximately 6 feet from the ligament of Treitz.

76. Sudeck's critical point is at:

(a) Between the junction of the sigmoid and superior hemorrhoidal arteries
(b) Midpoints between the middle colic and right colic arteries
(c) Between the middle colic and left colic arteries
(d) Between the left colic arteries and sigmoidal arteries

(Answer is A) Sudeck's critical point, which is located between the junction of the sigmoid and superior hemorrhoidal arteries.

77. The advantage of stomach over other intestinal segments for urinary intestinal diversion is all *except:*

(a) Thick seromuscular layer that can easily be separated from the mucosa should a submucosal ureteral reimplantation be necessary
(b) Patient with severe abdominal adhesions is that the area of the stomach is generally adhesion free and easily mobilized
(c) The incidence of bacteriuria has been reported to be as low as 25%
(d) It has a net absorption of chloride and protons rather than a net excretion

(Answer is D) The advantage of stomach over other intestinal segments for urinary intestinal diversion is that it is less permeable to urinary solutes, it has a net excretion of chloride and protons rather than a net absorption of them, and it produces less mucus.

78. Which statement regarding complication of ureteroileal anastomosis is not correct?

(a) Of the colonic antirefluxing procedures, the Pagano technique offers the lowest incidence of stricture
(b) With respect to small bowel antireflux procedures, the Le Due procedure seem to offer the lowest incidence of stricture
(c) With respect to stricture formation and leakage, Bricker technique has the best results

(d) The incidence of urinary intestinal leak is markedly reduced by the use of soft silastic stents

79. Which one of the following is not the ureterocolonic anastomosis?

(a) Leadbetter-Clark (b) Strickler
(c) Pagano (d) Le Duc

(Answer is D) Le Duc method establishes a nonrefluxing anastomosis by laying the ureter onto the interior of the bowel wall.

80. In which refluxing anastomosis end of the intestine is sutured to the end of the ureter?

(a) Wallace (b) Bricker
(c) Strickler (d) Pagano

(Answer is A) Frequently employed anastomotic technique is that of Wallace, in which the end of the intestine is sutured to the end of the ureter. This is a refluxing anastomosis.

81. The most common cause of death in patients who have had a ureterosigmoidostomy for more than 15 years is:

(a) Cirrhosis
(b) Electrolyte abnormalities
(c) Renal failure
(d) Malignancy

(Answer is C) The most common cause of death in patients who have had a ureterosigmoidostomy for more than 15 years is acquired renal disease (i.e., sepsis or renal failure).

82. All are suitable candidates for retentive diversion or for long segments of intestine *except:*

(a) Serum creatinine concentration exceeds 2.0 mg/dl
(b) Patient is able to achieve a urine pH of 5.8 or less after an ammonium chloride load
(c) Has a urine osmolality of 600 mOsm/kg or greater in response to water deprivation
(d) Has a GFR that exceeds 15 ml/min, and has minimal protein in the urine

(Answer is D) GFR that exceeds 35 ml/min, and has minimal protein in the urine, the patient may be considered for a retentive diversion.

83. Electrolyte disorders that occur when jejunum is used are:

(a) Hyponatremia, hypokalemia, hypochloremia and acidosis
(b) Hyponatremia, hyperkalemia, hypochloremia and acidosis
(c) Hyponatremia, hypokalemia, hyperchloremia and acidosis
(d) Hyponatremia, hypokalemia, hypochloremia and alkalosis

(Answer is B) Electrolyte disorders that occur when jejunum is used for urinary intestinal diversion, particularly when proximal jejunum is used, include hyponatremia, hypochloremia, hyperkalemia, azotemia and acidosis.

84. When stomach is used which electrolyte abnormality can occur?

(a) Hypochloremic, hypokalemic metabolic alkalosis
(b) Hypochloremic, hypokalemic metabolic acidosis
(c) Hyperchloremic, hypokalemic metabolic alkalosis
(d) Hypochloremic, hyperkalemic metabolic alkalosis

(Answer is A) When stomach is used, a hypochloremic, hypokalemic metabolic alkalosis may ensue.

85. Hypokalemia and total body depletion of potassium occurs most in:

(a) Ureterosigmoidostomies
(b) Illeal conduit
(c) Colon conduit
(d) Sigmoid conduit

(Answer is A) Hypokalemia and total body depletion of potassium may occur in patients with urinary intestinal diversion. This is more common in patients with ureterosigmoidostomies than it is in patients who have other types of urinary intestinal diversion.

86. Which statement regarding infections in urinary diversion is not true?

(a) Approximately three quarters of ileal conduit urine specimens are infected
(b) Deterioration of the upper tracts is more likely when the culture becomes dominant for Proteus or Pseudomonas
(c) Patients with relatively pure cultures of Proteus or Pseudomonas should be treated
(d) Asymptomatic mixed cultures generally require multiple antibiotics

(Answer is D) Mixed cultures may generally be observed, provided they are not symptomatic.

87. Majority of stones formed in patients with urinary intestinal diversions are composed:

(a) Uric acid
(b) Calcium, magnesium and ammonium phosphate
(c) Xanthine
(d) Cystine

(Answer is B) Great majority of stones formed in patients with urinary intestinal diversions are composed of calcium, magnesium and ammonium phosphate.

88. Which one of the following is the most technologically demanding of all the continence mechanisms, and it is associated with the highest complication and reoperation rates?

(a) Nipple valve
(b) Imbricated terminal ileum
(c) Appendiceal tunneling techniques
(d) T pouch

(Answer is A) The creation of nipple valves is by far the most technologically demanding of all the continence mechanisms, and it is associated with the highest complication and reoperation rates.

89. For appendiceal sphincters which is appropriate catheter?

(a) 14- to 16-Fr coudé tip catheter
(b) 18- to 20-Fr coudé tip catheter
(c) 14- to 16-Fr Foley tip catheter
(d) 18- to 20-Fr Foley tip catheter

(Answer is A) For appendiceal sphincters, a 14- to 16-Fr coudé tip catheter.

90. Which is the most reliable of all cathetrerizable reservoirs?

(a) Koch (b) Mainz
(c) Indiana (d) Penn

(Answer is C) The Indiana pouch remains one of the most reliable of all catheterizable reservoirs. It is among the easiest to construct, and it has very low short-term and long-term complications.

91. First continent diversion employing the Mitrofanoff principle:

(a) Koch (b) Mainz
(c) Indiana (d) Penn

(Answer is D) The Penn pouch was the first continent diversion employing the Mitrofanoff principle in which the appendix served as the continence mechanism.

92. A minimum creatinine clearance required before a continent form of urinary diversion is undertaken:

(a) 15 ml/min (b) 30 ml /min
(c) 45 ml/min (d) 60 ml/min

(Answer is D) A minimum creatinine clearance of 60 ml/min should be documented before a continent form of urinary diversion is undertaken.

93. Which form of neobladder may be more appropriate for patients with borderline renal function who otherwise would be candidates for lower urinary tract reconstruction?

(a) Stomach
(b) Jejunum
(c) Ileum
(d) Colon

(Answer is A) A gastric form of neobladder may be more appropriate for patients with borderline renal function who otherwise would be candidates for lower urinary tract reconstruction.

94. Rhabdosphincter is probably supplied primarily by the branches of:

(a) Cavernosal
(b) Crural
(c) Pudendal
(d) The autonomic innervation arising from the pelvic plexus

(Answer is C) Rhabdosphincter is probably supplied primarily by the branches of the pudendal nerve.

95. Which statement regarding orthotopic neobladders is not correct?

(a) The clinical goal of most orthotopic neobladders is to allow volitional voiding every 3 to 4 hours with a capacity range of 400 to 500 ml
(b) Nocturnal incontinence is observed in approximately 28% of patients undergoing orthotopic diversion
(c) Factors influencing continence rates include age, intestinal segment used, and possibly the application of a nerve-sparing technique
(d) Failure to empty or urinary retention has been reported to be more common in men

(Answer is D) Failure to empty or urinary retention has been reported in 4% to 25% of patients undergoing orthotopic reconstruction and is more common in women.

96. Which statement regarding urethral and pelvic recurrence in patients with bladder cancer after cystectomy is not true?

(a) The overall risk of a urethral recurrence of TCC after cystectomy is approximately 10% in men
(b) The two most important risk factors for a urethral tumor recurrence in men are invasive prostatic tumor involvement and the form of urinary diversion
(c) The two most important risk factors in women for urethral tumor recurrence are bladder neck involvement and anterior vaginal wall involvement with tumor
(d) A local pelvic recurrence rate of approximately 20% is seen in patients undergoing radical cystectomy for bladder cancer

(Answer is D) A local pelvic recurrence rate of approximately 10% is seen in patients undergoing radical cystectomy for bladder cancer and rarely interferes with the function of the neobladder.

97. Which statement regarding technique of making neobladder is not correct?

(a) In hautmann neobladder, segment of terminal ileum of approximately 70 cm is selected
(b) In studer neobladder, distal 40 cm segment of ileum is placed in a U shape and opened along the antimesenteric border
(c) In ghoneim pouch, 40 cm ileal segment is isolated from the distal ileum and arranged in a W configuration
(d) In Le Bag pouch, 40 cm segment of ascending colon and a corresponding length of terminal ileum is isolated

(Answer is D) The Le Bag ileocolonic bladder substitute was initially described by Light and Engelmann in 1986. A 20 cm segment of ascending colon and a corresponding length of terminal ileum are isolated, and bowel continuity is restored.

98. The tensile strength of the tunica albuginea is remarkable, resisting rupture until intracavernous pressures rise to more than:

(a) 500 mm of Hg

(b) 1000 mm of Hg

(c) 1500 mm of Hg

(d) 1800 mm of Hg

(Answer is C) The tensile strength of the tunica albuginea is remarkable, resisting rupture until intracavernous pressures rise to more than 1500 mm Hg.

99. Which statement regarding penile fracture is not correct?

(a) If Buck's fascia rupture, the penile hematoma results in a typical eggplant deformity

(b) The diagnosis of penile fracture is often straightforward and can be made reliably by history and physical examination alone

(c) MRI is a noninvasive and highly accurate in demonstrating disruption of the tunica albuginea

(d) Site of rupture is mostly distal to the suspensory ligament

(Answer is A) If Buck's fascia remains intact, the penile hematoma remains contained between the skin and tunica, resulting in a typical eggplant deformity.

100. Regarding penile revascularization which statement is not correct?

(a) Microscopic anastomosis of the dorsal artery with 11-0 nylon

(b) Microscopic dorsal vein repair with 9-0 nylon

(c) Microscopic epineural repair of dorsal nerve with 8-0 nylon

(d) Two-layer urethral closure over a catheter with 5-0 absorbable suture

(Answer is C) Microscopic epineural repair of dorsal nerve with 10-0 nylon.

101. Successful penile reimplantation is possible up to how many hours of cold ischemia and warm ischemia respectively?

(a) 16 and 6 (b) 12 and 4

(c) 8 and 3 (d) 20 and 8

(Answer is A) Successful reimplantation is possible after 16 hours of cold ischemia time or 6 hours of warm ischemia.

102. Which statement regarding testicular rupture is not correct?

(a) Degree of hematoma correlate with the severity of testis injury

(b) Absence of hematoma does not entirely rule out testis rupture

(c) Contusion without fracture can present with significant bleeding

(d) Ultrasound findings include heterogeneity of the testicular parenchymal texture

(Answer is A) Degree of hematoma does not correlate with the severity of testis injury; absence does not entirely rule out testis rupture, and contusion without fracture can present with significant bleeding. Ultrasound findings suggestive of testis fracture include inhomogeneity of the testicular parenchymal texture and disruption of the tunica albuginea.

103. Which type of skin graft is preferred for extensive penile reconstruction?

(a) Thick, meshed, split thickness

(b) Thin, meshed, full thickness

(c) Thin, nonmeshed, full thickness

(d) Thick, nonmeshed, split thickness

(Answer is D) Thick (0.010- to 0.015-inch), nonmeshed, split-thickness skin grafts are preferred for extensive penile reconstruction.

104. Relative indications for cystography after blunt trauma include all *except:*

(a) Pelvic fracture with gross hematuria

(b) Pelvic fracture with microhematuria

(c) Gross hematuria without pelvic fracture

(d) Isolated microscopic hematuria

(Answer is A) Relative indications for cystography after blunt trauma include gross hematuria without a pelvic fracture, microhematuria with pelvic fracture, and isolated microscopic hematuria. Conversely, penetrating injuries of the buttock, pelvis, or lower abdomen with any degree of hematuria warrant cystography.

105. Which statement is not true regarding cystography?

(a) Retrograde or stress cystography is nearly 100% accurate for bladder injury

(b) Dense, flame-shaped collection of contrast material in the pelvis is characteristic of extraperitoneal extravasation

(c) A three-film technique is recommended

(d) The amount of extravasation is proportional to the extent of bladder injury

(Answer is D) The amount of extravasation is not always proportional to the extent of bladder injury.

106. Which statement is not true regarding CT cystography?

(a) CT cystography is as accurate and reliable as plain film cystography to evaluate suspected bladder injury

(b) Drainage films are not required after CT cystography

(c) Dilution of the contrast material (2:1 with saline) is mandatory

(d) Clamping the urethral catheter to allow antegrade distention of the bladder is inadequate for diagnosis of bladder rupture

(Answer is C) Dilution of the contrast material (6:1 with saline) is mandatory.

107. Indication for immediate repair of bladder injury are all *except:*

(a) Intraperitoneal injury from external trauma

(b) Penetrating or iatrogenic non-urologic injury

(c) Inadequate bladder drainage or clots in urine

(d) Close pelvic fracture

(Answer is D) Indication of immediate repair of bladder injury:

- Intraperitoneal injury from external trauma.
- Penetrating or iatrogenic non-urologic injury.
- Inadequate bladder drainage or clots in urine.
- Open pelvic fracture.
- Pelvic fracture requiring OR +IF.
- Bladder neck/vaginal or rectal injury.

108. Bladder calculi due to urinary tract infection, most commonly involves:

(a) E coli (b) Proteus

(c) Pseudomonas (d) Enterococcus

(Answer is B) Between 22% and 34% of bladder calculi are associated with urinary tract infection, most commonly with proteus.

109. Which statement regarding bladder stone not correct?

(a) Most calculi that migrate out of the ureter into the bladder are smaller than 1 cm and, in adults, are easily passed per urethra

(b) Endemic bladder calculi are most commonly composed of ammonium acid urate alone or in combination with calcium oxalate

(c) Incomplete bladder emptying was identified as the greatest single factor in vesical stone formation

(d) Multiple stones are usually encountered in the bladder, but single stones are seen in 25% to 30% of cases

(Answer is D) Single stones are usually encountered in the bladder, but multiple stones are seen in 25% to 30% of cases.

110. Majority of calculi in augmentations and diversions are composed of:

(a) Cystine
(b) Magnesium ammonium phosphate
(c) Uric acid
(d) Oxalate

(Answer is B) The majority of calculi in augmentations and diversions are composed of magnesium ammonium phosphate or carbonate apatite, signifying that infection with urea-spitting bacteria plays a role in calculi formation.

111. Which group of patients has maximum risk for bladder stone?

(a) Patients with indwelling catheter
(b) Patients with intermittent catheterisation
(c) Patients with condom catheter
(d) Patients who are catheter free and had continent bladder control

(Answer is A) Patients managed with an indwelling urethral or suprapubic catheter had a nine-fold increased risk and those using intermittent catheterization or a condom catheter had a four-fold increased risk for development of a bladder stone compared with patients who were catheter free and had continent bladder control within the first year after injury.

112. Single most accurate examination to document bladder calculus is:

(a) USG
(b) CECT
(c) MCU
(d) Cystopan endoscopy (CPE)

(Answer is D) Cystoscopy is the single most accurate examination to document the presence of a bladder calculus.

113. Which one is not the contraindication for cystolitholapaxy?

(a) Large capacity bladder
(b) Bladder stones in children
(c) 3 cm calculi
(d) Hard stones

(Answer is A) Contraindications include small-capacity bladders, multiple stones or calculi larger than 2 cm that cannot be engaged, hard stones, bladder calculi in children, and small-caliber urethras.

114. Which statement regarding prostatic stones is not correct?

(a) Prostatic calculi are depositions of calcified material on corpora amylacea
(b) Prostatic calculi are primarily composed of calcium phosphate trihydrate and carbonate
(c) Cystoscopy will usually show stones protruding through the prostate
(d) No treatment is indicated for asymptomatic prostatic stones

(Answer is C) Cystoscopy is usually unremarkable.

115. To which group of lymph nodes do tumors at the anterior superior area of the bladder, first, drain?

(a) Hypogastric
(b) Internal iliac
(c) External iliac
(d) Lateral sacral

(Answer is C) External iliac

116. Adult size of bladder capacity is achieved at what age?

(a) 5 – 6 years
(b) 7 – 8 years
(c) 9 – 10 years
(d) 11 – 12 years

(Answer is C) 9 – 10 years

117. Which action of thigh muscles could be impaired if the obturator nerve was injured during endoscopic resection of bladder tumors?

(a) Adduction
(b) Abduction
(c) Flexion
(d) Extension

(Answer is A) Adduction

118. The manifestations of autonomic dysreflexia include:

(a) Hypotension and tachycardia

(b) Hypotension and bradycardia
(c) Hypertension and tachycardia
(d) Hypertension and bradycardia

(Answer is D) Hypertension and bradycardia

119. What could cause autonomic dysreflexia?

(a) Full bladder or rectum
(b) Tooth extraction
(c) Hypertension medications
(d) Uncontrolled diabetes mellitus

(Answer is A) Full bladder or rectum

120. What could render "red urine" workup, false positive for hematuria?

(a) Dehydration
(b) Myoglobinuria
(c) High doses of vitamin C
(d) All of the above

(Answer is D) All of the above

121. What do urine tests examine to detect hematuria?

(a) Catalase activity of erythrocytes
(b) Peroxidase activity of erythrocytes
(c) Lyase activity of erythrocytes
(d) None of the above

(Answer is B) Peroxidase activity of erythrocytes

122. Hematuria of glomerular origin is associated with:

(a) Significant proteinuria, dysmorphic RBCs, RBC casts
(b) Glycosuria, eumorphic RBCs, WBC casts
(c) Hypercalciuria, eumorphic RBCs, granular casts
(d) Proteinuria, dysmorphic RBCs, hyaline casts

(Answer is A) Significant proteinuria, dysmorphic RBCs, RBC casts

123. Which statement is false concerning the dipstick method for detecting hematuria?

(a) Depends on the ability of hemoglobin to oxidize a chromogen indicator
(b) Negative results need to be confirmed by microscopic examination
(c) Has a sensitivity of 95% and a specificity of 75%
(d) The presence of many epithelial cells suggests skin or vaginal contamination

(Answer is B) Negative results need to be confirmed by microscopic examination

124. Which statement is false concerning microhematuria?

(a) Malignancy is identified in patients presenting with microhematuria more than in patients presenting with gross hematuria
(b) Microscopic hematuria is defined as > 3 red blood cells per high powered field (RBC/hpf) on a single specimen
(c) Warrants full hematuria workup
(d) History of cigarette smoking is of significance

(Answer is A) Malignancy is identified in patients presenting with microhematuria more than in patients presenting with gross hematuria

125. Which drug does not result in urinary retention?

(a) Terazosin, antihypertensive
(b) Benzodiazepines, psychotropic medicine
(c) Levodopa, anti-Parkinsonism medicine
(d) Brimonidine, glaucoma eye drops

(Answer is A) Terazosin, antihypertensive

126. What is the most common cause of hematuria in men over 60 years?

(a) Kidney stones
(b) Glomerulonephritis
(c) BPH
(d) Bladder cancer

(Answer is C) BPH

127. What is false concerning the urinary bladder anatomy?

(a) As it distends, it peels off the peritoneum from the abdominal wall
(b) The interureteric ridge is located between the 2 ureteric orifices and the uvula vesicae
(c) Waldeyer's sheath covers only the distal ureter and forms the deep trigone
(d) In adults, it is percussible over the abdomen when contains at least 150 ml

(Answer is B) The interureteric ridge is located between the 2 ureteric orifices and the uvula vesicae

128. What nerve provides the major neural supply to the striated urinary sphincter and levator ani muscle?

(a) Somatic innervations
(b) Sympathetic fibers from T_{11} - L_2
(c) The pudendal nerve
(d) The obturator nerve

(Answer is C) The pudendal nerve

129. What is false concerning inverted papilloma of the bladder?

(a) It is an endophytic tumor of the transitional urothelium
(b) Harbors p53 gene mutations
(c) Presents with hematuria, dysuria and irritative voiding
(d) The lesion requires transurethral resection

(Answer is B) Harbors p53 gene mutations

130. What is true regarding nephrogenic adenoma of the bladder?

(a) Results from ectopic nephrogenic blastema cells in the detrusor muscle
(b) Might undergo malignant transformation in 15 – 40% of the cases
(c) Cystoscopy, it appears as a bladder mucosal irregularity or large intramural mass
(d) The preferred treatment is cystectomy and urinary diversion

(Answer is C) Cystoscopy, it appears as a bladder mucosal irregularity or large intramural mass

131. In what percentages do upper tract urothelial tumors develop in patients with a bladder urothelial cancer?

(a) 2 - 4% (b) 4 - 6%
(c) 6 - 8% (d) 8 - 10%

(Answer is A) 2 - 4%

132. What is false concerning upper tract urothelial tumors?

(a) Rarely diagnosed at autopsy
(b) The peak incidence occurs between ages 70 and 80
(c) They occur twice as frequently in men as in women
(d) None of the above

(Answer is D) None of the above

133. What is false regarding squamous metaplasia of the urinary bladder (non-keratinized) subtype?

(a) Only in females
(b) Associated with chronic irritation, polypoid cystitis and cystitis glandularis
(c) Risk for squamous cell carcinoma
(d) Treated with estrogen, if symptomatic

(Answer is B) Associated with chronic irritation, polypoid cystitis and cystitis glandularis

134. Regarding bladder neoplasia, squamous metaplasia differs from squamous dysplasia as the latter is/has:

(a) Well-differentiated tumor with broad-based invasive font
(b) Marked atypia distributed on wide areas of superficial urothelium
(c) Atypia is present

(d) Atypia but marked degenerative epithelial changes

(Answer is C) Atypia is present

135. During women's life span, what percentage of women will develop keratinizing squamous metaplasia of the bladder?

(a) 10% (b) 20%
(c) 30% (d) 40%

(Answer is D) 40%

136. What percntage of bladder cancers is squamous cell type in origin?

(a) 2% (b) 5%
(c) 70% (d) 90%

(Answer is B) 5%

137. What is true regarding inverted papilloma of the bladder?

(a) The standard treatment is transurethral resection
(b) The prognosis for inverted papilloma is pathetic, with a recurrence rate of approximately 65%
(c) The likelihood of synchronous urothelial carcinoma is 26%
(d) Has been shown to harbor p53 gene mutations

(Answer is A) The standard treatment is transurethral resection

138. What gene mutation is common in carcinoma *in situ* of urinary bladder?

(a) RB (b) Cyclin A
(c) HRAS (d) CD-44

(Answer is A) RB

139. Intravesical installation of BCG should not be given soon after bladder tumor resection (TURBT) because:

(a) There will be no target tumor tissue to work on
(b) Post-op. hematuria interacts unfavorably with BCG composition
(c) The risk of systemic absorption and sepsis
(d) The high risk of BCG reflux to kidneys while bladder irrigation

(Answer is C) The risk of systemic absorption and sepsis

140. On diagnosing bladder cancers, what advantage does urine cytology has over tumor markers?

(a) High specificity
(b) High sensitivity
(c) High reliability
(d) Strong validity

(Answer is A) High specificity

141. What might occur while resecting a bladder mass at the posterolateral wall?

(a) Bladder perforation
(b) Obturator nerve reflex
(c) Vesico-ureteral reflux
(d) Terrible bleeding

(Answer is B) Obturator nerve reflex

142. What is (are) the classic presentation(s) of bladder cancers?

(a) Irritative bladder symptoms
(b) Obstructive bladder symptoms
(c) Palpable suprapubic mass on physical examination
(d) Painless profuse hematuria

(Answer is D) Painless profuse hematuria

143. The treatment of muscle-invasive bladder cancer in men includes all of the following, *except:*

(a) Radical cysto-prostatectomy
(b) Anterior pelvic exenteration
(c) Bilateral pelvic lymphadenectomy
(d) Creation of a urinary diversion

(Answer is B) Anterior pelvic exenteration

144. The treatment of non-muscle-invasive bladder cancer begins with:

(a) Single intravesical chemotherapy
(b) TURBT
(c) Intravesical BCG vaccine
(d) Multiple bladder biopsies

(Answer is B) TURBT

145. What is false concerning carcinoma *in situ* (CIS) of urinary tract?

(a) Frequently found in association with high-grade or extensive TCC
(b) Has a rate of progression to muscle invasion of 10-25%
(c) Significant areas of CIS are easily missed by routine cystoscopy
(d) Treatment begins with TURBT

(Answer is B) Has a rate of progression to muscle invasion of 10-25%

146. What type of bladder cancers might be caused by Schistosoma hematobium infection?

(a) Transitional cell carcinoma
(b) Squamous cell carcinoma
(c) Adenocarcinoma
(d) Small cell carcinoma

(Answer is B) Squamous cell carcinoma

147. Which of the following cystoscopic descriptions of bladder tumors is false?

(a) Nodular or sessile lesions usually invade muscle
(b) Papillary bladder tumors are typical of low stage and grade
(c) Carcinoma in situ appears as a flat, velvety patch
(d) Sarcomas commonly invade bladder base and ureteral orifices causing obstructions

(Answer is D) Sarcomas commonly invade bladder base and ureteral orifices causing obstructions

148. What is the most common sarcoma of the bladder?

(a) Leiomyosarcoma (b) Rhabdosarcoma
(c) Carcinosarcoma (d) Neurosarcoma

(Answer is A) Leiomyosarcoma

149. Which of the following does not predispose to bladder cancer?

(a) Working with organic chemicals and dyes
(b) Abuse of pain-control medications especially phenacetin
(c) Exposure to arsenic and aromatic amines
(d) Schistosomiasis

(Answer is B) Abuse of pain-control medications especially phenacetin

150. The 5-year survival rates of non-muscle-invasive bladder cancer are:

(a) 40 - 55% (b) 55 - 70%
(c) 70 - 85% (d) 85 - 100%

(Answer is D) 85 - 100%

151. Risk factors for recurrence and progression of bladder cancers include the following:

(a) Multifocality
(b) High tumor grade and advanced stage
(c) Presence of CIS
(d) All of the above

(Answer is D) All of the above

152. Once muscle invasion is detected in bladder cancers, what percentage of occult metastasis is expected?

(a) 30% (b) 40%
(c) 50% (d) 60%

(Answer is C) 50%

153. Bladder tumors with hydronephrosis are:

(a) Often of high-grade sarcomas
(b) Often associated with muscularis propria invasion

(c) Due to vesical polyps occluding ureteric orifices
(d) Should be resected but not diathermized

(Answer is B) Often associated with muscularis propria invasion

154. What is the most effective adjuvant intravesical therapy for bladder tumors?

(a) Cisplatin (b) BCG
(c) Mitomycin C (d) 5-fluorouracil

(Answer is C) Mitomycin C

155. Bladder cancer patients who once failed BCG vaccine, should:

(a) Undergo cystectomy
(b) Try mitomycin c
(c) Take a second course of BCG
(d) Take a second course of BCG + quinolones

(Answer is C) Take a second course of BCG

156. What is not a contraindication to BCG treatment?

(a) History of pulmonary TB
(b) Total incontinence
(c) Immunosuppression
(d) Impaired renal function

(Answer is D) Impaired renal function

157. What is the ideal vesical tumor patient for bladder preservation?

(a) Patients with carcinoma in situ
(b) Patients with completely resected solitary tumor
(c) Patients with preserved kidney and liver functions after 2 courses of BCG
(d) Patients with leiomyosarcoma

(Answer is B) Patients with completely resected solitary tumor

158. Carcinoma *in situ* of the prostatic urethra mostly occurs at the:

(a) Mid prostate to the verumontanum at the 5 and 7 O'clock positions
(b) Lateral margins of the prostate at the 10 and 2 O'clock positions
(c) Entire area distal to the urethral crest
(d) Area between ejaculatory duct openings and prostatic utricle

(Answer is A) Mid prostate to the verumontanum at the 5 and 7 O'clock positions

159. Partial cystectomy for bladder tumors can be performed when the following criterion(a) is (are) met:

(a) The lesion is solitary and no associated CIS
(b) Physically, a surgical margin of 2 cm can be obtained
(c) The resected area should be far enough from ureteral orifices and the bladder neck
(d) All of the above

(Answer is D) All of the above

160. Immediately following transurethral resection of bladder tumors, intravesical installation of which material(s) is(are) contraindicated?

(a) Epirubicin
(b) Mitomycin C
(c) BCG
(d) None of the above

(Answer is C) BCG

161. For radical cystectomy, thromboembolism prophylaxis is required:

(a) Immediately before operation
(b) Immediately before incision and post-operative for 1 day
(c) Immediately before incision and post-operative for 15 days
(d) Immediately before incision and post-operative for 30 days

(Answer is D) Immediately before incision and post-operative for 30 days

162. While deeply resecting a large bladder tumor, the surgeon noted loss of bladder distension, what should next step be?

(a) Increase the irrigation fluid and pursue the procedure
(b) Abort the procedure and leave a urethral catheter
(c) Perform cystogram and manage accordingly
(d) Perform abdominal exploration and manage accordingly

(Answer is C) Perform cystogram and manage accordingly

163. While resecting a large bladder tumor located at the right lateral wall, the surgeon observes a bladder perforation, what should next step be?

(a) Continue the procedure as perforations at this site do no harm
(b) Abort the procedure and leave a urethral catheter
(c) Convert tumor removal to open method and repair the defect
(d) Perform abdominal exploration and manage accordingly

(Answer is B) Abort the procedure and leave a urethral catheter

164. What is the most common type of primary urethral tumors?

(a) Adenocarcinoma
(b) Transitional cell carcinoma
(c) Squamous cell carcinoma
(d) Basal cell carcinoma

(Answer is B) Transitional cell carcinoma

165. What is false regarding the symptomatology of urethral cancers?

(a) Obstructive LUTS are common presentations and occur in association with carcinoma in situ
(b) Might present as perineal abscesses and fistulae
(c) Could be asymptomatic
(d) Venereal diseases increase the risk of urethral cancers

(Answer is A) Obstructive LUTS are common presentations and occur in association with carcinoma in situ

166. What is the imaging modality of choice in the evaluation of a suspected urethral cancer?

(a) Ascending urethrography
(b) Boiding cystourethrography
(c) MRI
(d) IVU

(Answer is C) MRI

167. The treatment of $T_2/N_x/M_0$ prostatic urethral cancer is:

(a) Bloc resection involving total penectomy, cystoprostatectomy, resection of the pubic rami and urogenital diaphragm, with pelvic lymphadenectomy. In addition, creating a urinary diversion
(b) Total penectomy involving removal of the penis, urethra and penile root
(c) Partial penectomy involving excision of the malignant lesion with 2 cm margins
(d) Transurethral resection or fulguration

(Answer is A) Bloc resection involving total penectomy, cystoprostatectomy, resection of the pubic rami and urogenital diaphragm, with pelvic lymphadenectomy. In addition, creating a urinary diversion

168. Partial penectomy for urethral cancer is indicated in:

(a) Infiltrative proximal penile urethral carcinomas
(b) Infiltrative distal penile urethral carcinomas
(c) Recurrent proximal penile urethral carcinoma after laser resection
(d) $T_3/N_2/M_0$ at bulbar urethra

(Answer is B) Infiltrative distal penile urethral carcinomas

169. What is the most common type of tumor occurring in urethral diverticuli?

(a) Adenocarcinoma
(b) Transitional cell carcinoma
(c) Squamous cell carcinoma
(d) Basal cell carcinoma

(Answer is A) Adenocarcinoma

170. Common benign urethral tumors include all of the following, *except:*

(a) Leiomyoma
(b) Hemangioma
(c) Fibroepithelial polyp
(d) Lymphangioma

(Answer is D) Lymphangioma

171. What is the most common type of tumors occurring in the penile urethra?

(a) Adenocarcinoma
(b) Transitional cell carcinoma
(c) Squamous cell carcinoma
(d) Basal cell carcinoma

(Answer is C) Squamous cell carcinoma

172. What is the most common type of tumors occurring in the female urethra?

(a) Adenocarcinoma
(b) Transitional cell carcinoma
(c) Squamous cell carcinoma
(d) Comparable

(Answer is D) Comparable

173. Which of the following statements concerning lymphatic drainage of the male urethra is true?

(a) The anterior urethra drains into the inguinal and pelvic nodes
(b) The posterior urethra drains into the pelvic nodes
(c) The proximal two-thirds drain into the external and internal iliac nodes
(d) The distal one-third drains into the obturator nodes

(Answer is B) The posterior urethra drains into the pelvic nodes

174. In women, what is the most common type of cancers occurring in the proximal urethra?

(a) Adenocarcinoma
(b) Transitional cell carcinoma
(c) Squamous cell carcinoma
(d) Basal cell carcinoma

(Answer is C) Squamous cell carcinoma

175. The most significant prognostic factors for survival in female urethral cancers are:

(a) Sensitivity to chemotherapy and age at presentation
(b) Anatomic location and extent of the tumor
(c) Histologic type of the tumor and sensitivity to radiotherapy
(d) Tumor's stage and grade

(Answer is B) Anatomic location and extent of the tumor

176. The proper indication for surgical repair of a urethral diverticulum is when:

(a) The ostium is ≥ 5 mm wide located close to the sphincter
(b) Symptomatic
(c) Is evident on positive-pressure urethrography
(d) Harbors stones

(Answer is B) Symptomatic

177. Complications of urethral strictures include all of the following, *except:*

(a) Impotence
(b) Bladder stones
(c) Urethral fistula
(d) Periurethral abscess

(Answer is A) Impotence

178. Urethral strictures are, routinely, evaluated by all of the following, *except:*

(a) Cystoscopy
(b) Uroflowmetry
(c) Retrograde urethrography
(d) Urethral pressure profile

(Answer is D) Urethral pressure profile

179. The unlikely cause of weak urinary stream in a 65 years old man is:

(a) Urethral stricture
(b) BPH
(c) Large cystocele
(d) Detrusor under-activity

(Answer is C) Large cystocele

180. When compared to posterior urethral strictures, anterior strictures are amenable to:

(a) Urethroplasty by flaps or grafts
(b) Dilation by urethral sounds
(c) Visual internal urethrotomy
(d) Ablation by laser technology

(Answer is A) Urethroplasty by flaps or grafts

181. Up to what length can bulbar urethral strictures be excised and directly re-anastomosed without the need for tissue transfer?

(a) 1 cm (b) 1.5 cm
(c) 2 cm (d) 2.5 cm

(Answer is C) 2 cm

182. What is the most common cause of urethral strictures?

(a) Infections (b) Trauma
(c) Congenital (d) Malignancies

(Answer is B) Trauma

183. What is the most common pathogen that could result in a urethral stricture?

(a) Trichomonas vaginalis
(b) Chlamydia trachomatis
(c) Gonococcal urethritis
(d) HIV infection

(Answer is C) Gonococcal urethritis

184. What is the likelihood that urethral strictures present as retention of urine?

(a) Never (b) Unlikely
(c) Likely (d) Always

(Answer is C) Likely

185. Which of the following management options cannot treat a 6 mm bulbar urethral stricture?

(a) Medical treatment
(b) Permanent urethral stenting
(c) Dilation by urethral sounds
(d) Visual internal urethrotomy

(Answer is A) Medical treatment

186. The most common mechanism of blunt bladder trauma is:

(a) Motor vehicle accident
(b) Fall from a height
(c) Violence
(d) None of the above

(Answer is A) Motor vehicle accident

187. How common do patients with pelvic fractures have urethral injuries?

(a) 2 – 10% (b) 10 – 25%
(c) 25 – 35% (d) 35 – 45%

(Answer is B) 10 – 25 %

188. What is false concerning traumatic bladder rupture?

(a) Intraperitoneal are commoner than extraperitoneal bladder perforations
(b) Combined intra and extraperitoneal perforations occur in about 10% of the total
(c) Pediatrics, the incidence of intraperitoneal

bladder perforation is markedly higher than extraperitoneal perforations
(d) All idiopathic bladder perforations are intraperitoneal

(Answer is A) Intraperitoneal are commoner than extraperitoneal bladder perforations

189. What is false concerning intraperitoneal bladder rupture?

(a) Results of a direct blow to a distended bladder
(b) Hyperkalemia, hypernatremia, and renal failure might occur
(c) Cystogram, the contrast may outline loops of bowel, fill the paracolic gutters, and pool under the diaphragm
(d) Disruption of the puboprostatic ligaments might occur

(Answer is D) Disruption of the puboprostatic ligaments might occur

190. What is false concerning extraperitoneal bladder rupture?

(a) Typically, is an anterolateral perforation of the bladder due to fractured anterior rami of the pelvic bones
(b) The association with pelvic fracture is in > 90% of cases
(c) Cystogram, the contrast shapes like flames or feathers around the base of the bladder
(d) The bladder may assume a teardrop shape due to the extravasated urine from the dome

(Answer is D) The bladder may assume a teardrop shape due to the extravasated urine from the dome

191. What is false in managing bladder traumas?

(a) Minor intra or extraperitoneal perforations may be managed with bladder drainage alone
(b) The bladder should be drained for 10 - 14 days and then revaluated by static cystogram
(c) Minor extraperitoneal perforations should be primarily repaired if the patient is going for abdominal exploration for other injuries
(d) Cystogram should include AP, lateral, oblique and post drainage views

(Answer is C) Minor extraperitoneal perforations should be primarily repaired if the patient is going for abdominal exploration for other injuries

192. A 12 years boy falls down from a horse back and is overrun by the horse. He is brought to the casualty in pain and unable to void. No pelvic fracture is noted. A urethral catheter is introduced easily but no urine is drained. On filling the bladder, what is pushed in does not come out. What is the most likely diagnosis?

(a) Partial posterior urethral injury
(b) Intraperitoneal bladder injury
(c) Extraperitoneal bladder injury
(d) None of the above

(Answer is B) Intraperitoneal bladder injury

193. What is false concerning the mechanisms of urethral injuries?

(a) Anterior urethral injury occurs from a blunt blow to the perineum
(b) Posterior urethral injury occurs when a shearing force is exerted on the prostato-membranous junction
(c) Not uncommonly, inflating the Foley's catheter's balloon in the bulbous urethral results in anterior urethral injury
(d) Transurethral procedures, e.g., TURP could end in a posterior urethral thermal injury and stricture

(Answer is D) Transurethral procedures, e.g., TURP could end in a posterior urethral thermal injury and stricture

194. Which of the following signs does not indicate a urethral injury?

(a) Teardrop shaped bladder

(b) Pie-in-the sky bladder
(c) High-riding prostate on rectal examination
(d) Blood at external meatus

(Answer is A) Teardrop shaped bladder

195. In the acute setting, the proper procedure to diagnose urethral injury is:

(a) Descending urethrogram
(b) Ascending urethrogram
(c) Uroflowmetry
(d) Flexible cystoscopy

(Answer is B) Ascending urethrogram

196. If an early repair of a posterior urethral injury secondary to a pelvic fracture is desired, it should be:

(a) Soon after the accident
(b) Within one week of the accident
(c) 2–4 weeks after the accident
(d) Early realignment is not a treatment option

(Answer is B) Within one week of the accident

197. The conventional management of posterior urethral injury secondary to pelvic fracture is:

(a) Primary repair
(b) Placing a suprapubic catheter for drainage and repair in 3 months
(c) Clean intermittent catheterization (CIC), to prevent urethral stricture
(d) Delayed primary repair in 2–4 weeks

(Answer is B) Placing a suprapubic catheter for drainage and repair in 3 months

198. What is the most common long-term complication of urethral injuries?

(a) Erectile dysfunction
(b) Stress incontinence
(c) Recurrent strictures
(d) Repeated infections

(Answer is C) Recurrent strictures

199. What is the most common cause of iatrogenic urethral trauma?

(a) Transurethral surgery
(b) Cystectomy operation
(c) Cryotherapy procedure
(d) Foley's catheterization

(Answer is D) Foley's catheterization

200. What is true regarding penetrating injuries to the anterior urethra?

(a) Should be explored immediately
(b) Defects of up to 1.5 cm can be treated by spatulation and primary anastomosis
(c) Longer defects or infected wounds may be repaired in stages
(d) All of the above

(Answer is D) All of the above

201. What is the most telling radiologic examination in diagnosing bladder rupture?

(a) Contrast abdominopelvic CT
(b) A 30 min film of IVU
(c) Micturating cystography
(d) Static cystography

(Answer is D) Static cystography

202. What is the most telling radiologic examination in diagnosing urethral rupture?

(a) Ascending urethrography
(b) Post void film of IVU series
(c) Descending cystourethrography
(d) None of the above

(Answer is A) Ascending urethrography

203. What is the most likely diagnosis of blood at the external meatus in a case of pelvis fracture?

(a) Fracture of the penis
(b) Anterior urethral rupture
(c) Posterior urethral rupture
(d) Extraperitoneal bladder rupture

(Answer is C) Posterior urethral rupture

204. In a patient with stable hemodynamics, intraperitoneal bladder rupture is managed by:

(a) Suprapubic bladder drainage and a delayed repair in 6–12 weeks
(b) Immediate exploration for primary repair
(c) 2 weeks of intra-abdominal and suprapubic catheter drainage and then re-evaluate
(d) 2 weeks of urethral catheterization

(Answer is B) Immediate exploration for primary repair

205. What is true concerning the mechanism of penile fracture?

(a) Is a traumatic rupture of the corpus cavernosum
(b) Is a quick forceful bending of the penis while erection
(c) Is a traumatic fissure in the tunica albuginea
(d) All of the above

(Answer is D) All of the above

206. Penile fractures are basically diagnosed upon:

(a) History and physical examination
(b) Penile color Doppler ultrasonography
(c) Cavernosography
(d) MRI

(Answer is A) History and physical examination

207. What is false concerning penile fractures?

(a) Commonly, results in a 0.5-4 cm longitudinal tear of the tunica albuginea
(b) Associated urethral injuries are more noted in bilateral cavernosal tears
(c) During erection the tunica albuginea thins from 2 mm to 0.25-0.5 mm
(d) May present as an "eggplant" deformity

(Answer is A) Commonly, results in a 0.5-4 cm longitudinal tear of the tunica albuginea

208. What is false concerning physical examination of a fractured penis?

(a) "Butterfly" deformity suggest Colles fascia tear
(b) "Eggplant" deformity suggests Buck's fascia tear
(c) When hematoma is confined under Buck's fascia, the injury presents as a penile nodule
(d) The penis is often presented curved and deviated towards the site of the tear

(Answer is D) The penis is often presented curved and deviated towards the site of the tear

209. What is the likelihood that conservative management of penile fractures results in good outcomes?

(a) Never
(b) Unlikely
(c) Likely
(d) Always

(Answer is C) Likely

210. A 21 years man sustains a motor traffic accident. On examination, his right testis is found at the subcutaneous epifascial planes. What is the most likely diagnosis?

(a) Testicular fracture
(b) Retractile testis
(c) Testicular dislocation
(d) Testicular rupture

(Answer is C) Testicular dislocation

211. What is false concerning a testicular rupture?

(a) A force of around 50 kg is necessary to cause testicular rupture
(b) The vast majority of cases are related to direct blunt scrotal trauma
(c) Sufferers present in pain, nausea, vomiting and occasionally fainting
(d) Color Doppler ultrasonography, reliably, evaluates testicular perfusion in trauma cases

(Answer is B) The vast majority of cases are related to direct blunt scrotal trauma

212. What is true concerning injuries to the female genitalia?

(a) To 35% of cases occur during first sexual contact
(b) Associated pelvic and/or abdominal injuries might occur
(c) Most presentations are pain and swellings
(d) All of the above

(Answer is D) All of the above

213. What is the respective sensitivity and specificity of ultrasonography in diagnosing testicular trauma?

(a) 93.5% and 100%
(b) 88% and 90.4%
(c) 73.8% and 87%
(d) 68.2% and 76.2%

(Answer is A) 93.5% and 100%

214. What is the percentage of hematoceles associated with testicular ruptures?

(a) 20%
(b) 40%
(c) 60%
(d) 80%

(Answer is D) 80%

215. What type of scrotal injuries, typically, takes place while operating a heavy machinery:

(a) Penetrating
(b) Blunt
(c) Degloving
(d) Dislocation

(Answer is C) Degloving

216. What is false concerning ultrasonic findings in acute scrotal traumas?

(a) Contrast-enhanced ultrasonography provides no additional information
(b) The most telling finding of testicular rupture is a projecting testicular tissue outside its confinements
(c) Absence of blood flow indicates a torsion or a devascularization injury
(d) Aging scrotal hematoma appears as hypo-, iso- or hyperechoic area

(Answer is B) The most telling finding of testicular rupture is a projecting testicular tissue outside its confinements

217. What is emergently recommended in unilateral traumatic amputation of the testis?

(a) Microvascular re-implantation within 6 hours of the injury
(b) Sperm extraction for cryopreservation if re-implantation failed
(c) Placing a testicular prosthesis if re-implantation failed
(d) Concomitant injury to the vas deferens should be microsurgically repaired, even if re-implantation failed

(Answer is A) Microvascular re-implantation within 6 hours of the injury

218. What type of neurogenic bladder does manifest as an overactive detrusor, exaggerated sacral reflexes, detrusor-sphincter dyssynergia, thickened bladder wall, and closed bladder neck?

(a) Atonic neurogenic urinary bladder
(b) Automatic urinary bladder
(c) Autonomous urinary bladder
(d) Irritable urinary bladder

(Answer is B) Automatic urinary bladder

219. What are the normal voiding pressures in boys and in girls?

(a) 55 - 80 cm H_2O and 30 - 65 cm H_2O respectively
(b) 45 - 70 cm H_2O and 20 - 55 cm H_2O respectively
(c) 35 - 60 cm H_2O and 10 - 45 cm H_2O respectively
(d) 55 - 80 cm H_2O and 30 - 65 cm H_2O respectively

(Answer is A) 55 - 80 cm H_2O and 30 - 65 cm H_2O respectively

220. Below what limit should resting bladder pressure be maintained to prevent upper tract function deterioration?

(a) 30 cm H_2O (b) 35 cm H_2O
(c) 40 cm H_2O (d) 45 cm H_2O

(Answer is C) 40 cm H_2O

221. A 69 years diabetic man with a history of ischemic stroke and BPH complaining of urgency, intermittency, and poor stream of urine. Uroflowmetry shows a prolonged depressed curve with the following parameters: 280 ml prevoid volume, 130 ml postvoid residual, 11 ml/s maximum flow rate, 56 sec. voiding time. What could be the cause?

(a) Bladder outlet obstruction
(b) Over reflexive bladder
(c) Hypo active detrusor
(d) A combination of all

(Answer is D) A combination of all

222. What is false concerning myelodysplasia in girls?

(a) Urodynamic might exhibit synergy, dyssynergy, and/or complete denervation
(b) Serum cystatin C may be a better predictor of renal function when compared to creatinine
(c) They might achieve puberty 2 years earlier than controls
(d) Auto augmentation is the ideal surgical treatment

(Answer is D) Auto augmentation is the ideal surgical treatment

223. In a 5 years child with neurovesical dysfunction, detrusor-sphincter dyssynergia, and high-grade vesicoureteral reflux; initial management should be by:

(a) Watchful waiting for febrile UTIs for at least 6 months
(b) CIC and anticholinergics
(c) Ureteroneocystostomy
(d) Vesicostomy with or without antireflux subureteral injections

(Answer is B) CIC and anticholinergics

224. In a child with myelodysplasia, what is the most prognostic parameter in urodynamic studies that reflects upper tract dysfunction?

(a) Elevated leak-point pressure
(b) Elevated Valsalva leak-point pressure
(c) Declined maximum urethral closure pressure
(d) Declined urethral pressure profilometry

(Answer is A) Elevated leak-point pressure

225. What is false regarding bladder compliance?

(a) Urinary bladder is the most compliant organ in the body
(b) Is the ability of the bladder to expand at a low storage pressure
(c) Basically, it is an interaction between intracellular matrix and smooth muscle cells
(d) The autonomic nervous system contributes significantly to bladder tone

(Answer is C) Basically, it is an interaction between intracellular matrix and smooth muscle cells

226. What is false concerning the maximal urethral closure pressure (MUCP) in a 32 years woman complaining of stress incontinence?

(a) Is the maximum urethral pressure minus intravesical pressure
(b) MUCP of < 20 cm water implies that she is a good candidate for Burch colposus-pension
(c) The functional urethral length measures the distance along the urethra where urethral pressure exceeds bladder pressure
(d) Nearly all patients with stress urinary incontinence have somehow an element of intrinsic sphincter deficiency

(Answer are B and C) (b) MUCP of < 20 cm water implies that she is a good candidate for Burch colposuspension

(c) The functional urethral length measures the distance along the urethra where urethral pressure exceeds bladder pressure

227. What type of bladder dysfunctions do diabetic patients, initially, develop?

(a) Reflex neurogenic
(b) Sensory neurogenic
(c) Motor neurogenic
(d) Automatic neurogenic

(Answer is B) Sensory neurogenic

228. What type of bladder dysfunctions do symptomatic disc prolapse patients, commonly, develop?

(a) Hinman syndrome
(b) Detrusor areflexia
(c) Autonomic dysreflexia
(d) Upper motor neuron lesion

(Answer is B) Detrusor areflexia

229. Which of the following is not a feature of Prune-Belly syndrome?

(a) Defective abdominal musculature
(b) Bilateral intra-abdominal testes
(c) Epispadias
(d) Anomalous urinary tract

(Answer is C) Epispadias

230. How common do bladder exstrophy patients have vesicoureteral reflux?

(a) Uncommon
(b) Not uncommon
(c) Common
(d) Exceedingly common

(Answer is D) Exceedingly common

231. What is the least common feature of cloacal exstrophy?

(a) Spinal defects
(b) Complete phallic separation
(c) Imperforate anus
(d) Exstrophy of the terminal ileum

(Answer is A) Spinal defects

232. Which statement is false regarding detrusor under activity (DUA)?

(a) What factor for bladder power is not affected by increased outlet resistance
(b) Multisystem atrophy disease is frequently associated with DUA on urodynamic
(c) Intravesical electrotherapy works by direct stimulation of detrusor myocytes and to a lesser extent by inhibiting pathologic urethral afferent signaling
(d) Treatment plans involve timed voiding and CIC

(Answer is C) Intravesical electrotherapy works by direct stimulation of detrusor myocytes and to a lesser extent by inhibiting pathologic urethral afferent signaling

233. What type of bladder capacities best described as the largest volume of urine voided as per the urinary diary chart?

(a) Full bladder capacity
(b) Maximum anesthetic capacity
(c) Functional bladder capacity
(d) Maximum cystometric capacity

(Answer is C) Functional bladder capacity

234. What is the most telling cystometric sign of bladder outlet obstruction on conducting pressure flow studies for a BPH patient?

(a) Detrusor pressure at maximum flow > 100 cm H_2O
(b) Detrusor opening pressure > 80 cm H_2O
(c) Increased maximum urethral closure pressure
(d) Increased opening time

(Answer is A) Detrusor pressure at maximum flow > 100 cm H_2O

235. The luminal phenotype of carcinoma bladder is characterised by high levels of mutations in all *except:*

(a) FGFR3 (b) GATA3
(c) KRT20 (d) CK5

(Answer is D) CK5

236. False about cystoscopy:

(a) Blue light cystoscopy detects 40.8% more cis than white light cystoscopy
(b) In 26.7% patients cis is detected only by blue light cystoscopy
(c) Narrow band imaging doesn't use any dye
(d) Currently blue light cystoscopy is the standard of care for the diagnosis of a bladder tumor

(Answer is D) Currently blue light cystoscopy is the standard of care for the diagnosis of a bladder tumor

237. Lymphatic drainage of bulbar urethra:

(a) Superficial and deep inguinal lymph nodes
(b) Perianal nodes
(c) Directly to pelvic nodes
(d) Paraaortic nodes

(Answer is C) Directly to pelvic nodes

238. Use of stoamch in urinary diversion – false is:

(a) Stomach causes hypochloremic metabolic alkalosis
(b) Less mucus production
(c) More permeable to urinary solutes
(d) Hematuria dysuria syndrome is a specific complication

(Answer is C) More permeable to urinary solutes

239. False about use of intestine for urinary diversion is:

(a) Use of jejunum is avoided due to risk of hypokalemia
(b) Ileum has the advantage of constant blood supply
(c) In patients who have received pelvic irradiation, portions of the right, transverse, and descending colon may be used
(d) Use of colon is associated with less post operative bowel obstruction than ileum

(Answer is A) Use of jejunum is avoided due to risk of hypokalemia

240. Non refluxing type of ureterocolonic anastomosis is all *except:*

(a) Lead Better and Clarke
(b) Goodwin
(c) Strickler
(d) Cordonnier and Nesbit

(Answer is D) Cordonnier and Nesbit

241. False about Mainz 1 pouch:

(a) An ileocolonic pouch
(b) Uses Nipple valve mechanism
(c) A reasonably low pressure urinary reservoir
(d) A type of orthotopic neobladder

(Answer is C) A reasonably low pressure urinary reservoir

242. False about Indiana Pouch:

(a) Buttressed ileocaecal valve is used as continence mechanism
(b) An ileocolonic pouch
(c) More complications and difficult to construct compared to other pouches
(d) Most common cause of stone formation is insufficient pouch irrigation

(Answer is C) More complications and difficult to construct compared to other pouches

243. True about MAINZ III pouch:

(a) Continent cutaneous reservoir
(b) Ileal pouch
(c) Orthotopic neobladder
(d) Rectosigmoid pouch

(Answer is C) Orthotopic neobladder

244. False about TRUS:

(a) Multiple diffuse calcification is usually a normal age related change
(b) Normal volume of mature prostate is 20-25 g and is constant till 50 years
(c) Carcinoma usually appears hyperechoic
(d) Classical Zonal anatomy is not evident on TRUS

(Answer is C) Carcinoma usually appears hyperechoic

245. All are antimuscarinics in clinical use *except:*

(a) Oxybutinin (b) Fesoterodine
(c) Trospium (d) Mirabegeron

(Answer is D) Mirabegeron

246. False about Muscarinic antagonists:

(a) Tolterodine has less CNS penetration and low cognitive side effects
(b) No muscarinic receptor subtype selectivity for tolterodine
(c) Solifenacin has M3 receptor selectivity
(d) The pharmacologically active antimuscarinic component of Darifenacin is L-hyoscyamine

(Answer is D) The pharmacologically active antimuscarinic component of Darifenacin is L-hyoscyamine

247. False about oxybutynin:

(a) Dry mouth is a significant side effect
(b) Has direct muscle relaxant effect
(c) Has local anesthetic action
(d) The primary adverse effect of transdermal oxybutynin is arrhythmia

(Answer is D) The primary adverse effect of transdermal oxybutynin is arrhythmia

248. Causes for increased incidence of bladder tumor after UTUC are all *except:*

(a) More number of urothelial cells
(b) Longer exposure time
(c) Downstream seeding
(d) Renal failure

(Answer is D) Renal failure

249. All are true about primary bladder calculi *except:*

(a) Primary bladder calculi form without any predisposing cause
(b) Primary bladder calculi are associated with nutritional deficiency
(c) Peak age is 2-4 years
(d) Usually recurs after treatment

(Answer is D) Usually recurs after treatment

250. Cystolitholapaxy means:

(a) Intact removal of bladder calculi
(b) Fragmenting the stone with laser
(c) Fragmenting the stone with pneumatic energy
(d) Mechanical breakage of the stone

(Answer is D) Mechanical breakage of the stone

251. Energy modality of choice for management of bladder calculi:

(a) Pneumatic lithotripsy
(b) Laser with end firing probe
(c) Laser with side firing probe
(d) Ultrasound lithotripsy

(Answer is C) Laser with side firing probe

252. Latzko procedure for Vesicovaginal fistula is:

(a) Classical saucerization technique
(b) Flap splitting technique
(c) Partial colpocleisis technique

(d) Vaginal flap technique

(Answer is C) Partial colpocleisis technique

253. Preferential tissue for interposition for fistulae involving trigone, bladder neck and urethra is:

(a) Martius flap (b) Peritoneum
(c) Omentum (d) Gracilis flap

(Answer is A) Martius flap

254. Youssef syndrome occurs due to:

(a) Vesicouterine fistula
(b) Vesicovaginal fistula
(c) Ureterovascular fistula
(d) Pyelovascular fistula

(Answer is A) Vesicouterine fistula

255. Most common cause of vesicouterine fistula is:

(a) Radical hysterectomy
(b) Low segment caesarean section
(c) Transvaginal taping
(d) Laparoscopic hysterectomy

(Answer is B) Low segment caesarean section

256. Most common urodynamic finding in Parkinson's disease is:

(a) Detrusor underactivity
(b) Detrusor overactivity
(c) Smooth sphincter dyssynergia
(d) Bradykinesia of striated sphincter

(Answer is B) Detrusor overactivity

257. Current recommendation for acute pharmacologic treatment of autonomic dysreflexia is:

(a) Nitroglycerin paste above the level of the lesion
(b) Oral terazosin
(c) Intravenous nitroprusside
(d) Sublingual nifedipine

(Answer is A) Nitroglycerin paste above the level of the lesion

CHAPTER

16

Prostate

1. In patients with relapse following first-line docetaxel chemotherapy which is the first-choice option for second-line treatment:

(a) Cisplatin (b) Abiraterone
(c) Sipuleucel-T (d) Adriamycin

(Answer is B) In patients with relapse following first-line docetaxel chemotherapy–Cabazitaxel and Abiraterone is regarded as first-choice option for second-line treatment.

2. Which one of the following is not the sex accessory tissues?

(a) Seminal vesicle
(b) Ampullary glands
(c) Bulbourethral glands
(d) Ejaculatory ducts

(Answer is D) Sex accessory tissues include the prostate, seminal vesicles, ampullary glands, and bulbourethral glands, and they are believed to play a major but unknown role in the reproductive process.

3. Which statement regarding the embryology of genitourinary tract is not true?

(a) The developmental growth of the wolffian-derived sex accessory glands is completed by the 13th week
(b) Developmental growth of wolffian derived group of glands is stimulated by fetal testosterone
(c) Development of prostate starts from the urogenital sinus during the fifth month of fetal growth
(d) Prostate development is directed primarily by DHT and not testosterone

(Answer is C) The development of prostate starts from the urogenital sinus during the third month of fetal growth.

4. In the human male, neonatal surges in testosterone and progesterone is observed at:

(a) 2 days (b) 10 days
(c) 2 months (d) 10 months

(Answer is C) In the human male, neonatal surges in testosterone are observed to peak between 2 and 3 months of age. There is a second transient progesterone surge that occurs in humans at approximately 2 months of age.

5. Which is not the α1-adrenergic receptor?

(a) α1A (b) α1B
(c) α1C (d) α1D

(Answer is C) Recent work has demonstrated three subtypes of the α1-adrenergic receptor (α1A, α1B and α1D).

6. Which statement regarding the cell biology of prostate gland is not correct?

(a) With androgen ablation, the typical secretory cells decrease by 90% in number
(b) Neuroendocrine cells typically express chromogranin-A and neuron-specific enolase
(c) Basal cells are much smaller, have a low mitotic index, and are less abundant, accounting for less than 10% of the total cell number

(d) Androgen deprivation decreases stem cells by 40% in number

(Answer is D) Androgen deprivation does not affect stem cells but rather enriches for them, as the more terminally differentiated cells initiate apoptosis.

7. **Which statement is not correct?**

(a) Leydig cells of the testis are the major source of the testicular androgens
(b) Man undergoing bilateral simple orchiectomy in functionally castrate within 1 to 2 hours of surgery
(c) Only 2% of the total serum testosterone is unbound (free testosterone) in the plasma
(d) Testosterone is the major form of androgen found within the prostate gland

(Answer is D) DHT is the major form of androgen found within the prostate gland (5 ng/g tissue wet weight) and is five-fold higher than testosterone.

8. **Which statement regarding 5α-reductase enzyme is not correct?**

(a) The type 1 enzyme is in the skin and in the adult scalp and is believed to be involved in hair formation
(b) The type I enzyme is mutated in men with congenital 5α-reductase deficiency
(c) The type II enzyme appears in the basal cells of the epithelium and in the stromal cells
(d) The type II enzyme is absent in the secretory epithelial cells

(Answer is B) The type II enzyme is mutated in 5α-reductase deficiency and is the dominant isoform present in the prostate gland.

9. **Which statement regarding testosterone is not correct?**

(a) Serum albumin has a relatively low affinity for testosterone, but given its abundance, it has a high capacity
(b) The majority of testosterone bound to plasma protein is associated with albumin
(c) Free testosterone can be converted to estrogens, but estrogens cannot be converted to testosterone
(d) Administration of testosterone decreases SHBG (TeBG) levels in the plasma

(Answer is B) The majority of testosterone bound to plasma protein is associated with SHBG (TeBG).

10. **Which hormone can cause a florid squamous cell metaplasia in prostate growth that can be offset by androgens?**

(a) Progesterone (b) Estrogen
(c) Testosterone (d) Androsterone

(Answer is B) Estrogens can cause a florid squamous cell metaplasia in prostate growth that can be offset by androgens.

11. **Which cell adhesion molecule link the cell to carbohydrate moieties primarily on the vascular system?**

(a) Integrin (b) Cadherin
(c) Selectin (d) Immunoglobulin

(Answer is C) The cell adhesion molecules (CAM) are divided into four major types: (1) integrins, which link the cell to the basement membrane and extracellular matrix components through heterodimer interactions; (2) cadherins, which link the cell to neighbouring cells through homotypic polymers; (3) selectins, which link the cell to carbohydrate moieties primarily on the vascular system; and (4) immunoglobulin superfamily adhesion molecules.

12. **Androgen receptor gene is located on:**

(a) Short arm of the Y chromosome
(b) Long arm of the Y chromosome
(c) Short arm of the X chromosome
(d) Long arm of the X chromosome

(Answer is D) Androgen receptor gene is on the long arm of the X chromosome at position Xq 11.2-q12.

13. Which is a potent mitogen working on the stromal cells and involved in angiogenesis and cellular chemotaxis?

(a) EGF (b) TGF α
(c) β FGF (d) VEGF

(Answer is C) FGF-2 (βFGF) is a potent mitogen working on the stromal cells and involved in angiogenesis and cellular chemotaxis, but it is a weak epithelial mitogen.

14. Which two factors are important for maintaining the structural and functional integrity of BPH?

(a) FGF and TGF-α (b) VEGF and TGF-α
(c) EGF and FGF (d) EGF and TGF-α

(Answer is D) EGF and TGF-α are important for maintaining the structural and functional integrity of BPH.

15. Which statement regarding growth factors of prostate gland is not correct?

(a) Basic fibroblast growth factor is present in normal prostate and elevated in BPH
(b) EGF is otherwise called as urogastrone
(c) TGF-β stimulates the growth of fibroblasts and epithelium
(d) TGF-β2 elevated in benign prostatic hyperplasia

(Answer is C) TGF-β is inhibitor of epithelial growth.

16. True about normal human ejaculate are all *except:*

(a) Spermatozoa, represent less than 1% of the total ejaculate
(b) The major contribution to the volume of seminal plasma comes from the prostate
(c) The first fraction of the human ejaculate is rich in sperm and prostatic secretions
(d) Fructose, which represents a major secretory product of the seminal vesicles, is elevated in the later fraction of ejaculate

(Answer is B) The major contribution to the volume of seminal plasma (average 3 ml) comes from the seminal vesicle (1.5 to 2 ml).

17. The richest sources of prostaglandins in the human are:

(a) Prostate (b) Seminal vesicles
(c) Testis (d) Pituitary

(Answer is B) The richest sources of prostaglandins in the human are the seminal vesicles.

18. Which statement regarding PSA is not correct?

(a) PSA is a glycoprotein acting as a serine protease of molecular weight 33,000
(b) It contains 7% carbohydrate
(c) Found almost exclusively in the epithelial cells of the prostate
(d) The PSA gene *(hKLK3)* is a member of a human tissue kallikrein gene family

(Answer is D) The PSA gene *(hKLK3)* is a member of a human tissue kallikrein gene family.

19. Which statement regarding prostate secretions is not correct?

(a) Drugs whose concentrations in the prostatic secretion approach their concentrations in blood, includes erythromycin, sulfonamides and chloramphenicol
(b) Prostatic secretions are slightly alkaline
(c) pH of freshly ejaculated human semen is slightly alkaline (pH 7.3 to 7.7)
(d) On standing, semen with the loss of carbon dioxide becomes acidic owing to accumulation of lactic acid

(Answer is B) Prostatic secretions are slightly acidic (pH-6.6).

20. Which statement regarding effect of aging on androgens is not correct?

(a) Prostatic levels of DHT remains high
(b) Androgen receptor turns to low level
(c) Estradiol/bioavailable testosterone ratio is increased

(d) Peripheral levels of testosterone are decreasing

(Answer is B) Androgen receptor remain high.

21. In BPH growth stimulatory factors are all *except:*

(a) FGF (b) VEGF
(c) IGF (d) TGF-β

(Answer is D) If cellular proliferation is a component of the BPH process, it appears that growth stimulatory factors such as the FGF-1, -2, -7 and -17 families; VEGF; and LGF may play a role, with DHT augmenting or modulating the growth factor effects. In contrast, TGF-β, is known to inhibit epithelial cell proliferation.

22. Which statement is not true regarding prostate volume determination?

(a) DRE tends to overestimate true prostate size as determined by TRUS
(b) The magnitude of the false estimation by DRE increases with increasing prostate size
(c) TRUS volume measurements using the prostate ellipsoid volume formula are the most widely accepted measure of prostate volume
(d) Volume as assessed by TRUS has been found to increase slowly but steadily with advancing age

(Answer is A) DRE tends to underestimate true prostate size as determined by TRUS.

23. In MTOPS study endpoints are all *except:*

(a) Worsening of 4 points on the I-PSS score verified twice within 4 weeks
(b) Acute urinary retention
(c) Socially unacceptable incontinence
(d) Hematuria

(Answer is D) In MTOPS study the composite endpoint captured either a worsening of 4 points on the I-PSS score verified twice within 4 weeks, acute urinary retention, socially unacceptable incontinence, recurrent urinary tract infection, or renal insufficiency related to BPH.

24. In MTOPS incidence of 4 points worsening in the I-PSS over 4 years of follow-up in placebo-treated patients is:

(a) 7% (b) 14%
(c) 21% (d) 28%

(Answer is B) In MTOPS approximately 14% of placebo-treated patients experienced 4 points worsening in the I-PSS over 4 years of follow-up.

25. On the basis of TRUS, the growth of the prostate in the men 40 to 79 years old was estimated to be about:

(a) 0.2 ml per year (b) 0.4 ml per year
(c) 0.6 ml per year (d) 0.8 ml per year

(Answer is C) On the basis of TRUS, the growth of the prostate in the men 40 to 79 years old was estimated to be about 0.6 ml per year or 6 ml per decade of life.

26. Regarding complications related to BPH which statement is not true?

(a) Bladder stones were eight times higher in men with a histologic diagnosis of BPH than in control subjects
(b) The self-reported rate of hematuria is 2.5%
(c) In MTOPS, there was not a single case of renal insufficiency related to BPH in over 3000 men observed for over 4 years
(d) Following precipitated AUR, 15% of patients had another episode of spontaneous AUR and a total of 75% underwent surgery

(Answer is D) Following spontaneous AUR, 15% of patients had another episode of spontaneous AUR and a total of 75% underwent surgery, whereas after precipitated AUR only 9% had an episode of spontaneous AUR and 26% underwent surgery.

27. In PLESS study how many patients with enlarged prostate and moderate symptoms underwent episode of AUR?

(a) 1 .8 per 100 person-years
(b) 3.0 per 100 person-years
(c) 4.8 per 100 person-years
(d) 6.0 per 100 person-years

(Answer is A) In PLESS, 1376 placebo-treated men with enlarged prostates and moderate symptoms had complete follow-up over 4 years; 99 of the men experienced an episode of AUR for a calculated incidence rate of 1.8 per 100 person-years.

28. If a more accurate measurement of prostate volume is needed to determine whether to perform open prostatectomy rather than TURP which is more accurate?

(a) DRE (b) USG
(c) CPE (d) MRI

(Answer is B) If a more accurate measurement of prostate volume is needed to determine whether to perform open prostatectomy rather than transurethral resection of the prostate (TURP), ultrasound (transabdominal or transrectal) is more accurate than cystourethroscopy.

29. According to IPSS scoring system which signifies moderate symptoms?

(a) 8 to 19 (b) 8 to 18
(c) 9 to 18 (d) 9 to 19

(Answer is A) When the IPSS system is used, symptoms can be classified as mild (0 to 7), moderate (8 to 19), or severe (20 to 35).

30. Which statement regarding evaluation of BPH is not correct?

(a) A urinalysis should be done
(b) Routine creatinine measurement in the standard patient is not recommended
(c) Elevated serum creatinine in a patient with BPH is an indication for imaging studies
(d) Measurement of the serum PSA value should be done in all patients with BPH

(Answer is D) Measurement of the serum PSA value should be performed in patients in whom the identification of cancer would clearly alter BPH management.

31. Incidence of men with histologically proven, BPH, and having PSA greater than 4.0 ng/ml is:

(a) 7% (b) 14%
(c) 21% (d) 28%

(Answer is D) Twenty-eight percent of men with histologically proven BPH have a serum PSA greater than 4.0 ng/ml.

32. Which statement regarding flow rate is not correct?

(a) Flow rate measurements are inaccurate if the voided volume is less than 125 to 150 ml
(b) Flow rate recording is the single best noninvasive urodynamic test to detect lower urinary tract obstruction
(c) The peak flow rate more specifically identifies patients with BPH than does the average flow rate
(d) Patients with a Qmax greater than 15 ml/s appear to have better treatment outcomes after prostatectomy than patients with a Qmax of less than 15 ml/s

(Answer is D) Although considerable uncertainty exists, patients with a Qmax greater than 15 ml/s appear to have somewhat poorer treatment outcomes after prostatectomy than patients with a Qmax of less than 15 ml/s.

33. Which statement regarding PVR is not correct?

(a) Residual urine volume measurement has significant intraindividual variability that limits its clinical usefulness
(b) Residual urine volume does not correlate well with other signs or symptoms of clinical BPH

(c) Large residual urine volumes may predict a slightly higher failure rate with a strategy of watchful waiting
(d) Residual urine volume predicts the outcome of surgical treatment

(Answer is D) It is uncertain whether residual urine volume predicts the outcome of surgical treatment.

34. Which statement regarding CMG is not correct?

(a) The test may have value in the evaluation of patients with known or suspected neurologic lesions and LUTS
(b) OAB contractions are present in about 60% of men with LUTS
(c) Only about one fourth of patients who have an overactive bladder before treatment retain the problem afterward
(d) Patients whose symptoms do not improve after surgery are reliably identified by preoperative cystometrography

(Answer is D) Patients whose symptoms do not improve after surgery are more likely to have a persistently overactive bladder, but preoperative cystometrography does not reliably identify those patients.

35. Upper urinary tract imaging is recommended in evaluation of men with LUTS in all *except:*

(a) Hematuria
(b) History of urolithiasis
(c) History of urinary tract surgery
(d) Trabeculated bladder

(Answer is D) Upper urinary tract imaging is not recommended in the routine evaluation of men with LUTS unless they also have one or more of the following: hematuria, UTI, renal insufficiency (ultrasound recommended), history of urolithiasis, or history of urinary tract surgery.

36. AUA symptom score is decreased by 5 after medical therapy. It will be rated as what level of improvement?

(a) Marked (b) Moderate
(c) Mild (d) Slightly improved

(Answer is B) The group mean changes in AUA symptom Index for subjects rating their improvement as markedly, moderately, or slightly improved, unchanged, or worse were -8.8, -5.1, -3.0, -0.7 and +2.7, respectively.

37. Bladder overactivity is considered at what pressures of detrusor contraction when a bladder volume is less than 300 ml?

(a) 10 cm H_2O (b) 15 cm H_2O
(c) 20 cm H_2O (d) 25 cm H_2O

(Answer is B) The definition of bladder overactivity (detrusor instability) is the development of a detrusor contraction exceeding 15 cm H_2O at a bladder volume less than 300 ml.

38. Incidence of AUR was related to all *except:*

(a) Age
(b) Size of prostate
(c) Severity of symptoms
(d) PSA

(Answer is D) Incidence of AUR was related to age, severity of symptoms, and size of the prostate gland.

39. Which one of the following is not the long-acting α1?

(a) Prazosin (b) Terazosin
(c) Doxazosin (d) Alfuzosin SR

(Answer is A)

Long-Acting α1	
Terazosin	5 or 10 mg qd
Doxazosin	4 or 8 mg qd
Alfuzosin SR	10 mg qd

40. Which statement regarding medical therapy for BPH is not correct?

(a) The half-life of doxazosin is longer than that of terazosin (22 vs. 12 hours)

(b) Terazocin is the most potent available $\alpha 1$ antagonist
(c) With tamsulosin treatment-related incidence of abnormal ejaculation in the 0.8 mg group is 18%
(d) Because of the lack of adverse effects and blood pressure changes, alfuzosin has been described as a uroselective drug

(Answer is B) Tamsulosin is the most potent available $\alpha 1$ antagonist.

41. Major conclusions drawn from the ALFOO study are all *except:*

(a) Fifty-five percent of men randomized to the SR alfuzosin voided spontaneously after catheter removal
(b) Twenty-nine percent of men in placebo group voided spontaneously after catheter removal
(c) The clinical effect of alfuzosin was greatest in younger men
(d) Of the men who successfully completed the voiding trial, 12% ultimately experienced a second episode of AUR

(Answer is D) Fifty-five percent and 29% of men randomized to the SR alfuzosin and placebo groups voided spontaneously after catheter removal, respectively. The clinical effect was greatest in younger men. Of the men who successfully completed the voiding trial, 32% ultimately experienced a second episode of AUR or underwent prostatectomy.

42. Incidence of beneficial effect on the quality of life of men suffering from BPH in ALFORTI trial is:

(a) 15% (b) 25%
(c) 35% (d) 45%

(Answer is C) Alfuzosin has been shown to have a beneficial effect on the quality of life of men suffering from BPH. In the ALFUS study the quality of life index improved by 18% in both active groups compared with 8% in the placebo arm (P = .002). In an open extension of the ALFORTI trial there was a 35% improvement from baseline of quality of life.

43. Conclusion drawn from North American Finasteride Trial in which the subjects were randomized to receive placebo or 1 or 5 mg of finasteride for 1 year are all *except:*

(a) The difference between the group mean changes in PFR and prostate volume was statistically significant for both the 1 and the 5 mg finasteride groups versus the placebo group
(b) The difference between the group mean changes in symptom scores was statistically significant only for placebo versus 5 mg of finasteride
(c) Prostate volume regression was maximal at 6 months
(d) The greatest change in symptom scores and PFR occurred after 6 months of initiating active treatment

(Answer is D) The greatest change in symptom scores and PFR occurred within the first 2 months of initiating active treatment.

44. Which study represents the longest-duration multicenter, randomized, double-blind, placebo-controlled study reported to date in the medical therapy of BPH literature?

(a) North American Finasteride Trial
(b) International Finasteride Study
(c) PLESS
(d) MTOPS

(Answer is C) The Proscar Long-Term Efficacy and Safety Study (PLESS) represents the longest-duration multicenter, randomized, double-blind, placebo-controlled study reported to date in the medical therapy of BPH literature.

45. Which statement regarding dutasteride is not correct?

(a) Dutasteride is a dual inhibitor of 5α-reductase

(b) Serum dihydrotestosterone is reduced by approx 99%
(c) The risk reduction of AUR is 57%, and the risk reduction of BPH-related surgery is 48% compared with placebo
(d) Risk reduction of AUR and BPH-related surgery is durable over 4 years

(Answer is B) Serum dihydrotestosterone is reduced by approx 90%.

46. Finasteride reduces prostate volume by:

(a) 10% (b) 20%
(c) 40% (d) 50%

(Answer is B) Finasteride reduces prostate volume approximately 20%.

47. Which statement regarding MTOPS is not correct?

(a) Men who received combination therapy were significantly less likely to experience BPH progression than those with any monotherapy groups
(b) Invasive therapy and AUR risk were significantly reduced by doxazosin and combination therapy
(c) AUA symptom score and Qmax improved significantly more in the combination therapy group compared with the monotherapy groups
(d) The number needed to treat to prevent a case of BPH progression as defined in MTOPS in the overall population was 8.4 for the combination therapy group

(Answer is B) Invasive therapy and AUR risk were significantly reduced by finasteride and combination therapy.

48. The main mechanisms of action that have received the greatest attention for phytotherapeutic agents are all *except:*

(a) Anti-inflammatory effects
(b) 5α-reductase inhibition
(c) Growth factor alteration
(d) α-blocker action

(Answer is D) The three mechanisms of action that have received the greatest attention for phytotherapeutic agents are anti-inflammatory effects, 5α-reductase inhibition, and growth factor alteration.

49. Which one of the following is permanent stents?

(a) Urospiral and the prosta kath
(b) Memokath and the prosta coil
(c) Barnes stent and the trestle stent
(d) UroLume and Memotherm

(Answer is D) The UroLume endourethral prosthesis is a woven tubular mesh that maintains its position in the urethra by outward external pressure. The Memotherm is a heat-expandable stent of nickel-titanium alloy.

50. Which statement is not true regarding microwave?

(a) Microwaves treat a broad area than Radiofrequency (RF)
(b) Microwave penetrate tissue superficially than RF
(c) The central temperature with microwave is lower than with RF
(d) Treatment with microwaves takes longer than RF to produce coagulative necrosis

(Answer is B) There is a difference in the method of tissue heating brought about by RF and, for example, microwave application. Microwaves treat a broad area and can penetrate tissue more deeply than RF. The central temperature is therefore lower than with RF in order to maintain safe heat levels at the treatment rim. Therefore, treatment with microwaves takes longer than RF to produce coagulative necrosis.

51. Which statement regarding TUNA system is not correct?

(a) The generator produces a monopolar RF signal of 490 kHz

(b) TUNA system can create 1 cm necrotic lesions without difficulty in the prostate with no damage to rectum, bladder base, or distal prostatic urethra
(c) Nitric oxide synthase receptors were found to be most vulnerable to thermal damage, which occurred earliest
(d) Damage to the α-adrenergic receptors is maximal at 1 to 2 months

(Answer is D) Damage to the α-adrenergic receptors is maximal at 1 to 2 weeks.

52. Ho:YAG, Nd:YAG and KTP laser respectively emits light at a frequency of:

(a) 532 nm , 1064 nm, 2100 nm
(b) 532 nm, 2100 nm, 1064 nm
(c) 1064 nm, 532 nm , 2100 nm
(d) 2100 nm, 1064 nm , 532 nm

(Answer is D) The holmium:yttrium-aluminum-garnet (Ho:YAG) laser emits light at a frequency of 2100 nm. The neodymium:yttrium- aluminum-garnet (Nd:YAG) laser emits light at a wavelength of 1064 nm. (KTP) laser uses a KTP crystal to double the frequency of an Nd:YAG laser and produces a 532 nm wavelength.

53. Regarding TUR syndrome which statement is not correct?

(a) TUR syndrome occurred in 2% of the patients
(b) Risk is increased if the gland is larger than 45 g and the resection time is longer than 90 minutes
(c) The syndrome is characterized by mental confusion, nausea, vomiting, hypertension, tachycardia
(d) Usually, the patients do not become symptomatic until the serum sodium concentration reaches 125 mEq/dl

(Answer is C) The syndrome is characterized by mental confusion, nausea, vomiting, hypertension, bradycardia.

54. In TUIP incision is given at:

(a) 6 O'clock (b) 5 and 7 O'clock
(c) 3 and 9 O'clock (d) 12 O'clock

(Answer is B) Using a Collings knife, an incision is made at the 5 and 7 O'clock positions or on one side of the midline only. It starts just distal to the ureteral orifice and ends just proximal to the verumontanum.

55. When compared with TURP, open prostatectomy offers all the advantages *except:*

(a) Lower retreatment rate
(b) More complete removal of the prostatic adenoma under direct vision
(c) Avoids the risk of dilutional hyponatremia
(d) Decreased potential for perioperative hemorrhage

(Answer is D) The disadvantages of open prostatectomy compared with TURP include the need for a lower midline incision and a resultant longer hospitalization and convalescence period. In addition, there may be an increased potential for perioperative hemorrhage.

56. Suprapubic prostatectomy operation is ideally suited in all *except:*

(a) BPH in obese men
(b) BPH with 2-3 small bladder calculi
(c) Large median lobe protruding into the bladder
(d) Significant bladder diverticulum

(Answer is B) Suprapubic prostatectomy operation is ideally suited for patients with (1) a large median lobe protruding into the bladder, (2) a clinically significant bladder diverticulum, or (3) large bladder calculi. It may also be preferable for obese men, in whom it is difficult to gain direct access to the prostatic capsule and dorsal vein complex.

57. The indications for prostatectomy, by either open approach or TUR, include all *except:*

(a) Persistent urinary tract infections

(b) Recurrent gross hematuria of prostatic origin
(c) Pathophysiologic changes of the kidneys, ureters, or bladder secondary to prostatic obstruction
(d) Severely trabecuted bladder suggestive of severe obstruction

(Answer is D) The indications for prostatectomy, by either open approach or transurethral resection, include (1) acute urinary retention; (2) recurrent or persistent urinary tract infections; (3) significant symptoms from bladder outlet obstruction not responsive to medical therapy; (4) recurrent gross hematuria of prostatic origin; (5) pathophysiologic changes of the kidneys, ureters, or bladder secondary to prostatic obstruction; and (6) bladder calculi secondary to obstruction.

58. Management of large bladder diverticula with BPH is:

(a) Suprapubic prostatectomy followed by diverticulectomy after 3 months
(b) Retropubic prostatectomy followed by diverticulectomy after 3 months
(c) Diverticulectomy followed by suprapubic prostatectomy after 3 months
(d) Suprapubic prostatectomy and diverticulectomy concurrently

(Answer is D) If sizable bladder diverticula justify removal, suprapubic prostatectomy and diverticulectomy should be performed concurrently.

59. All *except* one is the disadvantage of suprapubic approach over retropubic approach:

(a) Direct visualization of the apical prostatic adenoma is reduced
(b) Apical enucleation is less precise
(c) Hemostasis may be more difficult
(d) Direct access to bladder not possible

(Answer is D) The disadvantage of suprapubic approach, compared with the retropubic approach, is that direct visualization of the apical prostatic adenoma is reduced. As a result, the apical enucleation is less precise, and this factor may affect postoperative urinary continence. Furthermore, hemostasis may be more difficult because of inadequate visualization of the entire prostatic fossa after enucleation.

60. Prostate cancer in men younger than 50 years, accounts for:

(a) 0.1% (b) 1%
(c) 5% (d) 10%

(Answer is A) Prostate cancer is rarely diagnosed in men younger than 50 years, accounting for less than 0.1% of all patients.

61. AJCC clinical stage T1c accounts for how many of the newly diagnosed carcinoma prostate?

(a) 25% (b) 50%
(c) 75% (d) 90%

(Answer is C) Nonpalpable cancers (AJCC clinical stage T1c) now account for 75% of newly diagnosed disease.

62. Which statement regarding expression of markers in carcinoma prostate is not correct?

(a) The expression of GSTP1, is absent in about 70% of prostate cancer and virtually all cases of PIN
(b) VEGF is expressed in a majority of prostate cancers
(c) E-cadherin expression is reduced in poorly differentiated tumors
(d) b-Methylacyl-CoA racemase is upregulated in virtually all prostate cancer

(Answer is A) The expression of GSTP1, is absent in about 70% of prostatic intraepithelial neoplasia and virtually all cases of prostate cancer.

63. All *except* one is the main findings of the PCPT:

(a) The prevalence of prostate cancer was reduced by 25% in those randomized to finasteride compared with placebo

(b) The prevalence of Gleason grade 7 to 10 tumors was lower in the finasteride group than in the placebo group
(c) The risk reductions associated with finasteride among risk groups defined by age, family history, race, and PSA level were of the same general magnitude
(d) Sexual side effects were more common with finasteride

(Answer is B) The main findings of the PCPT are as follows:

The prevalence of Gleason grade 7 to 10 tumors was higher in the finasteride group than in the placebo group (6.4% versus 5.1%; hazard rate = 1.27; 95% confidence interval, 1.07 to 1.50).

64. Benefit-to-risk ratio as defined by the number of cancers prevented for each excess high-grade cancer in those taking finasteride as shown by PCPT trial is:

(a) 3:1 (b) 1:3
(c) 5:1 (d) 1:5

(Answer is C) Mathematical model from PCPT suggests a baseline 5:1 benefit-to-risk ratio as defined by the number of cancers prevented for each excess high-grade cancer in those taking finasteride.

65. Which is associated with associated higher risk of prostate cancer?

(a) Vitamin E (b) Rich calcium diet
(c) Genistein (d) Green tea

(Answer is B) Dietary intake of dairy products rich in calcium, which depresses serum levels of vitamin D, are associated with a higher risk of prostate cancer.

66. Which statement regarding PIN is not correct?

(a) Low-grade PIN should not be commented on in diagnostic reports
(b) If low-grade PIN is diagnosed on needle biopsy, these patients are at no greater risk of having carcinoma on repeated biopsy
(c) High-grade PIN on needle biopsy with follow-up, the mean risk of cancer is 26.4%
(d) In patients with PIN, PSA levels, ORE and TRUS findings enhances the prediction of who is more likely to have carcinoma on repeat biopsy

(Answer is D) In the majority of studies, serum prostate-specific antigen (PSA) levels, results of digital rectal examination, and transrectal ultrasound findings do not enhance the prediction of who is more likely to have carcinoma on repeat biopsy.

67. Which parameter by itself in radical prostatectomy specimens does not worsen prognosis?

(a) Perineural invasion
(b) Lymphatic invasion
(c) Vascular invasion
(d) Seminal vesicle invasion

(Answer is A) Perineural invasion by itself in radical prostatectomy specimens does not worsen prognosis because perineural invasion merely represents extension of tumor along a plane of decreased resistance and not invasion into lymphatics.

68. Extraprostatic extension preferentially occurs:

(a) Posteriorly (b) Anteriorly
(c) Superiorly (d) Inferiorly

(Answer is A) Extraprostatic extension preferentially occurs posteriorly and posterolaterally, paralleling the location of most adenocarcinomas.

69. The most common route of seminal vesicle invasion is by:

(a) Tumor penetration out of the prostate at the base of the gland, with growth and extension into the peri-seminal vesicle soft tissue
(b) Direct extension through the ejaculatory ducts into the seminal vesicles
(c) Direct extension from the base of the prostate into the wall of the seminal vesicles

(d) Discrete metastases to the seminal vesicle

(Answer is A) The most common route of seminal vesicle invasion is by tumor penetration out of the prostate at the base of the gland, with growth and extension into the peri-seminal vesicle soft tissue and eventually into the seminal vesicles.

70. Following in frequency after lymph nodes and bones, the next most common regions of spread of prostate cancer at autopsy are:

(a) Lung (b) Bladder
(c) Liver (d) Adrenal gland

(Answer is A) Following in frequency after lymph nodes, bones and lung, the next most common regions of spread of prostate cancer at autopsy are bladder, liver and adrenal gland.

71. Which statement regarding Gleason grading is not correct?

(a) The Gleason system is based on the glandular pattern of the tumor as identified at relatively High magnification
(b) In Gleason system 1 being the most differentiated and 5 being the least diffeentiated
(c) Gleason scoring can be improved is by virtually never assigning Gleason score 2 to 4 for adenocarcinoma of the prostate on needle biopsy
(d) Tumors with Gleason score 4 + 3 = 7 have a worse prognosis than those with Gleason score 3 + 4 = 7

(Answer is A) The Gleason system is based on the glandular pattern of the tumor as identified at relatively Low magnification.

72. The likelihood of cancer after an atypical diagnosis on biopsy is:

(a) 6% to 13% (b) 22% to 29%
(c) 32% to 39% (d) 42% to 49%

(Answer is D) The likelihood of cancer after an atypical diagnosis is 42% or 49%, according to the two largest studies from the Mayo Clinic and The Johns Hopkins Hospital, respectively.

73. Incidence of men being biochemically progression-free at 10 years after radical prostatectomy with seminal vesicle invasion and lymph node metastasis respectively is:

(a) 60% and 45% (b) 45% and 30%
(c) 30% and 15% (d) 25% and 0%

(Answer is D) Only 25% of men with seminal vesicle invasion and none with lymph node metastases are biochemically progression-free at 10 years after radical prostatectomy, with grade and in some studies margins of resection influencing prognosis.

74. Which parameter in the radical prostatectomy specimen does not independently predict postsurgical progression?

(a) Tumor volume (b) Grade
(c) Pathological stage (d) Margins

(Answer is A) Tumor volume measured in the radical prostatectomy specimen does not independently predict postsurgical progression once grade, pathologic stage, and margins are accounted for and should not be required for routine pathologic analysis.

75. Which statement regarding histological variant of prostate cancer is not correct?

(a) Most prostatic duct adenocarcinomas are advanced stage at presentation and have an aggressive course
(b) Small cell carcinoma account for the majority of prostatic tumors with clinically evident ACTH or ADH production
(c) Rhabdomyosarcoma is the most frequent mesenchymal tumor within the prostate and is seen almost exclusively in childhood
(d) Squamous cell tumors develop osteoblastic metastases, respond to estrogen therapy, and develop elevated serum acid phosphatase levels with metastatic disease

(Answer is D) Squamous cell tumors develop osteolytic metastases, do not respond to estrogen therapy, and do not develop elevated serum acid phosphatase levels with metastatic disease.

76. Absence of which marker is specifc for prostate adenocarcinoma?

(a) CK7 (b) CK22
(c) 34βEI2 (d) Thrombomodulin

(Answer is C) The most specific is high-molecular-weight cytokeratin (34βE12), which is negative in prostate adenocarcinoma.

77. Which statement regarding endorectal probes used for TRUS is not true?

(a) The commonly used 7 MHz transducer produces a high resolution image
(b) Focal ranges from 1 to 4 cm with the 7 MHz transducer
(c) Lower frequency transducers improve anterior delineation of large glands, increasing the accuracy of volume measurements
(d) High frequency transducer provides poor internal architecture

(Answer is D) Lower frequency transducers improve anterior delineation of large glands, increasing the accuracy of volume measurements, but provide poor internal architecture.

78. Which statement regarding prostate cancer on conventional gray-scale TRUS is not true?

(a) Nearly 39% of all cancers are isoechoic
(b) A hypoechoic lesion i s malignant in 57% to 87% of cases
(c) Only 1% of tumors may be hyperechoic
(d) 7 MHz transducer is best to detect PZ cancer

(Answer is B) A hypoechoic lesion is malignant in 17% to 57% of cases.

79. Which statement regarding prostate cancer biopsy is not true?

(a) NSAIDs should be stopped 7 to 10 days before prostate biopsy
(b) Oral fluoroquinolone is given 30 to 60 minutes before biopsy and continued for 2 to 3 days
(c) The use of a second prostate biopsy in all cases of a negative finding on initial biopsy is not justified
(d) 18 gauge needle core biopsy device or biopsy gun, is most often used

(Answer is C) The use of a second prostate biopsy in all cases of a negative finding on initial biopsy appears justified. Third and fourth repeat biopsies, however, should only be obtained in very selected patients with high suspicion of cancer and /or poor prognostic factors on the first or second biopsy.

80. Which is the most common complication seen after prostate biopsy?

(a) Bleeding
(b) Infection
(c) Vasovagal syncope
(d) Acute urinary retention

(Answer is A) Even with normal coagulation parameters, bleeding is the most common complication seen after prostate biopsy.

81. Kallikerin gene is located on which chromosome?

(a) 13 (b) 15
(c) 17 (d) 19

(Answer is D) Located on the long arm of chromosome 19 within the region spanning q13.2-q13.4.

82. Regarding hK2 which statement is true?

(a) Elevated in well differentiated prostate cancer
(b) Elevated in poorly differentiated prostate cancer
(c) Low levels in poorly differentiated prostate cancer

(d) Low levels in well differentiated prostate cancer

(Answer is B) hK2 levels have been shown to be elevated in poorly differentiated prostate cancer.

83. Which statement regarding PSA is not true?

(a) The serum half-life of PSA, calculated after removal of all prostate tissue, is 2 to 3 days
(b) Uncomplexed PSA is cleared from the serum within 2 to 3 hours and is probably excreted by the kidney because of its smaller size
(c) Prostate cancer cells make less PSA than normal prostatic tissue
(d) Binding of free PSA to ACT inactivates the protease, and complex PSA-ACT remains undetectable by current assays

(Answer is D) Binding of free PSA to ACT inactivates the protease, but the complex PSA-ACT remains immunodetectable by current assays.

84. In men without BPH, the rate of change in PSA is:

(a) 0.02 ng/ml per year
(b) 0.04 ng/ml per year
(c) 0.06 ng/ml per year
(d) 0.08 ng/ml per year

(Answer is B) In men without BPH, the rate of change in PSA is 0.04 ng/ml per year.

85. Regarding factors influencing the serum level of PSA which statement is not true?

(a) Prostatic inflammation (acute and chronic) and urinary retention can cause PSA elevations
(b) Prostatic biopsy can result in a leak of PSA into the circulation that may require more than 8 weeks for return to baseline values
(c) After 48 hours of ejaculation, increase in PSA would be expected to return to baseline levels in most men
(d) 5α-reductase inhibitors for treatment of BPH have been shown to lower PSA levels by an average of 50% after 6 months

(Answer is B) Prostatic biopsy can result in a leak of PSA into the circulation that may require more than 4 weeks for return to baseline values.

86. All *except* one statement is true regarding prostate cancer:

(a) PSAD greater than 0.15 has been suggested as discriminatory for the presence of cancer
(b) PSA velocity more than 0.75 ng/ml per year was a specific marker for the presence of prostate cancer
(c) Free/total PSA cutoff of 0.18 significantly improved the ability to distinguish between subjects with and without cancer
(d) Minimal follow-up time over which changes in PSA should be adjusted for PSA velocity is 12 months

(Answer is D) Minimal follow-up time over which changes in PSA should be adjusted for PSA velocity to be useful in cancer detection has been calculated in separate studies to be 18 months.

87. In prostate which is more commonly expressed in benign epithelial and cancerous tissue respectively?

(a) hK2 in both
(b) PSA in both
(c) hK2 in benign and PSA in cancerous tissue
(d) PSA in benign and hK2 in cancerous tissue

(Answer is D) In benign epithelium, PSA is intensely expressed compared with the minimal immunoreactivity of hK2. In contrast, in cancerous tissue more intense expression of hK2 is seen.

88. PSMA has been identified in all *except:*

(a) Central nervous system
(b) Intestine
(c) Prostate
(d) Urinary bladder

(Answer is D) PSMA has been identified in central nervous system, intestine and prostate.

89. Expression of which marker in biopsy tissue may provide 97% sensitivity and 100% specificity for prostate cancer detection?

(a) α-Methylacyl coenzyme A racemase
(b) UROC28
(c) DD3PCA3
(d) NMP 48

(Answer is A) AMACR expression in biopsy tissue may provide 97% sensitivity and 100% specificity for prostate cancer detection.

90. Detection rate for carcinoma prostate is maximum when:

(a) DRE alone is used
(b) PSA and TRUS is used
(c) DRE and PSA is used
(d) DRE and TRUS is used

(Answer is C) When DRE and PSA are used as screening tests for prostate cancer detection, detection rates are higher with PSA than with DRE and highest with a combination of the two tests.

91. Which statement regarding prostate cancer is not correct?

(a) The pathologic features of prostate cancers detected with PSA testing are more favorable than those of cancers detected without PSA testing
(b) When a PSA cutoff of 4 ng/ml and an abnormal DRE were used together as screening criteria, pathologically organ-confined disease was found in 50% of men
(c) Addition of PSA testing to DRE leads to detection of a greater proportion of pathologically confined cancers compared with cancer detection by DRE alone
(d) With the widespread use of PSA, a stage shift favoring localized disease occurred because PSA increases the lead time for prostate cancer detection

(Answer is B) When a PSA cutoff of 4 ng/ ml and an abnormal DRE were used together as screening criteria, pathologically organ-confined disease was found in 71% of men.

92. Which test has the highest positive predictive value for prostate cancer?

(a) DRE (b) PSA
(c) TRUS (d) MRI

(Answer is B) If serum PSA is elevated, a greater proportion of men actually have cancer found at biopsy when compared with an abnormality on DRE or TRUS. Thus, an elevated PSA level has the highest positive predictive value for prostate cancer. In addition, whereas DRE and TRUS are dependent on the examiner, PSA is an objective measure of prostate cancer risk.

93. The American Cancer Society and the AUA recommend that prostate cancer screening be offered annually beginning at age:

(a) 45 years (b) 50 years
(c) 55 years (d) 60 years

(Answer is B) The American Cancer Society and the AUA recommend that prostate cancer screening be offered annually beginning at age 50 years and perhaps earlier for those at higher risk (family history of disease, black).

94. The upper age limit for enrolment in current randomized screening trials of prostate cancer is:

(a) 63 years (b) 74 years
(c) 81 years (d) 85 years

(Answer is B) The upper age limit for enrolment in current randomized screening trials of prostate cancer is 74 years.

95. According to TNM classification 1997 tumor involving more than one lobe is staged as:

(a) T2b (b) T2c
(c) T3a (d) T3b

(Answer is A) T2a–Tumor involves one lobe or less.

T2b–Tumor involved more than one lobe.

96. According to Whitmore classification hormone refractory disease is classified as:

(a) D0 (b) Dl
(c) D2 (d) D3

(Answer is D) D3 hormonal refractory disease.

97. Partin tables are based on all *except:*

(a) Clinical stage
(b) PSA
(c) Gleason score
(d) Number of cores positive

(Answer is D) Combination of prostate-specific antigen, clinical stage, and Gleason Score to predict pathologic stage of localized prostate cancer is Partin tables.

98. Incidence of pelvic lymph node involvement in patients with PSA greater than 20 ng/ml and 50 ng/ml respectively is:

(a) 5% and 20% (b) 20% and 50%
(c) 20% and 75% (d) 30 and 75%

(Answer is C) 20% of men with PSA greater than 20 ng/ml and 75% of those with PSA greater than 50 ng/ml are found to have pelvic lymph node involvement.

99. Bone survey films (skeletal radiography), require how much bone density to be replaced with tumor before they can identify distant spread?

(a) 20% (b) 40%
(c) 50% (d) 75%

(Answer is C) Bone survey films (skeletal radiography), which require more than 50% of the bone density to be replaced with tumor before they can identify distant spread.

100. As compare to Retropubic RP which is not true regarding perineal RP is:

(a) Less blood loss
(b) Longer operative time
(c) No access to lymph nodes
(d) Higher postoperative fecal incontinence

(Answer is B) The perineal approach is usually associated with less blood loss and a shorter operative time than the retropubic approach. The disadvantages are that it does not provide access for a pelvic lymph node dissection, there is a higher rate of rectal injury, and there is occasional postoperative fecal incontinence that does not occur commonly with other approaches.

101. After RP biochemical recurrence usually precedes:

(a) Clinical metastases by 3 years and cancer-specific mortality by about 5 years
(b) Clinical metastases by 5 years and cancer-specific mortality by about 8 years
(c) Clinical metastases by 8 years and cancer-specific mortality by about 13 years
(d) Clinical metastases by 13 years and cancer-specific mortality by about 15 years

(Answer is C) Depending on the Gleason score and the PSA doubling time, biochemical (PSA) evidence of recurrence usually precedes clinical metastases by mean of about 8 years and cancer-specific mortality by about 13 years.

102. The return of urinary continence is associated with:

(a) Age of patient
(b) Pre-op status
(c) Extent of nerve sparing surgery
(d) Era of surgery

(Answer is A) The return of urinary continence is associated with the patient's age.

103. Which statement regarding post-operative complication after RRP is not true?

(a) The return of erectile function after radical retropubic prostatectomy correlates with the age of the patient, preoperative potency status, extent of nerve-sparing surgery, and era of surgery

(b) In most patients erections usually begin to return as partial erections 3 to 6 months after surgery

(c) Maximum erection improvement is reached by-one year

(d) Erection rehabilitation programs using intracavernosal injection therapy or PDE-5 inhibitors might hasten the return of erections

(Answer is C) Erections may continue to improve for up to 3 years or more.

104. Which statement regarding complications after RP is not correct?

(a) To prevent thromboembolic and cardio-vascular events it is advisable routinely to use support stockings and to ensure early ambulation

(b) Without obturator nerve repair patients will have a significant thigh adductor deficit after the injury

(c) Rectal injury can occur and be repaired primarily by a multiple-layer closure

(d) Ureteral injury is a rare complication. A minor injury or ligation can be managed with removal of the ligature and ureteral stenting

(Answer is B) Inadvertent injury to the obturator nerve can occur during the pelvic lymphadenectomy. Even without a nerve repair, conservative management with physical therapy can compensate for the deficit, and therefore many patients do not have a significant thigh adductor deficit after the injury.

105. Relative contraindication to brachytherapy and EBRT includes all *except:*

(a) Prior TURP

(b) Inflammatory bowel disease

(c) Severe LUTS

(d) Irritable bowel disease

(Answer is D) Relative contraindication is inflammatory bowel disease, prior TURP and severe LUTS.

106. Which statement regarding PSA bounce is correct?

(a) Usually occurs during first 2 years after treatment and is more common with EBRT than with brachytherapy

(b) Usually occurs during first 2 years after treatment and is less common with EBRT than with brachytherapy

(c) Usually occurs in first year after treatment and is more common with EBRT than with brachytherapy

(d) Usually occurs in first year after treatment and is less common with EBRT than with brachytherapy

(Answer is B) Inflammation in the prostate gland can produce transient PSA elevations, called a PSA "bounce". PSA bounce usually occurs during the first 2 years after treatment and is less common with external beam therapy than with brachytherapy.

107. ASTRO definition includes:

(a) It requires two consecutive PSA increases measured 6 months apart and back-dates the time of cancer progression to halfway between the PSA nadir and the first rising PSA

(b) It requires three consecutive PSA increases measured 6 months apart and back-dates the time of cancer progression to halfway between the PSA nadir and the first rising PSA

(c) It requires two consecutive PSA increases measured 6 months apart and back-dates the time of cancer progression to halfway between the first rising PSA and the second rising PSA

(d) It requires three consecutive PSA increases measured 6 months apart and back-dates the time of cancer progression to halfway between the first rising PSA and the second rising PSA

(Answer is B) ASTRO definition: It requires three consecutive PSA increases measured 6 months apart and back-dates the time of cancer progression to halfway between the PSA nadir and the first rising PSA level.

108. According to phoenix definition of treatment failure is declared when rises to:

(a) 0.5 ng/ml
(b) 1.0 ng/ml
(c) 1.5 ng/ml
(d) 2.0 ng/ml

(Answer is D) Phoenix definition was proposed to replace the ASTRO definition. It eliminates back-dating but requires the PSA level to rise by 2 ng/ml before treatment failure is declared.

109. Which symptoms are more common after brachytherapy than after external beam radiotherapy?

(a) Urinary symptoms
(b) Erectile dysfunction
(c) Urinary symptoms and erectile dysfunction
(d) Proctitis and rectal injury

(Answer is C) Urinary symptoms are more common after brachytherapy than after external beam radiotherapy, especially in patients with prostatic hyperplasia. Proctitis and rectal injury are less common with brachytherapy than with external beam therapy, whereas erectile dysfunction occurs more commonly with brachytherapy than with external beam radiation.

110. Adjuvant radiotherapy after RP is most likely to benefit patients with:

(a) Negative surgical margins
(b) Extracapsular tumor extension without seminal vesicle invasion
(c) Extracapsular tumor extension with seminal vesicle invasion
(d) Lymph node involvement present

(Answer is B) Adjuvant radiotherapy after RP is most likely to benefit patients with positive surgical margins or extracapsular tumor extension without seminal vesicle invasion or lymph node involvement.

111. Patients most likely to have favorable responses to salvage radiotherapy are all these *except:*

(a) PSA <0.5 ng/ml
(b) PSA recurrence long after surgery
(c) Fast growing PSA level
(d) No seminal vesicle invasion or lymph node metastases

(Answer is C) If salvage radiotherapy is planned, it should be initiated before the PSA level rises much above 0.5 ng/ml. Patients most likely to have favorable responses to salvage radiotherapy are those with PSA recurrence long after surgery, slowly rising PSA level, low-grade tumor, and no seminal vesicle invasion or lymph node metastases.

112. Which statement is not true regarding watchful waiting?

(a) Aim is to avoid treatment
(b) Patients with any PSA any Gleason grade and any T stage can be candidates
(c) Treatment intent is palliative
(d) Treatment timing is delayed

(Answer is B) Any T stage, GS = 7, any PSA are candidates for watchful waiting.

113. Which statement is not true regarding active surveillance?

(a) Aim is to individualize treatment
(b) Treatment timing is early
(c) Treatment intent is palliative
(d) Indication for treatment is short PSADT

(Answer is C)

	Active Surveillance (AS)	*Watchful Waiting (WW)*
Aim	To individualize treatment	To avoid treatment
Patient characteristics	Fit for radical treatment with LE > 15 years	LE < 15 years
Tumor characteristics	**T1-T2, PSA <15 ng/ml, GS < 7**	**Any T stage, any PSA GS < 7**
Monitoring	Frequent PSA testing and biopsies	PSA and repeat biopsies unimportant
Indications for treatment	Short PSADT or increase in stage on biopsy	Symptomatic progression
Treatment timing	Early	Delayed
Treatment intent	Radical	Palliative

114. Kattan nomogram for prostate cancer includes all *except:*

(a) Post treatment PSA
(b) Secondary biopsy Gleason grade
(c) Mm of cancer
(d) Mm of non-cancer

(Answer is A) Pre treatment PSA is prognostic factor not post treatment PSA.

115. Intermediate-risk localized prostate cancer is classified as:

(a) PSA between 0 and 10 ng/ml, Gleason score 7, or clinical stage T2b
(b) PSA between 10 and 20 ng/ml, Gleason score 7, or clinical stage T2b
(c) PSA between 10 and 20 ng/ml, Gleason score 8, or clinical stage T2b
(d) PSA between 10 and 20 ng/ml, Gleason score 7, or clinical stage T2a

(Answer is B) Intermediate-risk localized prostate cancer (PSA between 10 and 20 ng/ml, Gleason score 7, or clinical stage T2b).

116. Surgery is deferred for how many weeks after needle biopsy of the prostate and after transurethral resection of the prostate?

(a) 4 to 6 weeks and 12 weeks respectively
(b) 6 to 8 weeks and 8 weeks respectively
(c) 6 to 8 weeks and 12 weeks respectively
(d) 8 to 12 weeks and 16 weeks respectively

(Answer is C) Surgery is deferred for 6 to 8 weeks after needle biopsy of the prostate and 12 weeks after transurethral resection of the prostate.

117. Prostate receives its blood supply mainly from:

(a) Superior vesical artery
(b) Inferior vesical artery
(c) Obturator artery
(d) Inferior gluteal artery

(Answer is B) The prostate receives arterial blood supply from the inferior vesical artery.

118. Which vessels serve as macroscopic landmark to aid in the identification of the microscopic branches of the pelvic plexus?

(a) Capsular arteries (b) Urethral arteries
(c) Pudendal artery (d) Cavernosal artery

(Answer is A) On histologic examination, the capsular arteries and veins are surrounded by an extensive network of nerves. These capsular vessels provide the macroscopic landmark to aid in the identification of the microscopic branches of the pelvic plexus that innervate the corpora cavernosa.

119. Which nerve provides the major nerve supply to the striated sphincter and levator ani?

(a) Pudendal nerve
(b) Obturator nerve
(c) Cavernosal nerve
(d) Neurovascular bundle

(Answer is A) The pudendal nerve provides the major nerve supply to the striated sphincter and levator ani.

120. The prostate receives its blood supply and autonomic innervation between the layers of:

(a) Denonvilliers' fascia and levator fascia
(b) Denonvilliers' fascia and prostatic fascia
(c) Prostatic fascia and levator fascia
(d) Anterior layer of Denonvilliers' fascia and posterior layer of Denonvilliers' fascia

(Answer is C) The prostate receives its blood supply and autonomic innervation between the layers of the levator fascia and prostatic fascia.

121. During radical prostatectomy:

(a) Both puboprostatic and pubourethral ligament are ligated
(b) Both puboprostatic and pubourethral ligament are left intact
(c) Puboprostatic ligament is remained intact and pubourethral ligament is ligated
(d) Pubourethral ligament is remained intact and puboprostatic ligament is ligated

(Answer is D) The pubourethral component of the complex must remain intact to preserve the anterior fixation of the striated urethral sphincter to the pubis.

122. Most common site for positive surgical margin after radical prostatectomy is:

(a) Neurovascular bundle
(b) Apex of prostate
(c) Posterior wall of prostate
(d) Posterolateral wall of prostate

(Answer is B) Neurovascular bundle is not the most common site for positive margins. Rather, the most common site is the apex, followed by posterior and then posterolateral.

123. If there is troublesome bleeding from the dorsal vein complex at any point, the surgeon should:

(a) Immediate blood tranfusions and abandon surgery
(b) Place 24 fr Foley catheter and apply traction
(c) Ligate internal iliac artery
(d) Completely divide the dorsal vein complex over the urethra

(Answer is D) If there is troublesome bleeding from the dorsal vein complex at any point, the surgeon should completely divide the dorsal vein complex over the urethra and oversew the end. This is the single best means to control bleeding from the dorsal vein complex. Any maneuver short of this only worsens the bleeding.

124. Which statement regarding bladder neck contracture after radical prostatectomy is not true?

(a) Bladder neck contractures occur in less than 10% of patients after radical prostatectomy
(b) They may arise from urinary extravasation
(c) The use of a Babcock clamp to approximate the bladder neck and urethra while the anastomotic sutures are tied has virtually eliminated bladder neck contractures
(d) Cold-knife incision of the bladder neck at 5 and 7 O'clock followed by intermittent self-catheterization for a limited time usually corrects the problem

(Answer is D) They arise from inadequate coaptation of the mucosal surfaces. This may be due to inadequate approximation at the time of surgery, urinary extravasation, or distraction of the bladder neck from a hematoma. If treatment with simple dilation fails, direct cold-knife incision of the bladder neck at 3, 6 and 9 O'clock followed by intermittent self-catheterization for a limited time usually corrects the problem.

125. Which statement regarding salvage prostatectomy is not true?

(a) Salvage prostatectomy is reserved for patients with excellent health and with a life expectancy of more than 15 years
(b) Patients must have no evidence of metastatic disease
(c) Salvage surgery should be offered only to men who at initial presentation had unequivocally clinically localized or locally advanced prostate cancer
(d) Prostate biopsy, histologic grade, clinical

examination findings, and serum PSA levels must be done before salvage prostatectomy

(Answer is C) Salvage surgery should be offered only to men who at initial presentation had unequivocally clinically localized prostate cancer.

126. Which complication is decreased with increasing experience in salvage prostatectomy?

(a) Blood loss
(b) Total incontinence
(c) Rectal injury
(d) Erectile dysfunction

(Answer is C) Summary of the published literature regarding salvage prostatectomy demonstrates that the length of hospital stay has dropped from 13 days to 3.2 days, mean estimated blood loss has remained stable around 1000 ml, overall incontinence (stress, total) rates have remained stable at nearly 50% and total incontinence rates have remained stable at 20% to 30%, rectal injury has decreased from 30% to nearly 6%, and bladder neck contracture has remained constant at 20% to 30%. Erectile dysfunction is nearly universal.

127. Who described the first radical perineal prostatectomy for treatment of prostate cancer?

(a) Walsh (b) Millin
(c) Freyer (d) Young

(Answer is D) Hugh Hampton Young described the first radical perineal prostatectomy for treatment of cancer in 1905.

128. Which statement regarding perineal RP is not correct?

(a) With perineal approach potency rate is comparable to that with RRP
(b) Perineal approach offers poor visualization of the urethral dissection and anastomosis, resulting in poor urinary continence
(c) Perineal prostatectomy demonstrates the proven long-term cancer control of RRP with low morbidity, rapid convalescence
(d) Perineal prostatectomy demonstrates lower operative times and lower hospital costs than with RRP

(Answer is B) Perineal approach offers unmatched visualization of the urethral dissection and anastomosis, resulting in excellent urinary continence.

129. Which statement regarding perineal RP is not correct?

(a) A nerve-sparing approach is accomplished for most of these patients
(b) A laparoscopic pelvic lymphadenectomy is deemed unnecessary if the biopsy Gleason score is below 7 and the serum PSA level is less than 10 ng/m
(c) When it is required, the laparoscopic lymphadenectomy is usually carried out immediately before prostatectomy
(d) Patients with common degenerative disk disease is contraindication to positioning

(Answer is D) Patients with severe ankylosis of the hips or spine and those with unstable artificial hip replacements may not tolerate the exaggerated lithotomy position. However, common degenerative disk disease is not a contraindication to positioning.

130. Contraindications to minimally invasive laparoscopic prostatectomy is:

(a) Uncorrectable bleeding diatheses
(b) Patients with a history of prior complex lower abdominal/pelvic surgery
(c) Patients with a history of prior transurethral resection of the prostate
(d) Morbid obesity with large prostate size (e.g., > 100 g)

(Answer is A) Contraindications to minimally invasive laparoscopic prostatectomy include uncorrectable bleeding diatheses or the inability to undergo general anesthesia due to severe cardiopulmonary compromise. Patients with a history of prior complex lower abdominal/pelvic surgery, morbid obesity, large prostate size (e.g., >100 g), prior pelvic irradiation, neoadjuvant hormonal therapy, or prior prostate surgery (e.g., transurethral resection of the prostate) are more challenging, but these features are not by themselves contraindications for laparoscopic or robotic prostatectomy.

131. There is greater risk of ongoing bleeding with the retrograde technique because:

(a) Both DVC and prostate pedicle is divided early in the operation
(b) Both DVC and prostate pedicle is divided late in the operation
(c) DVC is divided early in the operation and the prostatic pedicles late
(d) DVC is divided late in the operation and the prostatic pedicles early

(Answer is C) Because the DVC is divided early in the operation and the prostatic pedicles late, there is potentially a greater risk of ongoing bleeding with the retrograde technique.

132. Which statement regarding laparoscopic radical prostatectomy with extraperitoneal approach is not correct?

(a) Little or no difference in operative time and perioperative outcomes between transperitoneal and extraperitoneal approaches
(b) With the extraperitoneal approach, the peritoneum acts as a natural barrier, minimizing the potential for bowel injury and preventing the bowels from falling into the operative field and obscuring the surgeon's view
(c) Extraperitoneal approach helps to confine any urine leak that may occur from the vesicourethral anastomosis within the extraperitoneal space
(d) Extraperitoneal approach provides relatively larger working space

(Answer is D) One limitation with the extraperitoneal approach is the reduced working space as compared with the relatively larger working space of the peritoneal cavity gained with transperitoneal access.

133. LRP and RALP are better than open RP in:

(a) Operative time
(b) Pain
(c) Blood loss
(d) Hospital stay

(Answer is C) Because most of the blood loss that occurs during radical prostatectomy is from venous sinuses, the tamponade effect from the pneumoperitoneum helps diminish ongoing blood loss during LRP and RALP.

134. Which statement regarding laparoscopic pelvic lymphadenectomy is not true?

(a) It is deemed unnecessary if the biopsy Gleason score is below 7 and the serum PSA level is less than 10 ng/ml
(b) Usually carried out immediately before or after prostatectomy
(c) Prostatectomy is aborted if the lymph nodes are positive for metastatic disease
(d) With laparoscopic lymph node dissection, postoperative lymphoceles is very common

(Answer is D) With laparoscopic lymph node dissection, postoperative lymphoceles are less common.

135. PLND is to be performed under which circumstances?

(a) On DRE only one lobe is involved
(b) PSA of 8 ng/ml
(c) Gleason score of 6
(d) Tumor found in tissue removed at TUR; >5% is cancerous or histologic grade >7

(Answer is A) There are some patients in whom PLND may be unnecessary because of a low risk of nodal metastasis. Most studies show histologic evidence of nodal metastasis in fewer than 5% of patients with good risk features (cT1c, PSA <

10 ng/ml, Gleason score 6). If PLND is planned, it can be performed either before or after dissection of the prostate.

136. Which is likely to suggest malignant prostate after RT?

(a) Longer the time to nadir
(b) Lower the absolute nadir
(c) PSA nadir of 0.4 to 0.5 ng/ml
(d) Earlier the time to nadir

(Answer is D) The longer the time to nadir and the lower the absolute nadir, the more likely it is that only benign prostatic epithelium remains.

137. Optimal time to biopsy after radiotherapy in carcinoma prostate is:

(a) 24 to 30 months (b) 30 to 36 months
(c) 36 to 42 months (d) 42 to 48 months

(Answer is B) Optimal time to biopsy is 30 to 36 months after radiotherapy.

138. Which statement regarding ^{125}I is not correct?

(a) ^{125}I is the most commonly used isotope
(b) ^{125}I emits higher energy X-rays as compare to 103Pd
(c) ^{125}I has a longer half life as compare to ^{103}Pd
(d) Higher activity seeds are required for ^{125}I as compare to ^{103}Pd to deliver a similar tumoricidal dose

(Answer is D) ^{125}I is the most commonly used isotope. ^{125}I emits low-energy X-rays at 27 keV with a half-life of 59.6 days. The radiation from palladium has an energy spectrum similar to that of ^{125}I, with 21 keV X-rays, but with a significantly shorter half-life of 17 days. Therefore, higher activity seeds are required for ^{103}Pd versus ^{125}I to deliver a similar tumoricidal dose.

139. Not true regarding strontium therapy is:

(a) Strontium has half life of 50 days
(b) Response rate is approximately 60% to 70%
(c) Duration of response is 2 to 3 years
(d) Toxicity is mainly hematological

(Answer is C) Response duration is only 6 months.

140. Temperatures required to completely destroy cells in carcinoma prostate is:

(a) 0°C (b) –20°C
(c) –40°C (d) –178°C

(Answer is C) Complete cell death was unlikely to occur at temperatures higher than –20°C, and temperatures lower than –40°C were required to completely destroy cells.

141. Factors which will affect most in tissue destruction during cryotherapy:

(a) Velocity of cooling
(b) Velocity of thawing
(c) Lowest temperature achieved
(d) Number of freeze-thaw cycles

(Answer is D) In a clinical setting, the number of freezing cycles, the lowest temperature achieved, and the existence of any regional "heat sinks" may be important factors relating to cancer destruction. Double freeze-thaw cycles during cryotherapy for prostate cancer in humans have been associated with lower positive biopsy rates, as well as improved PSA results, when compared with a single freeze-thaw cycle, without an increase in the development of cryotherapy-related morbidities.

142. Primary cryotherapy is suitable for patients with:

(a) Clinical stage T1c-T4 disease of any tumor grade
(b) Clinical stage T1c-T3 disease with grade less than and equal to 9
(c) Clinical stage T1c-T4 disease with grade less than and equal to 9
(d) Clinical stage T1c-T3 disease of any tumor grade

(Answer is D) Primary cryotherapy is suitable for patients with clinical stage T1c-T3 disease of any tumor grade who are not potent or not interested in maintaining their potency. If the prostate size exceeds 50 cm^3, complete freezing of the prostate may be difficult and neoadjuvant hormone therapy is indicated to reduce the target volume and allow for more effective cryotherapy.

143. In cryotherapy freezing is started from:

(a) Laterally (b) Posteriorly
(c) Anterioly (d) Superiorly

(Answer is C) To maintain TRUS visibility, the freezing is started at the anterior probe layer and continued posteriorly.

144. Candidates which were unlikely to be successfully salvaged by cryotherapy are:

(a) PSA > 10 ng/ml and GS of the recurrent cancer greater than or equal to 9
(b) PSA >20 ng/ml and GS of the recurrent cancer greater than or equal to 9
(c) PSA > 10 ng/ml and GS of the recurrent cancer of 10
(d) PSA >20 ng/ml and GS of the recurrent cancer of 10

(Answer is A) PSA greater than 10 ng/ml and Gleason score of the recurrent cancer greater than or equal to 9 were unlikely to be successfully salvaged .

145. Most common complication after cryotherapy is:

(a) Urinary incontinence
(b) Erectile dysfunction
(c) Rectourethral fistula
(d) Urethral sloughing

(Answer is B) Erectile dysfunction after cryotherapy of the prostate is common. Although some series have reported rates ranging from 40% to 47%, more contemporary series report rates of more than 80%.

146. Which pathological parameter has highest risk of progression after radical prostatectomy?

(a) Seminal vesicle invasion
(b) LN involvement
(c) Extracapsular extension
(d) Positive surgical margins

(Answer is D) In multivariate analysis, pathologic parameters increasing the relative risk (RR) for progression included extracapsular extension (RR, 2.17 to 2.72), seminal vesicle involvement (RR, 2.61), and lymph node involvement (RR, 3.31). The presence of a positive surgical margin was associated with the greatest relative risk (4.37; range, 2.90 to 6.58).

147. Which statement regarding hormone therapy is correct?

(a) Estradiol is a thousand-fold more potent at suppressing LH and FSH compared with testosterone
(b) Estradiol is a ten-fold more potent at suppressing LH and FSH compared with testosterone
(c) Testosterone is a thousand-fold more potent at suppressing LH and FSH compared with estradiol
(d) Testosterone is a ten-fold more potent at suppressing LH and FSH compared with estradiol

(Answer is A) The first central inhibition of the axis exploited the potent negative feedback of estrogen on luteinizing hormone (LH) secretion. It is now known that estradiol is a thousand-fold more potent at suppressing LH and follicle-stimulating hormone (FSH) secretion by the pituitary compared with testosterone.

148. Which is the classic steroidal anti-androgen?

(a) Cyproterone (b) Leuprolide
(c) Ketoconazole (d) Flutamide

(Answer is A) Cyproterone Acetate is the classic steroidal antiandrogen with direct androgen receptor-blocking effects.

149. Which statement regarding nonsteroidal antiandrogen is not correct?

(a) Have no antigonadotropic effects
(b) Produce a paradoxical increase in LH and testosterone
(c) Peripheral conversion of this excessive testosterone to estrogen can lead to painful gynecomastia
(d) Block androgen action at the cellular level and also reduce circulating testosterone levels

(Answer is D) Steroidal antiandrogens block androgen action at the cellular level and also reduce circulating testosterone levels, leading to the classic side effects of hypogonadal state, such as loss of libido and erectile dysfunction.

150. Which statement regarding androgen withdrawal phenomenon is not correct?

(a) Declines in PSA level are seen within 4 to 6 weeks
(b) Between 15% and 30% of patients may have declines in PSA level of more than 50%
(c) Overall survival has been shown to be increased in those demonstrating the antiandrogen withdrawal phenomenon compared with those who have not
(d) Those with rapid PSA responses after androgen ablation have higher rates of antiandrogen withdrawal phenomenon

(Answer is C) Overall survival has not been shown to be increased in those demonstrating the antiandrogen withdrawal phenomenon compared with those who have not.

151. Which statement regarding bicalutamide is not true?

(a) Bicalutamide is non-steroidal antiandrogen with a long serum half-life (6 days)
(b) Bicalutamide is the most potent and the better tolerated antiandrogen
(c) The *S* isomer of bicalutamide has about a 30-fold higher binding affinity to the androgen receptor compared with the *R* isomer
(d) The pharmacokinetics of bicalutamide are not affected by age, renal insufficiency, or moderate hepatic impairment

(Answer is C) The *R* isomer of bicalutamide has about a 30-fold higher binding affinity to the androgen receptor compared with the *S* isomer.

152. Which statement regarding bicalutamide monotherapy is not true?

(a) Bicalutamide monotherapy at a dose of 50 mg/day was inferior to castration in survival of men with metastatic disease
(b) Dose of 150 mg/day, bicalutamide monotherapy appears to have efficacy equivalent to that of castration in men with metastatic or locally advanced disease
(c) Bicalutamide monotherapy with 150 mg/day had significantly better quality of life in the domains of sexual interest and physical capacity
(d) Men with low-risk, localized prostate cancer, bicalutamide was associated with improved survival compared with those on watchful waiting

(Answer is D) Men with low-risk, localized prostate cancer, bicalutamide was associated with significantly worse overall survival compared with those on watchful waiting.

153. Which antiandrogen is associated with delayed adaptation to darkness after exposure to bright illumination?

(a) Flutamide (b) Bicalutamide
(c) Cyproterone (d) Nilutamide

(Answer is D) About one quarter of men receiving nilutamide therapy will note a delayed adaptation to darkness after exposure to bright illumination.

154. Which statement regarding flare phenomenon with LHRH agonist is not correct?

(a) The initial exposure to more potent agonists of LHRH results in a flare of LH (10 times) and testosterone levels
(b) Can result in a severe, life-threatening exacerbation of symptoms
(c) Co-administration of an antiandrogen functionally blocks the increased levels of testosterone
(d) Co-administration of antiandrogens is required for only 1 to 2 days

(Answer is D) Given the predictable length of the flare phenomenon, co-administration of anti-androgens is required for only 21 to 28 days.

155. Abarelix is:

(a) Antiandrogen
(b) LHRH antagonist
(c) LHRH agonist
(d) Inhibition of androgen synthesis

(Answer is B) LHRH antagonist abarelix.

156. Which statement regarding LHRH antagonist is not correct?

(a) The LHRH antagonists bind immediately and competitively to the LHRH receptors in the pituitary
(b) The direct antagonistic activity eliminates the LH and testosterone flare
(c) No need for antiandrogen co-administration
(d) Severe allergic reactions does not occur, after previously uneventful treatment

(Answer is D) Severe allergic reactions can occur even after previously uneventful treatment.

157. Which statement regarding ADT is not true?

(a) 3 months of neoadjuvant ADT before radical prostatectomy improves biochemical outcomes
(b) There is considerable evidence that ADT combined with external beam radiation therapy improves overall survival
(c) The benefit of ADT appears to be in men with locally advanced disease or those with high-grade, high-risk disease
(d) Combined androgen blockade with non-steroidal antiandrogens provides about a 3% survival benefit at 5 years compared with standard ADT

(Answer is A) There is no evidence that 3 months of neoadjuvant ADT before radica l prostatectomy improves biochemical outcomes.

158. Which statement regarding ADT is not true?

(a) There is no overall survival benefit to immediate ADT in low-risk, localized prostate cancer
(b) In locally advanced, asymptomatic metastatic, immediate ADT results in significantly better overall survival
(c) In N+ disease without primary treatment, there is no significant advantage to immediate ADT
(d) In N+ disease with radical prostatectomy, there is a significant survival advantage favoring immediate ADT

(Answer is B) In locally advanced, asymptomatic-metastatic, immediate ADT results in significantly better prostate cancer-specific survival but not better overall survival.

159. Progression-free and overall survival figures of patients with metastatic disease with various methods of ADT have ranged from:

(a) 6 to 12 months and 24 to 36 months, respectively
(b) 12 to 20 months and 20 to 24 months, respectively
(c) 12 to 20 months and 24 to 36 months, respectively
(d) 20 to 24 months and 24 to 36 months, respectively

(Answer is C) Progression-free and overall survival figures of patients with metastatic disease with various methods of ADT have ranged from 12 to 20 months and 24 to 36 months, respectively.

160. In patients with hormone-refractory prostate cancer which drug has not been used?

(a) Bleomycin (b) Estramustine
(c) Etoposide (d) 5-Fluorouracil

(Answer is A) Bleomycin has not been tried for HRPC.

161. Agent of choice for HRPC:

(a) Mitoxantrone (b) Docetaxel
(c) Extramustine (d) Prednisone

(Answer is B) Docetaxel has become the agent of choice as of 2004 on the basis of a large phase III randomized trial, TAX 327 which demonstrated its superiority to the past standard, mitoxantrone and prednisone.

162. Which toxicity was most noticeable in the every 3-week versus weekly docetaxel arms?

(a) Hematological
(b) Nausea and vomiting
(c) Fatigue, nail changes, hyperlacrimation
(d) Diarrhea

(Answer is A) Toxicity in the every 3-week versus weekly docetaxel arms was notable for more hematological toxicity in the every 3-week arm (3% neutropenic fever versus 0%, and 32% grade 3-4 neutropenia versus 1.5%) but slightly lower rates of nausea and vomiting, fatigue, nail changes, hyperlacrimation, and diarrhea. Neuropathy was slightly mpre common in the every 3-week arm (grade 3-4 in 1.8% versus 0.9%).

163. All *except* one are the clinical characteristics of neuroendocrine subtype of carcinoma of prostate:

(a) Lytic bone metastasis
(b) Frequent brain metastasis
(c) Very high serum PSA
(d) Elevated plasma chromogranin levels

(Answer is C) Low serum PSA is characteristic of neuroendocine tumors.

164. Which is not true regarding intraoperative floppy iris syndrome:

(a) Association with the α1-adrenergic antagonist tamsulosin
(b) α1a is the predominant receptor subtype in the iris dilator muscle as well
(c) Occur until patients have been on tamsulosin therapy for 4 to 6 months
(d) IFIS stops immediately after discontinuation of tamsulosin.

(Answer is D) Intraoperative floppy iris syndrome (IFIS)

- The clinical manifestations are poor preoperative pupil dilation, iris billowing and prolapse, and progressive intraoperative miosis.
- Association with the α1-adrenergic antagonist tamsulosin has become well established.
- α1a is the predominant receptor subtype in the iris dilator muscle as well.
- Occur until patients have been on tamsulosin therapy for 4 to 6 months.

IFIS can also occur up to several years after discontinuation of tamsulosin.

165. Which zone of the prostate originates from the Wolffian duct tissue?

(a) Central zone
(b) Peripheral zone
(c) Transitional zone
(d) Periurethral glands

(Answer is A) Central zone

166. Which part of the prostate is traversed by the ejaculatory duct?

(a) Central zone

(b) Peripheral zone
(c) Transitional zone
(d) Fibromuscular stroma

(Answer is A) Central zone

167. What are the first and second most common zones from where prostate cancers arise?

(a) Central then transitional
(b) Peripheral then transitional
(c) Peripheral then central
(d) Transitional then central

(Answer is B) Peripheral then transitional

168. Which of the following does not increase PSA value?

(a) Trauma to the prostate
(b) Digital rectal examination
(c) Urinary retention
(d) Prostatitis

(Answer is B) Digital rectal examination

169. What is the function of PSA in semen?

(a) Increases semen volume
(b) Has antimicrobial activity
(c) Liquefies the seminal coagulum
(d) Decreases semen pH

(Answer is C) Liquefies the seminal coagulum

170. Which of the prostate medications could result in retrograde ejaculation?

(a) Tamsulosin (b) Doxazosin
(c) Dutasteride (d) Alfuzosin

(Answer is A) Tamsulosin

171. Which of the prostate medications could result in significant hypotension?

(a) Finasteride (b) Prazosin
(c) Silodosin (d) Vardenafil

(Answer is B) Prazosin

172. Which artery(ies) supply(ies) the prostate?

(a) Middle rectal (b) Inferior vesical
(c) A and B (c) None of the above

(Answer is C) A and B

173. What is false concerning PSA molecule?

(a) The free form of PSA exists in small proportions in the body, and found mainly in BPH and in the ejaculate
(b) α1-anti chymotrypsin binds to 3 epitopes of the PSA molecule to form a complexed PSA
(c) α2-macroglobulin binds to 5 epitopes of the PSA molecule to form a complexed PSA
(d) The purified PSA molecule has a molecular weight of 90 kDa

(Answer is D) The purified PSA molecule has a molecular weight of 90 kDa

174. When should a 70 years man with 40 ml prostate volume, and total PSA of 2.0 ng/ml, go for a prostate biopsy?

(a) If PSA reading had exceeded 2.7 ng/ml over 12 months
(b) If free PSA reading was less than 0.4 ng/ml
(c) If total PSA reading was greater than 8 ng/ml
(d) Any of the above

(Answer is D) Any of the above

175. In utero, which hormone stimulates the development of the prostate gland?

(a) Estradiol (b) DHT
(c) FSH (d) Testosterone

(Answer is B) DHT

176. Which α-adrenergic receptor subtype mediates smooth muscle contraction of the prostate?

(a) α1-a (b) α2-a
(c) α1-b (d) α2-b

(Answer is A) α1-a

177. The epithelial component of the prostate consists of all of the following, *except:*

(a) Basal cells
(b) Intermediate cells
(c) Tubulo-columnar cells
(d) Neuroendocrine cells

(Answer is C) Tubulo-columnar cells

178. Which of the following process(es) is (are) reversible?

(a) 5α-reductase enzyme reduces testosterone to DHT
(b) Aromatase enzyme reduces testosterone to estrogen
(c) PSA molecule binds to α1-antichymotrypsin and α2-macroglobulin
(d) None of the above

(Answer is D) None of the above

179. Which of the following does not increase in prostate cancer?

(a) Human kallikrein 2
(b) Pro-PSA
(c) Free PSA
(d) Complexed PSA

(Answer is C) Free PSA

180. What vessels are located in the prostate neurovascular bundle?

(a) Watson plexus
(b) Capsular arteries and veins
(c) Inferior vesical and midrectal vessels
(d) Santorini plexus

(Answer is B) Capsular arteries and veins

181. What fascial layer(s) cover(s) the prostate?

(a) Denonvilliers fascia
(b) Prostatic fascia
(c) Levator fascia
(d) All of the above

(Answer is D) All of the above

182. What is true concerning epithelial and stromal cells in BPH?

(a) There is an increase in the number of epithelial and stromal cells
(b) There is an increase in the size of epithelial and stromal cells
(c) BPH, epithelial to stromal cells ratio is 1:2
(d) All of the above

(Answer is A) There is an increase in the number of epithelial and stromal cells

183. What is false concerning BPH and androgenic hormones?

(a) The most potent androgenic hormones in BPH development is DHT
(b) Type-2 steroid 5 α-reductase, is most commonly found in the prostate
(c) Castrated individuals before puberty will not develop BPH
(d) A man ages, the number of androgen receptors in the prostate decreases

(Answer is D) A man ages, the number of androgen receptors in the prostate decreases

184. What is true regarding BPH and androgens?

(a) A man ages, the responsiveness of prostate cells to androgenic stimuli decreases
(b) Adrenal androgens have no role in BPH development
(c) Type-1 steroid 5 α-reductase is functionally active in the hair follicle
(d) All of the above

(Answer is C) Type-1 steroid 5 α-reductase is functionally active in the hair follicle

185. What is false concerning bladder and prostate histology in BPH?

(a) Obstruction results in bladder smooth muscle hypertrophy and myofibroblasts deposition

(b) BPH occurs chiefly in the transitional zone and periurethral tissues
(c) BPH microscopical changes begin in early thirties
(d) Histologic findings of chronic prostatitis are common in BPH

(Answer is A) Obstruction results in bladder smooth muscle hypertrophy and myofibroblasts deposition

186. What is false regarding BPH genetics?

(a) BPH is an inheritable and progressive disease
(b) Familial BPH presents at an older age when compared to sporadic cases
(c) Approximately 90% of men in their 80s have histologic evidence of BPH
(d) BPH tends to be more severe and progressive in black men when compared to whites

(Answer is B) Familial BPH presents at an older age when compared to sporadic cases

187. What class(es) of medications decrease(s) IPSS questionnaire points?

(a) Calcium channel blockers
(b) Antihistamines
(c) Antidepressants
(d) Cold medications containing pseudo-ephedrine

(Answer is A) Calcium channel blockers

188. What is false concerning IPSS questionnaire?

(a) Specific for prostate symptom
(b) A seven-question, self-administered questionnaire that yields a total score that ranges from 0 to 35
(c) A sum of 20 on IPSS scale is "severe"
(d) Covers both voiding and storage symptomatology

(Answer is A) Specific for prostate symptom

189. What is (are) true concerning IPSS questionnaire?

(a) Focuses on last month's symptoms
(b) Scores of moderate symptoms suggest surgical treatment if the patient's quality of life was poor
(c) Has been validated and translated to many languages
(d) All of the above

(Answer is D) All of the above

190. What is false regarding BPH symptomatology?

(a) The size of the prostate correlates well to the degree of obstruction
(b) A decrease of 3 points in IPSS is associated with a subjective perception of improvement
(c) Median lobe enlargement gives rise to serious obstructive symptoms
(d) Bladder trabeculation is not specific for an obstructing prostate

(Answer is A) The size of the prostate correlates well to the degree of obstruction

191. In BPH patients, total PSA level correlates to:

(a) The glandular component of the prostate
(b) The IPSS questionnaire points
(c) The PVR
(d) The transitional zone volume

(Answer is A) The glandular component of the prostate

192. What is the likelihood that PSA level in men with acute urinary retention due to urethral stricture will decrease after catheterization?

(a) Never (b) Unlikely
(c) Likely (d) Always

(Answer is D) Always

193. IPSS decreases after successful TURP because:

(a) PSA decreases
(b) The prostate size decreases

(c) The complaints resolve
(d) The Q.O.L. improves

(Answer is C) The complaints resolve

194. The probability of developing acute urinary retention is related to:

(a) The neurological status of the patient
(b) PVR
(c) Severity of obstructive LUTS
(d) All of the above

(Answer is D) All of the above

195. Smooth muscle tension in the prostate is mediated by which receptors?

(a) α1-a (b) α1-b
(c) α2-a (d) α2-b

(Answer is A) α1-a

196. A 50% reduction of prostate size is expected after a 6-month therapy with:

(a) Alfuzosin (b) Silodosin
(c) Finasteride (d) Tamsulosin

(Answer is C) Finasteride

197. Open prostatectomy is preferred in treating BPH with:

(a) Sizable bladder stones
(b) Hutch diverticulum
(c) A suspicion of cancer
(d) A and B

(Answer is D) A and B

198. A 55 years male patient with familial BPH, IPSS 9, PSA 23 ng/ml, prostate size 31 cc, PVR 54 cc, on watchful waiting management. Next step should be:

(a) Tamsulosin 0.8 mg
(b) Reassurance
(c) Repeat total and free PSA
(d) Diagnostic cystoscopy

(Answer is C) Repeat total and free PSA

199. An ED patient on low-dose tadalafil develops BPH. What medication should he avoid?

(a) Tamsulosin (b) Alfuzosin
(c) Doxazosin (d) Silodosin

(Answer is C) Doxazosin

200. A BPH patient presents with retention of urine. He is catheterized. Later, he underwent TURP. When would the highest PSA value be?

(a) Before catheterization
(b) After catheterization and before TURP
(c) Immediately after TURP
(d) 2 weeks after TURP

(Answer is C) Immediately after TURP

201. In an 80 years diabetic man on insulin for 35 years, what would be the proper sequence of developing the following obstructing BPH/LUTS?

(a) Frequency, over-flow incontinence, straining, retention
(b) Straining, frequency, over-flow incontinence, retention
(c) Straining, frequency, retention, over-flow incontinence
(d) Frequency, straining, retention, over-flow incontinence

(Answer is D) Frequency, straining, retention, over-flow incontinence

202. What prostatic lobe(s) can be assessed during DRE?

(a) Anterior (b) Median
(c) Left lateral (d) All of the above

(Answer is C) Left lateral

203. Complications related to obstructive BPH/LUTS include all of the following, *except:*

(a) Bladder stones
(b) Prostate cancer
(c) Renal insufficiency

(d) Bladder diverticula

(Answer is B) Prostate cancer

204. BPH patients with severe irritative symptoms or microscopic hematuria should:

(a) For urine cytology testing
(b) For PSA testing
(c) For TRUS
(d) Use anticholinergic medication

(Answer is A) For urine cytology testing

205. Anticholinergic medications work best with BPH patients who have:

(a) Small prostate
(b) Mainly median lobe hypertrophy
(c) History of urinary retention
(d) Mainly irritative symptoms

(Answer is D) Mainly irritative symptoms

206. The most serious drawback of anticholinergic drugs on BPH patients is:

(a) Renal insufficiency
(b) Urinary retention
(c) Dry mouth
(d) Painless hematuria

(Answer is B) Urinary retention

207. In BPH patients, follow up PSA is of value because:

(a) Helps predict the response to 5α-reductase inhibitors
(b) Monitors LUTS/BPH progression
(c) BPH patients are at higher risk of developing prostate cancer
(d) A and B

(Answer is D) A and B

208. In BPH patients, which of the following measures reduces PSA value by one-half?

(a) 2 weeks after performing prostatic urethral lift
(b) 6-month treatment with 5α-reductase inhibitors
(c) After placing a stent in the prostatic urethra
(d) Immediately after removing one-half of the prostate by TURP

(Answer is B) 6-month treatment with 5α-reductase inhibitors

209. Prostatic nodules palpated on DRE might indicate:

(a) Tuberculous prostatitis
(b) Prostatic cancer
(c) Inspissated prostatic abscess
(d) Any of the above

(Answer is D) Any of the above

210. PSA value has a strong correlation with:

(a) IPSS
(b) Post void residual
(c) Prostate volume
(d) Q-max at uroflowmetry

(Answer is C) Prostate volume

211. What cannot be assessed during DRE?

(a) Sacral cord integrity
(b) Pelvic hematoma
(c) Pelvic floor muscle tenderness
(d) Prostatic median lobe hypertrophy

(Answer is D) Prostatic median lobe hypertrophy

212. BPH/LUTS patients when present with mild creatinine elevation, are advised to do:

(a) Total and free PSA
(b) Renal ultrasonography
(c) Creatinine clearance
(d) Uroflowmetry

(Answer is B) Renal ultrasonography

213. In men with obstructive BPH, what will not resolve after TURP?

(a) Bladder trabeculation

(b) Significant PVR
(c) Low peak flow rate
(d) High IPSS

(Answer is A) Bladder trabeculation

214. What is (are) the favorite criterion (criteria) to prescribe 5α-reductase inhibitors for BPH cases?

(a) PSA > 1.5 ng/dl
(b) Prostate volume > 40 ml
(c) IPSS > 19
(d) A and B

(Answer is D) A and B

215. What is (are) the indication(s) to prescribe α-adrenergic inhibitors for BPH patients?

(a) Peak flow rate of ≤ 12 ml/sec
(b) Prostate volume > 40 ml
(c) Psa > 1.5 ng/dl
(d) B and C

(Answer is A) Peak flow rate of ≤ 12 ml/sec

216. What is (are) the indication(s) of upper urinary tract imaging in men with LUTS?

(a) Hematuria
(b) Recurrent urinary tract infection
(c) Renal insufficiency
(d) All of the above

(Answer is D) All of the above

217. In men with LUTS, which of the following is not a compelling indication for upper urinary tract imaging?

(a) Urolithiasis
(b) Receiving chemotherapy
(c) Upper tract surgery
(d) Painless hematuria

(Answer is B) Receiving chemotherapy

218. What drug prevents recurrent gross hematuria secondary to BPH?

(a) Enoxaparin (b) Silodosin
(c) Finasteride (d) Tolterodine

(Answer is C) Finasteride

219. Which statement is false regarding TURP syndrome?

(a) Occurs because of absorption of non-sodium-containing irrigating fluid
(b) Occurs only on using unipolar TURP
(c) Results in brain edema due to dilutional hyponatremia
(d) Positioning the patient in anti-Trendelenburg helps prevent the syndrome

(Answer is D) Positioning the patient in anti-Trendelenburg helps prevent the syndrome

220. What is false concerning TURP syndrome?

(a) Symptoms begin with a serum sodium of less than 120 mEq/l
(b) The mortality is 2.7-5.8%
(c) Manifestations rely on acute changes in the intravascular volume and plasma solute concentrations
(d) The preferred height of irrigating fluid is 60 cm above the patient

(Answer is B) The mortality is 2.7-5.8%

221. What is false concerning needle ablation therapy of the prostate (TUNA)?

(a) Prostate sizes of up to 70 ml can be treated
(b) Not recommended in patients with metallic artificial hip
(c) Retreatment rates are lower than for TURP
(d) Can be performed in an office-based setting

(Answer is C) Retreatment rates are lower than for TURP

222. Transurethral incision of the prostate (TUIP):

(a) Only indicated in small prostates
(b) Complications are related to the amount of lost blood and removed chips

(c) A minimal procedure where no risk of rectal injury or retrograde ejaculation have been reported
(d) Entails making 1 or 2 incisions along all prostate lobes except the apical

(Answer is A) Only indicated in small prostates

223. Which statement is false concerning transurethral microwave therapy (TUMT) for BPH treatment:

(a) Induces nerve degeneration in the prostate and tissue necrosis
(b) Frequently results in transient urinary retention
(c) Frequently leads to erectile dysfunction
(d) The high-energy platform is superior to the low-energy with regard to clinical efficacy

(Answer is C) Frequently leads to erectile dysfunction

224. Which statement is false regarding laser enucleation of the prostate (HoLEP)?

(a) Provides tissue preservation for pathological examination
(b) Treats any size of prostatic adenoma
(c) Follows anatomic planes to remove the prostate in lobes
(d) Urinary incontinence is a significant drawback after HoLEP

(Answer is D) Urinary incontinence is a significant drawback after HoLEP

225. On treating BPH, which procedure provides the best tissue preservation for pathological examination?

(a) TURP (b) TUIP
(c) HoLEP (d) HoLRP

(Answer is C) HoLEP

226. On treating BPH, which procedure carries the risk of morcellator injury to the bladder?

(a) PVP (b) HoLEP
(c) HoLRP (d) TUMT

(Answer is B) HoLEP

227. To achieve better hemostasis in prostate laser surgery, what is the ideal wavelength that is easily absorbed by hemoglobin?

(a) 532 nm (b) 694 nm
(c) 755 nm (d) 1064 nm

(Answer is A) 532 nm

228. What is false regarding prostate embolization for BPH?

(a) The aim is to occlude the internal iliac vessels
(b) There is a considerable radiation risk during the procedure
(c) Bilateral embolization provides better results
(d) Eye protection is not required

(Answer is A) The aim is to occlude the internal iliac vessels

229. What is (are) the possible complication(s) of prostate stents?

(a) Hematuria and infections
(b) Migration and encrustation of the stent
(c) Irritative urinary symptoms and painful ejaculation
(d) All of the above

(Answer is D) All of the above

230. Preferably, what is the last part of the prostate to be removed while performing TURP?

(a) Bladder neck (b) Apex
(c) Median lobe (d) Para-collecular

(Answer is B) Apex

231. How to manage priapism that occurs during endoscopic surgery?

(a) Corporal aspiration

(b) Corpora injection with an α-adrenergic agent
(c) Corpora injection with an α-adrenergic blocker
(d) Treatment required

(Answer is B) Corpora injection with an α-adrenergic agent

232. On measuring the prostate volume during endoscopy:

(a) Each centimeter over the normal 2 cm prostate urethral length equates to an additional 12 g in prostate weight
(b) Each centimeter over the normal 2.5 cm prostate urethral length equates to an additional 10 g in prostate weight
(c) Each centimeter over the normal 2.5 cm prostate urethral length equates to an additional 15 g in prostate weight
(d) Each centimeter over the normal 1.5 cm prostate urethral length equates to an additional 5 g in prostate weight

(Answer is B) Each centimeter over the normal 2.5 cm prostate urethral length equates to an additional 10 g in prostate weight

233. When comparing suprapubic to retropubic prostatectomy for removing prostatic adenoma, the former allows:

(a) Management of concomitant Hutch diverticulum
(b) Removing small bladder stones
(c) Better access to prostatic fossa
(d) Technically, easier trigonization

(Answer is A) Management of concomitant Hutch diverticulum

234. When comparing retropubic to suprapubic prostatectomy for removing prostatic adenoma, the former has the advantage of:

(a) Lesser chance of post-operative urethral stricture
(b) Milder postoperative hematuria
(c) Tension-free bladder closure
(d) Extra-peritoneal approach

(Answer is B) Milder postoperative hematuria

235. When comparing TURP to open prostatectomy for removing prostatic adenoma, the latter has the following advantages, *except:*

(a) Risk of dilutional hyponatremia
(b) Operating on patients with multiple bladder diverticula
(c) Operating on patients who cannot flex their hips and/or knees
(d) Unfavorable tissue preservation for pathological examination

(Answer is D) Unfavorable tissue preservation for pathological examination

236. What is (are) the contraindication(s) to open prostatectomy for prostatic adenoma?

(a) Small fibrous glands
(b) The presence of prostate cancer
(c) Previous prostatectomy
(d) All of the above

(Answer is D) All of the above

237. Robot-assisted laparoscopic prostatectomy for prostatic adenoma has the following advantage over TURP:

(a) Operation cost
(b) Smaller incisions with a shorter hospital stay
(c) Lower risk for blood transfusion
(d) None of the above

(Answer is C) Lower risk for blood transfusion

238. What is the first-line management of uncomplicated LUTS due to large prostate?

(a) α-adrenergic blocker
(b) Combination of α-adrenergic blocker and 5α-reductase inhibitor
(c) Watchful waiting

(d) TURP

(Answer is B) Combination of α-adrenergic blocker and 5α-reductase inhibitor

239. What is the most common cause of LUTS in men beyond middle age?

(a) Urethral stricture
(b) Bladder stones
(c) BPH
(d) Prostatitis syndrome

(Answer is C) BPH

240. What is (are) the indication(s) of antimuscarinic agents and PDE is as adjuncts therapy in BPH cases?

(a) Men with storage symptoms
(b) Men with ED
(c) Failed combination of α-adrenergic blocker and 5α-reductase inhibitor
(d) A and B

(Answer is D) A and B

241. Which statement(s) describe(s) the bladder's response to an obstructing prostate?

(a) May develop detrusor instability with irritative LUTS
(b) May develop poor compliance with frequency and urgency symptoms
(c) May develop poor detrusor contractility with obstructive LUTS
(d) All of the above

(Answer is D) All of the above

242. What is the initial response of the detrusor muscle to obstruction?

(a) Increased intravesical pressure
(b) Increased detrusor pressure
(c) Increase collagen deposition in the detrusor
(d) Detrusor smooth muscle hypertrophy

(Answer is D) Detrusor smooth muscle hypertrophy

243. What is false concerning the pathogenesis of BPH?

(a) Intra-prostatic levels of estrogen decrease in men with BPH
(b) Stimulation of the adrenergic nervous system results in a dynamic increase in prostatic urethral resistance
(c) Inflammation may play a role through cytokines to promote cell growth
(d) Hyperplasia occurs due to an imbalance between cell death and cell proliferation

(Answer is A) Intra-prostatic levels of estrogen decrease in men with BPH

244. In BPH, the etiology of acute urinary retention includes:

(a) Prostatic infarction
(b) Prostate infection
(c) Bladder overdistention
(d) All of the above

(Answer is D) All of the above

245. Which statement best describes the natural history of BPH?

(a) Worsening of LUTS and BPH over time
(b) Patients die of other reasons before serious complications occur
(c) Physically, the space of prostatic fossa limits the gland enlargement
(d) Ultimately, the gland will degenerate and undergo apoptosis

(Answer is A) Worsening of LUTS and BPH over time

246. What is false concerning the diagnosis of BPH?

(a) IPSS cannot be used to establish the diagnosis of BPH/LUTS
(b) Prostate biopsy is essential in diagnosing BPH and excluding cancers
(c) PSA and uroflowmetry help diagnose the condition
(d) None of the above

(Answer is B) Prostate biopsy is essential in diagnosing BPH and excluding cancers

247. What statement is true regarding post-void residual of urine (PVR)?

(a) Nearly all men have PVR of less than 12 ml
(b) Predicts the outcome of surgical treatment
(c) Correlates well with BPH/LUTS
(d) Is diagnostic for bladder outlet obstruction

(Answer is A) Nearly all men have PVR of less than 12 ml

248. What is true regarding the use of α-blockers and the development of "Intraoperative Floppy Iris Syndrome" (IFIS)?

(a) Complicates approximately 0.7% of cataract surgery cases
(b) Manifests as poor preoperative pupil dilation, iris prolapse and progressive intraoperative miosis
(c) Could persist long after the discontinuation of tamsulosin
(d) Intraoperative lidocaine reduces its incidence in patients taking α-adrenergic inhibitors

(Answer is A) Complicates approximately 0.7% of cataract surgery cases

249. What is true regarding mirabegron, the β3 agonist, in treating BPH?

(a) Achieves better results when combined with antimuscarinic
(b) Enhances detrusor contractility resulting in higher Q-max
(c) Enhance detrusor relaxation during bladder-filling phase
(d) Increases voiding pressure that poses risk on renal function

(Answer is C) Enhance detrusor relaxation during bladder-filling phase

250. Which drug reduces the incidence of prostate cancer by 23% with a small increase in high-grade tumor incidence?

(a) Cetrorelix (b) Flutamide
(c) Dutasteride (d) Zanoterone

(Answer is C) Dutasteride

251. Which of the following is not classified as a "complicated LUTS"?

(a) LUTS with neurologic disease
(b) LUTS with post-void dribble
(c) LUTS with suspicious DRE
(d) LUTS with hematuria

(Answer is B) LUTS with post-void dribble

252. "TURP syndrome" is more likely to occur when:

(a) The irrigating fluid is at a pressure exceeding 10 mm Hg
(b) The prostate volume is > 45 cc
(c) The resection time is > 90 minutes
(d) All of the above

(Answer is D) All of the above

253. The most serious complication of TURP is:

(a) Damage to the internal sphincter
(b) Damage to the external sphincter
(c) Bladder perforation
(d) Damage to a ureteral orifice

(Answer is B) Damage to the external sphincter

254. TURP carries an incidence of retrograde ejaculation of:

(a) 62 - 78% (b) 48 - 61%
(c) 79 - 93% (d) 34 - 47%

(Answer is A) 62 - 78%

255. The lowest re-treatment rate of BPH is for:

(a) TUIP (b) TURP
(c) HoLEP (d) HoLRP

(Answer is C) HoLEP

256. When comparing HoLEP to open prostatectomy for a 70 g prostatic adenoma removal; what parameter goes in favor of the latter?

(a) Operation time
(b) Duration of in-hospital stay
(c) Amount of blood transfused
(d) Time to catheter removal

(Answer is A) Operation time

257. What is the capsular perforation rate in prostate vaporization surgery?

(a) 0.2 – 1%
(b) 1.2 – 2.1%
(c) 2.3 – 3.4%
(d) 3.7 – 5.6%

(Answer is A) 0.2 – 1%

258. When comparing Thulium laser (Tm:YAG) to TURP for prostatic adenoma resection, which parameter is in favor of the former?

(a) Operation time and time to catheter removal
(b) Changes in symptom scoring and urodynamic findings
(c) Amount of blood transfused and duration of in-hospital stay
(d) None of the above

(Answer is D) None of the above

259. Screening for prostate cancer is recommended for men who are:

(a) Average risk, aging 50 years, and have at least a 10-year life expectancy
(b) Aging 40 years, and had a first-degree relative diagnosed with prostate cancer before age 65
(c) Aging 40 years, African Americans
(d) All of the above

(Answer is D) All of the above

260. What is false regarding the diagnosis of prostate cancer?

(a) Most cases are identified by screening asymptomatic men
(b) Physical examination alone cannot reliably differentiate benign prostatic conditions from cancer
(c) Most diagnosed cases have normal DRE and PSA values
(d) Prostate biopsy establishes the diagnosis

(Answer is C) Most diagnosed cases have normal DRE and PSA values

261. Genetically, increased risk of prostate cancer has been found in men with:

(a) Variants in the 8q24 region on chromosome 8, in sporadic cases
(b) Alterations on chromosome 1, chromosome 17, and the X chromosome, in some familial cases
(c) The human prostate cancer gene is on the X chromosome
(d) All are true

(Answer is D) All are true

262. Genetically, what are the changes associated with poor survival in prostate cancer patients?

(a) Loss of one or both copies of the tumor suppressor gene PTEN
(b) TMPRSS2–ERG chromosome fusion
(c) P53 mutations and overexpression of MYC
(d) All of the above

(Answer is D) All of the above

263. In which of the following cases PSA testing is not indicated:

(a) 72 years man newly diagnosed BPH with normal DRE
(b) 2 weeks post TURP for obstructing cancerous prostate
(c) Screening for prostate cancer in 75 years old Caucasian man

(d) 43 years man with obstructive LUTS, who had a first-degree relative diagnosed with prostate cancer before age 65

(Answer is C) Screening for prostate cancer in 75 years old Caucasian man

264. In which of the following PSA readings prostate cancer is least suspected?

(a) PSA velocity of 0.35 ng/ml/y, when the PSA is $\leq$ 2.5 ng/ml
(b) PSA velocity of 0.75 ng/ml/y, when the PSA is 4 – 10 ng/ml
(c) t-PSA is 2.8 ng/ml, f-PSA 0.94 ng/ml
(d) t-PSA is 3.7 ng/ml, f-PSA 0.51 ng/ml

(Answer is C) t-PSA is 2.8 ng/ml, f-PSA 0.94 ng/ml

265. In which of the following situations prostate biopsy is most indicated?

(a) Normal DRE, abnormal PSA
(b) Abnormal DRE, abnormal PSA
(c) Abnormal DRE, normal PSA
(d) Hyperechoic areas on TRUS

(Answer is B) Abnormal DRE, abnormal PSA

266. What is false concerning Gleason scoring system for prostate cancers?

(a) Ranges from 0-10 based on a histologic evaluation of tumor specimens
(b) Based on the 2 most common histologic patterns
(c) Greatly relies on the skills and experience of the pathologist
(d) A score of 7 indicates a moderate-grade or moderately differentiated tumor

(Answer is A) Ranges from 0 -10 based on a histologic evaluation of tumor specimens

267. What class of prostate cancer medications causes an initial increase in LH, FSH levels and consequently a rise in testosterone level for few weeks?

(a) GnRH agonists (b) Antiandrogens
(c) Antimicrotubular (d) Bisphosphonates

(Answer is A) GnRH agonists

268. What is false concerning antiandrogen class of prostate cancer medications?

(a) Commonly used in combination with a GnRH agonist
(b) Less effective than medical or surgical castration
(c) Not recommended for localized prostate cancer
(d) Inhibits various cytochrome P-450 enzymes

(Answer is D) Inhibits various cytochrome P-450 enzymes

269. What is true regarding prostatic tissue levels of hK_2?

(a) Intensely expressed in benign prostatic epithelium
(b) Increased in poorly differentiated prostate cancer tissue
(c) Helps differentiate benign from malignant causes of high t-PSA
(d) An organ but not pathology specific marker

(Answer is B) Increased in poorly differentiated prostate cancer tissue

270. What if false concerning the prostate cancer marker PCA_3?

(a) Entails a genetic analysis of cells in the voided urine
(b) Urine sample is collected after a firm massage of the prostate
(c) Helps screen patients who are at intermediate risk of cancer
(d) Helps avoid the inconvenience of prostate biopsy

(Answer is C) Helps screen patients who are at intermediate risk of cancer

271. BPH patients on finasteride longer than 6 months are expected to have:

(a) Decreased t-PSA but increased f-PSA
(b) Decreased t-PSA but unaltered f-PSA
(c) Decreased t-PSA and decreased f-PSA
(d) Any of the above

(Answer is C) Decreased t-PSA and decreased f-PSA

272. Prostate-specific membrane antigen has been detected in:

(a) The prostate gland only
(b) The central nervous system, intestine and the prostate
(c) Malignant ovarian cysts, skeletal muscles, and the prostate
(d) Thyroid glands, adrenals, and the prostate

(Answer is B) The central nervous system, intestine, and the prostate

273. Ectopic expression of PSA occurs in all of the following, *except:*

(a) Thyroid gland (b) Breast tissue
(c) Adrenal glands (d) Renal carcinomas

(Answer is A) Thyroid gland

274. What is false concerning prostate cancer?

(a) The most common cause of mortality in men with prostate cancer is cardiac disease
(b) The second most common cause of cancer death in males
(c) Androgens have a pivotal role in prostate cancer development
(d) Low protein and high carbohydrate diet play a role in the development of prostate cancer

(Answer is D) Low protein and high carbohydrate diet play a role in the development of prostate cancer

275. What is true surrounding PSA?

(a) Black individuals produce more PSA than whites
(b) Ejaculation can lead to a false decrease in PSA
(c) Pro-PSA is the serum proactive form of PSA molecule
(d) Prostate cancer cells make more PSA than normal prostate tissues do

(Answer is A) Black individuals produce more PSA than whites

276. What condition does not appear as a hypoechoic lesion in the prostate on TRUS?

(a) Prostate cancer
(b) Corpora amylacea
(c) Transitional zone
(d) Tuberculous prostatitis

(Answer is B) Corpora amylacea

277. What is true concerning TRUS prostatic biopsy?

(a) Hematospermia might persist for 4 – 6 weeks after taking biopsies
(b) Quinolone antibiotics prophylaxis eliminate possible infections
(c) The right lateral decubitus position is commonly preferred
(d) Only hypoechoic lesions should be biopsied

(Answer is A) Hematospermia might persist for 4 – 6 weeks after taking biopsies

278. Solid lesions in the seminal vesicles are most likely to be a result of:

(a) Imperfect prostate biopsies
(b) Immature teratoma
(c) Schistosomiasis
(d) Liposarcoma

(Answer is C) Schistosomiasis

279. What is false concerning TRUS prostatic biopsy?

(a) A 12-core biopsy is the standard
(b) Preparation for the procedure, a self-administered enema is suggested

(c) Sepsis might complicate the procedure
(d) The biopsy path is best visualized in the coronal plane

(Answer is D) The biopsy path is best visualized in the coronal plane

280. What is true about the usefulness of Gleason scoring system?

(a) Used to stage prostate cancer
(b) A specimen of grade 3 + 4 is worse than 4 + 3
(c) A sum of 6 suggests an intermediate risk for aggressive cancer
(d) Has a role in guiding the appropriate treatment options

(Answer is D) Has a role in guiding the appropriate treatment options

281. What is false concerning the interpretation of Gleason scoring system?

(a) A low score means the cancer tissue is similar to normal prostate tissue
(b) Indicates how likely the tumor will spread
(c) The more cellular atypia observed the higher scoring will be
(d) Relies only on the glandular architectural pattern

(Answer is C) The more cellular atypia observed the higher scoring will be

282. What is false regarding prostate adenocarcinoma in the peripheral zone?

(a) 85% of prostate adenocarcinomas are located in the peripheral zone
(b) 15% of them are multifocal
(c) They tend to extend outside the prostate through the perineural space
(d) The presence of perineural invasion does not worsen the prognosis

(Answer is B) 15% of them are multifocal

283. In descending order, to where do prostate cancers metastasize?

(a) Lymph nodes, bone, lung, bladder, liver and adrenal glands
(b) Bone, lung, lymph nodes, liver, bladder and adrenal glands
(c) Lung, liver, lymph nodes, bone, adrenal glands and bladder
(d) Liver, lung, bone, lymph nodes, bladder and adrenal glands

(Answer is A) Lymph nodes, bone, lung, bladder, liver and adrenal glands

284. What is true regarding seminal vesicles' involvement in prostate cancer?

(a) Almost always due to direct extension (T2c)
(b) Is involved in 85% of positive surgical margins following radical prostatectomy
(c) Carries a poor prognosis
(d) None of the above

(Answer is C) Carries a poor prognosis

285. What is false regarding the histology of prostatic cancers?

(a) Benign glands are different from malignant glands, as they contain basal cells
(b) Adenosis in the transitional zone carries 15% increase in cancer risk
(c) The prostate has no discrete histologic capsule
(d) Intraductal carcinoma is morphologically worse than high-grade PIN and is typically associated with high-grade carcinoma

(Answer is B) Adenosis in the transitional zone carries 15% increase in cancer risk

286. Which of the following tests has the highest positive predictive value for prostate cancer?

(a) PSA
(b) Digital rectal examination

(c) Transrectal ultrasonography
(d) Human kallikrein 2

(Answer is A) PSA

287. What pathologic findings after radical prostatectomy are predictive for occult metastases?

(a) Seminal vesicle invasion and lymph node metastases
(b) Positive surgical margins and seminal vesicle involvement
(c) Capsular penetration and lymph node metastases
(d) Rectal and bladder neck involvement

(Answer is A) Seminal vesicle invasion and lymph node metastases

288. What fraction of men with a PSA value between 4 and 10 ng/ml has an organ-confined prostate cancer?

(a) 1/3 (b) 1/4
(c) 1/2 (d) 2/3

(Answer is D) 2/3

289. Which PSA value interpretation is incorrect?

(a) > 50% of men with PSA > 10 ng/ml have the disease beyond the prostate
(b) Pelvic lymph node involvement is found in PSA > 20 ng/ml
(c) 70% of men with a PSA between 4 and 10 ng/ml have organ-confined disease
(d) 80% of men with PSA < 4 ng/ml have organ-confined disease

(Answer is B) Pelvic lymph node involvement is found in PSA > 20 ng/ml

290. Partin tables are probability tables for the determination of pathologic stages of prostatic cancers based on:

(a) Preoperative clinical stage, PSA level, and Gleason sum
(b) Seminal vesicle invasion, lymph node metastases and Gleason sum
(c) Positive surgical margins, capsular penetration and PSA level
(d) PSA level, perineural invasion, vascular metastasis and Gleason sum

(Answer is A) Preoperative clinical stage, PSA level and Gleason sum

291. For prostate cancer patients, what do Partin tables predict?

(a) Survival rate
(b) Pathologic stage
(c) Extracapsular extension
(d) Lymph node involvement

(Answer is B) Pathologic stage

292. Which factor is closely related to the return to urinary continence function after radical retropubic prostatectomy?

(a) Pathologic tumor stage
(b) Performing nerve-sparing surgery
(c) Patient's age
(d) Performing internal sphincter micro-dissection

(Answer is C) Patient's age

293. Which factor(s) determine(s) the return to normal erectile function after radical retropubic prostatectomy?

(a) The age of the patient
(b) Preoperative potency status
(c) Extent of nerve-sparing surgery
(d) All of the above

(Answer is D) All of the above

294. What is the likelihood that patients with positive surgical margins after radical prostatectomy will be cured for prostate cancer?

(a) Never (b) Unlikely

(c) Likely (d) Always

(Answer is C) Likely

295. Fill the blanks: "On treating prostate cancer patients, the median time from PSA failure to the development of metastatic disease after radical prostatectomy is approximately … years and from the time of metastases to death is approximately … years".

(a) 4, 2 respectively (b) 8, 5 respectively
(c) 6, 3 respectively (d) 7, 4 respectively

(Answer is B) 8, 5 respectively

296. Regarding treating prostate cancer patients, watchful waiting is a reasonable option for:

(a) Patients who have a life expectancy ≤ 10 years and/or well to moderately differentiated cancer
(b) ≥ 70 years of age
(c) PSA < 10 ng/ml, ratio < 0.22
(d) Patients with good performance status

(Answer is A) Patients who have a life expectancy $\leq$ 10 years and/or well to moderately differentiated cancer

297. Regarding treating prostate cancer patients, watchful waiting strategy involves:

(a) Periodic PSA testing
(b) Periodic TRUS
(c) All of the above
(d) None of the above

(Answer is D) None of the above

298. During retropubic radical prostatectomy, what complication could be encountered on dividing the dorsal vein complex anteriorly?

(a) Incontinence
(b) Retrograde ejaculation
(c) Impotence
(d) An ejaculation

(Answer is A) Incontinence

299. Regarding radical prostatectomy, the most common site of positive surgical margins is the:

(a) Apex (b) Posterior
(c) Posterolateral (d) Anterior

(Answer is A) Apex

300. What advantage does laparoscopic/robotic prostatectomy has over open surgery in treating prostate cancers?

(a) Preserving potency
(b) Avoiding incontinence
(c) Less bleeding
(d) All of the above

(Answer is C) Less bleeding

301. What are the possible complications of CO_2 pneumoperitoneum during laparoscopic/robotic prostatectomy?

(a) Hypoxia and acidosis
(b) Tachycardia and tachypnea
(c) Bradycardia and hypotension
(d) Hypercarbia and oliguria

(Answer is D) Hypercarbia and oliguria

302. In descending order, the most common complications of external beam radiation therapy for prostate cancer are:

(a) Urethral stricture, impotence and rectal bleeding
(b) Impotence, rectal bleeding and urethral stricture
(c) Impotence, urethral stricture and rectal bleeding
(d) Rectal bleeding, impotence and urethral stricture

(Answer is B) Impotence, rectal bleeding and urethral stricture

303. What is the proper pre-treatment risk stratification of prostate cancer for a patient with T2a, PSA < 11 ng/ml, and no Gleason score > 6?

(a) Low risk (b) Intermediate risk
(c) High risk (d) Data not adequate

(Answer is A) Low risk

304. Concerning prostate cancers, a pre-treatment PSA velocity of > 2 ng/ml/yr is associated with an increased risk of:

(a) Pathological bone fractures
(b) Biochemical failure following radiation therapy
(c) Hepato-renal disease following chemotherapy
(d) Upgrading the pre-treatment risk stratification

(Answer is B) Biochemical failure following radiation therapy

305. What are the clinical parameters of tissue ablation achieved by cryotherapy for cancer cells destruction?

(a) The number of freezing cycles
(b) The lowest temperature achieved
(c) The existence of regional "heat sinks"
(d) All of the above

(Answer is D) All of the above

306. What is the likelihood that prostate cells die in a single freeze cycle of cryotherapy when tissue temperature reaches colder than - 40°C?

(a) Never (b) Unlikely
(c) Likely (d) Always

(Answer is D) Always

307. What is the primary mechanism of prostate tissue ablation using high-intensity focused ultrasound?

(a) Disruption of protein synthesis
(b) Coagulative necrosis
(c) Cell wall destruction
(d) DNA damage

(Answer is B) Coagulative necrosis

308. What is the most common complication of high-intensity focused ultrasound on treating localized prostate cancer?

(a) Temporary incontinence
(b) Vasculogenic impotence
(c) Urinary retention
(d) Hyper-reflexive detrusor

(Answer is C) Urinary retention

309. What is against using TRUS-guided therapy for focal prostate cancer?

(a) Overdiagnoses clinically insignificant cancers
(b) Misses clinically significant cancers in the anterior or apical regions
(c) May underrepresent true cancer burden
(d) All of the above

(Answer is D) All of the above

310. Clinically significant prostate cancer is defined as:

(a) Volume ≥ 0.5 ml and/or a Gleason score of $\geq 3+4$
(b) Volume ≥ 0.8 ml and/or a Gleason score of $\geq 4+4$
(c) Volume ≥ 1.5 ml and/or a Gleason score of $\geq 4+3$
(d) Volume ≥ 1.0 ml and/or a Gleason score of $\geq 3+3$

(Answer is A) Volume ≥ 0.5 ml and/or a Gleason score of $\geq 3+4$

311. What is false concerning thawing procedure to treat prostate cancer cells?

(a) Slow thawing is more effective than rapid thawing
(b) The most common complication is erectile dysfunction
(c) For effective thawing a minimum temperature of –25°C and a double freeze/thaw cycle with urethral warming are recommended

(d) The two most common modalities employed in focal therapy are high-intensity focused ultrasound and cryosurgery

(Answer is C) For effective thawing a minimum temperature of –25°C and a double freeze/thaw cycle with urethral warming are recommended

312. All of the following modalities are used as salvage therapies after failing radiation therapy for prostate cancer treatment, *except:*

(a) Cryotherapy
(b) Chemotherapy
(c) Brachytherapy
(d) Radical prostatectomy

(Answer is B) Chemotherapy

313. What is the major advantage of neoadjuvant androgen deprivation before radical prostatectomy on treating clinical stages (cT1-T2) prostate cancers?

(a) Reduces positive surgical margins
(b) Reduces local recurrence
(c) Has no proven advantage
(d) Reduces cardiac complications

(Answer is A) Reduces positive surgical margins

314. Regarding radiotherapy for prostate cancer, what is the lowest recommended dose for salvage therapy?

(a) 54 Gy (b) 64 Gy
(c) 74 Gy (d) 84 Gy

(Answer is B) 64 Gy

315. Regarding chemotherapy for prostate cancers, nonsteroidal antiandrogens will result in:

(a) Elevated LH, elevated testosterone, elevated estrogen
(b) Elevated LH, elevated testosterone, declined estrogen
(c) Declined LH, declined testosterone, elevated estrogen
(d) Declined LH, elevated testosterone, declined estrogen

(Answer is A) Elevated LH, elevated testosterone, elevated estrogen

316. Following bilateral orchiectomy for prostate cancer, testosterone will:

(a) Initially drop to nadir, and then recover over 2 weeks
(b) Decline by 50% within 2 weeks and then normalize
(c) Decline by 90% within 24 hours
(d) Decline by 70%

(Answer is C) Decline by 90% within 24 hours

317. What is the first-line chemotherapeutic agent for metastatic castration-resistant prostate cancer?

(a) Bisphosphonate (b) Docetaxel
(c) Sipuleucel-T (d) Enzalutamide

(Answer is B) Docetaxel

318. False about bipolar TURP:

(a) Avoids risk of TUR syndrome
(b) Normal saline is used as irrigant
(c) Improved hemostasis compared with monopolar TURP
(d) Contraindicated in <80 cc gland

(Answer is D) Contraindicated in <80 cc gland

319. False about TUIP- transurethral incision of the prostate:

(a) Disrupts prostate capsule to alleviate voiding symptoms
(b) Ideally for prostate <30 cc
(c) More incidence of retrograde ejaculation than other surgical modalities
(d) Ideally for younger patients

(Answer is C) More incidence of retrograde ejaculation than other surgical modalities

320. All are contraindications to prostate biopsy *except:*

(a) Severe immunosuppression
(b) Coagulopathy
(c) Acute prostatitis
(d) Prostatodynia

(Answer is D) Prostatodynia

321. False about prostate biopsy:

(a) Extended core biopsy needs GA
(b) TRUS guided biopsy needs peroperative antibiotic prophylaxis for upto 24 hours
(c) Sextant biopsy is inadequate
(d) AUA recommendation is for minimum 12 core systematic biopsy

(Answer is A) Extended core biopsy needs GA

322. False about castration for Ca Prostate:

(a) Within 6 hours of orchidectomy testosterone becomes castrate level
(b) Median testosterone after orchidectomy is 15 ng/dl
(c) With Bicalutamide putative antiandrogen activity occurs without hypogonadism
(d) Most potent and best tolerated first generation antiandrogen is flutamide

(Answer is D) Most potent and best tolerated first generation antiandrogen is flutamide

323. False about enzalutamide:

(a) More potent than bicalutamide
(b) Inhibits nuclear translocation of androgen receptor
(c) Doesn't cross blood brain barrier
(d) FDA approved for entire spectrum of CRPC

(Answer is C) Doesn't cross blood brain barrier

324. All are true about prostatic calculi *except:*

(a) Prostatic urethral calculus is always migratory
(b) Most commonly calcium oxalate
(c) Secondary prostatic calculi are caused by reflux of urine
(d) Increased incidence in BPH

(Answer is B) Most commonly calcium oxalate

325. All are true about prostatic calculi *except:*

(a) Increased risk of carcinoma prostate
(b) Increased incidence in patients with prostatitis
(c) Type A calculi are discrete and multiple and throughout the gland
(d) X-ray show calculi in 14%

(Answer is A) Increased risk of carcinoma prostate

326. True about management of prostatic calculi:

(a) If identified during TURP then requires open removal
(b) They act as surrogate marker for prostatic capsule during TURP
(c) Removal of calculi doesn't give any significant symptomatic relief
(d) Presence of calculi mandates screening for carcinoma

(Answer is B) They act as surrogate marker for prostatic capsule during TURP

CHAPTER

17

Pediatric Urology

1. Primary determinant of the normal distribution of water between the ECF and ICF is:

(a) Osmolarity (b) Osmolality
(c) Specific gravity (d) Serum protein

(Answer is B) Serum osmolality is primary determinant of the normal distribution of water between the ECF and ICF in a 1:2 ratio.

2. Kidney develops from:

(a) Pronephros (b) Mesonephros
(c) Metanephros (d) All of the above

(Answer is C) The embryonic kidneys are, in order of their appearance, the pronephros, the mesonephros, and the metanephros. The first two kidneys regress in utero, and the third becomes the permanent kidney. Embryologically, all three kidneys develop from the intermediate mesoderm.

3. Ureteric bud comes in contact with the condensing blastema of metanephric mesenchyme at about:

(a) 7th day (b) 14th day
(c) 21st day (d) 28th day

(Answer is D) The definitive kidney, or the metanephros, forms in the sacral region as a pair of new structures, called the ureteric bud, sprouts from the distal portion of the nephric duct, and comes in contact with the condensing blastema of metanephric mesenchyme at about the 28th day.

4. Which is not derived from the metanephric mesenchyme?

(a) Glomerulus (b) Distal tubule
(c) Loop of Henle (d) Collecting duct

(Answer is D) The nephron, which consists of the glomerulus, proximal tubule, loop of Henle, and distal tubule, is thought to derive from the metanephric mesenchyme; and the collecting system, consisting of collecting ducts, calyces, pelvis, and ureter, is formed from the ureteric bud.

5. Renal ascent to a lumbar site just below the adrenal glands occurs between:

(a) 3rd and 6th weeks
(b) 6th and 9th weeks
(c) 9th and 11th weeks
(d) 11th and 14th weeks

(Answer is B) Between the 6th and 9th weeks, the kidneys ascend to a lumbar site just below the adrenal glands.

6. During ascent in horseshoe kidney, the fused lower pole becomes trapped under:

(a) Superior mesenteric artery
(b) Inferior mesenteric artery
(c) Celiac plexus
(d) Renal artery

(Answer is B) During ascent, the fused lower pole becomes trapped under the inferior mesenteric artery and thus does not reach its normal site.

7. Bladder body and trigone are derived respectively from:

(a) Both from endoderm
(b) Both from mesoderm
(c) Bladder body from mesoderm and trigone
(d) Trigone from mesoderm and bladder body from endoderm

(Answer is D) The bladder body is derived from the endoderm-lined vesicourethral canal and the surrounding mesenchyme. The trigone has a different embryologic origin (mesodermal) in that it develops from the incorporation of the common excretory ducts (the portion of nephric ducts caudal to the origin of the ureteric bud) into the base of the developing bladder.

8. The male and female genital structures are virtually identical through the:

(a) 5th week (b) 6th week
(c) 7th week (d) 8th week

(Answer is C) The male and female genital structures are virtually identical through the 7th week.

9. Which one of the following is not derived from mesonephric duct?

(a) Appendix epididymis
(b) Paradidymis
(c) Appendix testis
(d) Gartner's duct cysts

(Answer is C) The remnants of the mesonephric ducts are found in the ovarian mesentery as the epoöphoron and paroöphoron and in the anterolateral vaginal wall as the Gartner's duct cysts. Appendix epididymis and paradidymis arise from the mesonephric ducts. MIS hormone produced by the Sertoli cells then causes the paramesonephric ducts to regress, leaving behind appendix testis and prostatic utricle as remnants.

10. Primitive sex cords are formed by:

(a) 5th week (b) 6th week
(c) 7th week (d) 8th week

(Answer is B) During the 6th week, the cells of the genital ridge invade the mesenchyme in the region of future gonads to form aggregates of supporting cells called the primitive sex cords.

11. Bulbourethral glands originates from:

(a) Vesico-urethral canal
(b) Uro-genital sinus
(c) Mesonephric duct
(d) Paramesonephic duct

(Answer is B) The seminal vesicles sprout from the distal nephric ducts, whereas the prostate and bulbourethral glands develop from the urogenital sinus.

12. Neprogenesis is completed by:

(a) 34 weeks of gestation
(b) 28 weeks of gestation
(c) 6 weeks after birth
(d) 16 weeks after birth

(Answer is A) The metanephros begins its inductive phase after 5 weeks of gestation; and, in the human, nephrogenesis follows a sigmoidal curve, with most rapid increase in mid gestation, and is completed by 34 to 36 weeks.

13. Urine production in the human kidney begins by:

(a) 6 to 8 weeks (b) 10 to 12 weeks
(c) 14 to 16 weeks (d) 16 to 18 weeks

(Answer is B) Urine prbduction in the human kidney is· known to begin around 10 to 12 weeks.

14. Fetal urine is:

(a) Hypertonic with low sodium content
(b) Hypertonic with high sodium content
(c) Hypotonic with low sodium content
(d) Hypotonic with high sodium content

(Answer is D) The fetus produces hypotonic urine with high sodium content and in large volumes.

15. Urine production at 40 weeks of gestation is:

(a) 1 ml/hr (b) 10 ml/hr
(c) 50 ml/hr (d) 100 ml/hr

(Answer is C) Hourly human fetal urine production increases from 5 ml/hr at 20 weeks' gestation to 50 ml/hr at 40 weeks' gestation.

16. After what age oliguria is generally defined as a urine flow rate less than 1 ml/kg/hr?

(a) Immediately after birth
(b) After 2 days of birth
(c) After 2 months of birth
(d) After 2 years of birth

(Answer is B) After the first 2 days of life, oliguria is generally defined as a urine flow rate less than 1 ml/kg/ hr.

17. By how many days in a term infant, P Cr concentration becomes less than 0.5 mg/dl?

(a) Immediately after birth
(b) After 7 days of birth
(c) After 6 months of birth
(d) After 2 years of birth

(Answer is B) By 7 days in the term infant, P Cr concentration is normally less than 0.5 mg/dl.

18. Acid-base regulation in the neonate is characterized by:

(a) Reduced threshold for bicarbonate reabsorption
(b) Increased threshold for bicarbonate reabsorption
(c) Reduced threshold for acid reabsorption
(d) Increased threshold for acid reabsorption

(Answer is A) Acid-base regulation in the neonate is characterized by a reduced threshold for bicarbonate reabsorption.

19. Hazards to overhydration of the neonate include all *except:*

(a) Opening of a symptomatic patent ductus arteriosus
(b) Cerebral intraventricular hemorrhage
(c) Necrotizing enterocolitis
(d) Hyperbilirubinemia

(Answer is D) There are significant hazards to overhydration of the neonate, including the opening of a symptomatic patent ductus arteriosus, cerebral intraventricular hemorrhage, and necrotizing enterocolitis. Severe under-hydration, on the other hand, may lead to hypoglycemia, hyperbilirubinemia, and hyper-osmolality.

20. Mothers treated with ACE inhibitors during pregnancy have increased rates of all *except:*

(a) Fetal loss (b) Polyhydramnios
(c) Hypotension (d) Anuria

(Answer is B) Infants born to mothers treated with ACE inhibitors during pregnancy have increased rates of oligohydramnios, hypotension and anuria.

21. ANP has been shown to possess a number of systemic hemodynamic and renal effects *except:*

(a) Increase in GFR
(b) Natriuresis and diuresis
(c) Inhibition of renin and aldosterone release
(d) Decrease in vascular permeability

(Answer is D) ANP secreted by cardiac myocytes, has been shown to possess a number of systemic hemodynamic and renal effects, including an increase in GFR, natriuresis, diuresis, inhibition of renin and aldosterone release, vasorelaxation, and increase in vascular permeability.

22. Histologic hallmarks of renal dysplasia is the presence of:

(a) Primitive ducts
(b) Fibrosis
(c) Glomerular cyst
(d) Presence of abnormal tubules and glomeruli

(Answer is A) One of the histologic hallmarks of renal dysplasia is the presence of fibromuscular collars around tubular structures, so-called primitive ducts.

23. Which statement regarding recovery of renal function is not true?

(a) The functional salvageability of a unilateral

obstructed fetal kidney is dependent on the duration of obstruction and gestational age

(b) Measures of urinary sodium, chloride, osmolarity, and calcium have been correlated with fetal renal functional potential

(c) When fetal urine approaches the character of serum, irreversible damage appears to have been done to the developing kidney

(d) Thin parenchyma in the setting of hydronephrosis clearly predict decreased function

(Answer is D) Thickness of the parenchyma in the setting of hydronephrosis is important to note but does not clearly predict decreased function. Often this thinning is simply due to stretching of the parenchyma around a dilated collecting system.

24. The echolucent pyramids first become evident at about how many weeks of gestation?

(a) 12 weeks (b) 16 weeks
(c) 20 weeks (d) 24 weeks

(Answer is C) The echolucent pyramids should not be confused for dilated calyces and first become evident at about 20 weeks. Their absence later in gestation is abnormal.

25. Amniotic fluid is mostly derived from urine by how many weeks?

(a) 14-16 weeks (b) 20-22 weeks
(c) 30-32 weeks (d) 36-38 weeks

(Answer is B) The time of onset of changes in the AF is critical and reflects a normal shift from where most of the AF is a placental transudate to where it becomes predominantly a product of fetal urine. This occurs after 16 weeks, and by 20 or 22 weeks most AF is fetal urine.

26. "Keyhole" sign, is strongly suggestive of:

(a) PUV (b) VUR
(c) PUJO (d) Bladder extrophy

(Answer is A) Dilation of the posterior urethral, the "keyhole" sign, is strongly suggestive of posterior urethral valves (PUV).

27. Multiple small cysts not resolved on US and appear as a very bright, large, and echogenic kidney, is seen with:

(a) ADPKD
(b) ARPKD
(c) MCDK
(d) Congenital multilocular nephroma

(Answer is B) Multiple small cysts not resolved on US appear as a very bright, large, and echogenic kidney, as seen with autosomal recessive polycystic kidney disease (ARPKD).

28. In absence of which structure male gender cannot be finalized?

(a) Penis (b) Testis
(c) Scrotum (d) Vas

(Answer is B) Without the presence of scrotal testes one cannot finalize a male assignment.

29. All *except* one suggest the possibility of ureterocele:

(a) Presence of upper pole hydronephrosis and a dilated ureter that may be traced to the bladder

(b) Intravesical, thin-walled cystic structure associated with the base of the bladder

(c) Cystic dysplastic upper pole without obvious hydronephrosis

(d) Intravesical, thick-walled cystic structure

(Answer is D) An ectopic ureter, associated with a dilated upper pole, may give the false appearance of an intravesical ureterocele, but the ureterovesical wall is much thicker.

30. Classic US appearance of an MCDK includes all *except:*

(a) Reniform structure

(b) Multiple non-communicating fluid-filled cystic spaces

(c) No central large cyst
(d) Minimal to no recognizable renal parenchyma

(Answer is A) Classic US appearance of an MCDK was initially defined by Sanders as being a non-reniform structure, with multiple non-communicating fluid-filled cystic spaces, no central large cyst, and minimal to no recognizable renal parenchyma.

31. ARPKD (infantile polycystic kidney disease) is identified as all *except:*

(a) Kidneys appear large and cystic
(b) ARPKD is associated with various mutations on the PKHD1 gene on chromosome 6p12
(c) Most of these infants die of pulmonary insufficiency with Potter's syndrome
(d) Kidneys on USG are brightly echogenic kidneys

(Answer is A) ARPKD does not appear cystic but is characterized by markedly enlarged, brightly echogenic kidneys.

32. Most common renal mass in fetal urinary tract is:

(a) Wilms' tumor
(b) Congenital mesoblastic nephroma
(c) Renal cell carcinoma
(d) Congenital multilocular nephroma

(Answer is B) Renal masses are unusual in the fetal urinary tract and the most common is congenital mesoblastic nephroma.

33. Which statement regarding pathophysiology of congenital obstruction is not true?

(a) Congenital obstruction is different from postnatal obstruction
(b) There is association between renal agenesis, oligohydramnios, and pulmonary hypoplasia
(c) Late-onset oligohydramnios was not associated with pulmonary insufficiency, with a threshold at about 30 weeks
(d) Hydronephrosis of all etiologies is more common in females

(Answer is D) Hydronephrosis of all etiologies is four to five times more common in males.

34. Most common cause of hydronephrosis in fetal urinary tract is:

(a) PUJO (b) VUR
(c) PUV (d) Megaureter

(Answer is A) PUJ obstruction is the largest single entity producing hydronephrosis, followed by reflux, valves and megaureter.

35. The diagnosis of an upper pole renal cyst in a fetus indicates the presence of a:

(a) Simple cyst
(b) Duplication anomaly
(c) Ureterocele
(d) Megaureter

(Answer is B) The diagnosis of an upper pole renal cyst in a fetus indicates the presence of a duplication anomaly with hydronephrosis rather than a cyst.

36. Indications for in utero urinary decompression are all *except:*

(a) Evidence of bladder outlet obstruction
(b) Male fetus
(c) Singleton
(d) Polyhydramnios

(Answer is D) Oligohydramnios and not Polyhydramnios is indication for decompression.

37. Favorable urinary indices for in uretero decompression are all *except:*

(a) Na < 100
(b) Cl < 110
(c) Osm < 210
(d) β2-microglobulin in > 10 to 20

(Answer is D) Favorable urinary indices for in uretero

decompression is -Na < 100, Cl < 110, Osm < 210; or serial samplings trending toward normal; β2-microglobulin is < 10 to 20.

38. The association of a massively dilated thin wall and smooth bladder, hydroureteronephrosis, bilateral VUR is associated with:

(a) PUV
(b) Megacystis-megaureter
(c) BOO
(d) Primary megaureter

(Answer is B) The association of a massively dilated bladder, hydroureteronephrosis, and bilateral VUR has been termed the megacystis-megaureter association. The constant recycling of bladder urine into the upper tracts effectively prevents true bladder emptying. The US appearance, both prenatally and postnatally, may mimic that of PUV, yet the bladders in these children are typically thin walled and smooth.

39. When the diagnosis of MCDK is uncertain which renal scan is the most effective?

(a) MAG-3
(b) DTPA
(c) DMSA
(d) Gallium scan

(Answer is C) When the diagnosis of MCDK is uncertain and severe hydronephrosis may be present, a DMSA renal scan is the most effective means of confirming the diagnosis. MCDK can be expected to demonstrate no uptake on DMSA scanning.

40. The most common entity producing protuberant mass in the perineum of a newborn girl is a:

(a) Periurethral cyst
(b) Imperforate hymen
(c) Prolapse ectopic ureterocele
(d) Urethral prolapse

(Answer is A) The appearance of a protuberant mass in the perineum of a newborn girl should suggest four principal diagnoses. The most common entity producing this general finding in a newborn is a periurethral cyst.

41. Most common cause of abdominal mass in newborns is:

(a) PUJO (b) MCKD
(c) Wilms' tumor (d) ARPCKD

(Answer is B)

Pathology	*No.*	*%*
Urinary tract	186	68
MCDK	65	35
Hydronephrosis (non-specified)	38	20
UPJO	20	11
PUVs	18	10
UDEC	11	6
ARPKD	12	6
Wilms' tumor (also CMN)	8	4
RVT	5	3
Miscellaneous	9	5

42. Most common non genitourinary cause of abdominal mass in newborns is:

(a) Ovarian cyst
(b) Hydrometrocolpos
(c) Neuroblastoma
(d) GI duplication

(Answer is C)

Pathology	*No.*	*%*
Neuroblastoma	22	25
GI duplication	16	18
Hydrometrocolpos	13	15
Ovarian cysts	9	10
Miscellaneous	28	32

43. Neonate with enlarged kidneys, hematuria, anemia, and thrombocytopenia, often with a history of a prolonged delivery and prematurity is suggestive of:

(a) Renal artery thrombosis
(b) Renal vein thrombosis
(c) Adrenal hemorrhage
(d) Urinary tract infection

(Answer is B) Renal vein thrombosis (RVT) is suggested in the neonate with enlarged kidneys, hematuria, anemia, and thrombocytopenia, often with a history of a prolonged delivery and prematurity.

44. Egg shell calcifications is suggestive of:

(a) Adrenal hemorrhage
(b) Neuroblastoma
(c) Renal artery thrombosis
(d) Renal vein thrombosis

(Answer is A) The late appearance of an adrenal hemorrhage is that of peripheral egg shell calcifications in contrast to stippled calcifications of neuroblastoma.

45. All newborns need to be seen on emergent basis *except:*

(a) Newborns with bilateral hydronephrosis or a solitary kidney
(b) Newborns with gross hematuria, urinary tract infections
(c) Boys with priapism
(d) Nephrolithiasis

(Answer is D)

Emergent (as soon as possible)

- Trauma.
- Suspected child abuse.
- Acute postoperative problem.
- Newborns with bilateral hydronephrosis or a solitary kidney.
- Newborns with gross hematuria, urinary tract infections.
- Newborns with ambiguous genitalia, bladder or cloacal exstrophy, posterior urethral valves, prune-belly syndrome, spina bifida.
- Children with acute abdominal or scrotal pain.
- Boys with priapism.

46. A child with acute scrotal pain regardless of age until proven otherwise must be presumed to have:

(a) Spermatic cord torsion
(b) Testicular torsion
(c) Epididymitis
(d) Orchitis

(Answer is A) A child with acute scrotal pain must be presumed to have spermatic cord torsion regardless of age until proven otherwise.

47. Beckwith-Wiedemann syndrome includes all *except:*

(a) Hepatosplenomegaly
(b) Nephromegaly
(c) Macroglossia
(d) Hyperglycemia

(Answer is D) Macroglossia can be associated with the Beckwith-Wiedemann syndrome, which also includes hepatosplenomegaly, nephromegaly, and hypoglycemia secondary to pancreatic beta cell hyperplasia in a large gestational age infant.

48. Regarding "atypical" presacral dimple all are true *except:*

(a) Dimple is off center
(b) More than 2.5 cm from the anal verge at birth
(c) Deeper than 1.0 mm
(d) 40% of patients with atypical dimples were found to have occult spinal dysraphism

(Answer is C) An "atypical" presacral dimple may indicate spina bifida or cord tethering if the dimple is off center, more than 2.5 cm from the anal verge at birth or deeper than 0.5 cm. 40% of patients with atypical dimples were found to have occult spinal dysraphism.

49. Optimal timing of the spinal ultrasound in spinal dysraphism is:

(a) At birth
(b) At 6 months of age
(c) At puberty
(d) Any age

(Answer is B) When used as a first-line test in suspected occult spinal dysraphism, optimal timing of the spinal ultrasound is before 6 months of age. Ossification of the posterior elements after 6 months of age prevents an acoustic window.

50. Which statement regarding Ga 67 and In 111 is not true?

(a) Ga 67or In 111-labelled leukocytes is helpful to diagnose and localize site of UTI
(b) Used to identify and guide therapy for children with focal segmental bacterial pyelonephritis
(c) More sensitive than DMSA scans in the diagnosis of acute pyelonephritis, especially in differentiating older lesions
(d) Useful in patients with abnormal renal anatomy or in patients with diminished renal function

(Answer is C) Renal scintigraphy scans using gallium 67 renal scans were more sensitive than DMSA scans in the diagnosis of acute pyelonephritis, especially in differentiating new lesions from old ones.

51. Most common cause of primary nephrotic syndrome in children is:

(a) Minimal change disease
(b) Focal segmental glomerulosclerosis
(c) Membranous nephropathy
(d) Postinfectious glomerulonephritis

(Answer is A) The most common cause of primary nephrotic syndrome in children is minimal change disease, also referred to as steroid-responsive nephrotic syndrome.

52. Hypercalciuria is not seen in:

(a) Distal renal tubular acidosis
(b) Bartter's syndrome
(c) Gitelman's syndrome
(d) Proximal renal tubular acidosis

(Answer is C) Hypocalciuria is a unique feature distinguishing Gitelman's syndrome from the Bartter's syndrome.

53. Which statement regarding HUS is not correct?

(a) The diagnosis of HUS is based on clinical features at presentation, because renal biopsies are not usually performed
(b) Severity of renal involvement is related to the severity of anemia, it does not appear to be related to the severity of the gastro-intestinal prodrome
(c) The prodrome of diarrhea-associated HUS is enterocolitis, typically bloody diarrhea
(d) It is defined by the triad of (1) hemolytic microangiopathic anemia (2) thrombo-cytopenia and (3) renal insufficiency

(Answer is B) Severity of renal involvement is not related to the severity of anemia, it does appear to be related to the severity of the gastrointestinal prodrome.

54. Nephrogenic diabetes insipidus is characterized by all *except:*

(a) The most common is autosomal recessive mutation of the vasopressin receptor
(b) Occurs at a median age of 9 months and mean age of 25 months
(c) UOsm < 300
(d) Presence of hypernatremic dehydration

(Answer is A) The most common form is X-linked recessive mutation of the vasopressin receptor.

55. Estimation of the GFR by creatinine clearance using the Schwartz formula in male >70 kg is:

(a) Height (cm) × 0.45 / creatinine (mg/dl)
(b) Height (cm) × 0.55 / creatinine (mg/dl)
(c) Height (cm) × 0.70 / creatinine (mg/dl)
(d) Creatinine (mg/dl) × 0.45 / Height (cm)

(Answer is C) Schwartz formula-Height (cm) × 0.70 / creatinine (mg/dl).

56. In which duration of life males have more UTIs than females?

(a) First year (b) Prepubertal
(c) Postpubertal (d) Elderly

(Answer is A) The first year of life is the only year during which males have more UTis than females.

57. In order of least to most reliable for UTI diagnosis is:

(a) (1) Suprapubic bladder aspirate (2) midstream void (3) catheterization (4) plastic bag attached to the perineum, a "bagged specimen"
(b) (1) Bagged specimen (2) catheterization (3) midstream void (4) suprapubic bladder aspirate
(c) (1) Midstream void (2) bagged specimen (3) catheterization (4) suprapubic bladder aspirate
(d) (1) Bagged specimen (2) midstream void (3) catheterization (4) suprapubic bladder aspirate

(Answer is D) In order of least to most reliable for UTI diagnosis, they are (1) plastic bag attached to the perineum, a "bagged specimen"; (2) midstream void; (3) catheterization; or (4) suprapubic bladder aspirate.

58. Which statement regarding urinary nitrite test is not correct?

(a) Dietary nitrates are reduced to nitrite by many gram-negative urinary bacteria
(b) First morning voided urinary specimens should be avoided for this test
(c) Many gram-positive bacteria do not perform this reduction
(d) Combination of positive leukocyte esterase and nitrite testing and microscopic confirmation of bacteria has almost 100% sensitivity for detection of UTI

(Answer is B) First morning voided urinary specimens should be used for this test because bacterial reduction of nitrate can take several hours.

59. The ideal prophylactic agent should have all *except:*

(a) High serum concentrations
(b) High urinary concentrations
(c) Have minimal effect on the normal fecal flora
(d) Easily administered and tolerated, and be cost-effective

(Answer is A) The ideal prophylactic agent should have low serum and high urinary concentrations, have minimal effect on the normal fecal flora, be easily administered and tolerated, and be cost-effective.

60. Regarding probiotic which statement is not true?

(a) Probiotic therapy refers to a concept in which live organisms are given to patients for therapeutic benefit
(b) This is based upon the possible mechanism that competitive colonization may create a barrier to colonization with potential pathogens
(c) Gram-negative strains is used most commonly
(d) Probiotic therapy may have efficacy in infants with necrotizing enterocolitis

(Answer is C) Strains of gram-positive lactobacillus is used most commonly.

61. The main advantage of radionuclide VCUG are all *except:*

(a) Lower radiation exposure
(b) More sensitive for reflux detection
(c) Most useful for periodic reflux reevaluation or for screening siblings who have a low risk of reflux
(d) Offers better spatial resolution

(Answer is D) The radionuclide VCUG should not be used to evaluate first infections in infants or young boys in whom risk of genitourinary abnormality is high and urethral visualization important or in any child in whom high-resolution imaging of the lower urinary tract is important. Little anatomic detail afforded by radionuclide. It is ideal both for screening and for monitoring rational history.

62. **All are associated with bilateral renal agenesis *except:***
   (a) Forty percent of the affected infants are stillborn
   (b) Most of the children who are born alive do not survive beyond 48 hours
   (c) The adrenal glands are usually absent
   (d) The characteristic potter facies and the presence of oligohydramnios are pathognomonic

(Answer is C) The adrenal glands are usually normally positioned.

63. **All are associated with unilateral renal agenesis *except:***
   (a) Ipsilateral adrenal agenesis is rarely encountered
   (b) Reproductive organ abnormalities occur with more frequency in males
   (c) Most commonly involved organ system is cardiovascular (30%)
   (d) The ipsilateral ureter is completely absent in about half of the patients

(Answer is B) Despite the predominance of male infants with URA, reproductive organ abnormalities occur with more frequency in females, occurring in 25% to 50% of cases, compared with 10% to 15% in males.

64. **All are associated with unilateral renal agenesis *except:***
   (a) The contralateral kidney appear to be more prone to disease
   (b) On physical examination vas deferens or body and tail of the epididymis is missing
   (c) Absent, septate, or hypoplastic vagina is associated with a unicornuate or bicornuate uterus
   (d) Complete absence of one kidney occurs more commonly than does BRA

(Answer is A) The contralateral kidney does not appear to be more prone to disease.

65. **All are associated with supernumerary kidney *except:***
   (a) The supernumerary kidney is truly an accessory organ with its own collecting system and blood supply
   (b) The supernumerary kidney is a distinct parenchymatous mass that may be either completely separate or only loosely attached to the major kidney
   (c) The supernumerary kidney is nonreniform and larger than the main ipsilateral organ
   (d) Usually the ipsilateral and contralateral kidneys are normal

(Answer is C) The supernumerary kidney is reniform and is generally smaller than the main ipsilateral organ.

66. **The developing metanephric tissue and ureteral bud migrate:**
   (a) Cephalad, rotating medially on its long axis
   (b) Cephalad, rotating laterally on its long axis
   (c) Caudad, rotating medially on its long axis
   (d) Caudad, rotating laterally on its long axis

(Answer is A) The developing metanephric tissue and ureteral bud migrate cephalad, rotating medially on its long axis as it does so.

67. **Most common anomaly associated with renal ectopia is:**
   (a) PUJO (b) VUJO
   (c) VUR (d) Malrotation

(Answer is A) Renal pelvis is usually anterior (instead of medial) to the parenchyma because the kidney has incompletely rotated. As a result, 56% of ectopic kidneys have a hydronephrotic collecting system. Half of these cases result from obstruction at either the ureteropelvic or the ureterovesical junction (70% and 30%, respectively); 25% from reflux grade 3 or greater, and 25% from the malrotation alone.

68. Regarding renal ectopia which statement is not true?

(a) The left side is affected slightly more than the right
(b) The ureter usually enters the bladder on the ipsilateral side with its orifice situated normally
(c) Rarely, the adrenal gland is absent or abnormally positioned
(d) The ectopic kidney is more susceptible to disease than the normally positioned kidney

(Answer is D) The ectopic kidney is no more susceptible to disease than the normally positioned kidney.

69. Regarding thoracic kidney all statements are true *except:*

(a) There appears to be a left-sided predominance, and the sex ratio favors male
(b) Kidney is situated in the posterior mediastinum and usually has completed the normal rotation process
(c) Kidney is within the pleural space
(d) The ureter is elongated and it never enters ectopically into the bladder

(Answer is C) The kidney usually lies in the posterolateral aspect of the diaphragm in the foramen of Bochdalek. The diaphragm at this point thins out, and a flimsy membrane surrounds the protruding portion of kidney. Therefore, the kidney is not within the pleural space.

70. Least common renal fusion anomalies associated with ectopia is:

(a) Unilateral fused kidney with inferior ectopia
(b) Sigmoid or S-shaped
(c) L-shaped or tandem
(d) Unilateral fused kidneys with superior ectopia

(Answer is D) Unilaterally fused kidney with inferior ectopia is the most common variety, whereas fusion with superior ectopia is the least common.

71. About horseshoe kidney all the following is true *except:*

(a) PUJO causes significant hydronephrosis in as many as one third of individuals
(b) The horseshoe kidney is probably the most common of all renal fusion anomalies
(c) Isthmus is located adjacent to the L3 or L4 vertebra just below the origin of the superior mesenteric artery from the aorta
(d) In 95% of patients, the kidneys join at the lower pole

(Answer is C) Isthmus is located adjacent to the L3 or L4 vertebra just below the origin of the inferior mesenteric artery from the aorta.

72. Which statement regarding horseshoe kidney is not true?

(a) The isthmus most often lies anterior to the aorta and vena cava
(b) Lower ureter usually enters the bladder in ectopic position
(c) Calyces point posteriorly
(d) The ureter may insert high on the renal pelvis and lie laterally

(Answer is B) Despite upper ureteral angulation, the lower ureter usually enters the bladder normally and rarely is ectopic.

73. How does kidney and renal pelvis rotate during ascent?

(a) 90 degrees ventromedially
(b) 90 degrees ventrolaterally

(c) 90 degrees dorsomedially
(d) 90 degrees dorsolaterally

(Answer is A) The kidney and renal pelvis normally rotate 90 degrees ventromedially during ascent.

74. Regarding vascular supply of renal parenchma which statement is not true?

(a) On the basis of vascular supply, the renal parenchyma is divided into five segments
(b) The anterior branch almost always supplies the upper, middle and lower segments of the kidney
(c) The posterior branch invariably nourishes the posterior and lower segments
(d) The vessel to the lower segment has the greatest variation in origin

(Answer is D) The vessel to the apical segment has the greatest variation in origin.

75. Endourologic incision of an obstructed UPJ should be done at:

(a) Laterally and posteriorly
(b) Laterally and anteriorly
(c) Medially and posteriorly
(d) Medially and anteriorly

(Answer is A) Endourologic incision of an obstructed UPJ should be done laterally and posteriorly instead of anteriorly to avoid injury to this vessel.

76. Excision of renal artery aneurysms are done for all *except:*

(a) The hypertension cannot be easily controlled
(b) In complete ring like calcification is present
(c) Aneurysm is larger than 1.0 cm
(d) Patient is female and of child-bearing age

(Answer is C) Any aneurysm larger than 2.5 cm is repaired and 1.0 cm in younger women with the potential for child bearing should be repaired.

77. Regarding renal arteriovenous fistulas which statement is not true?

(a) More than 75% of all arteriovenous fistulas are of the congenital type
(b) Rarely present clinically before the third or fourth decade
(c) May result in left ventricular hypetrophy and eventually in high-output cardiac failure
(d) Women are affected more often as men, and the right kidney is involved more often than the left

(Answer is A) Fewer than 25% of all arteriovenous fistulas are of the congenital type.

78. Dilation of the upper calyx due to obstruction of the upper infundibulum by vessels or stenosis has been described:

(a) Fraley syndrome
(b) Fraser syndrome
(c) Simpson-Golabi-Behmel syndrome
(d) Townes-Brocks syndrome

(Answer is A) Dilation of the upper calyx due to obstruction of the upper infundibulum by vessels or stenosis has been described in Fraley syndrome.

79. Regarding megacalycosis which statement is not true?

(a) Megacalycosis is most likely congenital
(b) Occurs predominantly in males in a ratio of 6 : 1
(c) Obstructive enlargement of calyces resulting from malformation of the renal papillae
(d) Bilateral disease has been seen almost exclusively in males

(Answer is C) Megacalycosis is nonobstructive enlargement of calyces resulting from malformation of the renal papillae and has been diagnosed prenatally.

80. Which of the following is correct?

(a) VHL is located on chromosome 3
(b) TSC2 is located on chromosome 14
(c) PKD1 is located on chromosome 4

(d) PKD2 is located on chromosome 16

(Answer is A) One tuberous sclerosis gene, TSCl, is located on chromosome 2 and the second, TSC2, on chromosome 16. The PKD1 gene is located on chromosome 16, and the PKD2 gene is on chromosome 4.

81. Regarding Ask-Upmark kidney which statement is not true?

(a) Most patients are 10 years of age or younger at diagnosis
(b) It is defined as segmental hypoplasia
(c) The Ask-Upmark kidney is smaller than normal–12 to 35 g
(d) In patients with unilateral disease, nephrectomy may control the hypertension

(Answer is A) Most patients are 10 years of age or older at diagnosis.

82. Most common sites in the body for cysts:

(a) Epididymis (b) Bladder
(c) Kidney (d) Prostate

(Answer is C) The kidney is one of the most common sites in the body for cysts.

83. All *except* one have cysts with hyperplastic lining, sometimes with nodules of hyperplasia or polyps that project into the cyst lumen:

(a) ADPKD (b) ARPKD
(c) VHL (d) ARCD

(Answer is B) ADPKD, tuberous sclerosis, VHL disease, and acquired renal cystic disease (ARCD), the cysts have a hyperplastic lining, sometimes with nodules of hyperplasia or polyps that project into the cyst lumen.

84. Most renal cystic conditions arise from the nephrons and collecting ducts after they have formed *except:*

(a) ADPKD
(b) ARPKD
(c) Medullary cystic disease
(d) MCKD

(Answer is D) Multicystic dysplasia is an exception in that it arises before formation of the nephron, from abnormal induction of metanephric development, a primary abnormality of the nephrogenic blastema, or obstruction occurring early in renal development.

85. Bilateral renal cystic disease occurs in all *except:*

(a) ARPKD (b) MSK
(c) ARCD (d) VHL

(Answer is B) Bilateral renal cystic disease creates a dilemma in diagnosis at any age. The differential diagnosis includes ARPKD, ADPKD, tuberous sclerosis, VHL disease, bilateral simple cysts and ARCD.

86. Homogenous, hyperechogenic kidneys without macrocysts is seen in all *except:*

(a) Autosomal recessive polycystic kidney disease
(b) Sporadic glomerulocystic kidney disease
(c) Contrast nephropathy
(d) Tuberous sclerosis

(Answer is D) Autosomal dominant polycystic kidney disease, sporadic glomerulocystic kidney disease, tuberous sclerosis has diffuse macrocysts.

87. Regarding ARPKD which statement is not true?

(a) 50% of affected newborns die in the first few hours or days of life
(b) All patients have varying degrees of congenital hepatic fibrosis
(c) Younger the patient at presentation with ARPKD, the more the liver disease
(d) Younger the patient who presents with congenital hepatic fibrosis, the milder the renal cystic disease

(Answer is C) Younger the patient at presentation with ARPKD, the milder the liver disease; and, conversely, the younger the patient who presents with congenital hepatic fibrosis, the milder the renal cystic disease.

88. Intravenous urography showing characteristic radial or medullary streaking (sunburst pattern) caused by dilated collecting tubules filled with contrast medium is seen in:

(a) ARPKD (b) ADPKD
(c) MSK (d) ARCD

(Answer is A) Intravenous urography with delayed films may show functioning kidneys with characteristic radial or medullary streaking (sunburst pattern) caused by dilated collecting tubules filled with contrast medium. This picture can persist for as long as 48 hours after the study in ARPKD.

89. Regarding ADPKD which statement is not true?

(a) Possibility of making the diagnosis in affected individuals before 25 years of age is at least 85%
(b) Men tend to have more renal involvement than women
(c) All intracranial hemorrhages in patients with ADPKD represent subarachnoid bleeding secondary to berry aneurysms
(d) Disease can manifest asymmetrically, with cysts on only one side at first or with a unilateral renal mass

(Answer is C) Not all intracranial hemorrhages in patients with ADPKD represent subarachnoid bleeding secondary to berry aneurysms; in some patients, hemorrhage follows the rupture of intracerebral arteries.

90. Incidence of RCC in patients with ADPKD is:

(a) No higher (b) 2 folds increase
(c) 5 folds increase (d) 10 folds increase

(Answer is A) The incidence of RCC in patients with ADPKD is no higher than that in the general population.

91. Which disease is usually discovered because of an enormously enlarged and edematous placenta, which accounts for more than 25% of the birth weight?

(a) Congenital nephrosis (CNF)
(b) Diffuse mesangial sclerosis
(c) ADPKD
(d) Juvenile nephronophthisis

(Answer is A) CNF usually is discovered because of an enormously enlarged and edematous placenta, which accounts for more than 25% of the birth weight.

92. Regarding tuberous sclerosis (TS) which statement is not true?

(a) The hallmark lesion of the central nervous system is a superficial cortical hamartoma of the cerebrum
(b) RCC in patients with tuberous sclerosis may be as frequent as 20%
(c) Renal cysts develop in approximately 20% of patients
(d) Angiomyolipomas occur in 40% to 80% of patients

(Answer is B) Tuberous sclerosis complex is an autosomal dominant condition that includes the triad of epilepsy, mental retardation, and adenoma sebaceum. It is associated with renal cysts (20% of patients), renal angiomyolipoma (40% to 80%) and RCC (2%).

93. Contiguous gene syndrome is seen among:

(a) PKD and ARCD (b) PKD and TS
(c) PKD and VHL (d) VHL and TS

(Answer is B) When severe polycystic kidneys are present in patients, particularly infants, with tuberous sclerosis, the condition represents a contiguous gene syndrome (i.e., defects in both *TSC2* and *PKD1*).

94. In which entity renal cyst lining is of hypertrophic, hyperplastic eosinophilic cells?

(a) TS (b) ARPKD
(c) VHL (d) MSK

(Answer is A) In tuberous sclerosis the renal cysts are of a unique histologic type in that they have a lining of hypertrophic, hyperplastic eosinophilic cells.

95. Regarding VHL which statement is not true?

(a) When present, renal cysts and tumors often are multiple and bilateral

(b) Renal cysts, the most common and often earliest manifestation

(c) The gene associated with the transmission of VHL disease is located on chromosome 3

(d) Most common cause of death is pheochromocytoma

(Answer is D) VHL disease is an AR condition associated with cerebellar and retinal hemangioblastomas; cysts of the pancreas, kidney and epididymis; pheochromocytoma (10% to 12%); and clear cell RCC (50% incidence, 30%-40% of death).

96. Which is the most common type of renal cystic disease?

(a) MCKD

(b) ADPKD

(c) VHL

(d) Medullary sponge kidney

(Answer is A) Multicystic dysplasia is the most common type of renal cystic disease.

97. Regarding MCKD which statement is not true?

(a) The kidney does not have a reniform configuration, and no calyceal drainage system is present

(b) The contralateral system frequently is abnormal as well

(c) Multicystic kidney has a haphazard distribution of cysts of various sizes without a larger central or medial cyst

(d) Multicystic kidney should be removed as it has high chances of transforming into malignancy

(Answer is D) There is no clear indication for removal of the kidney unless an increased amount of solid tissue is identified.

98. Hydronephrotic kidneys can be differentiated from MCKD by which scan?

(a) DMSA (b) DTPA

(c) Ga (d) MIBI

(Answer is A) Hydronephrotic kidneys usually show some function on a dimercaptosuccinic acid (DMSA) scan, whereas renal uptake is seldom seen in multicystic kidneys.

99. Regarding cystic nephroma which statement is not true?

(a) Patient is twice as likely to be male if younger than 4 years and eight times as likely to be female if older than 30 years of age

(b) A benign multilocular cyst is a benign, nondysplastic, neoplastic lesion

(c) In children an abdominal pain is the most common finding

(d) Adults present with either a flank mass, abdominal pain, or hematuria

(Answer is C) In children, an asymptomatic flank mass is the most common finding.

100. Diagnosis of a benign simple cyst on sonography, includes all *except:*

(a) Sharply defined

(b) Thin distinct smooth wall

(c) No internal echoes

(d) Poor transmission of sound waves

(Answer is D) To make the diagnosis of a benign simple cyst on sonography, it should have a sharply defined, thin distinct smooth wall, be spherical or oval with no internal echoes, and have good transmission of sound waves with acoustic enhancement behind the cyst.

101. Cyst with thin calcification and septa with minimal enhancement falls into which Bosniak's category?

(a) Category I (b) Category II
(c) Category IIF (d) Category III

(Answer is C) Calcification in wall of cyst thicker and more nodular than in category II, septa with minimal enhancement, especially those with calcium falls in category IIF.

102. Regarding simple renal cyst which statement is not true?

(a) Renal cyst is lined by cuboidal epithelium
(b) By 50 years of age, 50% patients will have renal cyst
(c) Cysts have no blood vessels and do not communicate directly with nephrons
(d) The density of renal cyst always ranges from – 10 to +20 HU

(Answer is D) When the cyst fluid is hyperdense (i.e., between 20 and 90 HU), it still is likely to be a simple cyst if no enhancement occurs when intravenous contrast agent is injected and if the other criteria of CT and sonography are met.

103. Regarding unilateral renal cystic disease which statement is not true?

(a) Large renal cysts of varying size appearing side by side, often more numerous at one pole
(b) Long-term follow-up demonstrate absence of cyst development in the contralateral kidney
(c) Family members should be affected with cystic disease
(d) Considered as a variation of the presentation of simple cysts

(Answer is C) No family members should be affected with cystic disease.

104. Collecting ducts are ectatic and are filled with calcifications, giving an appearance suggestive of a "bouquet of flowers":

(a) MSK (b) ARPKD
(c) VHL (d) TS

(Answer is A) Collecting ducts are more ectatic and are filled with calcifications, giving an appearance suggestive of a "bouquet of flowers".

105. Regarding medullary sponge kidney which statement is not true?

(a) Dilated collecting ducts that appear as bristles on a brush on IVU
(b) The most common presentation is urinary tract infection
(c) One third to one half of the patients with MSK have hypercalcemia
(d) For patients with renal lithiasis, thiazides should be administered even if hypercalciuria is not present

(Answer is B) The most common presentation is renal colic (50% to 60%), followed by urinary tract infection (20% to 33%) and gross hematuria (10% to 18%).

106. RCC occurring in ESRD is different biologically in a number of ways from classic RCC *except:*

(a) When RCC develops in ESRD, 80% of the time it is associated with ARCD
(b) RCC is associated with ARCD, it frequently occurs at an earlier age
(c) The incidence of RCC in ESRD is twice that of general population
(d) The male-to-female ratio is significantly greater in ESRD patients with RCC than in the general population with RCC

(Answer is C) The incidence of RCC in ESRD is 3 to 6 times that of the general population and may be as high as 10 times the incidence in blacks.

107. Regarding ARCD which statement is not true?

(a) It is associated with CRF and often seen in patients on long-term hemodialysis
(b) It consists of hyperplastic renal cysts and frequently adenomas; either can progress to RCC
(c) If RCC develops, it mostly does so after 10 years of dialysis

(d) The cysts usually regress with transplantation

(Answer is C) If RCC develops, it mostly does so before 10 years of dialysis.

108. Renal sinus cyst is not derived from:

(a) Renal parenchyma (b) Arteries
(c) Lymphatics (d) Fat

(Answer is A) The term renal sinus cyst should be reserved for all other cysts in the hilum, that is, those that are not derived from the renal parenchyma but rather from the other structures of the sinus, such as arteries, lymphatics and fat.

109. Regarding renal sinus cyst which statement is not true?

(a) The predominant type appears to be derived from the lymphatics
(b) Most often these cysts are solitary, and often they are unilateral
(c) Majority appear after the fifth decade
(d) May be associated with inflammation, obstruction, or a calculus

(Answer is B) The predominant type of renal sinus cyst appears to be one derived from the lymphatics. Most often these cysts are multiple, and often they are bilateral.

110. Regarding PUJO which statement is not true?

(a) Bilateral UPJ obstruction is present in 10% to 40% of cases
(b) An aberrant vessel pass anteriorly to the UPJ and contribute to mechanical obstruction
(c) UPJ obstruction may also be seen with severe VUR; these conditions coexist in 10% of cases
(d) In PUJO secondary to VUR, the reflux needs to be corrected initially

(Answer is D) In PUJO secondary to VUR, obstructive lesion needs to be corrected initially, even though the VUR contributed to the initial problem.

111. In PUJO which congenital anomaly is most commonly seen in contralateral kidney?

(a) PUJO (b) MCKD
(c) VUR (d) Renal dysplasia

(Answer is A) UPJ obstruction is the most common anomaly encountered in the opposite kidney.

112. Maturation of renal parenchyma occurs at what age?

(a) At birth (b) 1 month
(c) 3 months (d) 6 months

(Answer is C) The fetal and neonatal kidney may appear to be hydronephrotic on ultrasonography secondary to the sonolucent appearance of the medullary area and pyramids. This appearance tends to resolve after parenchymal maturation, which occurs at 3 months of age.

113. What ratio of parenchyma-pelvicaliceal area suggests obstructive process and need for pyeloplasty?

(a) <0.6 (b) <1.6
(c) <2.0 (d) <2.6

(Answer is B) To improve diagnostic accuracy of UPJO on ultrasonography, the renal parenchyma-pelvicaliceal area has been measured and compared with the result of conventional diuretic renography. A ratio of less than 1.6 correlates well with an obstructive process and need for pyeloplasty, whereas patients with a ratio greater than 1.6 can be safely observed.

114. Term F +20 is used in which study?

(a) CECT (b) MRI
(c) PET (d) DTPA

(Answer is D) When diuretic is given prior to tracer in dynamic scan it is F -15, some with the tracer it is F 0, and if diuretic is given when the renal pelvis is full of tracer it is F +20.

115. To assess urinary tract obstruction which is the most superior investigation?

(a) USG (b) MRU

(c) Whitaker test (d) Dynamic scan

(Answer is B) MRI urography is being investigated to define urinary tract anatomy, calculate differential renal function, and assess urinary tract obstruction. In comparison with ultrasonography and nuclear renography, dynamic contrast enhanced MRI is superior.

116. Indication of performing transperitoneal laparoscopic pyeloplasty rather than by retroperitoneal approach is:

(a) Hydronephrosis secondary to low UPJ
(b) Horseshoe kidney
(c) Retrocaval ureter
(d) Situation demanding ureterocalyceal anastomosis

(Answer is B) The retroperitoneal lateral approach provides the advantage of dealing with most situations requiring a pyeloplasty. Thus far, the only indications for performing a transperitoneal approach are the horseshoe kidney and the ectopic kidney.

117. Acucise is used for the treatment of:

(a) VUR (b) BPH
(c) PUV (d) PUJO

(Answer is D) Acucise balloon is inflated across the ureteropelvic junction narrowing for treatment of PUJO.

118. Bifid ureters are defined as:

(a) The ureters join at the level of the ureteropelvic junction
(b) The ureters join more distally but are still proximal to the bladder level
(c) Ureters that drain their respective poles and empty separately into the genitourinary tract
(d) Two separate pelvicalyceal systems

(Answer is B) A *duplex kidney* is one that has two separate pelvicalyceal systems. A duplex kidney has an upper pole and a lower pole. The ureters may join at any point. If they join at the level of the ureteropelvic junction, the configuration is termed a *bifid system.* If the ureters join more distally but are still proximal to the bladder level, the configuration is termed *bifid ureters.* Double ureters are ureters that drain their respective poles and empty separately into the genitourinary tract.

119. Cecoureterocele is defined as:

(a) Ureterocele with narrowed or pinpoint opening inside the bladder
(b) Ureterocele with orifice distal to the bladder neck
(c) Ureterocele with orifice that is stenotic and distal to the bladder neck
(d) Ureterocele with intravesical orifice and a submucosal extension that dips into the urethra

(Answer is D) Cecoureterocele has an intravesical orifice and a submucosal extension that dips into the urethra.

120. Which statement regarding embryology of genitourinary tract is not correct?

(a) At 4 weeks' gestation, an outpouching arises from the distal mesonephric duct
(b) The segment of mesonephric duct distal to the ureteric bud is the common excretory duct
(c) The point of origin of the ureteric bud is the ureteral orifice
(d) When the ureteral orifice enters the bladder it begins to migrate in the bladder in a cranial and medial direction

(Answer is D) When the ureteral orifice enters the bladder it begins to migrate in the bladder in a cranial and lateral direction.

121. Ectopic ureter in females can drain at all *except:*

(a) Ovary (b) Fallopian tube

(c) Uterus (d) Upper vagina

(Answer is A) An ectopic ureter draining into any of these female structures can rupture into the adjoining fallopian tube, uterus, upper vagina or vestibule.

122. Weigert-Meyer rule is for:

(a) Vesicourteric reflux
(b) Ureterocele
(c) Complete duplicated systems
(d) Posterior urethral valve

(Answer is C) Weigert-Meyer rule of complete duplicated systems yields a fairly constant anatomy that is important for radiologic, cystoscopic, and reconstructive considerations.

123. Which statement regarding ectopic ureter is not true?

(a) Of all ectopic orifices, 80% are associated with a duplicated collecting system
(b) Between 5% and 17% of ectopic ureters appear bilaterally
(c) In females, more than 80% are duplicated, but in males, most ectopic ureters drain single systems
(d) Ectopic ureters appear more commonly in males clinically

(Answer is D) Ectopic ureters appear more commonly in females clinically, from 2 to 12 times more frequently.

124. In male, the most common site of termination of an ectopic ureter is:

(a) Posterior urethra (b) Seminal vesicle
(c) Ejaculatory duct (d) Vas deferens

(Answer is A) In the male, the posterior urethra is the most common site of termination of an ectopic ureter.

125. In female, the most common site of termination of an ectopic ureter is:

(a) Urethra and vestibule
(b) Vestibule and vagina
(c) Vagina and cervix
(d) Cervix and uterus

(Answer is A) In the female, the urethra and vestibule are the most common sites.

126. Continuous incontinence in a girl with an otherwise normal voiding pattern after toilet training is the classic symptom of:

(a) Functional
(b) Ectopic ureteral orifice
(c) Ureterocele
(d) Urethrocele

(Answer is B) Continuous incontinence in a girl with an otherwise normal voiding pattern after toilet training is the classic symptom of an ectopic ureteral orifice and ureterovaginal fistula.

127. Ureterocele incision is recommended in all *except:*

(a) Intravesical ureterocele
(b) Ureterocele associated with a functioning upper pole
(c) Single-system ureterocele
(d) Ectopic ureterocele

(Answer is D) Ureterocele incision is recommended in all neonates as well as in older children with either an intravesical ureterocele, a ureterocele associated with a functioning upper pole, or a single-system ureterocele.

128. Patient with ectopic ureterocele with non-functioning upper pole with high-grade reflux into the ipsilateral lower pole ureter, best management policy is:

(a) Upper pole partial nephrectomy
(b) Upper pole nephrectomy, ureterocele excision, and lower pole ureteral reimplantation
(c) Upper pole nephroureterectomy, ureterocele excision, and lower pole ureteral reimplantation

(d) Ureteropyelostomy

(Answer is C) This combined approach would be recommended because these severe degrees of reflux are less likely to disappear spontaneously and would probably require a second procedure.

129. Most common areas of the ureter that is particularly liable to ureteral stenosis is:

(a) Ureteropelvic junction
(b) Distal ureter just above the extravesical junction
(c) Mid ureter at the pelvic brim
(d) All above three sites have same frequency

(Answer is A) Areas of the ureter liable to ureteral stenosis. In order of decreasing frequency, they are the ureteropelvic junction, the distal ureter just above the extravesical junction, and, rarely, the mid ureter at the pelvic brim.

130. Which statement regarding VUR in children is not true?

(a) Prevalence of VUR in siblings to be approximately 32%
(b) Reflux may be present in up to 70% of infants with UTI
(c) There is a tendency for an autosomal dominant pattern of inheritance
(d) Prevalence of reflux in children remains same with or without infection

(Answer is D) The prevalence of reflux was estimated to be approximately 30% in children with UTI and 17% in those without infection.

131. Paquin's ratio of tunnel length to ureteral diameter in normal UVJ is:

(a) 1.4 : 1 (b) 3 : 1
(c) 5 : 1 (d) 1 : 3

(Answer is C) Paquin's early dissections of the UVJ in children revealed an approximate 5:1 ratio of tunnel length to ureteral diameter in nonrefluxing junctions versus a 1.4:1 ratio in refluxing UVJs.

132. According to IRSC mild dilatation of the ureter with minimal blunting of the fornices is classified as which grade of VUR?

(a) Grade I (b) Grade II
(c) Grade III (d) Grade IV

(Answer is C)

III Mild to moderate dilatation of the ureter, renal pelvis, and calyces with minimal blunting of the fornices.

133. Which statement regarding diagnosis and evaluation of VUR is not correct?

(a) Radiologic studies should be tailored to age, gender, and mode of manifestation
(b) Direct cystography for the diagnosis of reflux requires bladder catheterization
(c) Nuclear cystograms, though more sensitive, provide much less anatomic detail than a VCUG does
(d) Routine cystoscopy is indicated in reflux management

(Answer is D) Modern management of reflux does not include routine cystoscopy. Cystoscopy can provide useful information immediately before open surgery.

134. Which scan has high sensitivity and specificity for scar detection?

(a) DMSA (b) DTPA
(c) MAG (d) Gallium scan

(Answer is A) DMSA scanning provided 98% sensitivity and 92% specificity for scar detection.

135. Which statement regarding management of VUR is not correct?

(a) Spontaneous resolution of reflux is very common
(b) High-grade reflux is more likely to resolve spontaneously
(c) Sterile reflux is benign
(d) The success rate with surgical correction is very high

(Answer is B) High-grade reflux is less likely to resolve spontaneously.

136. In which surgical technique supra-hiatal tunnel is formed?

(a) Politano-Leadbetter technique
(b) Glenn-Anderson technique
(c) Cohen Cross-Trigonal technique
(d) Lich-Gregoir technique

(Answer is A) Politano-Leadbetter Technique is a supra-hiatal technique.

137. Which is the technique of choice for ureter reimplant in bladder neck reconstructive procedures?

(a) Politano-Leadbetter technique
(b) Glenn-Anderson technique
(c) Cohen Cross-Trigonal technique
(d) Lich-Gregoir technique

(Answer is C) Cross-trigonal reimplantation is the procedure of choice in conjunction with bladder neck reconstructive procedures because the superior displacement of the ureters provides room for adequate elongation of the bladder neck.

138. In which surgical technique extravesical ureter reimplant is done?

(a) Politano-Leadbetter technique
(b) Glenn-Anderson technique
(c) Cohen Cross-Trigonal technique
(d) Lich-Gregoir technique

(Answer is D) Lich and colleagues (1961) in the United States and Gregoir (1964) in Europe independently described the extravesical approach to ureteral reimplantation.

139. STING technique is used for the treatment of:

(a) PUV
(b) Megaureter
(c) PUJO
(d) VUR

(Answer is D) O'Donnell and Puri who popularized the technique of endoscopic correction of primary VUR with a success rate of 75% after one injection. They coined the term STING (subureteric Teflon injection).

140. Which is currently the preferred agent for endoscopic correction for VUR?

(a) PTFE
(b) Deflux
(c) Cross-linked collagen
(d) Macroplastique

(Answer is B) Deflux is currently the preferred agent for endoscopic correction in most centers.

141. Which statement regarding prune belly syndrome is not correct?

(a) Unilateral intra-abdominal testes
(b) Urinary bladder is massively enlarged
(c) The ureters are typically dilated and tortuous
(d) Posterior urethra is dilated

(Answer is A) Bilateral intra-abdominal testes lying over the iliac vessels are the most typical findings.

142. Incomplete form of PBS includes all *except:*

(a) Many of these patients may go on to renal failure
(b) Cryptorchidism
(c) Deficiency of the abdominal musculature
(d) Anomalous urinary tract

(Answer is C) Incomplete forms of the syndrome would lack the typical abdominal wall features but have the common uropathy and cryptorchidism. Many of these patients may go on to renal failure.

143. Incidence of refluxin closed bladder exstrophy is:

(a) 70%
(b) 80%
(c) 90%
(d) 100%

(Answer is D) Reflux in the closed exstrophy bladder occurs in 100% of cases, and subsequent surgery is usually required at the time of bladder neck reconstruction.

144. In modern stage reconstruction of bladder exstrophy, epispadias repair is done at what age?

(a) Immediately after birth
(b) Before 6 months of age
(c) 6 to 12 months of age
(d) 4 to 5 years of age

(Answer is C) Typically, epispadias repair is now performed between 6 months and 12 months of age, after testosterone stimulation. Bladder neck repair usually occurs when the child is 4 to 5 years of age.

145. Which statement regarding variants of exstrophy repair is not true?

(a) In pseudoexstrophy, presence of musculoskeletal defect of the exstrophy anomaly with no major defect in the urinary tract has been named
(b) In superior vesical fissure, persistent cloacal membrane ruptures only at the lowermost portion
(c) Duplicate exstrophy occurs when a superior vesical fissure opens but there is later fusion of the abdominal wall and a portion of the bladder elements (mucosa) remains outside
(d) Covered exstrophy has also been referred to as split symphysis variant

(Answer is B) In superior vesical fissure, persistent cloacal membrane ruptures only at the uppermost portion.

146. Which is the most common urachal anomaly?

(a) Patent urachus
(b) Umbilical-urachus sinus
(c) Urachal cyst
(d) Vesicourachal diverticulum

(Answer is A) Patent urachus forms 50% of urachal anomaly.

147. Which statement regarding primary paraureteral diverticula is not correct?

(a) It is smooth walled
(b) Multiple
(c) Occurs mostly in children
(d) No infravesical obstruction

(Answer is B) Primary paraureteral diverticula are seen in smooth-walled bladders, occur isolated with no other diverticula, are intermittent, and occur in children with no infravesical obstruction.

148. Which type of PUV is most common?

(a) Type III (b) Type I
(c) Type II (d) Type IV

(Answer is B) Young's type I valves make up 95% of all posterior urethral obstructions.

149. Which statement regarding PUV I is not correct?

(a) The valve itself is made of a fibrous stroma covered on each side by transitional epithelium
(b) There is hypertrophy of muscle within the valve
(c) It may be related to an abnormal insertion of the mesonephric ducts into the fetal cloaca
(d) Lack plicae colliculi

(Answer is B) There is no muscle within the PUV I.

150. Embryologic origin of which type of valve has been attributed to incomplete dissolution of the urogenital portion of the cloacal membrane?

(a) Type I (b) Type II
(c) Type III (d) Type IV

(Answer is C) The embryologic origin of type III valves has been attributed to incomplete dissolution of the urogenital portion of the cloacal membrane.

151. Regarding initial management of patients with PUV all are true *except:*

(a) PUV requires the immediate establishment of urinary catheter drainage

(b) Before catheter drainage diagnosis should always be confirmed by VCUG
(c) Neonates can be catheterized with a 3.5 or 5 French pediatric feeding tube
(d) One-shot cystogram is often advisable to aid and document proper catheter placement

(Answer is B) Initial management of all patients with PUV requires the immediate catheter drainage from the bladder. This should be performed even if the diagnosis has not been confirmed by YCUG.

152. Regarding valve bladder which is not true?

(a) Despite successful valve ablation, intrinsic bladder dysfunction persist
(b) Poor sensation
(c) Poor compliance
(d) Poor bladder capacity

(Answer is D) Valve bladder has combination of poor sensation, high bladder volumes, and poor compliance producing storage pressures high enough to prevent adequate drainage of the upper tracts.

153. Isosthenuria implies:

(a) Similar pH
(b) Similar glucose
(c) Similar protein
(d) Similar specific gravity

(Answer is D) Isosthenuria defines as excretion of urine with fixed specific gravity. It may occur in terminal renal disease when the specific gravity reaches that of the glomerular filtrate, 1.010.

154. Most common cause for need for renal transplant in children is:

(a) PUJO (b) MCKD
(c) VUR (d) PUV

(Answer is D) The most common condition reqiuring the need for renal transplant is posterior urethral valves.

155. All are true regarding Hinman's syndrome *except:*

(a) Also termed as neurogenic bladder syndrome
(b) Combination of bladder decompensation with incontinence and poor emptying
(c) Most children also have significant bowel dysfunction
(d) Nearly every patient has a grossly trabeculated, large-capacity bladder with a considerable volume of postmicturition residual urine

(Answer is A) Hinman first coined the terms nonneurogenic neurogenic bladder or subclinical neurogenic bladder, and later Hinman syndrome.

156. Augmentation with an intestinal segment leads to:

(a) Decrease in serum chloride and serum bicarbonate level
(b) Increase in serum chloride and serum bicarbonate level
(c) Increase in serum chloride and a decrease in serum bicarbonate level
(d) Decrease in serum chloride and an increase in serum bicarbonate level

(Answer is C) Augmentation with an intestinal segment had an increase in serum chloride and a decrease in serum bicarbonate level, although full acidosis was rare if renal function was normal.

157. With which segment of bowel most and least rhythmic contractions have been noted after bladder augmentation?

(a) Ileum and stomach
(b) Stomach and ileum
(c) Stomach and colon
(d) Colon and ileum

(Answer is B) Rhythmic contractions have been noted postoperatively after bladder augmentation, with all bowel segments, although ileum seems the least likely to demonstrate remarkable urodynamic abnormalities and stomach the most.

158. Which segment of bowel is most likely to require reaugmentation?

(a) Sigmoid colon (b) Stomach
(c) Ileum (d) Jejunum

(Answer is A) Sigmoid colon followed by stomach and then ileum were more likely to require reaugmentation.

159. Hematuria-dysuria syndrome occurs with the use of which bowel segment?

(a) Colon (b) Ileum
(c) Jejunum (d) Stomach

(Answer is D) Acid secretion by gastric mucosa may result in another unique problem after gastrocystoplasty, the hematuria-dysuria syndrome.

160. Which type of stones are formed in patients with augmentation cystoplasty?

(a) Uric acid
(b) Calcium oxalate monohydrate
(c) Calcium oxalate dihydrate
(d) Struvite

(Answer is D) The majority of bladder stones in this population of patients are struvite in composition, and bacteriuria has been thought to be an important risk factor.

161. Most common type of hypospadias is:

(a) Distal (b) Middle
(c) Posterior (d) Proximal

(Answer is A) Overall rates of approximately 50%, 30% and 20 % for distal, middle, and posterior/proximal hypospadias, respectively.

162. The best time for surgery for hypospadias is:

(a) Immediately after birth
(b) Before 6 months
(c) Between 6 and 12 months
(d) Between 1 and 5 years

(Answer is C) The best time for surgery for hypospadias is between 6 and 12 months of age.

163. Closure of neourethra is best done with which suture?

(a) Silk (b) Prolene
(c) PDS (d) Chromic

(Answer is D) There is four-fold increase in urethral stricture rate after hypospadias repair with polydioxanone suture (PDS) compared with chromic or polyglycolic acid suture.

164. MAGPI technique is used for the repair of:

(a) Distal hypospadias
(b) Middle hypospadias
(c) Proximal hypospadias
(d) Distal and middle hypospadias

(Answer is A) Glanular and some coronal hypospadias defects are amenable to the meatoplasty and glanuloplasty (MAGPI) technique.

165. Ideal techniques for repair of middle hypospadias is the:

(a) Mathieu, perimeatal-based flap
(b) MAGPI
(c) Onlay island flap
(d) Transverse preputial island flap (TPIF)

(Answer is C) The onlay island flap technique is ideal for middle hypospadias defects. Among the most commonly used techniques for repair of middle hypospadias is the onlay island flap (OIF) technique.

166. Most common complication of hypospadias repair:

(a) Infection
(b) Meatal stenosis
(c) Urethrocutaneous fistula
(d) Bleeding

(Answer is D) Bleeding is the most common complication of hypospadias repair. Infection is an uncommon complication of hypospadias repair.

167. Skin deficient hypospadias requiring reoperation, which is the best material for reconstruction?

(a) FTG from skin (b) Bladder mucosa
(c) Rectal mucosa (d) Buccal mucosa

(Answer is D) Skin deficient hypospadias requiring reoperation, buccal mucosa has become the preferred material for reconstruction.

168. Which is not the correct pair?

(a) Genital tubercle in male–glans penis
(b) Genital tubercle in female–clitoris
(c) Genital swellings in male–scrotum
(d) Genital swellings in female–labia minora

(Answer is D) In the female, because of the absence of testosterone and DHT, the genital tubercle develops passively into the clitoris, the genital folds become the labia minora, and the genital swellings become the labia majora.

169. Incidence of urological malformation, in patients with congenital anorectal malformation is:

(a) 40% (b) 50%
(c) 60% (d) 70%

(Answer is B) As many as 50% of children with congenital anorectal malformations also have an associated urologic malformation, and the external genitalia are frequently involved.

170. Micropenis is defined as below how many standard deviations?

(a) 1.5 (b) 2.0
(c) 2.5 (d) 3.0

(Answer is C) Micropenis is a normally formed penis that is at l east 2.5 standard deviations (SD) below the mean in size.

171. The most common cause of micropenis is:

(a) Hypogonadotropic hypogonadism
(b) Primary hypogonadism
(c) Defect in testosterone secretion
(d) Developmental anomalies

(Answer is A) The most common cause of micropenis is failure of the hypothalamus to produce an adequate amount of gonadotropin-releasing hormone (GnRH). This condition, termed hypogonadotropic hypogonadism.

172. Midline brain defects is associated with which urological abnormality?

(a) Undescended testis
(b) Renal agenesis
(c) Ectopic ureter
(d) Micropenis

(Answer is D) Micropenis is associated with congenital pituitary aplasia and midline brain defects, such as agenesis of the corpus callosum and occipital encephalocele.

173. Regarding penile torsion which statement is not true?

(a) Almost always, the shaft is rotated in a counterclockwise direction
(b) In most cases, penile size is small
(c) Correction is unnecessary if the rotation is less than 60 to 90 degrees from the midline
(d) Orientation of the corporal bodies and the corpus spongiosum at the base of the penis is normal

(Answer is B) Penile size is normal and the condition is unrecognized until circumcision is performed or until the foreskin is retracted.

174. The gubernaculum appears at which week of embryologic development?

(a) Five weeks (b) Seven weeks
(c) Nine weeks (d) Eleven weeks

(Answer is B) The gubernaculum appears at the seventh week of embryologic development.

175. SRY gene is located at which week?

(a) Short arm of Y (b) Long arm of Y
(c) Short arm of X (d) Long arm of X

(Answer is A) The *SRY* gene, located in a 35 kb region on the short arm of the Y chromosome, appears to be primarily responsible for male sexual differentiation.

176. Factors that predict complete spontaneous descent by 3 months of age are all *except:*

(a) Low birth weight
(b) Bilateral cryptorchidism
(c) Abnormal scrotal anatomy
(d) Testis that are positioned lower along the normal path of descent

(Answer is C) Factors that predict complete spontaneous descent by 3 months of age include low birth weight, bilateral cryptorchidism, normal scrotal anatomy, and testis that are positioned lower along the normal path of descent.

177. The most common ectopic location of testis is:

(a) Transverse scrotal
(b) Femoral
(c) Perineal
(d) Denis-Browne pouch

(Answer is D) The most common ectopic location is within a superficial pouch between the external oblique fascia and Scarpa's fascia, a structure that has been termed the Denis-Browne pouch.

178. Regarding retractile testis which statement is not true?

(a) Testis withdraws spontaneously out of the scrotum toward the inguinal canal
(b) Retractile testes are most commonly encountered below the age of 3 years
(c) Children with retractile testes should be monitored regularly (yearly), at least up to puberty
(d) The retractability of the testes is caused by an overactive cremasteric reflex

(Answer is B) Retractile testes are most commonly encountered between the ages of 3 and 7 years. The retractability of the testes is caused by an overactive cremasteric reflex.

179. The histopathologic hallmarks associated with cryptorchidism are all *except:*

(a) Decreased numbers of Leydig cells, degeneration of Sertoli cells
(b) Delayed appearance of gonocytes
(c) Delayed appearance of adult dark (AD) spermatogonia
(d) Failure of primary spermatocytes to develop

(Answer is B) The histopathologic hallmarks associated with cryptorchidism are evident between 1 and 2 years of age and include decreased numbers of Leydig cells, degeneration of Sertoli cells, delayed disappearance of gonocytes, delayed appearance of adult dark (AD) spermatogonia, failure of primary spermatocytes to develop, and reduced total germ cell counts.

180. Current treatment recommendations of orchidopexy is at what age?

(a) Immediately after birth
(b) At 6 months
(c) Between 6 and 12 months
(d) Before child goes to school

(Answer is C) Definitive treatment of an undescended testis should take place between 6 and 12 months of age.

181. What is the incidence of testicular tumors from an undescended testis (UDT)?

(a) 1% (b) 10%
(c) 20% (d) 25%

(Answer is B) Approximately 10% of testicular tumors arise from an undescended testis.

182. The most common tumor that develops from a cryptorchid testis is:

(a) Teratoma (b) Lymphoma
(c) Leydig cell tumor (d) Seminoma

(Answer is D) The most common tumor that develops from a cryptorchid testis is seminoma.

183. Patent processus vaginalis is found in how many patients with undescended testis?

(a) 0% (b) 50%
(c) 90% (d) 100%

(Answer is C) Patent processus vaginalis is found in more than 90% of patients with an undescended testis.

184. Hormonal treatment in UDT can be tried in patients with:

(a) Previously operated testes
(b) Ectopic testes
(c) Retractile testis
(d) Those with an inguinal hernia

(Answer is C) Successful results are more commonly reported in older groups of children and in testis that were retractile or below the external inguinal ring.

185. Best success rate of orchiopexy is seen with:

(a) Microvascular orchiopexy
(b) Standard abdominal orchiopexy
(c) Fowler-Stephens orchiopexy
(d) Standard Fowler-Stephens orchiopexy

(Answer is A) Success rate of 92% for testes below the external ring, 89% for inguinal testes, 84% for· microvascular orchiopexy, 81% for standard abdominal orchiopexy, 77% for staged Fowler-Stephens orchiopexy, and 67% for standard Fowler-Stephens orchiopexy.

186. Which is the best modality for assessment of UDT?

(a) USG
(b) CT scan
(c) MRI
(d) Diagnostic laparoscopy

(Answer is D) Diagnostic laparoscopy is commonly used for the assessment of a nonpalpable testis, with the accuracy of testicular localization reported to be greater than 95%.

187. Regarding torsion of spermatic cord which statement is not true?

(a) Irreversible ischemic injury to the testicular parenchyma may begin as soon as 4 hours after occlusion of the cord
(b) The absence of a cremasteric reflex is a good indicator of torsion of the cord
(c) Exploration of the contralateral hemiscrotum should be carried out only if there is evidence of torsion on that side
(d) Color Doppler ultrasound examination has become the adjunctive investigation of choice

(Answer is C) When torsion of the spermatic cord is found, exploration of the contralateral hemiscrotum must be carried out. In almost all cases a bell-clapper deformity is found. The contralateral testis must be fixed to prevent subsequent torsion.

188. Regarding torsion of testicular appendages which statement is not true?

(a) Color Doppler studies may show normal or decreased flow
(b) Infarcted appendage is visible through the skin as a "blue dot sign"
(c) The cremasteric reflex should be present
(d) Nonoperative management allows most cases to resolve spontaneously

(Answer is A) Radionuclide scans or color Doppler studies may show normal or increased flow, and ultrasound imaging may delineate the swollen appendage.

189. Testosterone and estrogen secretion is detected by what weeks of gestation respectively?

(a) 9th and 10th (b) 10th and 9th
(c) 8th and 9th (d) 9th and 8th

(Answer is D) Testosterone secretion by the fetal testes is detectable shortly after the formation of Leydig cells in the interstitium at approximately 9 weeks' gestation. Estrogen synthesis is detectable in the female embryo just after 8 weeks of gestation.

190. Most common structural abnormality seen in Turner's syndrome is:

(a) Horseshoe kidney
(b) Renal agenesis
(c) Multiple renal arteries
(d) Malrotation

(Answer is C) Between 33% and 60% of patients with Turner's syndrome have structure or positional abnormalities of the kidney. HSK accounts for 10%, duplication or renal agenesis for 20%, malrotation for 15% and multiple renal arteries have been noted in 90% of patients with Turner's syndrome.

191. Most common cause of ambiguous genitalia is:

(a) Mixed gonadal dysgenesis
(b) CAH
(c) Pure gonadal dysgenesis
(d) Klinefelter's syndrome

(Answer is B) In the newborn period, mixed gonadal dysgenesis is the second most common cause of ambiguous genitalia (after CAH) and must be in the differential diagnosis.

192. A deficiency of which enzyme is mostly responsible for CAH?

(a) 21-hydroxylase
(b) 11 β-hydroxylase
(c) 3β-hydroxysteroid dehydrogenase
(d) 17, 20 lysase

(Answer is A) A deficiency of steroid 21-hydroxylase is responsible for 95% of cases of CAH.

193. All are cause of female pseudohermaphroditism *except:*

(a) 21-hydroxylase
(b) 11β-hydroxylase
(c) 3β-hydroxysteroid dehydrogenase
(d) 17, 20 lysase

(Answer is D) Masculinized Female (Female Pseudohermaphroditism) causes are: Congenital adrenal hyperplasia (21-hydroxylase, 11β-hydroxylase, 3β-hydroxysteroid dehydrogenase deficiencies).

194. Which is the most common cause of primary amenorrhea?

(a) Gonadal dysgenesis
(b) MRKH
(c) CAH
(d) Klinefelter's syndrome

(Answer is A) MRKH syndrome is in fact second only to gonadal dysgenesis as a cause of primary amenorrhea.

195. What is the incidence of skeletal abnormalities in MRKH syndrome?

(a) 0 to 10% (b) 10% to 20%
(c) 20% to 30% (d) 30% to 40%

(Answer is B) Associated congenital abnormalities of the skeletal system have been described in 10% to 20% of cases.

196. Which statement is not true about MRKH syndrome?

(a) Results from failure of sinovaginal bulbs to develop and form the vaginal plate
(b) The karyotype is that of a normal 46,XX woman
(c) In the typical form of MRKH syndrome (type A), the patient has symmetrical uterine remnants and normal fallopian tubes

(d) Renal anomalies are present almost exclusively in type A patients

(Answer is D) Renal anomalies are present almost exclusively in patients with the atypical subtype of vaginal agenesis (type B).

197. Most common extracranial solid tumor of childhood:

(a) Rhabdomyosarcoma
(b) Wilms
(c) Neuroblastoma
(d) Yolk sac tumor

(Answer is C) Neuroblastoma is the most common extracranial solid tumor of childhood.

198. Which statement is not true about neuroblastoma?

(a) More than 95% of cases are diagnosed in children by 10 years of age
(b) Twenty-five of these children have metastatic disease at diagnosis
(c) Seventy-five percent arise in the retroperitoneum
(d) It is the most common malignant tumor of infancy

(Answer is B) Over half of these children have metastatic disease at diagnosis.

199. Poor prognostic factors for neuroblastoma are all *except:*

(a) Age less than 1 year
(b) Adrenal tumor
(c) N-myc namplification
(d) DNA index greater than 1

(Answer is A) Children 1 year or younger have better survival than older children do.

200. Which statement is not true about rhabdomyosarcoma (RMS)?

(a) Fifteen percent to 20% of all cases of RMS arise from the genitourinary system
(b) The most common genitourinary sites are the prostate and bladder
(c) Prostate and bladder region having a better prognosis than vagina/uterus primaries
(d) The botryoid and spindle cell variants of embryonal RMS are associated with excellent survival

(Answer is C) Vagina and paratesticular region having a better prognosis than bladder/prostate primaries.

201. Which is the most common primary malignant renal tumor of childhood?

(a) Neuroblastoma
(b) Nephroblastoma
(c) Renal cell carcinoma
(d) Rhabdomyosarcoma

(Answer is B) Wilms' tumor, or nephroblastoma, is the most common primary malignant renal tumor of childhood.

202. Chromosomal abnormalities associated with Wilms' tumor are all *except:*

(a) 11p13 (b) 11p15
(c) 11p17 (d) 16q

(Answer is C) 11p13-WT1, 11p15-WT2 are associated with Wilms' tumor.

203. Loss of the short arm of chromosome 1 is associated with which malignancy?

(a) Angiomyolipoma
(b) Rhabdomyosarcoma
(c) Neuroblastoma
(d) Wilms' tumor

(Answer is C) Deletion of the short arm of chromosome 1 is found in 70% to 80% of patients with neuroblastoma and is an adverse prognostic marker.

204. Children with bilateral Wilms' is staged as:

(a) Stage 2 (b) Stage 4

(c) Stage 5 (d) Stage 6

(Answer is C)

V Bilateral renal involvement at diagnosis.

205. According to NWTS-5 all are candidates for radiotherapy *except:*

(a) Stage 2 FH
(b) Stage 2 diffuse anaplasia
(c) Clear cell sarcoma kidney any stage
(d) Rhabdoid tumour kidney any stage

(Answer is A) All except stage 2 FH and stage 1 any anaplasia should receive radiotherapy.

206. In patients with Wilms' disease preoperative chemotherapy is recommended *except:*

(a) Bilateral Wilms' tumors
(b) Tumor inoperable at surgical exploration
(c) Tumor extension into inferior vena cava above the hepatic veins
(d) Tumor demonstrating diffuse anaplasia

(Answer is D) Preoperative chemotherapy is routinely recommended, including children with bilateral Wilms' tumors, tumors inoperable at surgical exploration, and tumor extension into inferior vena cava above the hepatic veins.

207. Which is the most aggressive and lethal childhood renal tumor?

(a) Clear cell sarcoma
(b) Rhabdoid tumor (RTK)
(c) Congenital mesoblastic nephroma
(d) Nephroblastoma

(Answer is B) RTK is the most aggressive and lethal childhood renal tumor.

208. Which is the most common renal tumor in infants?

(a) Wilms' tumor
(b) Congential mesoblastic nephroma (CMN)
(c) Renal cell carcinoma
(d) Congenital multilocular nephroma

(Answer is B) CMN is the most common renal tumor in infants.

209. Most common renal malignancy in the second decade of life:

(a) Wilms' tumor
(b) Congenital mesoblastic nephroma
(c) Renal cell carcinoma
(d) Rhabdoid tumor

(Answer is C) Renal cell carcinoma is the most common renal malignancy in the second decade of life.

210. Radiographic assessment of the genitourinary tract for a possible injury in pediatric patient should occur in all *except:*

(a) All penetrating abdominal trauma
(b) History of a significant deceleration or high-velocity injury
(c) Significant trauma that has resulted in fractures
(d) All patients with microscopic hematuria

(Answer is D) Radiographic assessment of the GUT for a possible injury should occur after all penetrating abdominal trauma as well as in blunt trauma victims who have one of four criteria: (1) a history of a significant deceleration; (2) significant trauma that has resulted in fractures or signs of peritonitis; (3) gross hematuria; and (4) microscopic hematuria associated with shock.

211. Which statement regarding PUJ disruption is not true?

(a) 30% will have a completely normal urinalysis
(b) Presentation can be delayed for more than 36 hours in more than 50% of patients
(c) In delayed diagnosis of UPJ disruption, repair is done at 12 weeks
(d) Diagnosis made 2nd day after the traumatic insult, placement of a nephrostomy tube is preferred

(Answer is D) In the clinically stable patient in whom the diagnosis is made within 5 days after the traumatic insult immediate surgical repair with debridement of any devitalized tissue, spatulation and reanastomosis of the ureter over a stent, and placement of an intraoperative nephrostomy tube and retroperitoneal drain is preferred.

212. Children with a posterior urethral injury will differ from adults with urethral injury by all the following *except:*

(a) More likely to be unstable
(b) More likely to be severely and permanently displaced prostatic urethra
(c) Complete posterior urethral disruption more common in adult
(d) Coexisting anterior longitudinal tears though the bladder neck and sphincteric complex being more common in boys

(Answer is C) The severe displacement of the prostate off the pelvic floor makes a complete posterior urethral disruption more common in boys than men.

213. Patient with karyotype-46 XY with symmetrical anatomy will be:

(a) Undervirilized male
(b) Mixed gonadal dysgenesis
(c) Overvirilized female
(d) Ovotesticular disorder or sex differentiation

(Answer is A) Diagnoses based on karyotype and anatomic symmetry

Karyotype-46XY Symmetric anatomy-
Undervirilized male
Asymmetric anatomy-
Mixed gonadal dysgenesis
Karyotype-46XX- Symmetric anatomy-
Overvirilized female
Asymmetric anatomy-
Ovotesticular disorder of sex differentiation

214. What is the most likely cause of large scrotal hematoma in neonates?

(a) Clotting factor VIII deficiency
(b) Clotting factor IX deficiency
(c) Breech delivery
(d) Scrotal cavernous hemangioma

(Answer is C) Breech delivery

215. What is the most frequent anomaly associated with multicystic renal dysplasia?

(a) Ureteral atresia
(b) Vesicoureteral reflux
(c) Ureteropelvic junction obstruction
(d) Ureteral duplication

(Answer is A) Ureteral atresia

216. What is the approximated bladder capacity of an 8 years girl?

(a) 150 ml (b) 200 ml
(c) 250 ml (d) 300 ml

(Answer is D) 300 ml

217. Two weeks of prolonged wound drainage after a non-stented Anderson-Hynes pyeloplasty. What would be next step in the management?

(a) Watchful waiting
(b) Open surgical correction
(c) IVU with possible endoscopic ureteral stenting
(d) Perc. nephrostomy tube insertion

(Answer is C) IVU with possible endoscopic ureteral stenting

218. What is false concerning neonatal nephrolithiasis?

(a) Frequently caused by loop diuretics
(b) Stones are often radiolucent
(c) May be reversed by the use of thiazides
(d) Low calcium-to-creatinine ratio predicts stones resolution

(Answer is B) Stones are often radiolucent

219. Patients with "bladder pain syndrome" have:

(a) A history of repeated urologic and/or gynecologic procedures

(b) 10-fold higher incidence of childhood voiding problems

(c) 4-fold higher incidence of anxiety-depression syndrome

(d) 6-fold higher incidence of psychosomatic disorders

(Answer is B) 10-fold higher incidence of childhood voiding problems

220. What is the most common cause of genetic ESRD in children?

(a) Autosomal recessive polycystic kidney disease

(b) Autosomal dominant polycystic kidney disease

(c) Multicystic dysplastic kidney disease

(d) Juvenile nephronophthisis

(Answer is D) Juvenile nephronophthisis

221. What is the most common testicular cancer in infants and young children?

(a) Choriocarcinoma

(b) Yolk cell tumor

(c) Embryonal carcinoma

(d) Seminoma

(Answer is B) Yolk cell tumor

222. What is the most common para-testicular tumor in children?

(a) Rhabdomyosarcoma

(b) Liposarcoma

(c) Sarcomatoid tumor

(d) Angiosarcoma

(Answer is A) Rhabdomyosarcoma

223. What is false concerning the pathophysiology of posterior urethral valve (PUV)?

(a) They are formed at about the 4th week of gestation

(b) They are formed by the fusion of the Wolffian duct with the cloaca

(c) Almost all patients born with PUVs progress to end-stage renal disease

(d) Type I- PUV accounts for 95% of cases

(Answer is C) Almost all patients born with PUVs progress to end-stage renal disease

224. What is false concerning the pathophysiology of detrusor muscle in posterior urethral valve cases?

(a) The obstructive process leads to increased collagen deposition and detrusor hypertrophy

(b) During filling, hypertrophy the detrusor muscle along with increases in connective tissue limit bladder compliance

(c) As patients grow up, bladder decompensation may occur, resulting in detrusor failure and spacious bladder

(d) During infancy, bladder emptying occurs at low intravesical pressures

(Answer is D) During infancy, bladder emptying occurs at low intravesical pressures

225. In modern medical practice, the most common presentation of posterior urethral valve is:

(a) Recurrent UTI in infancy

(b) Antenatal hydronephrosis

(c) Childhood voiding dysfunction

(d) Childhood enuresis

(Answer is B) Antenatal hydronephrosis

226. A newborn with posterior urethral valve may have the following manifestations, *except:*

(a) Bladder rupture (b) Forniceal rupture

(c) Pulmonary distress (d) Limb deformities

(Answer is A) Bladder rupture

227. What is not a clinical feature of posterior urethral valve fetus?

(a) Pulmonary hypoplasia
(b) Thickened bladder wall
(c) Bilateral upper urinary tract dilation
(d) Polyhydramnios

(Answer is D) Polyhydramnios

228. The most common cause of neonatal fatality in posterior urethral valve neonates is:

(a) Uremic encephalopathy due to renal failure
(b) Sepsis due to urinary tract infections
(c) Respiratory failure due to pulmonary hypoplasia
(d) Cardiac arrhythmia due to electrolytes imbalance

(Answer is C) Respiratory failure due to pulmonary hypoplasia

229. A toddler boy presents with urinary incontinence, abdominal pain, repeated UTIs. Renal ultrasonography shows moderate bilateral hydroureteronephroses. Next step in the management would be:

(a) Voiding cystourethrography
(b) Uroflowmetry
(c) Cystoscopy and retrograde ureterography
(d) Ascending urethrocystography

(Answer is A) Voiding cystourethrography

230. What condition(s), radiologically, mimic(s) antenatal fetal hydronephrosis?

(a) Obstructed megaureter
(b) Multicystic kidney
(c) Renal cystic disease
(d) All of the above

(Answer is D) All of the above

231. Up to what size of neonatal renal pelvis diameter is normal?

(a) 8mm (b) 10mm
(c) 12mm (d) 14mm

(Answer is C) 12 mm

232. In a suspected case of UPJ obstruction, beyond what intrarenal pelvis pressure is high?

(a) 16 cm H_2O (b) 18 cm H_2O
(c) 20 cm H_2O (d) 22 cm H_2O

(Answer is D) 22 cm H_2O

233. What imaging study is diagnostic for posterior urethral valve?

(a) Ascending urethrocystography
(b) Voiding cystourethrography
(c) Intravenous urography
(d) Tc-dimercaptosuccinic acid

(Answer is B) Voiding cystourethrography

234. What are the diagnostic signs of posterior urethral valve on voiding cystourethrography?

(a) Visualization of the valve leaflets
(b) Thickened trabeculated bladder and hypertrophied bladder neck
(c) Dilated or elongated posterior urethra
(d) All of the above

(Answer is D) All of the above

235. What renal scintigraphy helps judge the renal cortical function in a child with posterior urethral valve, and when combined with furosemide provides information about renal drainage and possible obstruction?

(a) Tc-dimercaptosuccinic acid (DMSA)
(b) Diethylene triamine pentaacetic acid (DTPA)
(c) All of the above
(d) Mercaptoacetyltriglycine (MAG-3)

(Answer is D) Mercaptoacetyltriglycine (MAG-3)

236. A newborn with a suspected posterior urethral valve, the first step in management is to:

(a) Set a baseline renal function
(b) Relief obstruction by passing a urethral catheter
(c) Confirm the diagnosis by performing voiding cystourethrography
(d) Repeat ultrasonography and compare it to the antenatal image

(Answer is B) Relief obstruction by passing a urethral catheter

237. What is improper in managing a newborn with posterior urethral valve?

(a) The valve can be incised at the 12, 5 and 7 O'clock positions, with either a cold knife or an electrocautery
(b) Cutaneous ureterostomies are reserved only for patients with ureterovesical junction obstruction
(c) Vesicostomy always help relief upper tract dilations
(d) While awaiting surgery, placing a 5-Fr urethral catheter and initiating a prophylactic antibiotic are advised

(Answer is C) Vesicostomy always help relief upper tract dilations

238. Potential complications following augmentation cystoplasty for a posterior urethral valve child include all of the following, *except:*

(a) Bladder rupture
(b) High voiding pressure
(c) Electrolyte disturbances
(d) Mucus production

(Answer is B) High voiding pressure

239. An antenatal ultrasonography reveals signs of posterior urethral valve, fetal bladder drainage will:

(a) Improve lung function in neonates
(b) Eliminate the need for vesicostomy
(c) Mandate prophylactic antibiotics
(d) Predispose to amniotic fluid aspiration

(Answer is A) Improve lung function in neonates

240. All of the following ailments are related to the "valve bladder syndrome", *except:*

(a) Hyper reflexive detrusor
(b) Vesicoureteral obstruction
(c) Narrow proximal urethra
(d) Renal tubular and glomerular impairment

(Answer is C) Narrow proximal urethra

241. What is the most common type of posterior urethral valve?

(a) Type I (b) Type II
(c) Type III (d) Comparable

(Answer is A) Type I

242. What type of posterior urethral valves is a membrane in nature that transversely crosses the urethra?

(a) Type I
(b) Type II
(c) Type III
(d) All fit this description

(Answer is C) Type III

243. What is the likelihood that posterior urethral valve patients have hydroureteronephrosis?

(a) Never (b) Unlikely
(c) Likely (d) Always

(Answer is D) Always

244. Concerning posterior urethral valve patients, what is the likelihood that ablation of the valve and/or vesicostomy will treat vesicoureteral reflux?

(a) Never (b) Unlikely
(c) Likely (d) Always

(Answer is C) Likely

245. Anterior urethral valve anomaly often occurs in the form of a:

(a) Membrane (b) Fold
(c) Diverticulum (d) Stenosis

(Answer is C) Diverticulum

246. In valve bladder patients, polyuria is due to:

(a) Nephrogenic diabetes insipidus
(b) Overflow incontinence
(c) Hyper reflexive detrusor
(d) None of the above

(Answer is A) Nephrogenic diabetes insipidus

247. In urethral duplication anomaly, the ventral urethra is usually:

(a) Blind ended
(b) The functional urethra
(c) Hypoplastic
(d) Wide calibre

(Answer is B) The functional urethra

248. Management of a newborn with hypospadias and cryptorchidism should:

(a) At the same operative session
(b) Include karyotyping
(c) Deferred until the child is 2 years
(d) Handled by a plastic surgeon

(Answer is B) Include karyotyping

249. What is the most common reason for difficult urethral catheterization during hypospadias repair?

(a) Enlarged prostatic utricle
(b) Elevated uvula vesica
(c) Associated posterior urethral valve anomaly
(d) Associated cecoureterocele anomaly

(Answer is A) Enlarged prostatic utricle

250. Which of the following does not reduce the incidence of fistula development after hypospadias repair?

(a) Stenting the urethra until scabs fall
(b) Closing up the corpus spongiosum edges over the neourethra
(c) Using monofilament stitches
(d) Avoiding overlapping suture lines

(Answer is C) Using monofilament stitches

251. Following hypospadias repair:

(a) The meatus should calibrate to 8 to 10 Fr
(b) Topical antibiotics should be applied over sutures
(c) Scabs should be removed under local anesthesia
(d) Repeat uroflowmetry should reveal better results than pre op.

(Answer is A) The meatus should calibrate to 8 to 10 Fr

252. What is not a potential long-term complication after hypospadias repair?

(a) Uneasiness with the cosmetic appearance
(b) Dissatisfaction with sexual function
(c) Ejaculatory dysfunctions
(d) Suture breakdown

(Answer is D) Suture breakdown

253. Penile curvature of greater than 30° can be straightened by:

(a) Single dorsal plication
(b) Ventral corporal grafting
(c) Penile degloving and urethrolysis
(d) Any of the above

(Answer is B) Ventral corporal grafting

254. The most common location of hypospadias is:

(a) Distal shaft (b) Mid shaft
(c) Proximal shaft (d) Penoscrotal

(Answer is A) Distal shaft

255. What is (are) technically crucial on repairing hypospadias?

(a) Careful tissue handling
(b) Using vascularised tissues
(c) Tension-free anastomosis
(d) All of the above

(Answer is D) All of the above

256. During hypospadias surgery, the following consideration(s) is (are) technically essential:

(a) Meticulous hemostasis preferably by using bipolar diathermy
(b) Avoiding overlapping suture line
(c) Placement of a dartos flap over the neourethra
(d) All of the above

(Answer is D) All of the above

257. In a family with no history of hypospadias, if a child was born with the anomaly, what would be the risk of next child having hypospadias?

(a) 12% (b) 18%
(c) 24% (d) 30%

(Answer is A) 12%

258. Which of the following anomalies cannot be explained as a failure of the cloacal membrane to migrate caudally?

(a) Hypospadias (b) Epispadias
(c) Bladder extrophy (d) All of the above

(Answer is A) Hypospadias

259. The principals of epispadias repair include all of the following, *except:*

(a) Urethroplasty
(b) Corporoplasty
(c) Penile lengthening
(d) Chordee correction

(Answer is B) Corporoplasty

260. The following factors impose risks on hypospadias development, *except:*

(a) In vitro fertilization
(b) Black race
(c) Family history of hypospadias
(d) Mutations in the 5-α reductase enzyme

(Answer is B) Black race

261. What is the preferred age for hypospadias repair?

(a) After 2 years
(b) Between 8 and 18 months
(c) Before school age
(d) Depends on the surgical technique

(Answer is B) between 8 and 18 months

262. What are the possible karyotype results of a newborn with a severe degree of hypospadias and probably has a "disorder of sex development"?

(a) XX virilization
(b) Mixed gonadal dysgenesis XY/XO
(c) XY under virilization
(d) Any of the above

(Answer is B) Mixed gonadal dysgenesis XY/XO

263. The most common presentation of urethral diverticulum in women is:

(a) Urinary frequency, dysuria and urgency
(b) Post-micturition dribbling
(c) Dyspareunia
(d) Urinary incontinence

(Answer is A) Urinary frequency, dysuria and urgency

264. The differential diagnosis of urethral diverticulum includes:

(a) Skene gland abscess
(b) Gartner duct cyst

(c) Ectopic ureter with ureterocele
(d) All of the above

(Answer is D) All of the above

265. A proper pre op. evaluation of a urethral diverticulum should be performed by:

(a) Performing a positive - pressure urethroscopy
(b) Assessing the number, size and location of the diverticulum
(c) Applying the L/N/S/C3 system
(d) Ensuring the absence of stones and active infections

(Answer is C) Applying the L/N/S/C3 system

266. The preferred operation(s) for urethral diverticulum is (are):

(a) Marsupialization
(b) Partial ablation
(c) Diverticulectomy
(d) Any of the above

(Answer is D) Any of the above

267. Which of the following criteria does not line up with the diagnosis of monosymptomatic primary enuresis in a 6 years girl?

(a) Diurnal incontinence
(b) Positive family history
(c) Gradual resolution of the symptoms over years
(d) She has never achieved a satisfactory period of night time dryness

(Answer is A) Diurnal incontinence

268. What is the least important issue to inquire about while taking a history of bed wetting in pediatrics?

(a) Bowel habits
(b) Daytime incontinence
(c) Prematurity
(d) Major motor seizures

(Answer is C) Prematurity

269. What is the prevalence of monosymptomatic nocturnal enuresis at the age of 10?

(a) 1 – 3%
(b) 3 – 7%
(c) 7 – 9%
(d) 9 – 12%

(Answer is B) 3 – 7%

270. Dysfunctional voiding in pediatrics is suspected in:

(a) Girls with diurnal enuresis
(b) Infrequent voiders
(c) Children assuming squatting behaviour
(d) All of the above

(Answer is D) All of the above

271. What is false concerning the management of enuresis in childhood?

(a) Rare instances, the treatment could be surgical
(b) The most important point is to raise the child's self-esteem and to resolve psychological and/or behavioral problems
(c) The most common drawback is family incompliance
(d) The reported natural history is spontaneous cure at a rate of 15% per annum

(Answer is C) The most common drawback is family incompliance

272. Which of the following physical examinations is least related to enuresis in children?

(a) Proximal penile hypospadias
(b) Dimples on either side of the sacrum
(c) The inability to stand on the toes
(d) The presence of hair tuft or skin discoloration over the lower back

(Answer is A) Proximal penile hypospadias

273. In childhood enuresis, MRI of the spine is indicated with the following finding(s):

(a) Abnormal neurologic findings of the lower extremities

(b) The presence of dimples on either side of the sacrum or hair tuft, skin discoloration over the lower back

(c) The presence of gait abnormality, encopresis and daytime enuresis

(d) Any of the above

(Answer is D) Any of the above

274. What is false concerning "alarm therapy" on treating enuresis in children?

(a) Works best with deep sleepers

(b) Reduces nocturnal urine output

(c) Should be continued for a month after achieving full dryness

(d) Should be considered for every patient of primary type

(Answer is B) Reduces nocturnal urine output

275. Which of the following anti-enuresis medications could result in serious hyponatremia?

(a) Desmopressin acetate

(b) Oxybutynin chloride

(c) Imipramine

(d) Botulinum toxin A

(Answer is A) Desmopressin acetate

276. Which of the following is the least to cause adult enuresis?

(a) HTN medications

(b) Sleep apnea

(c) Senile prostatic enlargement

(d) End-stage renal disease

(Answer is D) End-stage renal disease

277. False about neuroblastoma:

(a) Most common extracranial solid neoplasm in children

(b) Better survival in >18 months child

(c) Complete surgical resection is curative for low stage disease

(d) MYCN gene amplification carries poor prognosis

(Answer is B) Better survival in >18 months child

278. False about Wilms' tumor:

(a) Most common primary malignant renal tumor of childhood

(b) The Birt Hogg Dube syndrome is the specific association of male pseudohermaphroditism, renal mesangial sclerosis and nephroblastoma

(c) Wilms tumor is characterized by wide histologic diversity

(d) Favourable histology Wilms' tumor has a pseudocapsule

(Answer is B) The Birt Hogg Dube syndrome is the specific association of male pseudohermaphroditism, renal mesangial sclerosis, and nephroblastoma

279. WAGR syndrome comprises all *except:*

(a) Wilm's tumor (b) Anosmia

(c) Genital anomalies (d) Mental retardation

(Answer is B) Anosmia

280. False about retrocaval ureter:

(a) Occurs almost always on the right side

(b) Characteristic S shaped deformity on IVU

(c) Standard repair is pyelopyelostomy

(d) Unlike PUJO no stenotic segment of ureter occurs

(Answer is D) Unlike PUJO no stenotic segment of ureter occurs

CHAPTER

18

Uro-Imaging

1. **During fluoroscopy, what is the main source of radiation hazards that urologists could be exposed to?**
   (a) Scattered radiation from the unleaded wall
   (b) Scattered radiation from the patient
   (c) Scattered radiation from the floor and ceiling
   (d) Radiation from the primary beam

(Answer is B) Scattered radiation from the patient

2. **Which of the following does asymptomatic hematuria workup include?**
   (a) Cystoscopy (b) CT urography
   (c) Urine cytology (d) All of the above

(Answer is D) All of the above

3. **On tracing the IVU dye down, in a dilated ureter, the dilation stops at a level then continues as a normal calibre ureter. What could the pathology be?**
   (a) Lower ureteral stricture
   (b) Ureteral valve
   (c) Modified Lich-Gregoire ureteral reimplantation
   (d) Residual dilation of hydroureter

(Answer is B) Ureteral valve

4. **What is the optimal time for viewing the renal parenchyma after injecting a contrast material during IVU study?**
   (a) 0 minute
   (b) 5 minutes
   (c) 10 minutes
   (d) Renal parenchyma does not appear on IVU

(Answer is A) 0 minute

5. **What is the emergency treatment of intravenous contrast allergy?**
   (a) Epinephrine (b) Atropine
   (c) Hydrocortisone (d) Antihistamine

(Answer is A) Epinephrine

6. **To which class of Bosniak system of renal cysts does an oval renal parenchymal cyst of uniform water density filling, with attenuation of ≤ 20 HU, thin, non-calcified wall, and no contrast enhancement; belong to?**
   (a) Class 1 (b) Class 2
   (c) Class 3 (d) Class 4

(Answer is A) Class 1

7. **Ultrasonic 3.5 MHz curved array probe is suitable to detect:**
   (a) Epididymal cysts
   (b) Testicular tumors
   (c) Renal stones
   (d) Penile vasculature

(Answer is C) Renal stones

8. **Which condition does not show a false positive result for hydronephrosis on ultrasonic examination?**
   (a) Hydrocalicosis
   (b) Extrarenal pelvis

(c) Parapelvic cyst
(d) Class 2 Bosniak renal cyst

(Answer is D) Class 2 Bosniak renal cyst

9. **Which condition does not show a false negative result for hydronephrosis on ultrasonic examination?**
(a) Forniceal rupture
(b) Drained renal pelvis
(c) High urine output
(d) Acute obstruction

(Answer is C) High urine output

10. **Which statement is true concerning renal ultrasonography?**
(a) End-stage renal failure kidneys look small and hypoechoic
(b) Is more accurate on diagnosing cystic lesions than solid masses
(c) Is able to detect tumors as small as 2 mm
(d) Cortical carbuncle might be mistaken for hydronephrosis

(Answer is B) Is more accurate on diagnosing cystic lesions than solid masses

11. **Which radiological modality carries the highest radiation hazard?**
(a) Nuclear medicine
(b) Ultrasonography
(c) X-ray fluoroscopy
(d) Intravenous urography

(Answer is C) X-ray fluoroscopy

12. **What is the improper usage of TRUS?**
(a) Evaluate ejaculatory duct obstruction in infertility case
(b) Screen for prostate cancers
(c) Take prostate biopsies
(d) Place interstitial radiotherapy seeds

(Answer is B) Screen for prostate cancers

13. **Which condition could present as a filling defect in the bladder on IVU study?**
(a) Blood clot
(b) Fibro-epithelial polyp
(c) Sloughed renal papilla
(d) All of the above

(Answer is D) All of the above

14. **What should type II diabetic patients on metformin do when going for intravenous contrast urography to avoid biguanide lactic acidosis?**
(a) Take urine acidifiers
(b) Withhold metformin the day before the study and restart 48 hours later
(c) Get premedicated by steroids and anti-histamines
(d) Decrease metformin dose and turn to insulin

(Answer is B) Withhold metformin the day before the study and restart 48 hours later

15. **What is the minimum estimate of GFR to take gadolinium-based contrast agents?**
(a) More than 30 ml/min/1.73 m^2
(b) More than 60 ml/min/1.73 m^2
(c) More than 90 ml/min/1.73 m^2
(d) None of the above

(Answer is A) More than 30 ml/min/1.73 m^2

16. **How does fluid appear on T_2-weighted MR images?**
(a) Dark
(b) Intermediate
(c) Bright
(d) None of the above

(Answer is C) Bright

17. **What matter does correspond to zero Hounsfield units?**
(a) Air
(b) Water
(c) Fat
(d) Bone

(Answer is B) Water

18. What imaging modality is superior in detecting undescended testis in the abdomen?

(a) MRI (b) CT
(c) Ultrasound (d) All are comparable

(Answer is A) MRI

19. By ultrasonography, when kidneys appear darker than the liver, they are:

(a) Hypoechoic (b) Hyperechoic
(c) Anechoic (d) Isoechoic

(Answer is A) Hypoechoic

20. What is correct concerning sound waves?

(a) The higher the frequency, the deeper tissue penetration
(b) The higher the frequency, the better the axial resolution
(c) Low-frequency transducers are of 6 to 10 MHz
(d) The deeper tissue penetration, the better axial resolution

(Answer is B) The higher the frequency, the better the axial resolution

21. Which USG mode is able to depict motion direction and flow velocity?

(a) Grey-scale
(b) Simultaneous bilateral views
(c) Color Doppler
(d) Power Doppler

(Answer is C) Color Doppler

22. How does a full bladder appear on ultrasonography?

(a) Hyperechoic (b) Hypoechoic
(c) Isoechoic (d) Anechoic

(Answer is D) Anechoic

23. Which of the following is not an indication of retrograde pyelography?

(a) Evaluation of probable ureteral obstruction
(b) Conjunction with ureteroscopy
(c) Evaluation of hematuria
(d) Evaluation of probable ureterovesical reflux

(Answer is D) Evaluation of probable ureterovesical reflux

24. Which of the following is false concerning retrograde urethrogram?

(a) Coning at the bulbar urethra is normal
(b) Segmental narrowing at bulbar urethra is normal
(c) Multiple round filling defects could be air bubbles
(d) Indicated in urethral trauma cases

(Answer is B) Segmental narrowing at bulbar urethra is normal

25. Which of the following is not an indication of static cystography?

(a) Evaluating a probable bladder rupture
(b) Evaluating a probable colovesical or vesicovaginal fistulae
(c) Evaluating a probable intravesical pathology
(d) Evaluating a probable bladder diverticula

(Answer is B) Evaluating a probable colovesical or vesicovaginal fistulae

26. Which of the following is an indication of VCUG?

(a) Repeated febrile UTI in children
(b) Evaluating a probable posterior urethral valve
(c) A and B
(d) None of the above

(Answer is C) A and B

27. Which statement is false concerning diuretic nuclear scintigraphy renogram?

(a) Elimination T½ < 10 minutes indicates obstructed system

(b) The diuretic must be given at the maximum kidney activity
(c) If ureteral stents are in place, the bladder catheter must be unclamped
(d) ^{99}mTc-MAG$_3$ is the agent of choice to study differential renal function and obstruction

(Answer is A) Elimination T½ < 10 minutes indicates obstructed system

28. Which statement concerning phlebolith is false?

(a) Can be mistaken for a ureteral stone
(b) A small single, usually spiky, calcification within a vein
(c) The amount of phleboliths increases with age
(d) Appears more often on the left than on the right side of the pelvis

(Answer is B) A small single, usually spiky, calcification within a vein

29. What is (are) the characteristic finding(s) of testicular torsion on color Doppler ultrasonography?

(a) The classic blue dot sign
(b) Thick, short, edematous spermatic cord
(c) Absence of intratesticular blood flow
(d) Increased epididymal blood flow

(Answer is C) Absence of intratesticular blood flow

30. What is the poorest method of measuring the amount of urine in the bladder of a 65 years old man?

(a) Using bladder scanner
(b) Measuring the voided urine
(c) Using abdominal ultrasonography
(d) Performing urinary catheterization

(Answer is B) Measuring the voided urine

31. On sagittal plane of midline TRUS, which structure might not be visible?

(a) Peripheral zone of the prostate
(b) Ejaculatory duct
(c) Tip of the right seminal vesicle
(d) Tip of the left lateral lobe of the prostate

(Answer is C) Tip of the right seminal vesicle

32. Which structure cannot be assessed by TRUS of the prostate?

(a) Ejaculatory duct
(b) Vas deferens
(c) Seminal vesicles
(d) Rectal wall

(Answer is B) Vas deferens

33. Ultrasonic waves, in nature, are:

(a) Mechanical waves
(b) Radar waves
(c) Microwaves
(d) Radio waves

(Answer is A) Mechanical waves

34. What is false concerning "ureteric jets"?

(a) Obstruction of the upper urinary tract may increase renal pelvis pressure and delay or decrease pelvis peristaltic rates
(b) Measured by color Doppler flow mapping in transverse scans at the suprapubic region
(c) Patients with ureteral stents are the ideal
(d) Adequate hydration is necessary

(Answer is C) Patients with ureteral stents are the ideal

35. What is the signal characteristic of renal stones on MRU?

(a) High signal on T_1-weighted images
(b) High signal on T_2-weighted images
(c) Low signal on T_1-weighted images
(d) None of the above

(Answer is D) None of the above

36. **Using ultrasonography, which testicular lesion is described as a solid, round, homogeneous, low-reflectivity tumor mass, with no calcification?**
    (a) Seminoma
    (b) Embryonal cell tumor
    (c) Mixed germ cell tumor
    (d) Epidermoid cyst

(Answer is A) Seminoma

37. **Using ultrasonography, which testicular lesion is of low reflectivity with irregular borders, hypervascular rims but no internal vascularity to mention?**
    (a) Intratesticular hematoma
    (b) Testicular abscess
    (c) Orchitis
    (d) Sex cord stromal tumors

(Answer is B) Testicular abscess

38. **Using ultrasonography, which testicular lesion is cystic with heterogeneous echoes representing a mixture of mucinous and/or sebaceous material with or without hair follicles, cartilages and bones?**
    (a) Non-seminomatous germ cell tumors
    (b) Acute bleed on top of old hematoma
    (c) Mature teratoma
    (d) Sex cord stromal tumors

(Answer is C) Mature teratoma

39. **Using CT scanning, which solid kidney mass is well-defined, heterogeneous tumor, located in the renal cortex and containing areas of fat density of -20 HU or less. No calcifications, but some areas of enhancement?**
    (a) RCC (b) Metastases
    (c) Angiomyolipoma (d) Oncocytoma

(Answer is C) Angiomyolipoma

40. **Using CT scanning, which solid kidney mass is sharply demarcated with uniform enhancement and often has a central scar?**
    (a) RCC (b) Metastases
    (c) Angiomyolipoma (d) Oncocytoma

(Answer is D) Oncocytoma

41. **Using CT, which solid kidney mass is like a bulge of the renal contour characterized by normal corticomedullary patterns?**
    (a) Prominent columns of Bertin
    (b) Xanthogranulomatous pyelonephritis
    (c) Lymphoma
    (d) Renal infarction

(Answer is A) Prominent columns of Bertin

42. **On staging left kidney RCC using enhanced CT, the radiologist must look for:**
    (a) Extension of the tumor to the diaphragm
    (b) Extension of the tumor to the right atrium
    (c) The density of calcifications
    (d) The amount and bilaterality of cysts formation

(Answer is B) Extension of the tumor to the right atrium

43. **Which of the following is not an indication of renal arteriography?**
    (a) Preparation for donor nephrectomy
    (b) Advanced RCC in the right kidney
    (c) Renal artery stenosis
    (d) Oncocytoma in the left kidney

(Answer is D) Oncocytoma in the left kidney

44. **What is (are) the indication(s) of renal artery embolization?**
    (a) Bleeding angiomyolipomas
    (b) Alternative to nephrectomy in severe uncontrolled hypertension among patients with end-stage renal disease

(c) Renal artery aneurysms or symptomatic AV malformations
(d) All of the above

(Answer is D) All of the above

45. Which statement is false concerning complications of left renal artery embolization?

(a) Embolizing the non-target artery might occur
(b) Severe pain at the renal area could occur
(c) Complications depend on the embolic agent
(d) Reactive left pulmonary edema

(Answer is D) Reactive left pulmonary edema

46. Which statement is false regarding magnetic resonance urography (MRU)?

(a) Small non-obstructive calculi might be missed at MRU performed for the evaluation of hematuria
(b) Pediatrics, performing a dynamic contrast-enhanced imaging helps in evaluating crossing vessels in the setting of UPJ obstruction
(c) The success of static-fluid MR urography depends on the presence of fluid within the urinary system regardless of renal function
(d) MRU at 3T, carries the risk of nephrogenic systemic fibrosis

(Answer is D) MRU at 3T, carries the risk of nephrogenic systemic fibrosis

47. Which statement is false concerning plain KUB film?

(a) Reliable tool to exclude urinary calculi
(b) Calcifications at renal area might lead to the discovery of renal cancers
(c) Can detect soft tissues
(d) Fecoliths and phleboliths could be mistaken for calculi

(Answer is A) Reliable tool to exclude urinary calculi

48. What is false concerning Tc-99m DMSA?

(a) Diseases affecting the proximal convoluted tubules inhibit DMSA uptake
(b) Is ideal to assess UPJ obstruction in adults
(c) Gentamicin and cisplatin inhibit the DMSA uptake
(d) Allows better assessment of differential renal function

(Answer is B) Is ideal to assess UPJ obstruction in adults

49. What is true concerning Tc-99m DTPA?

(a) Its uptake by glomerular filtration is almost 100%
(b) It helps evaluate cortical structure and morphology
(c) It provides a static picture of kidneys when compared to MAG_3
(d) Binds to the sulfhydryl groups in proximal tubules resulting in much higher resolution pinhole SPECT imaging

(Answer is A) Its uptake by glomerular filtration is almost 100%

50. What is false on comparing Tc-99m DTPA to Tc-99m MAG_3?

(a) DTPA provides better quality images with renal insufficiency
(b) Giving captopril, MAG_3 plasma clearance declines in hypertensive patients with renal artery stenosis but rises in those who do not have the disease
(c) DTPA provides an excellent measurement of GFR
(d) Pediatrics, MAG_3 provides better quality images than DTPA

(Answer is A) DTPA provides better quality images with renal insufficiency

51. **In routine practice, when do urologists request plain skull X-ray?**
    (a) Advanced prostatic cancer
    (b) Central diabetes insipidus
    (c) Pituitary adenoma
    (d) A and C

(Answer is D) A and C

52. **What is the hallmark finding on plain KUB of bladder exstrophy?**
    (a) Malunion of lumbar and/or sacral vertebral bodies
    (b) Pelvic bone diastasis
    (c) Sacral agenesis
    (d) Fracture of anterior pubic rami

(Answer is B) Pelvic bone diastasis

53. **Which condition tops the differential diagnoses list of CT picture of Xanthogranulomatous pyelonephritis?**
    (a) Renal tuberculosis
    (b) Renal abscess
    (c) Renal cell carcinoma
    (d) Angiomyolipoma

(Answer is A) Renal tuberculosis

54. **What nuclear medicine study can diagnose interstitial nephritis?**
    (a) DTPA (b) DMSA
    (c) Gallium-67 (d) MAG-3

(Answer is C) Gallium-67

55. **Regarding acute renal infections, what is the least diagnostic radionuclide study for detecting an inflammatory focus?**
    (a) Hippuran I-131
    (b) Technetium-99 m
    (c) Gallium-67
    (d) Indium-111–labelled WBC

(Answer is D) Indium-111–labelled WBC

56. **What is the Hounsfield density range of uric acid stones?**
    (a) 400 – 600 HU
    (b) 600 – 800 HU
    (c) 800 – 1000 HU
    (d) 1000 – 1200 HU

(Answer is A) 400 – 600 HU

57. **What is false concerning radiation exposure to a pregnant woman with a kidney stone?**
    (a) One or two films of IVU are acceptable
    (b) CT is absolutely discouraged
    (c) MRI is the diagnostic modality of choice
    (d) Ultrasonography is the safest

(Answer is C) MRI is the diagnostic modality of choice

58. **What is false concerning radiation cystitis?**
    (a) The average time from the beginning of radiation therapy to initial symptoms could be 2–4 weeks
    (b) Treatment with stationary radiation, portals carry a higher risk of morbidity than treatment with rotating portals do
    (c) Occurs in about 10% of patients treated with definitive irradiation therapy for prostate cancer after 10 years
    (d) Most cases are mildly affected and require no specific therapy

(Answer is A) The average time from the beginning of radiation therapy to initial symptoms could be 2–4 weeks

59. **On an ascending urethrogram, what anatomical structure could be mistaken for urethral stricture?**
    (a) Verumontanum
    (b) Membranous urethra
    (c) Prostatic utricle
    (d) Uvula vesicae

(Answer is B) Membranous urethra

60. Causes for filling defects in upper tract in urogram are all *except*:

(a) Blood clot (b) Urothelial cis
(c) Papillary necrosis (d) Stone

(Answer is B) Urothelial cis

61. False about DTPA scan:

(a) Can be used to assess relative renal plasma flow
(b) Can be used to evaluate functional obstruction
(c) Can be used to calculate GFR
(d) Ideally suited for imaging cortical disease

(Answer is D) Ideally suited for imaging cortical disease

62. False about MAG_3 scan:

(a) Can be used to assess split renal function
(b) Can be used to assess functional obstruction
(c) Excreted entirely by glomerular filtration
(d) Cheaper than DTPA

(Answer is C) Excreted entirely by glomerular filtration

63. Captopril scintigraphy is used for diagnosing:

(a) Renovascular hypertension
(b) Renal cortical scar
(c) Reflux nephropathy
(d) Reninoma

(Answer is A) Renovascular hypertension